AF518357

Textbook on
Meat, Poultry and Fish Technology

ABOUT THE BOOK

The book entitled "**Textbook on Meat, Poultry and Fish Technology**" contains Part I Fresh Meat technology Chapter 1-11 containing History and development; Structure and chemistry of animal tissues; Postmortem changes- rigor mortis; Effect of transport on meat quality; PSE and DFD in meat quality; Composition, essential nutrients in meat and poultry meat; General quality characterization; Meat microbiology; Factors affecting; Tenderization; and Chemical residues. Part II Poultry and Fish Technology Chapter 12-30 contains History and development; Anti-nutrients and antibiotics effect on egg and meat; Quality identification and quality maintenance of poultry meat; Structure, chemical, nutritional and microbiological quality of poultry meat; Nutritive value, preservation and packaging techniques; Quality identification and factors influencing the quality; Pre-slaughter care, transportation, resting, fasting, ante-mortem examination; Methods of slaughter and slaughtering procedure-postmortem inspection; Yield and loss in poultry carcass component parts; Structure, nutritive value, compositional chemistry, microbiology and functional properties of eggs; Low cholesterol-cum-designer eggs; GMP, HACCP, Codex regulation for food products safety, WTO/GOI regulations; National and international regulations, Utilization of fish processing waste; Fishery resources, fishes, transportation, processing, preservation, grading standards; Post-processing value added meat for export-integration, poultry and fish processing and marketing; Storage, packaging, preservation methods; Cooking and preparation of further processed poultry and fish products.

This is a dependable text book not only for the students of all Veterinary Colleges of India, but also it serves as a helpful guide to the teaching faculty who are engaged in teaching in the area of Livestock Products Technology/Animal Products Technology/ Meat Science and Technology/Food Science and Technology.

ABOUT THE AUTHORS

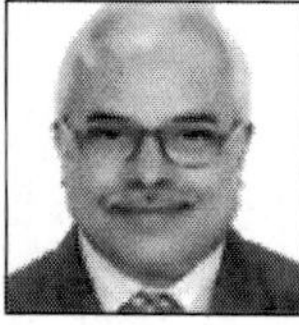

Dr. Jhari Sahoo, obtained his M.V. Sc. (APT) from HAU, Hisar and Ph.D. (LPT) from IVRI, Izatnagar. He has about 32 years of experience as teaching faculty. He served for a long period of 21years at Department of Animal Products technology, CCSHAU, Hisar in the capacity of Assistant professor, Associate professor and Professor. Later on he joined to the post of professor on dt.22.12.2003 at PAU, Ludhiana and remained Professor-cum-Head from dt.06.01.2004 to dt.12.08.2012 in the Department of Livestock Products Technology at PAU/GADVASU.

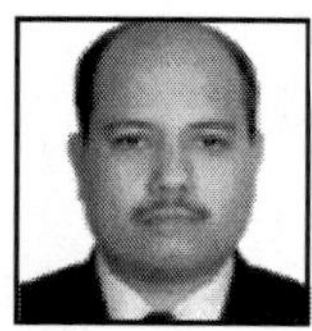

Dr. Manish Kumar Chatli, has more than 16 year experience in industry, teaching, research and extension in the area of Livestock Products Technology. He worked as Dairy Manager, Bombay and Assistant Professor at CSK HPKV, Palampur. He has joined PAU as Associate Professor in 2003 and subsequently promoted to Professor in 2009 and Head position in 2012.

Textbook on
Meat, Poultry and Fish Technology

Jhari Sahoo

Manish Kumar Chatli

Department of Livestock Products Technology
College of Veterinary Science
Guru Angad Dev Veterinary and Animal Sciences University
Ludhiana – 141004 (Punjab)

2022

Daya Publishing House®
A Division of
Astral International Pvt. Ltd.
New Delhi – 110 002

First Published, 2015

ISBN 978-93-5124-344-1 (Hardbound)

Published by : **Daya Publishing House®**
A Division of
Astral International Pvt. Ltd.
– ISO 9001:2015 Certified Company –
4736/23, Ansari Road, Darya Ganj
New Delhi-110 002
Ph. 011-43549197, 23278134
E-mail: info@astralint.com
Website: www.astralint.com

Digitally Printed at : **Replika Press Pvt. Ltd.**

Preface

The Expert Committee of the Indian Council of Medical Research (ICMR) has recommended 60 g of protein per day with net protein utilization (NPU) of 65. A minimum requirement of animal protein would be targeted at 20 g per person per day compared to the present availability of 10.8 g and the world average of 25 g. Demand for meat and poultry products is also expected to grow in tune with the population growth, rising incomes and increasing urbanization. In view of this, supplying wholesome, safe and acceptable meat foods to the ever increasing non-vegetarian consumers must be ensured.

There are 30 export-oriented modern abattoirs and 77 meat processing plants registered with APEDA exporting raw meat (chilled and frozen) to about 56 countries. The present production of meat is estimated at 6.27 million tons in 2010 (FAO, 2012), which is 2.21 per cent of the world's meat production. The contribution of meat from buffalo is about 23.33 per cent, while cattle contributes about 17.34 per cent, sheep 4.61 per cent, goat 9.36 per cent, pig 5.31 per cent, poultry 36.68 per cent and other species 3.37 per cent. The meat production has increased from 764,000 tonnes in 1970-71 to 6.27 million tons in 2010. The compounded average growth rate (CAGR) during the last two decades works out to be 4.5 per cent. It is noticed that about 10.6 per cent cattle, 10.6 per cent buffaloes, 24.1 per cent sheep, 58.7 per cent goats, 95.0 per cent pigs and 190.0 per cent chicken are slaughtered each year. The value of meat and by-products is Rs 79,889 crore including skin and hides, while the export value of meat and meat products work outs to be more than Rs 6,000 crore in the year 2009-10. The contribution of buffalo meat accounts for more than 75 per cent of total exports/ foreign earnings. The poultry has gaining the widely acceptance by consumers and growing 10-15 per cent annually. The chicken meat contributes about 37 per cent meat to total production and number one contributors. The growth is expected more in near future. This might be due to popularity, price, easy availability, no religious taboos and much more characteristics in poultry.

There is a changing trend in consumer priorities. Today, the consumer looks out for the Safety of the products, Animal Welfare, Ethics of the trade, Reliability and Zero Risk. With a view to this, The Food Safety and Standards Authority of India (FSSAI) has been established under Food Safety and Standards Act, 2006 which consolidates various acts and orders that have hitherto handled food related issues in various Ministries and Departments. FSSAI has been created for laying down science based standards for articles of food and to regulate their manufacture, storage, distribution, sale and import to ensure availability of safe and wholesome food for human consumption.

The conditions of domestic meat market in India is very precarious with acute problems of environmental pollution, animal welfare issues, lack of ante mortem and postmortem meat inspection, unhygienic slaughter practices, unhygienic transport of dressed carcasses from slaughter houses to the retail shops and very unhygienic substandard retail meat shops.

It is the need of the hour to awake and aware the all concerned persons including students and faculty to improve the aforementioned prevalent situations of the country. Prevention of postharvest loss of meat in terms of both quantity and quality is indirectly increasing of meat production. This is possible only if the persons involved directly/ or indirectly should have knowledge about the meat production, processing, preservation, packaging and marketing safely of meat and poultry products till it reaches the consumer table. The students and teachers are at foundation level for this. Keeping in view the above matter, very sincere efforts were made by the authors to publish this book **"Textbook on Meat, Poultry and Fish Technology".** The first author of the book Dr. Jhari Sahoo has been associated with industry, teaching, research, training and quality control in the field of meat and poultry products technology for more than 32 years, who has been aware of their problems and needs. He also helped Secretary, Veterinary Council of India while developing course curriculum both in the old and new VCI Syllabus pertaining to the subject discipline of Livestock Products Technology. This book has incorporated the Veterinary Council of India(VCI) New Syllabus 2008 Course No. LPT-321 Course Title: Meat Science prescribed for B.V. Sc. and A.H. degree programme and BSMA (ICAR) syllabus for Course No. LPT 601 Course Title: Fresh meat technology and LPT 603 title: Poultry and fish products technology. This book can be used as a dependable primary textbook for B.V. Sc. and A.H., M.V.Sc. and Ph.D. students of different veterinary colleges of the country. Besides, this book is of immense help to the teaching faculty of State Agricultural Universities(SAUs) and Veterinary Universities of the country who are engaged in teaching in the area of Livestock Products Technology/Animal Products Technology/Meat Science and Technology/Food Science and Technology.

I am thankful to the co-author Dr. Manish Kumar Chatli for his contribution in some chapters of the book.

I am dedicating this book to my darling wife Pravasini, for her constant support, cooperation and encouragement in every step while writing the book.

Dr. J. Sahoo

Department of Livestock Products Technology,
College of Veterinary Science,
Guru Angad Dev Veterinary and Animal Sciences University,
Ludhiana – 141004 (Punjab), India

Phone: +91-161-2414025 Fax: +91-161-2400822 Mobile: +91-9417463926

E-mail: j.sahoolptgadvasu354@gmail.com,
sahoo_j1203@yahoo.com; jsahoogadvasu@rediffmail.com

Contents

Part II–Poultry and Fish Technology

— Part I —

Fresh Meat Technology

– Chapter 1 –

History and Development of Meat Science and Meat Industry, Current Trends and Prospects of Meat Industry

Development of Meat Industry in India

Introduction

The meat industry is the collective of diverse businesses that together supply much of the food energy consumed by the world population. Food processing industry is widely recognized as a **'sunrise industry'** having huge potential for uplifting agricultural economy, creation of large scale processed food manufacturing and food chain facilities, and the resultant generation of employment and export earnings. India has enormous growth potential from its current status of being the world's second largest producer to be the world's number one producer.

Share of Agriculture and Livestock Sector in GDP

Rearing of livestock has been an integral component of India's agriculture and rural economy since time immemorial and India's livestock sector is one of the largest in the world. India has 56.7 per cent of world's buffaloes, 12.5 per cent cattle, 20.4 per cent small ruminants, 2.4 per cent camel, 1.4 per cent equine, 1.5 per cent pigs and 3.1 per cent poultry. The share of livestock in the agricultural GDP improved consistently from 15 per cent in 1981-82 to 26 per cent in 2010-11.

Development of Meat Industry

Man and animal relationship is as old as history of mankind. Even the Palaeolithic man was killing the animals for meat purpose and for various other economic benefits including using of animal skin as clothes. Both animal husbandry and meat industry are ancillary to each other and has great impact on the socioeconomic and cultural life of mankind. Meat is a food of high biological value and provides all the nutrients required for the body, but its production, processing and distribution tends to generate controversy due to religious and other sentiments of certain sections of the society. The social prejudice against it is the root cause of many of the problems that this age old industry faces in its healthy growth, scientific improvement and contribution to the livestock industry.

India is endowed with rich flora and vast livestock resources. Livestock rearing is considered as vital avenue for rural employment, income generation, social and gender equity, agricultural sustainability, diversification and foreign exchange earnings. India has 66 per cent of economically active population engaged in agriculture. Livestock has a great complementary, supplementary and sustainability role under mixed farming systems prevalent in the country. The contribution of livestock sector to the food basket in the form of milk, eggs and meat has been immense in fulfilling the animal protein requirement of ever-growing human population. The livestock sector is an important component of Indian agriculture. India has a huge livestock population (Table 1.2) and efficient utilisation of these resources including production and utilization of livestock products is important to earn increased returns and sustain livestock production activities. Following the sustained economic growth and rising domestic incomes and moreover increasing population has lead to increased demand of livestock products. During the last three to four decades, India has witnessed the green, white, yellow and blue revolutions and now the time has come to realize one more revolution *i.e.* red/pink revolution in the form of meat production. In fact, in spite of big potential because of large livestock population, the meat industry in India has not taken its due share. There are many reasons for the slow growth rate of the Indian meat industry, including the negative attitude of public towards meat on account of misinformation campaign and socio-political considerations.

Table 1.1: Share of Agriculture and Livestock Sector in GDP

Year	*GDP Total*	*GDP (Agriculture)*		*GDP (Livestock Sector)*	
		Rs. Crores	*Per cent Share*	*Rs. Crores*	*Per cent Share*
2006-07	3,953,276	604,672	15.3	142,695	3.6
2007-08	4,582,086	716,276	15.6	169,296	3.7
2008-09	5,303,567	806,646	15.2	200,440	3.8
2009-10	6,091,485	924,581	15.2	232,815	3.8
2010-11	7,157,412	1,093,806	15.3	260,300	3.6

Source: Ministry of Statistics, Govt. of India, 2012.

Current Status of Livestock Population

India has been bestowed with abundant livestock resources in terms of number of animals. India ranks first in the world in cattle, goats and buffalo population. India possesses 56.57 per cent of world's buffalo population and 13.90 per cent of cattle, 6.02 per cent of sheep, 1.50 per cent of pigs and 15.38 per cent of goats of the world. The livestock number has increased significantly irrespective of the species. Especially the poultry industry which has come up from the backyard farming to most organized industry. The figures are mind blowing in poultry industry. It has increased from a mere figure of 73.5 millions in 1951 to 711.54 millions in 2004 almost hundred times. Indian livestock population has increased almost by 6.16 per cent annually in the decade 1994 to 2004. Since 1994, the population of sheep, buffaloes and pigs has increased by double figure. The maximum increase in number was recorded for sheep (28.31 per cent) followed by pigs (26.58 per cent) and buffaloes (17.6 per cent). However, there was slight decline in cattle population (FAO, 2004) by 7.48 per cent in the last decade. The poultry population also increased around 35 per cent in the last recorded decade. In addition mithun is also recognised as a source of meat in north east and Sikkim while in Kerala, Andhra, Himachal Pradesh and Karnatka rabbit, quail and duck are emerging as other sources of meat.

Table 1.2: Scenario of Livestock Population of India Since 1951

Species	*Million Animals/Birds in Year*									
	1951	*1961*	*1972*	*1978*	*1982*	*1987*	*1992*	*1997*	*2002*	*2004*
Cattle	155.30	175.60	178.30	180.00	192.49	195.87	192.65	196.70	189.302	185.50
			(1.5)	(1.0)	(6.9)	(1.8)	(1.6)	(2.06)	(-3.90)	(-2.04)
Buffaloes	43.40	51.20	57.40	62.00	69.80	76.77	78.55	80.34	95.48	97.70
			(12.0)	(8.0)	(12.6)	(10.0)	(2.3)	(2.23)	(15.86)	(2.27)
Sheep	39.10	40.20	40.00	41.00	48.80	44.84	44.40	45.65	61.10	62.50
			(-0.5)	(2.5)	(19.0)	(-8.1)	(-1.0)	(2.74)	(25.29)	(2.24)
Goats	47.20	60.90	67.50	75.60	95.20	99.41	117.00	120.36	120.50	120.00
			(10.8)	(12.0)	(25.9)	(4.4)	(17.7)	(2.79)	(0.12)	(-0.41)
Pigs	4.40	5.20	6.90	7.60	10.10	10.76	10.50	15.42	14.00	14.30
			(32.7)	(10.1)	(32.9)	(6.5)	(-2.4)	(31.91)	(-10.14)	(2.1)
Poultry	73.50	114.20	138.50	59.20	107.70	258.34	410.00	570.00	682.81	711.54
			(21.3)	(-57.3)	(81.9)	(139.9)	(58.7)	(28.10)	(16.52)	(4.4)

India, with about 11 per cent of the world livestock population, occupies a significant place numerically in respect of livestock wealth. With 2.4 per cent of the land area of the world, and only 4.2 per cent of the world's freshwater, it maintains 1.21 billion human population which is more than 18 per cent of world's human population and about 529.70 million livestock and 648 million poultry (Table 1.4). The cattle, buffalo, sheep, goat and pigs population which was 185.20, 97.90, 61.50, 124.4, 13.50 millions in 2003 reached to 199.10, 105.30, 71.60, 140.5, 11.1 millions,

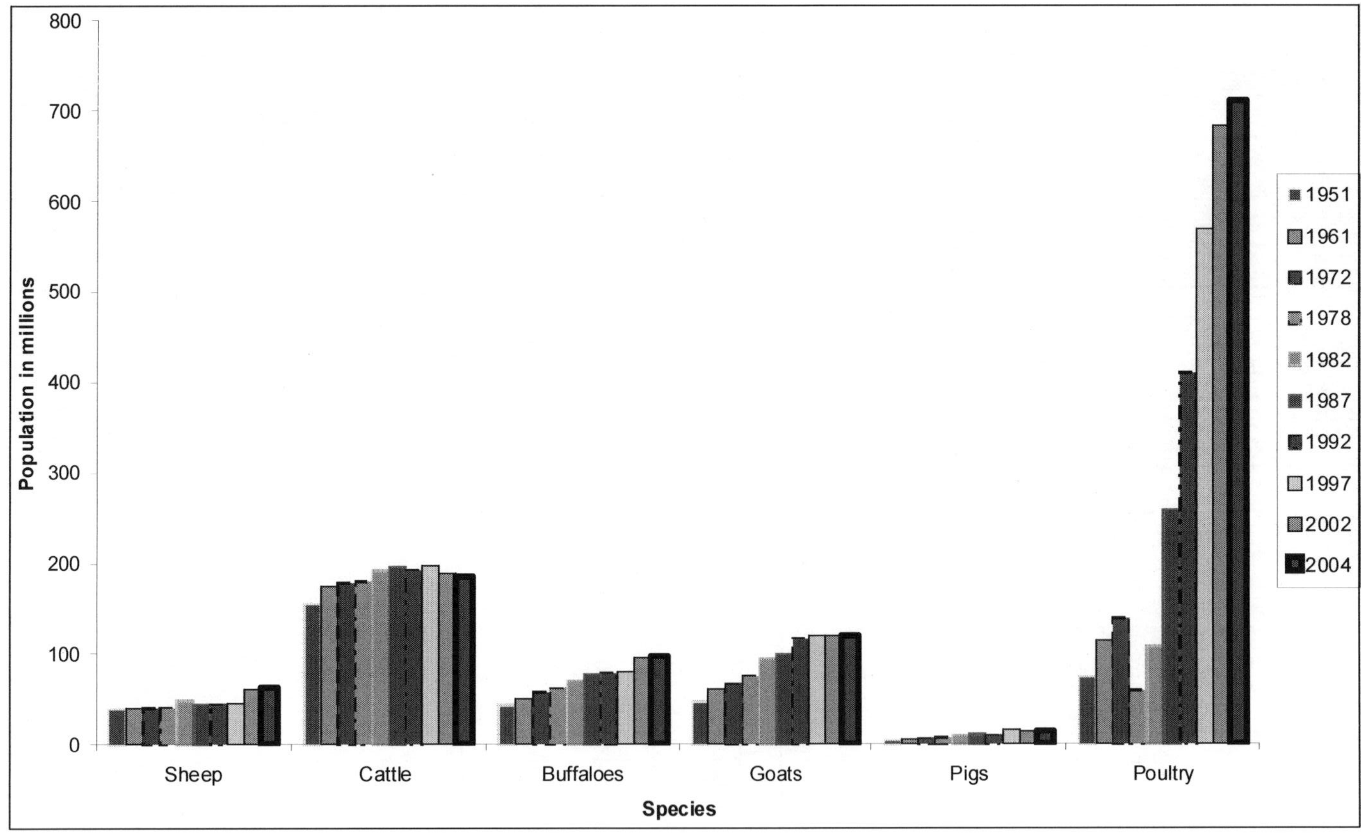

Figure 1.1: Scenario of Indian Livestock Population since Independence.

Table 1.3: Population of Various Livestock (in million) 2004 (FAO, 2004)

	India	World	Percent of World's Population	Rank in World
Cattle	185.50	1334.51	13.90	1
Buffaloes	97.70	172.72	56.57	1
Goats	120.00	780.10	15.38	1
Sheep	62.50	1038.78	6.02	4
Pigs	14.30	951.78	1.50	–
Total	480.00	4277.89	11.22	1
Poultry	711.54	–	–	–

respectively in 2007 (18th Livestock census, DADF, M/o Agriculture). The average annual growth rate in population of these species during the corresponding period was 1.83, 1.84, 3.87, 3.10, (-) 4.74 percent. Buffalo has surpassed the cattle population growth rate for various reasons *viz.*, use for milk, meat and draft purposes as well as PFA standards for per cent fat and SNF favoring buffalo milk rather than cow milk production. Though the country possesses about 57 per cent of buffaloes, 14 per cent of cattle, 16 per cent of goat, 6 per cent of sheep and 1.5 per cent of world pig population but on production front the progress in yield/animal does not match with even world averages. Country has the largest livestock population, with most milk production, 6th in Meat Production and 3rd in egg and fish production, yet has high incidence of malnutrition, food insecurity, and rural poverty. India's food security situation continues to rank as "alarming"(IFPRI, 2011).

Table 1.4: Livestock and Poultry Resources in the Country

Species	Population in 2003 (Millions)	Population in 2007 (Millions)	Average Annual Growth Rate (Per cent)	Per cent of World Population	World Ranking
Cattle	185.20	199.10*	1.83	14	2nd
Buffalo	97.90	105.30	1.84	57	1st
Sheep	61.50	71.60	3.87	6	3rd
Goat	124.4	140.50	3.10	16	2nd
Pigs	13.50	11.10	(-)4.74	1.50	–
Total Livestock	485.0	529.70	2.23	11.0	–
Poultry	489.0	648.0	7.33	–	5th

The meat animals include mainly the cattle, buffalo, sheep, goat, pigs and the poultry. Out of these, buffalo meat is the main contributor to the meat industry. The poultry contribution is also significant. Population of different livestock species is illustrated below as per FAO, 2010 (Figure 1.2).

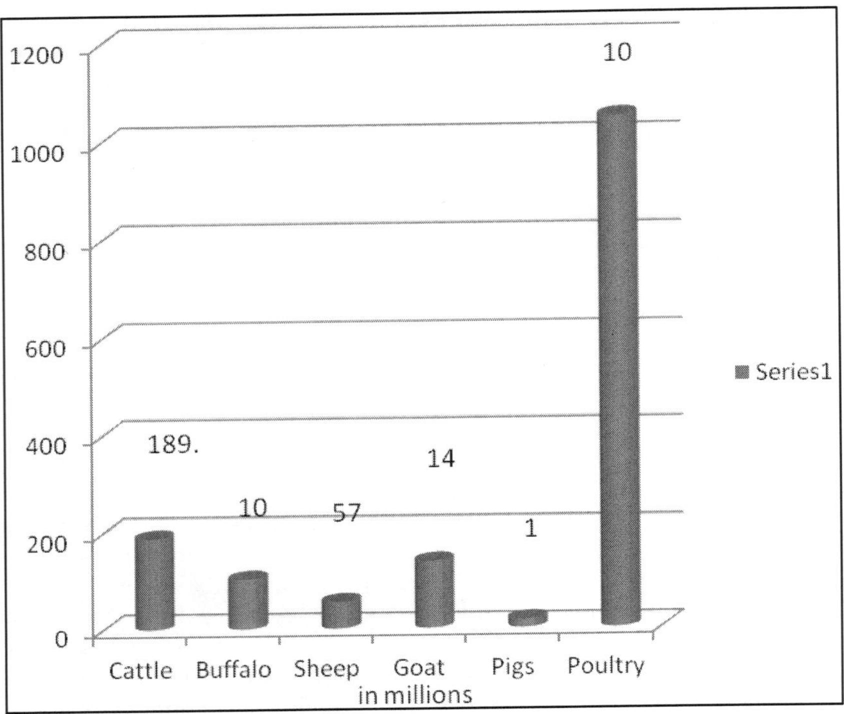

Figure 1.2: Livestock Population of different Species.
***Source*: Department of Animal Husbandry and Dairying, GOI, FAO-2010.**

Meat Production

No doubt that animal husbandry in India has made a great stride in different parts of the country. This has not been portrayed by the meat industry. However milk and egg production was justified to some extent. The animal protein supply to vast human population is only 10 kg as against the world average of 25 kg and Asian average of over 16 kg. This is due to lack of focused development efforts for improvement. On an average an India gets only 5.7 kg meat annually as against 11.0 kg recommended intake. It is estimated that to meet the requirement of non-vegetarian population which is estimated as 70.0 per cent, country requires to produce over 10 million tonnes of meat.

In India meat is obtained mainly from dual purpose livestock or unproductive ones after their usefulness for draft, milk, wool or reproduction is over. The social and religious taboos are attached to meat from large ruminants and pigs. Pig and poultry industry competes directly with human food for their better performance. Sheep and goat meat is most preferred among all livestock meat and free from religious and social taboos. There are about 5 million families are estimated to be engaged in rearing of sheep and goat and utilizing their products.

Table 1.5: Scenario in the Decade 1994-2004 (millions)

Species	*1994*				*2004*				*Per cent Increase/Decrease*		
	No.	*Slaughter Head*	*Extraction Rate (Per cent)*	*Meat Production (MT)*	*No.*	*Slaughter Head*	*Extraction Rate (per cent)*	*Meat Production (MT)*	*No.*	*Extraction Rate*	*Meat Production*
Cattle	192.98	11.89	6.16	1.29	185.50	14.40	7.76	1.48	–7.48	1.6	12.83
Buffalo	78.83	8.59	10.9	1.204	95.70	10.75	11.23	1.48	17.63	0.33	18.65
Sheep	44.81	14.03	31.3	0.16	62.50	19.90	31.84	0.24	28.31	0.54	33.33
Goats	118.35	46.16	39.0	0.47	120.0	47.50	39.58	0.48	1.34	0.58	2.08
Pigs	11.78	11.72	99.5	0.41	14.30	14.20	99.3	0.50	17.62	–0.2	18.0
Poultry	467.00	–	–	1.04	711.54	–	–	1.72	34.36	–	39.53
Total				**4.57**				**5.76**			**20.66**

The total meat production in India is 5.76 million tonnes. Majority of which is made available through about 3600 recognized slaughter houses in the country. As per FAO estimates (FAO, 2004) about 47.5 million goats, 19.9 million sheep, 25.2 million bovines (cattle and buffaloes), 14.2 million pigs were slaughtered leading to extraction rate of about 39.6 per cent goats, 31.84 per cent sheep and 11.24 per cent bovines and 98 per cent for the pigs. Perusal of these figures shows that though livestock population is highest in India, the slaughter rate is very low when compared to Europe or world average. In Europe the slaughter rate of sheep and goat is as high as 73 per cent and cattle are also above 45 per cent. The world average of sheep and goat slaughter is also above 50 per cent. Even in the last decade there is no change in the extraction rate of the animals. The slight fluctuation in increase in number of cattle slaughter head of about 1.6 per cent is observed. As it is expected that meat production is highly correlated with number of animals but the higher meat production in developed nation, Australia, Oceania and North Central America is due to higher carcass weight compared to African countries and India. Even if we compare among SAARC countries, under similar agroclimatic conditions and adopting similar production systems the average carcass weight in Pakistan for goat is 21.0 kg and sheep 24.0 kg as against 10 and 12.0 kg in India. The maximum bite of meat is contributed by poultry which accounts for 1.72 million MT. It contributes 29.86 per cent of total meat production of the country. The bovines (cattle and buffaloes) combined contributes more than 51 per cent of total meat production of the country. In the world meat scenario India accounts for only 2.23 per cent of total meat production, but it has an distinction of production of 46.7 per cent of 'carabeef' of the total world's production. It is quite evident that pig meat and chicken meat predominates world's total meat followed by beef.

Table 1.6: Meat Production from Various Livestock Resources–World and India 2004 (in MTs)

Species	*World*	*Percent of Total*	*India*	*Percent of Total*	*Percent of World's Total*
Beef and Veal	58.70	22.80	1.48	25.69	2.52
Buffalo Meat	3.17	1.27	1.48	25.69	46.69
Mutton and lamb	7.89	3.06	0.24	4.17	3.04
Goat Meat	10.04	3.90	0.48	8.33	4.78
Pig Meat	67.72	26.30	0.50	8.68	0.74
Chicken	70.96	27.56	1.72	29.86	2.42
Total	257.51		5.76		2.23

The meat produced from various species is given in the Table 1.8. As evident from the table, maximum contribution in the total meat is from bovines. The sheep contribution is least of all. The contribution from the goats is relatively less in consideration with its population.

Table 1.7: Meat Production (Tonnes) Year 2008 (India)

Species	*Poupulation (Million)*	*Slaughter Head (million)*	*Per cent Slaughter Rate*	*Production (Tonnes)*	*World Percentage (Per cent)*
Buffalo meat	106.63	10.34	10.0	1496748	44.56
Cattle meat	172.45	8.60	5.0	1258248	2.01
Chicken meat	613.0	–		2490000	36.63
Duck meat	–	–		72800	1.92
Goat meat	126.01	47.88	38.00	544000	11.05
Pig meat	13.84	13.74	99.27	497000	0.48
Sheep meat	65.72	19.98	30.40	237120	2.87
Meat nes (Others)	–	–		200000	2.94
Total				**6795916**	

Table 1.8: Meat Production (India) FAO 2010

Livestock Species	*Population (million)*	*Animal Slaughtered (million)*	*Percentage Slaughtered*	*Carcass Weight, kg*	*Meat Produced (Million tonnes)*	*Share in Total Meat Production (per cent)*
Cattle	189.4	14.2	8	103	1.49	31.1
Buffalo	105	10.3	10	138	1.85	30.5
Sheep	57	19.2	47.9	12	0.25	4.9
Goats	140	47	37.9	10	0.57	10
Pigs	18	16	88.9	31	0.6	10
Poultry	1049	604	73.6	0.8	1.6	13.4
Total					**6.09**	**100**

Source: Department of Animal Husbandry and Dairying, GOI, FAO-2010.

Production of Major Livestock Products

The White Revolution in the country simultaneous to Green Revolution has trebled milk production, now exceeding 127 million tons (2010-11). The egg production has increased significantly from 30.44 billion in 2000 to about 65.50 billion in 2010-11. The egg production has just doubled in ten years but our share in world total was only 2.13 per cent. On meat production front, with production of 6.18 million tons meat annually, country ranks 6th in the world contributing about 2.00 per cent to the world total meat production of about 295 million tons (FAO, 2012). India is the 6th largest producer of poultry meat (2.22 million tons) in the world, yet percentage share in world total was only 2.61 per cent. Despite having largest livestock population, the volume of global trade in leather stands at US$ 137.96 billion (2011-12), with India contributing only US $ 4.86 billion (3.52 per cent) (Council for Leather Exports, India, 2010).

Economic Contributions

Value of output from livestock sector on the basis of current prices (2010-11) was Rs. 4, 61,434 crore which is about 28.40 per cent of value of output of Rs.16,23,968 crore from total Agriculture and allied sector. Sector contributes approximately 4 per cent to National GDP and 25 per cent to Agricultural. The Economic contribution of meat was Rs.72, 444.22 crore. The economic contribution of milk (Rs.2, 62,215 crore) is higher than paddy, wheat and sugarcane. It not only provides high quality animal products but also utilizes non-edible agricultural by- products to convert them into quality proteins. It also provides skin as raw material base for the leather sector as well as fat, bones, bristles, blood, wool, fibers, hairs for the cottage industry. Meat industry in India has great economic potential but received limited attention for its growth and development. Yet the value of output from meat group is Rs. Rs.72, 444.22 crore. It is envisaged to achieve 10 per cent growth rate in meat sector during 12th Five Year Plan period. The earnings through meat and meat products export during 2010-11 were Rs. 9033.53 crore.

Slaughter Rate

As per FAO (2011) estimates, 10.60 million cattle, 10.89 million buffaloes, 24.45 million sheep, 59.66 million goats, and 9.40 million pigs were slaughtered for meat production.

Availability is Lower than Requirements

The per capita consumption of meat in the country was about 13.70 g/day *i.e.* 6.0 kg annually as against the 11 kg recommended. World average is 106.85 g. In USA, it is 337g, the highest followed by 331 g in Spain, 323 g in Australia. In China, it is about 148g/caput/day. Animal protein has its special significance in daily human diet because of its high biological value and being balanced and rich in essential amino acids, B-vitamins and certain essential minerals. The livestock products provide almost one third of protein intake by the people. However, keeping in view the growing population, the animal protein availability has to increase at least three fold (Table 1.10) for maintaining the nutritional level of growing children and nursing mothers in India. By increasing the production, it will serve as potential remedy for widely prevalent malnutrition in children and pregnant and nursing mothers. The price of meat, chicken, and eggs has also gone very high in the domestic market. This shows that there is significant short supply of these items in the market which is due to spurt in demands owing to increased purchasing power and growing nutrition consciousness in people.

Demand Projections by 2020

Assuming that national economy would continue to grow above 7 per cent GDP (High income growth), Dastagiri (2004) estimated that by 2020 country would require about 227.17 million tons of milk, 47.37 million tons of mutton and goat meat, 1.45 million tons of beef and buffalo meat, 1.23 million tons of chicken and 79.10 billion of eggs. Considering 1993 as base year, during 1993-2020, the demand will grow at the annual compound growth rate of 6.71 per cent for milk, 20.01 per cent for mutton and goat meat, 4.41 per cent beef and buffalo meat, 6.47 per cent for chicken, and 8.48 per cent for eggs. The demand for mutton and goat meat will grow much faster among livestock products followed by eggs.

Table 1.9: Production* of Major Livestock Products

Year	*Milk (million tons)*	*Eggs (billion Nos.)*	*Meat (million tons)***
1999-2000	78.30	30.44	3.99
2010-2011	127.30	65.5	6.18
Rank in World	1st	3rd	6th
Per cent Growth rate in 2009-10 over 1999-2000	63.0	115.0	28.0

Extracted from Basic Animal Husbandry Statistics Report (2012), DADF.

*: Anticipated; **: Plus poultry.

Table 1.10: Demand Projections for High Value Livestock Product Commodities by 2030 (in million tons)

Commodities	*Year*		*Expected increase*
	2000	*2030*	
Meat	4.5	15	3.3 times
Fish	6	16	2.67 times
Eggs	17	57	3.35 times
Milk	76	182	2.4 times

Source: Vision 2030, ICAR (2011).

Table 1.11: Growth Rate in Meat Sector during XI Plan

1.	Meat	4.1 per cent
2.	Buffalo meat	8.0 per cent
3.	Milk	4.1 per cent
4.	Eggs	5.56 per cent

Table 1.12: Meat Yield from Various Livestock in India

Sl.No.	*Species*	*Average Carcass Weight/per Animal (kg)*	
		India	*World*
1.	Cattle	103	202
2.	Buffalo	138	140
3.	Sheep	12	16
4.	Goat	10	12
5.	Pig	35	79

Table 1.13: Demand Projections for Livestock Products (in million tons) in India by 2020

Livestock Product	*Year*		*Growth Rates (per cent) from1993 to 2020*
	1993	*2020*	
Milk	45.02	277.17	6.71
Mutton and Goat meat	0.78	47.37	20.01
Beef and Buffalo meat	0.49	1.45	4.41
Chicken	0.25	1.23	6.47
Egg *	9.30	79.10	8.48

* Billion numbers in case of egg.

Growth rate of total is weighted average growth rate.

1993 is considered as base year.

The present production of meat is estimated at 6.27 million tons in 2010 (FAO, 2012), which is 2.21 per cent of the world's meat production. The contribution of meat from buffalo is about 23.33 per cent, while cattle contributes about 17.34 per cent, sheep 4.61 per cent, goat 9.36 per cent, pig 5.31 per cent, poultry 36.68 per cent and other species 3.37 per cent. The meat production has increased from 764,000 tonnes in 1970-71 to 6.27 million tons in 2010. The compounded average growth rate (CAGR) during the last two decades works out to be 4.5 per cent. It is noticed that about 10.6 per cent cattle, 10.6 per cent buffaloes, 24.1 per cent sheep, 58.7 per cent goats, 95.0 per cent pigs and 190.0 per cent chicken are slaughtered each year. The value of meat and by-products is Rs 79,889 crore including skin and hides, while the export value of meat and meat products work outs to be more than Rs 6,000 crore in the year 2009-10. The contribution of buffalo meat accounts for more than 75 per cent of total exports/ foreign earnings.

The poultry has gaining the widely acceptance by consumers and growing 10-15 per cent annually. The chicken meat contributes about 37 per cent meat to total production and number one contributors. The growth is expected more in near future. This might be due to popularity, price, easy availability, no religious taboos and much more characteristics in poultry.

Quality meat production depends on the hygienic harvesting of meat in the slaughter houses. Indian meat traders are still in stone age and using primitive, outdated, unhygienic and cruel practices. At present there are 3600 licensed or registered slaughter houses under civic bodies are very old and the hygienic conditions are very poor and not upto the standards except few plants under private/public sector management. First modern abattoir was established at Deonar in Mumbai in 1973. In the fourth five year plan 8 bacon factories were established at different parts of the country under foreign assistance. A central sector scheme for the modernization of slaughter house in major cities of the country was proposed during the fifth Five year plan. Few Export Oriented Units (EOU) were established by private sectors which are engaged in harvesting the quality meat and exporting to a large number of countries. In India most of the meat is sold as raw or served at restaurants and hotels and less than 2 per cent of the meat is processed. This figure is as high as 70 per cent in Russia, Netherlands, USA and other developed countries.

Meat Production Potential

In spite of big potential, the Indian meat industry has not taken its due share. The major constraints for the meat industry are lack of scientific approach to rearing of meat animals, unorganised nature of meat production and marketing, socio-economic taboos associated with meat eating, inadequate infrastructure facilities and poor post-harvest management. The situation is further compounded by insistence of domestic consumers to buy freshly cut meat from the wet market, rather than processed or frozen. A majority of these abattoirs have outdated, primitive slaughtering facilities, use unhygienic practices and lack basic facilities for the production of wholesome and safe meat for domestic consumers. Further, most of the meat for domestic consumption comes from poultry, sheep and goat that are slaughtered in unorganised/unregistered premises/meat shops. Livestock development is not in coherence with the requirements of meat consumption and meat business. Productivity of meat breeds has not tapped adequately. Livestock farmers are unaware of the potential of meat business. Many middle men are involved in livestock marketing. Livestock marketing is not well organised. There is no integration of animal farming, meat producers, processors and marketing. Potentiality of male buffalo for meat production is not realised.

Meat Production Practices

The meat animals are slaughtered in specially constructed establishment/place/premises/building wherein food animals are slaughtered for production of meat and slaughter by-products with licensing from the concerned authority is called as slaughter-house. Modern abattoir is also a slaughter-house where animals are slaughtered under humane and hygienic conditions for production of wholesome and safe meat for human consumption. Recently, "meat plant" is the word which has been introduced in the place of "slaughter houses" and "abattoirs" for two reasons: to obviate the bad feelings about animal slaughter and to denote factory system of operations by which the animals are handled humanely and the total operations are done hygienically and methodologically and, many a times, in a forward integration manner which include operations like carcass cutting, production of custom-designed retail and lean cuts, their packaging and dispatch. Initially, slaughtering was a backyard proposition. Every meat trader used to slaughter his food animals in the space adjacent to his selling premises. Slaughter operations produced lot of blood and animal wastes and, if these are not cleaned properly, they would stink because they are all perishable materials of organic origin. As awareness about the implications of meat on human health grew and the deleterious effects on the environment were realised more and more, governments considered "meat inspection" as one of their obligations to the society. Centralised premises were constructed for slaughter of food animals. Acts and ordinances were promulgated on meat inspection to the effect that sale of carcasses and offal's meant for human consumption should have been produced only from animals slaughtered in these special premises and passed through meat inspection procedures. Backyard slaughtering was banned and slaughter houses came into existence. In India, there are about 4,000 registered slaughter houses with the local bodies and more than 25,000 unregistered premises, where animals are slaughtered to fulfil the demands of domestic consumers. There are about 20 integrated abattoirs-cum-meat processing plants with state-of-the-art facilities for hygienic meat production to meet the export demands, where animals are received from the suppliers who procure the animals from the weekly markets.

Supply Chain

Production and supply of meat for local consumption is one of the most neglected and poorly organized sectors in the country. The local slaughterhouses operate as service abattoirs where butchers slaughter the animals for a fee/wages or get some edible/inedible by-products as a part of daily remuneration. Meat produced in municipal slaughter houses following ante and post-mortem inspection and declared fit for human consumption is transported to shops and sold "hot" for local consumption. The consumers prefer fresh carcass meat instead of chilled or frozen due to lack of confidence on cold chain maintained during transit and storage. Though the consumption of meat and meat products is on rise, hygiene, safety and quality aspects have not changed much. Except poultry (20 per cent), less than 1 per cent of meat produced from buffalo, small ruminants, and pigs is under organized sector. In private sector, there are 37 modern integrated approved abattoirs-cum-meat processing plants where quality de-boned frozen meat is produced for exports adopting OIE guidelines and international quality standards. These plants follow all the sanitary and phytosanitary (SPS) measures required by the International Animal Heath Code of OIE. In addition, 40 meat processing and packaging units that receive dressed carcasses from approved municipal slaughter houses across the states are also licensed under APEDA for exports.

Existing Conditions of Slaughter-Houses for Domestic Supply

The existing condition in the majority of the traditionally slaughter-houses is far from satisfactory. Most of the slaughter-houses are lacking basic facilities like water, electricity, ventilation, drainage, ceramic flooring, overhead rails and waste disposal. Animals are slaughtered in traditional ways on the open ground with/without further processing or dressing on the floor/rails are the common practices in a majority of the slaughter-houses. Carcasses are exposed to heavy contamination from dung and soil. Situation is further aggravated by inadequate ante-and post-mortem inspection practices. The quality of meat produced in these existing slaughterhouses is unhygienic and carries high levels of microbial contamination. Though cooking may kill many of the microorganisms in meat, cross-contamination of the products eventually occurs under the prevailing conditions of meat-handling. Enormous quantities of by-products are not utilised efficiently and economically. These existing slaughter houses are mostly under the local governmental authority and no one bother about their 'upgradation' and consumer/public health point of view. The authority is concerned for the collection of money in such type of slaughter houses. There is urgent need to upgrade these slaughter-houses with minimum basic facilities.

India is bestowed with a major share of the global livestock population comprising of 205 million cattle, 100 million buffaloes, 65 million sheep, 126 million goats, 14 million pigs and 621 million poultry. There are about 3,600 licensed slaughter houses in India to produce meat for human consumption. These are primary meat processing houses and are administered by local authorities. Most of them are use primitive technologies for the production of hygienic meat and lack facilities for value addition and efficient byproducts utilization. There are about 31 modern slaughterhouses involved mostly in slaughter and processing of buffalo and few in sheep and goat and poultry. In addition, a large proportion of meat is obtained from animals slaughtered or small unlicensed establishments. When meat animal is slaughtered and processed, only one third is meat and the rest comprise co-products and byproducts, which need to be adequately processed in order to recover useful products of human utility, economic significance and meet the environmental regulations. The animal byproducts (including organs, fat, skin, feet, abdominal and intestinal contents, bone and blood) of cattle, pigs and lambs represent 66.0, 52.0 and 68.0 per cent of the live weight, respectively. At the moment the industry focuses on selling carcass parts. This includes the muscle being sold as meat cuts and other parts are used for rendering (not fully/economically). Therefore, efforts are needed for proper collection, process and utilization of slaughter house byproducts to improve economic value and address environmental concerns.

The livestock sector is growing at 4.5 per cent annually, as against the crop sector which is growing at 2.5 per cent. The contribution of meat output to the total agriculture and livestock is about 4 per cent and 15 per cent respectively. The value of meat and related byproducts is Rs. 79,889 crores (US $ 16,997 million), including skin and hides. India is the largest buffalo meat exporting country (Carabeef) globally, with smaller amounts of other animal meat. Production and export of meat from India commenced in the year 1969. During the last 41 years, the quantity of meat exported from India has been increasing and so also the number of countries to which it is exported. Currently India is exporting quality and safe meat to about 64 countries. In India in 2009, 10344000 buffaloes were slaughtered and 1427472 tonnes of meat are produced (FAO, 2011), while the remaining about 2172240 tonnes of byproducts (excluding skin) are not properly utilized. Similarly 47880000 goats were slaughtered and 478800 tonnes of meat are produced, while the remaining about 718200 tonnes of byproducts (excluding skin) are not properly utilized, and 756000000 chickens were slaughtered and 680400 tonnes of meat are produced, while the remaining about 529200 tonnes of byproducts are not properly utilized. Hence, there is a huge potential for developing value addition technologies to byproducts and to develop a business model for by-product utilization for the growth of organized meat industry.

Export of Meat

Meat ranks first in the international trade. The pattern of the world meat production has changed with first position by poultry and closely followed by pork and buffalo meat. However at world meat trade scenario pork and beef has dominance. Despite India's vast livestock resources and huge share in the world livestock population, the export of meat and meat products are very meagre that is <2 per cent of the total world meat trade of more than 18 million tonnes. The major exporter of the world market and their share are USA (14 per cent), Netherlands (13 per cent), France (10 per cent) and Australia (9.0 per cent). India made a modest beginning in exports of meat in the year 1973-74 with about 2000 tonnes consisting mainly of buffalo meat. Since then our meat exports have grown substantially and buffalo is emerging as the future meat animal of the world and recognised as 'black gold' due to the fact that it is price competitive and lean without much of fat. The bulk of meat is exported as deboned frozen meat which accounts for 75 per cent of the total meat exported.The export of bovine meat, mutton, chevon and processed meat has increased almost 94-97 per cent by quantity and it is growing at the rate of 10 per cent annually. Abundance of livestock resources and central geographical location of India to Gulf and Far East countries hold a bright future for this trade. Moreover, Asia including India is emerging as the future heartland of meat production with the highest annual growth rate of 4.5 per cent in the world.

Table 1.14: Meat Exports from India

Year	*Quantity (Metric tonnes)*	*Value(Rs. in crores)*
1991-92	95000	230.00
1992-93	100000	330.00
1993-94	116180	361.54
1994-95	127400	391.80
1995-96	168317	611.43
1996-97	166265	690.08
1997-98	182900	791.03
2003-04	370466.81	2933.67
2004-05 (Apr-Jun)	73266.51	1638.78

Table 1.15: Slaughter Houses and Meat Processing Plants in India

Slaughter houses under civic/local bodies	3600
Modern Abattoirs	5
Integrated abattoir meat processing plant	1
Meat processing plants engaged in export of meat products	24
Approved export oriented units of meat processing	11
Bacon factories	7
Meat complex	1
Pork processing plant (public sector)	1
Modern integrated poultry processing plant	7

In 2005, the global meat production is expected to reach 270 million MT, an increase of 4.5 per cent than the previous year. International trade in meat is expected around 19 million MT. In the developing countries the meat production is stepping at

Table 1.16: Category-wise Export of Meat and Meat Products (Quantity and Rs in Millions)

	1995-96		1996-97		1997-98		2003-04		Growth per cent 1994-2004
	Tons	Rs	Tons	Rs	Tons	Rs	Tons	Rs	
Meat of Bovine animals	15970	5550	15757	6190	17633	7233	34381.76	15367.77	95.36
Mutton and Chevon	861	564	869	710	754	627	1682.53	1103.85	91.88
Processed Meat	48	41	51	44	26	22	159.57	89.97	96.98

the rate of 8 per cent whereas in developed countries it is expected to increase by 1 per cent. The poultry meat is expanding at the faster rate among the various meat categories, China and India will be next world player. Improved access to international markets following GATT/WTO agreement will contribute further expansion in world meat trade.

The largest share of export in India is from buffalo meat which rose almost three times in the last decade. Still total buffalo meat exports constitute only 10 per cent of buffalo meat production in the country and 90 per cent is consumed domestically. Our export has developed a niche in countries like Philippines, Malaysia, Iran, Egypt, Gulf, Middle East and CIS countries.

If we consider goat in particular this scenario takes on more significance when we consider that goat populations and goat meat production figures in developed countries are negligible compared to India. For example Australia has a very small goat population (2.3 million) compared to India (120 million), but it is the world's largest exporter (worth more than $ 15 million) of goat meat with over 90 per cent of its goat meat production being exported. On the other hand India's export earnings from goat meat are a meagre $0.7 million. The contribution of goat meat to total meat exported from India (mainly to Middle Eastern countries) accounts for less than 7 per cent compared to 70-80 per cent for buffaloes and 20 per cent for mutton. One could argue that in India most of the goat meat produced is consumed locally, thereby leaving little for export, but this is the only explanation for poor status of meat industry in India.

Table 1.17: The Meat Exports from India

Livestock Species	*2005-06*	*2006-07*	*2007-08*	*2008-09*	*2009-10*
Buffalo	460,593	494,111	482,925	460,031	513,668
Sheep/Goat	7,144	5,482	7,985	37,113	52,868
Total	**467,114**	**499,593**	**490,910**	**497,144**	**566,536**

Source: APEDA 2009-10.

Quantity in million metric tons.

Out of all the species, buffalo meat is the main contributor to the export business. Given ample buffalo populations and competitive Indian prices, the Indian buffalo meat industry has become one of the largest bovine meat producers in the world, with growth almost uniquely focused on the export market.

There is a preference for meat exported from India because of certain inherent merits such as its lean character, relative freedom from toxic feed additive residues, OIE 'negligible risk' classification for BSE, eradication of RP and CBPP, cheap, and near organic meat production. Currently India has been exporting meat to more than 60 countries. Buffalo meat is exported in frozen bone-less and de-glanded form and is free from FMD virus due to its ageing for minimum of 24 hrs at 2°C to bring down the meat pH below 6.0. Meat is available at very competitive prices. The Indian buffalo and lamb meat has established itself in the markets' of South-East Asia, Middle-East and African countries. India is the 6th largest producer of meat. The top five meat producing countries are China (80.75 million tons, 27.37 per cent), USA (42.17 million tons, 14.29 per cent), Brazil (23.45 million tons, 7.95 per cent), Germany (8.22 million tons, 2.78 per cent and India (6.18 million tons, 2.00 per cent). The world total buffalo meat production is about 3.32 million tons. Out of that, India contributes about 1.50 million tons. With this much production of buffalo meat, India ranks first, followed by Pakistan (0.63 million tons) and China (0.31 million tons). Country is 5th largest exporter of bovine (buffalo) meat out of the 9.45 million tons bovine meat traded internationally. The top five bovine meat exporting countries are Brazil (1.96 million tons), Australia (1.28 million tons), USA (0.60 million tons), Ireland (0.53 million tons) and India (0.48 million tons). Buffalo meat is one of the major commodities, among livestock products, exported from the country. Among the animal products exported from India, meat and meat products account for more than 90 per cent of the total exports volume. Remaining 10 per cent are dairy products and honey.

Table 1.18: Export of Animal Products from India

Quantity in M.Ts | Value in Rs. Crore

Products	*Year*					
	2008-09		*2009-10*		*2010-11*	
	Qty.	*Value*	*Qty.*	*Value*	*Qty.*	*Value*
Buffalo meat	462749	4839.70	495019	5480.60	709437	8412.68
Sheep and goat meat	37790	493.37	52868	747.20	11908	253.18
Poultry products	1057016	422.05	1016783	372.11	619150	301.32
Animal casings	1823	8.84	2020	31.52	1809	35.14
Processed meat	857	10.14	716	9.58	1366	21.05
Swine meat	817	9.17	1117	10.34	1115	10.51
Dairy Products	70146	980.96	34380	402. 68	36867	533.89
Natural Honey	15587	148.96	13311	146.65	31675	249.58
Total	**1646790**	**6913**	**1616216**	**7201**	**1413330**	**9817**

Source: APEDA 2012.

Export Potential

The meat exported from the country is simply chilled, de-boned, packed, and frozen for exports. In real terms there is no value addition as hardly 3 per cent of the total meat produced is processed and converted to various value added ready-to-eat/ready-to-cook products such as cured and canned products, sausages, ham, bacon, burgers, tikka, patties, kababs, pickle, cutlets etc. The consumption pattern of meat and poultry is quite promising for the processing industry but lacks proper organization and quality assurance. Under MFPO, 1973 there were 330 licensed meat processing units in the country as on 31-12-2010. The meat processed in these units mainly comprised of cured products, sausages and canned products. Several traditional meat products like meat kabab, chicken biryani, tandoori chicken, meat curry, etc. are already quite popular. Now-a-days other products like samosa, meat tikka, meat kofta, meat pickle are also in demand. Various region specific meat products like Nihari (Delhi), Goa sausage (Goa), pork pickle (HP), Gustaba and Nate Yakhni (Kashmir), Rapka (Arunachal Pradesh) are gaining wider acceptability. Western meat products like cured ham, bacon, sausages, frankfurters, hotdog, luncheon meat etc. have also registered an increase in demand in big cities. In view of the demand of Indian delicacies across the world, processing and export of processed meat products should be emphasized rather than export of live animals and fresh meat to fetch better profit and generating more employment. Major meat production centers in the country for exports are- Aurangabad, Nanded, Mumbai and Satara in Maharashtra; Goa; Zaherabad and Medak in Andhra Pradesh; Derabassi in Punjab; Barabanki, Unnao, Aligarh, Meerut, Saharanpur, Noida and Ghaziabad. in UP; Mourigram in West Bengal and Gurgaon in Haryana. State of UP is the largest producer and exporter of buffalo meat. Malaysia, Philippines, Saudi Arabia, Egypt, Angola, Jordan, UAE, Kuwait are major destinations for buffalo meat. Though there is no religious biasness for buffalo meat, its demand in domestic market is very limited due to limited consumer preference. Therefore, buffalo meat offers great potential for exports especially from male buffalo calves. During 2011, on carcass weight equivalence basis, around 1.15 million tons of buffalo meat was exported. The EU is expected to import large volume of bovine meat, over the next few years, as abolition of subsidies might lead to rapid decrease in production of livestock products.The Central America and the Caribbean, Russia, Middle East, East Asia and most of the African countries are the bovine meat deficit regions. The major demand for bovine meat is expected to come from these areas and also from the EU. South America, Oceania (Australia and New Zealand) and India are emerging as the major bovine and buffalo meat surplus countries. The continuous drought has been affecting Australia's herd building during the last few years and BSE issue limits the potential of North America. There are also serious concerns that Brazilian bovine meat supply may not be able to keep pace with sharply increased export projections for bovine meat. This offers a great opportunity for India, to grow its international trade volume in meat.

India Meat Export Surge-USDA' 2012

Indian buffalo meat exports have grown to a record level in the last two years, making India the fourth country in the world to export more than 1 million tons of bovine meat annually. As a result, 2013 buffalo meat exports are forecast at 2.15 million tons, around 30 per cent over 1.66 million tons in 2012. India's bovine herd continues to grow as a result of strong demand for dairy products, with calendar year 2013 combined stocks forecast at 327 million head and 2012 combined stocks estimated at 323.74 million head. Indian per capita consumption remains at 2 kg, reflection a preference for pulses, dairy, dairy and poultry.

- ✰ In 2013 Indian buffalo meat production is forecast to raise a record 4.16 million tons, up 10 per cent from 2012. In 2012 buffalo meat production is estimated at 3.64 million tons (up 12 per cent from 2011) and 2011 production has been slightly revised up to 3.24 million tons.

- India now accounts for nearly a quarter on world beef trade compared to a mere 8 per cent in 2009, while Brazil, Australia and US could made marginal increase in volume. This rapid expansion is fuelled by demand for low-cost product in many smaller, emerging and price sensitive markets (Middle East, Africa, South-east Asia).
- Expanding markets for processed Halal meat product provide a real opportunity for Indian meat export.

Advantages of India in the Export Market

1. Excellent Veterinary Infrastructure
   - Vet Hospitals/Polyclinics 1,715
   - Vet Dispensaries 14,473
   - Vet aid centers 23,682
   - Veterinarians 50,000
   - Para vets 45,000
   - Exclusive Veterinary Universities 4
   - Veterinary colleges 65
2. One National and four regional disease diagnostic labs working as referral labs.
3. India is strategically located.
4. Animals are fed on natural feeds- reared free from growth promoters and hormones.
5. Indian buffalo meat is produced according to Halal standards.
6. It is also characterized as a 93 per cent lean meat with positive blending characteristics.
7. Industry sources place significant weight on India's disease status, which includes OIE negligible risk classification for Bovine Spongiform Encephalopathy (BSE).
8. OIE free recognition for Rinderpest and CBP (Contagious Bovine Pleuropneumonia).
9. The meat is free from Radiation.

Various Export Companies in India

1. Allanasons

India's largest exporter of processed food products and agro commodities. The Company has been designated as the Five Star Trading House by the Government of India. Allana Group has achieved enviable growth in its exports, clocking 44 per cent over the last two years. They are the World's Largest Producer and Exporter of Frozen Halal Boneless Buffalo Meat. Allanasons is also India's single largest exporter of frozen meat, processed/frozen fruit and vegetable products. The Group has made substantial investments in creating world-class integrated food processing complexes.

Facilities have been certified for quality and product safety systems under ISO 9001:2000 and HACCP and ISO 14001 (Environment Management System). They have OHSAS 18000 towards an international occupational health and safety management system specification.The Allana Group enjoys the distinction of being the pioneer (1969) in the export of deboned and deglanded frozen Buffalo meat, exporting its products currently to 64 countries world-wide, including South East Asia, Middle East, CIS, Africa and Pacific Basin Nations, singularly accounting for about 60 per cent of meat exports from India. They are the World's Largest Producer and Exporter of Frozen Halal Boneless Buffalo Meat. Range of products:

- Fresh, frozen boneless Buffalo Halal meat.
- Chilled boneless Buffalo meat Compensated boneless Buffalo meat is supplied in natural proportion of the cuts and is guaranteed 93 per cent chemically lean.
- Canned corned meat.
- Full range of fresh quick frozen offal (fancy/ variety meat).

2. Darshan Foods Pvt. Ltd.

(Established in 1996) operating HACCP and ISO 9001:2008 certified processing plants at Haryana. The company maintains an excellent in-house Quality Control Laboratory which is fully equipped to test its product quality. All products are packed in virgin grade packaging materials and pass through stringent quality control checks and metal detection before being dispatched to customers in India and overseas.Delicatessen Stores in company owned company operated format along with shop-in-shop concept are also being operated by the company in major metro cities.

3. Hind Agro Industries Limited

Hind Agro Industries Limited is the first company in India to have Asia's one of the most modern abattoir-cum-meat processing plant at Aligarh in the State of Uttar Pradesh in North India. It is a joint venture of Hind Industries Limited, Govt. of Uttar Pradesh and assisted by Govt. of India. This plant at Aligarh is approved by the Agricultural and Processed Food Products Export Development Authority (APEDA), Ministry of Commerce, Govt. of India for export of meat and meat products. HAIL is the only company in the country to have the unique facilities of slaughtering the animals which have been bred and reared on strict guidelines set by the O.*I.E.* Paris. Farmers are encouraged to rear male buffalo calves specially for supplying to the company under the contractual farming. Company has also intensive feed lot to raise male buffalo calves on organic farming with natural feeds. The source and traceability of the animals are documented from the farm to the finished product. In turn, the company provides assistance to the farmers by supplying feed and veterinary services from the experts belonging to it. Qualified Veterinary Doctors conduct ante-mortem and post-mortem examinations on the animals procured from disease-free zones recognized by the U.P. Government's Veterinary Department, India. Halal is strictly

Table 1.19: List of Other Exporters from India

Sl.No.	Company	State	Products
1.	**Al Habib Food Exports**	Mysore, Karnataka India	Processed non vegetarian food, mutton samosa, chicken samosa, chicken burger patty, mutton kebab, mutton kofta, chicken kebab, chicken kofta, chicken fingers, chicken nuggets, chicken spring rolls
2.	**ALFA CHEM L CO - India**	Mumbai, Maharashtra India	Frozen cheek meat and meat product. frozen chicken feet, eggs, chicken
3.	**Al- Rabee Food Company - India**	New Delhi India	Buffalo meat, beef meat, frozen meat, meat and poultry, meat products
4.	**Ayaan International - India**	Navi Mumbai, Maharashtra India	Meat product,boneless meat, buffalo meat, red meat, halal meat, fresh meat, frozen meat etc.
5.	**Al Nasir Frozen Food Export - India**	Ghaziabad, Uttar Pradesh India	All Product of Frozen Buffalo Meat, Buffalo, Frozen Veal Meat Products, Meat Products, Meat Food Products, Canned Meat Products etc.
6.	**Suguna Poultry Farm Limited - India**	Coimbatore(tn), Tamil Nadu India	Frozen buffalo meat, shell eggs, fresh fish, poultry products, meat poultry, meat products, frozen seafood,
7.	**Muhawala Exporters - India**	Palakkad, Kerala India	Meat products
8.	**Qureshi Frozen Food - India**	Mumbai, Maharashtra India	Frozen meat, frozen boneless buffalo meat, crushed bone, beef hooves, poultry egg, tendon meat, poultry meat products
9.	**Fatimah Exports - India**	Ahmedabad, Gujarat India	Meat Products, Beef

carried out by Islamic Shariyath Procedures and is supervised by representative of Jamiath-Ulama-I-Hind, who issues certificate to that effect. THE HAIL plant has production capacity of 400 MT, certified by APEDA.

All the Plant machinery and equipments used are sourced from AUS/NZ/ EUROPE. Strictly hygiene and sanitation norms conforming to international standards are followed. Products are certified as quality produce of India by APEDA. The company has annual turnover in access of Rs 350 Crores. Focused area for exports to countries like Behrain, Egypt, Indonesia, Iran, Jordan, Kuwait, Lebanon, Malaysia, Mauritus, Oman, Oman, Phillipines, Qatar, Saudi Arabia, Thailand, UAE, Yemen, East and West African countries and CIS countries.

Prospects of Meat Industry

The prospects for the Indian meat industry seem bright in the years to come. This is primarily because of the improving livestock health situation in India, Dun and Bradstreet said in its latest study. India has always been free from mad cow disease and Rinderpest since 1995. With greater thrust on value addition and processed products, India's meat exports are likely to move up the value chain in a significant manner, the study said. Asian region is the largest importer of Indian meat with Malaysia and the Philippines being the most favored export markets, followed by the Middle East. Similarly, the African region has also emerged as a strong export destination for Indian meat exports in the last few years. Countries such as Angola, Congo and Gabon have grown significantly in the last five years. Even exports to the CIS countries have substantially improved over the years, the study added. According to the statistics, Asia accounts for 40.2 per cent of meat exports, followed by the Middle East (38.5 per cent) and Africa (12.1 per cent). Amongst the Asian region, Malaysia imports half of its $249 million worth meat from India alone. India is considered to be the single largest exporter of meat to the Philippines.

Government's Role

1. National Meat and Poultry Processing Board (NMPPB)

In this regard, in order to synergize the energies and efforts of every one related to the growth and development of meat and poultry processing in the country, the Ministry of Food processing Industries had formed a **National Meat and Poultry Processing Board (NMPPB)** as an autonomous body under the societies act and is functioning under the Ministry of Food Processing Industries. The NMPPB aims at boosting the growth of the sector for the benefit of the producers and processors. The Board will provide help to the industry in setting up or modernization of abattoirs by providing technical consultancy for the production of wholesome meat and meat products, value added meat food products and utilization of slaughterhouse by products. Immediate needs of the sector are to take advantage of liberalized world trade to benefit the Indian meat industry by harmonization of standards, giving incentives to farmer for quality livestock production and to adopt stringent quality control measures, to develop long term strategies for export, popularize and develop traditional products technology, and regularly monitoring for chemical residues and microbial quality and produce international standard meat products. The Board plans for modernization of Abattoirs in next five years by standardizing size, technologies, equipments, cost etc./bench marking of Abattoirs, establishing a full-fledged self financing Consultancy Division and providing consultancy to 10 large Abattoirs and 10 class 'B' city Abattoirs to be set up. Consultancy will be provided for setting up 50 large and 110 small Abattoirs. The Board will cater to the backward linkages- disease free zone/Traceability etc by organizing meetings with the Department of Animal Husbandry regarding.

2. Production Policy

A **National Project on Cattle and Buffalo Breeding (NPCBB)** was launched by the government in October 2000 for a period of 10 years. The project envisaged genetic improvements of indigenous cattle and buffaloes, development and conservation of important indigenous breeds and the building of a sustainable breeding policy, with a focus on increasing milk production. The government of India (GOI) has decided to continue this program through the 11th Five Year Plan period (2007 -2012). The nationwide animal mortality rate due to diseases as well as undefined reasons in India is reportedly at 7.5 percent in cattle and 9.6 percent in buffaloes. An estimated 40 million animals die every year in the country due to natural causes, disease and other problems. Livestock diseases constrain production and productivity of Indian cattle although a major pillar of the GOI's livestock development strategy recently has been the subsidized public delivery of veterinary services. Although Rinderpest has been eradicated, other cattle diseases still continue to pose a threat to livestock production. Diseases such as Foot-and Mouth Disease, New Castle Disease (Ranikhet Disease) are causing economic losses. Over time, the government has built up networks of physical and human infrastructure to provide veterinary services to millions of farmers. However, the quality of services provided by these institutions is sometimes inadequate. In response, the Department of Animal Husbandry, Dairying and Fisheries (DAHD), Ministry of Agriculture, GOI, is implementing the 2009 "**Livestock Health and Disease Control**" program in collaboration with various state governments (animal husbandry is a state subject), which aims to improve diagnosis of a series of common diseases. The various components of the program are: (a) Assistance to States for Control of Animal diseases; (b) National Project on Rinderpest Eradication; (c) Professional Efficiency Development; and (d) Foot and Mouth Disease Control Program. The DAHD has recently added some additional components to the program, which include The National Control Program of Peste des Petits Ruminants; The National Animal Disease Reporting System; Establishment and strengthening of existing veterinary hospitals/dispensaries; and a National Control Program of Brucellosis. At the World Organization of Animal Health 78th General Session, held in Paris, India was recognized as having negligible risk for Bovine Spongiform Encephalopathy (BSE). This recognition has been hailed by India's livestock sector in general and by the export-oriented meat industry in particular, which exports about 500,000 tons of bovine meat annually to over sixty countries. Based on the assessments and recommendations made by the GOI Standing Committee of Parliament and the Planning Commission, DAHD launched the program "Salvaging and Rearing of Male Buffalo Calves", which envisages utilizing male buffalo calves by rearing them for meat production and developing linkages with export-oriented slaughter-houses in several potential states. The Utilization of Fallen Animals scheme proposes to establish carcass utilization centers in animal density matrix areas and is expected to provide employment to the rural poor.

3. Govt's Role in Buffalo Meat Industry

One of the most important virtues of Indian Buffalo meat, we must emphasize, is its competitive price. It's a real value for money product and is also its Unique Selling Proposition (USP). For continued success, competitive price must be maintained. A number of issues from time to time affect the economics of the meat export industry detrimentally and are immediately taken up with the Authorities concerned. Issues which persist and currently affect the industry, many of which were projected at the first meeting of the Monitoring Committee on Agriculture held on 27th December 2004, are listed below. Inclusion of meat as an eligible item in the "Vishesh Krishi Upaj Yojana" (Special Agricultural Produce Scheme)

- ✰ Restoration of APEDA Financial Assistance for up gradation of export oriented abattoirs/processing plants as was applicable during 1997-2002.
- ✰ Inclusion of Buffalo meat under APEDA's Transport Assistance Scheme for new markets in Africa/CIS where freight cost from India for reefer containers is much higher than from competing countries.
- ✰ Restoration of DEPB rates for frozen Buffalo meat.
- ✰ Exemption from Service Tax on transportation of meat products processed for exports. This is presently applicable only for fruits, vegetables, eggs or milk even for domestic consumption.
- ✰ Ministry of Food Processing Industry's grants as per their published Schemes (currently being denied).

Most of these points pertain to steps which would help Indian Buffalo meat retain its competitive price. It will be seen that the meat export industry does not desire any special or out of the way benefits/subsidies. What it seeks is legitimate application (and non-denial) of existing schemes/policies to the meat export sector, wherever it is logical.

4. Processing

The processed meat sector, formerly regulated by the Ministry of Food Processing Industries MOFPI), is now regulated by the **Food Safety and Standards Authority of India (FSSAI)** through the Food Safety and Standards Rules and Regulation 2011. These regulations were enforced nationwide with effect from August 5, 2011, repealing the Meat and Meat Products Order (MFPO), 1973. The Food Safety and Standards Regulations (FSSR), 2011 contain standards and regulations for meat and meat products. The FSSR 2011 requires registration and licensing of meat processors and other food operators in the meat value chain. It also enforces sanitary maintenance and controls at all stages of meat (including fish and poultry) products production. These standards equally apply to domestic and imported meat and meat products. There are around 4000 municipal slaughter houses in the country and 30 abattoirs/meat processing plants. These 30 abattoirs/meat processing plants are 100 per cent export oriented units and are registered with the **Agricultural and Processed Food**

Export Development Authority (APEDA). Additionally, 74 meat processing and packaging units are also registered with APEDA. These meat processing and packaging units receive dressed carcasses from approved municipal slaughter houses for the export of meat. According to industry sources, approximately 7 slaughter houses are expected to be added by the end of 2012.

Existing Supply Chain and Value Chain

In India processed meat is sold primarily in two forms- frozen and chilled. Frozen meat is mainly meant for export while chilled meat is consumed in the domestic market. Municipal slaughter houses sell meat to the domestic market. Only 100 per cent export-oriented facilities, registered with the APEDA, are eligible to produce and process meat for export purposes. Export oriented processed meat is transported in refrigerated vans/containers from processing units to port locations and is stored in cold storage near port locations, from where the product is shipped to destination markets.

The Ministry of Food Processing Industries launched the comprehensive financial scheme, modernization of existing abattoirs/establishment of modern abattoirs, under the 11th five year plan (2007-2012). The program is expected to continue in the 12th five year plan period (2012-2017). MOFPI is also administering another scheme for technology upgrading, establishment and modernization of processing plants. In order to improve abattoir conditions, the National Meat and Poultry Processing Board http://nmppb.gov.in/), under the ministry of food processing industries (MoFPI), has taken up an initiative to provide consultancy to build around 160 modern abattoirs across the country. The first abattoir to be set up under the initiative has already started working in the Dholpur district of Rajasthan.

Pink Revolution

Harnessing buffalo for Quality meat production comes under Pink Revolution. When buffaloes are used for work and are sent to slaughter house at retirement age, the meat derived is definitely tough and of inferior quality. Comparison of meat from young buffalo and young cattle has clearly shown that buffalo meat is indeed as good as cattle meat (Heintz, 2001).

Future Strategies

The Government of India has given "Sun Rise Industry" status to Indian food processing industry under the Ministry of Food Processing and Industries. There is a lot of emphasis on the regularization and quality assurance of production, processing, packaging, storage, transportation and marketing of meat and meat products domestic as well as for export trade. Various programmes and policies were formulated for the development of meat industries in India. To circumvent the constraints and to achieve the targets of earnings, three pronged priorities are proposed.

Short Term Priorities (1st 5 Years)

1. Though meat has been recognised as important commodity and a thrust area, under recent five year plans, yet the required allocation of resources and practical implementation of the policy leave a big question mark along with several other issues crying for proper attention.

2. There is an urgent need to change the attitude and mindset of consumers as well as policy makers for the acceptance of meat as "maha prashad (grand blessings)" not "satan food (devil food)".
3. Ensuring the production of wholesome and safe meat, which can be accomplished by implementing uniform code of meat inspection (Ante mortem and post mortem), hygienic measures throughout the country with legal authority to bring corrective measures.
4. Regularization of disease control (FMD, Rinderpest) and to set up control points to check movements of the animals.
5. There is an urgent need for the technology upgradation, sanitary measures and modernization of our existing civic body's slaughterhouses and meat processing plant. A nationwide research survey on sanitary/hygienic status of fresh meat production and marketing chain including other factors effecting wholesomeness and safety of meat and byproducts be undertaken. Improvements suggested by this survey for quality assurance and safety programmes should be implemented.
6. Research and Development programmes should be established to focus on post harvest technology and value addition of meat and meat products for higher returns.
7. Commercial farming of meat animals should be encouraged in organised manner with appropriate animal husbandry practices and health care services. The programmes such as utilization of male calves by a feeder calf programme for meat purpose should be introduced and strongly implemented.
8. Improvement in the infrastructural facilities such as fast track refrigerated road and rail transport of commodities. The unfailing cold chains throughout the country connecting all major export points and processing units should be provided.

Medium Term Priorities (upto 10 years)

1. Eradication of diseases such as Avian influenza, BSE, Rinder pest and FMD etc. and setting up of disease free zones.
2. Development of meat breeds for different species which will give better yield and healthy animals for wholesome meat production.
3. Newer meat sources such as rabbit, yak, mithun, emu, duck, quail etc should get priority as regional or newer meat sources.
4. The programmes with strong R and D support for the economic utilization of byproducts and waste disposal for slaughter houses should be formulated and implemented. It will circumvent the cost escalation of meat and meat products.
5. There is a strong need for R and D in engineering inputs for the sector as the meat production and processing facilities are capital intensive.

6. The marketing of meat and meat products in domestic as well as international market should be deeply studied and socio-economic impact of the growth of the sector may be analysed from time to time.
7. The trained technical and supportive human resources should be harmonised with the institutes.

Long Term Priorities (Beyond ten years)

1. The role of biotechnology in processing and preservation of meat and egg products including development of newer, safe and healthy value added products should be explored on priority.
2. Genetic improvements through cross breeding programmes for intensive meat production. Development of tailor made and genetically modified meat and meat products with various nutritional and health positives.
3. Development of modernized meat industry which operate on 'state of the art' technologies in abattoirs, processing, preservation, packaging and marketing of meat and meat products.
4. Development of computer networking systems for the assessment of quality, shelf life and marketing of meat and meat products.
5. Development of health meat foods with natural preservative ingredients and bio-active compounds
6. Extension of shelf life of meat and meat products with innovative packa ging materials and methods with special emphasis to bio-active edible films.
7. Application of nanotechnology for improvement in the quality of meat and meat products.

The implementation of these strategies should be in true spirit with open and clear mind will augment the meat export. It will bring more foreign exchanges as well as generate large employment opportunities to the people in lower strata for better and prosperous life. It will also bring nutritional security to the people with animal proteins. The main reasons of poor productivity such as poor exploitation of genetic potential, inadequate resources of feed and fodder, insufficient health cover, inadequate marketing and credit support etc. should be curbed. All these efforts will make India ***'The Oyster'*** of global meat industry.

List of Major Programmes for the Promotion of Indian Meat Industry by different Agencies

Ministry of Food Processing Industries

Mega Food Parks

☆ The scheme envisages a onetime capital grant of 50 per cent of the project cost (excluding land cost) subject to a maximum of Rs. 50 crore in general areas and 75 per cent of the project cost (excluding land cost)subject to a ceiling of Rs. 50 crore in difficult and hilly areas *i.e.* North East Region including Sikkim, J&K, Himachal Pradesh, Uttarakhand and ITDP notified areas of the States.

- ☆ A Program Management Agency (PMA) is appointed by the Ministry to provide management, capacity building, coordination and monitoring support. For meeting the cost of the above and also other promotional activities by the Ministry, a separate amount, to the extent of 5 per cent of the overall grants available, is earmarked.

Cold Chain

The objective of the scheme of Cold Chain, Value Addition and Preservation Infrastructure is to provide integrated cold chain and preservation infrastructure facilities without any break from the farm gate to the consumer. It covers pre–cooling facilities at production sites, reefer vans, mobile cooling units as well as value addition centres which includes infrastructural facilities like Processing/Multi-line Processing/Collection Centres, etc. for horticulture, organic produce, marine, dairy, meat and poultry etc. Individual or group of entrepreneurs can set up integrated cold chain and preservation infrastructure with business interest in cold chain solutions. It can also be set up by those who manage supply chain enabling linking groups of producers to the processors and market through well-equipped supply chain and cold chain.

Financial assistance(grant-in-aid) of 50 per cent the total cost of plant and machinery and technical civil works in General areas and 75 per cent for NE region including Sikkim and difficult areas (J&K, Himachal Pradesh and Uttarakhand) subject to a maximum of Rs.10 crore.

Modernization of Abattoirs

The main objective of the scheme is for setting upof new and modernization of existing Abattoirs with a view to ensure applicationof modern technology for slaughtering of animal, supply of quality meat and meat products,efficient waste management and control of pollution,better utilization ofby-products,/value addition. The scheme is implemented preferably under PPPmode with the involvement of local bodies (Municipal Corporations andPanchayats)/Public Sector Undertakings/Co-operatives/Boards under Governmentand will have flexibility for involvement of private investors/exporters on aBuild-Operate–Own (BOO)/Build-Operate-Transfer(BOT)/Joint Venture (JV)basis.

The scheme envisages a grant of 50 per cent of the cost of plant and machinery and technical civil work and other eligible items subject to a maximum of Rs.15.00 Crores in general areas and 75 per cent of the cost of plant and machinery and technical civil work and other eligible items subject to a maximum of Rs. 15.00 Crores in difficult areas (NE states including Sikkim, Jammu and Kashmir, Himachal Pradesh, Uttarakhand and Integrated Tribal Development [ITDP] notified areas of the States) per abattoir.

R and D, QA, Codex and Promotional Activities

Quality and Food Safety have become competitive edge in the global market for the enterprises producing and marketing foods products. For a successful food processing sector in the country, various aspect of Total Quality Management (TQM) such as quality control, quality system and quality assurance should function in a horizontal fashion for total success. Further, in the processed Food Sector, R and D is an important area where focused attention is required as it is related to improvement of production, quality, consumer safety and public health. There is need for R and D for development and up-gradation of products, processes and technologies in the processed food sector.

The Scheme has the following components:

1. Setting Up/Up-gradation of Quality Control/Food Testing Laboratory
2. Implementation of HACCP/ISO 22000, ISO 14000/GHP/GMP Etc
3. Research and Development in the Food Processing Sector
4. Promotional Activities

National Mission on Food Processing

Ministry of Food Processing Industries (MOFPI) launched a new Centrally Sponsored Scheme (CSS) - National Mission- on Food Processing (NMFP) on 1st April 2012 for implementation through State/UT Governments. With the commissioning of NMFP, a number of schemes which were implemented by MOFPI during XI Plan period were subsumed with the Mission. The NMFP envisages establishment of a National Mission as well as corresponding Missions in the State and District level. The basic objective of NMFP is decentralization of implementation of food processing related schemes for ensuring substantial participation of State/UT Governments. The mission is expected to improve the Ministry's outreach significantly in terms of planning, supervision, monitoring of various schemes apart from playing a more meaningful role in policy formation.

Funding Pattern

NMFP implemented as anew centrally sponsored scheme in all the States in the ratio of 75:25 (Govt.of India and States) except for North Eastern States, where the ratio is 90:10.All the UTs are funded on 100 per cent grant basis.

Allocation and Release of Funds

Allocation of funds to state/UTs is based on population,area subject to minimum floor rate. MOFPI has already released its share for2012-13. GOI share for 2013-14 will be released to the extent of 50 per cent allocation meant for the states/UTs, after deducting the opening balance with the states/UT as on 01.04.2013. GOI share will be released in the corresponding years after deducting the balance in the previous financial year.

Second/subsequent installments in the respective financial year are released to the states on submission of the following documents:

GOI share will be released in the corresponding years after deducting the balance in the previous financial year.

- Proposal for release in prescribed format **(Annexure-I).**
- Utilization certificate of 50 per cent of the amount including the opening balance duly certified by Financial Authority of the State **(Annexure-II).**

Agricultural and Processed Food Products Export Development Authority (APEDA)

The Agricultural and Processed Food Products Export Development Authority (APEDA) was established by the Government of India under the Agricultural and Processed Food Products Export Development Authority Act passed by the Parliament in December, 1985. The Act (2 of 1986) came into effect from 13th February, 1986 by a notification issued in the Gazette of India: Extraordinary: Part-II [Sec. 3(ii): 13.2.1986). The Authority replaced the Processed Food Export Promotion Council (PFEPC). It is working under Ministry of Commerce and Industries.

APEDA provides financial assistance to its registered member exporters under the following schemes:

- Scheme for Market Development
- Scheme for Infrastructure Development
- Scheme for Quality Development
- Scheme for Research and Development
- Scheme for Transport Assistance

The details of the Financial Assistance Schemes along with check list for availing financial assistance can be accessed from APEDA website under icon **Financial Assistance Schemes** in section **Trade Information**.

Dept. of Animal Husbandry, Dairying and Fisheries, Govt. of India

Animal Husbandry Schemes

Centrally Sponsored

- Compendium of Salvaging and rearing of Male buffalo calves scheme
- Compendium of Pig Development
- Assistance for Modernisation of Slaughter Houses and Carcass Utilization Plants
- Conservation of Threatened Breeds of Small Ruminants, Rabbits, Pigs, Pack Animals and Equines
- Livestock Insurance
- Establishment/Modernisation of Rural Slaughterhouses

Conclusion

From the present status of the meat industry and the growth seen in this decade and the growing income of the people, it's clear that the scope of the meat industry is very bright in the coming years. Besides adding to the Indian financial status, it will also provide employment to lakhs of people thus improving the economy of the country. Also, the meat prepared and processed in the most hygienic conditions will help the people to overcome the deficiencies of various nutrients. But, this will happen only if the government takes the meat industry as seriously as the other industries.

SWOT Analysis of Indian Meat Industry

The overall acceleration of the pace of life, constraints of free time, the nuclear families and rapid urbanization besides global specialization has had a profound impact on the lifestyle of mankind. In the era of WTO/GATT regime we are now looking at the concept of global markets with each country identifying itself as either a consumer or a producer in a given industry. The food industry is no exception and with its scope, the meat industry.

Indian meat industry had a modest beginning in export in 1973-74 and even after 30 years it did not achieved 'adolescent' age. It is still considered as a kid in the global meat trade. However, it has its potential as a major foreign exchange earner. So, there is an urgent need for the crystal gazing of Indian Meat Industry and corrective steps should be taken to metamorphose it to adulthood. It will offers opportunities to galore entrepreneurs world wide and bring foreign exchange to the country. The complete and thorough evaluation of an industry is carried on the basis of **SWOT** formula which accounts for Strengths, Weaknesses, Opportunities and Threats.

Strengths

The strengths of Indian meat industry are:

1. Livestock Resources

India is a vast country and bestowed with abundant livestock resources in terms of number. The country has highest bovine population of the world. It possesses 185.5 million cattle and 95.7 million buffaloes which accounts for 13.9 per cent and 56.57 per cent of total world's, 50 per cent and 54 per cent of the Asian population respectively. India ranks first with respect to cattle, buffalo, goat population and fourth in sheep population. Small ruminants (sheep and goat) population estimates 21.4 per cent of the world. As per FAO estimate 2004, India posses 120 million goats, 62.5 million sheep and 14.30 million pigs (Table 1). The poultry industry is also growing at a very faster rate and increased 100 times in number since independence. The total poultry population is estimated to be 711.54 millions.

The annual growth rate in cattle, buffaloes, goat, sheep and pigs during the last two decade has been 0.1, 0.8, 2.5, 0.6, and 2.0 respectively.

2. Variety

India has varying agro-climatic conditions which have resulted in development of a number of breeds. The country has 26 breeds of cattle, 7 of buffaloes, 40 of sheep, 20 of goats, 4 of camels, 3 of pigs and 18 of poultry. Many high yielding breeds are also developed with cross breeding programme. In addition mithun, rabbit, quail, turkey and duck farming is also getting popular in few of the Indian states such as North eastern states, Kerala, Andhra Pradesh, Himachal Pradesh etc.

3. Organic Farming/Meat

In India, the animals utilized for meat purposes are generally reared either on pasture grazing or agricultural industry byproducts or crop residues. There is a less use of inorganic fertilizers, insecticides on these grass lands. No growth hormones are used for raising the animals and the animals are free from general toxic residues. Moreover Indian breeds are adaptable to tropical heat and diseases. So, there is less usage of drugs. Therefore, Indian meat is classified as organic meat free from various inorganic residues.

4. Price Competitive

The traditional and cost effective methods of rearing the livestock, lack of mechanized farming system lead to reduction in the cost of production of meat. Therefore, Indian meat cost is lesser than meat of other countries in the international market averaging US$1000-1500 per tonne depending on quality and type of meat. However, the world meat prices ranges from US$ 3,000-3,200. The FOB (Free on Board) prices of buffalo meat over the last five years have not shown any marked changes. The price of buffalo meat is ½ to 1/3 as compared to the world price of beef.

5. Cheap Labour

The cost of production of animals as well as meat and meat products are cheaper because of cheap human labour available in the country. The comparative labour cost (US dollars per hours) in India $0.40 and other countries (USA/Germany $6.7, Taiwan $4.0, South Korea $3.2, Mexico $1.8, China $0.6, Thailand $0.6, Indonesia $0.4) indicates advantageous position of India as the export of meat and meat products is labour intensive activity.

6. Geographical Position of India

The central geographical location of India to Gulf, African and Far East countries which are the major importer of meat is an added advantage. Whereas the other exporting countries USA, Australia, France, Germany are at distance. The proximity of India to the countries reduces transportation cost and ultimately the price of meat.

7. Acceptance of Indian Meat

The quality of Indian buffalo meat or mutton is well accepted in importing countries. It is devoid of much fat and is leaner. It has low cholesterol content. It is obtained from animals raised on natural pastures or green fodder thus has better flavour.

8. Free from Zoonotic Diseases

India is still **free from zoonotic** diseases such as Bovine Spongiform Encephalopathy (BSE) or 'mad cow disease' and Avian Influenza. These two diseases have created a panic in meat eating world.

9. Encouragement for Meat Export

The exports are the thrust area of Indian Government and several advantages are available in the new liberalised economic policies for establishing more number of processing units for export of meat and meat products. Government of India has given "Sun Rise Industry" status to Indian food processing industry under the Ministry of Food Processing and Industries. MOFPI is providing assistance upto 75 per cent to NGOs, co-operatives, civic bodies, govt. organizations, PSU/Joint sector in the form of grant or loan for establishing unit for meat and meat products. The Ministry of Agriculture and Agricultural and Processed Food Export Development Authority (APEDA) also promoting directly or indirectly the exports of meat by introducing various schemes.

Weaknesses

The second important aspect of SWOT analysis is to know the weaknesses of the industry. Indian meat industry is maligned with one or other abuse which weakens the image and growth of the industry. These weak links are following:

1. Prevalence of Livestock Diseases

The importing countries always demand meat from disease free herd especially the diseases listed as per O.I.E list "A", major animal diseases of the list are FMD, Contagious Bovine Pleuropneumonia (CBPP), PPR, Blue Tongue, Rinderpest, Blue Tongue, Vesicular Stomatistis etc. So, there is an urgent need to control and eradicate these diseases. The disease free zones should be established to promote the meat export at higher unit value realization.

2. Facilities in Abattoirs

Sanitary conditions and technology followed by most of the slaughter houses and meat plants are not desirable. Presently, there are about 3600 licensed slaughter houses which are controlled by civic bodies lacks basic amenities, hygienic measures and equipments. There are very few organized slaughter houses. A major quantity of meat is produced by unorganised sector or clandestine slaughter. There is preference for hot meat in India so mostly, poultry is slaughtered in front of customers without any veterinary inspection. There is an urgent need to improve the domestic slaughter houses in order to improve the image of Indian meat sector.

3. Lack of Effective Centralised and Uniform Meat Inspection

Procedures warrants the importing countries to keep their veterinarian to oversee the production and processing of meats in India. There is an urgent need for implementation of inspection procedures (ante mortem and post mortem inspection) by the trained qualified veterinarians. Presently, due to lack of infrastructural facilities and lack of trained man power the inspections are loosely monitored. The inspection procedures need to be strictly enforced. The meat stamped and passed after thorough inspection should only be sent to the market.

4. Productivity and Practices

The productivity levels of our meat livestock except poultry are much below as compared to those in the developed world. The average carcass weight for cattle 103 kg, buffalo 138 kg, goat 10 kg, sheep 12 kg and pigs 35 kg. However these figures are much higher in Oceania and Central America. Even if we compare among SAARC countries under similar agro-climatic conditions and adopting similar production systems. The average carcass weight for cattle/buffaloes, sheep and goat is taken as 220 kg 24.0 kg and 21 kg respectively. The poor productivity is mainly due to lack of high yielding meat breeds, poor exploitation of genetic potential, inadequate resources of feed and fodder, insufficient health cover, inadequate marketing and credit support system etc.

5. Lack of Cold Chain System

Meat is highly perishable commodity and needs chilled or frozen handling during transportation, storage and exports. However cold chains including refrigerated/frozen vans are not much developed in the country and thus danger of quality deterioration and public health risks remain high in our tropical climatic conditions. So, there is an urgent need to establish unfailing cold chains throughout the country connecting all major export points and processing units.

6. Lower Slaughter Rate

The slaughter percentages in India are poor especially large animals *i.e.* buffalo and cattle even compared to some Asian countries. The average extraction rate of cattle, buffaloes, sheep and goat is 7.76, 11.23, 31.84 and 39.58 per cent respectively. The Asian average of slaughter rate for buffaloes 12.40 per cent, cattle 19.90 per cent, goats 51.30 per cent and sheep 60.40 per cent (Table). This is due to lack of national slaughter policy for effective and efficient utilization of livestock resources. The government should formulate such a slaughter policy which promotes sustainable livestock production for maintaining growth trends in exports.

7. Grading Systems

Sometimes the importing countries specify their grades and their standards while placing orders create problem to comply with their requirements due to lack of proper grading system in Indian meat trade especially for live meat animals and carcass grades. Hence there is an urgent need to develop grading system in Indian meat trade both for quality meat animals and meeting the export market requirements.

8. Low Value Addition/Processed Meat

Major portion of Indian meat export is raw/boneless frozen meat. The share of the processed meat products/value added products is very little or negligible. The poor processing facilities for meat into value added products are another major constraint for better earnings of foreign exchange. We should give more emphasis on the exports of value added products based on scientific studies of eating habits and preparations liked in importing countries. Indian meat culinaries and many other products may be used to build brand image and to fetch higher foreign exchange.

9. High Capital Costs of Abattoirs and Processing Plant

The establishment of modern abattoir/meat processing plant requires high capital cost as most of the equipments/machineries are imported ones. There is a strong need to develop cost effective indigenous slaughtering, dressing and processing equipments to reduce the capital cost for the establishment of modern abattoirs and processing plants. This will ultimately reduce the cost of production of meat and add to the profits.

10. Religious and Ethnic Groups

Hinder the development of meat industry by their agitational approach. Negative propaganda of some social groups against meat exports, establishment of slaughter houses and promotion of non vegetarianism is seriously affecting meat trade. This need to be countered with facts and developmental requirements.

11. Poor Utilization of Slaughter House Byproducts

Non or under utilization of byproducts is big set back to Indian meat industry. It makes meat cost higher to the consumers and also deprives the trade and the nation of high valuable resources. Moreover it creates environmental pollution and 'bird hit' problems.

12. Lack of Food Retail Chains

In most of the developed countries the efficient marketing of meat, poultry and their products is developed by organized retail food chains. These organized retail chains develop their own cold chains and bring efficient supply chain management and develop market for food products.

Opportunities

In the era of WTO/GATT regime the opportunities for trade are abundant.

1. India's Liberalised Economic Policy

Thrust to export attracted large capital investments by NRI/foreign investments. The foreign investors recognising India as potential market as well as utilizing cheap land, raw materials and labour for setting their units. The export earnings through meat and meat products are increasing year by year @ 30 per cent. Earlier the major importing countries were United Arab Emirates (UAE), Kuwait, Saudi Arabia, Oman, Bahrain, Qatar and Yemen. Now many other countries such as Iran, Philippines, Malaysia, Egypt etc. also included in the list. The quantity of the meat exported is increased by 95-98 per cent in the last decade.

The opening of foreign direct investment (FDI) in food retailing if permitted, will lead to fast and efficient development of cold chain and supply chain management. The consumer will get better quality and variety of meat products and expansion of domestic and export market.

2. Buffalo- Black Gold

Buffalo is considered as future meat animals of the world. It is termed as "Black Gold" and it is emerging as animal of choice for Indian meat industry. India possesses 56.57 per cent of total world's buffalo population. The contribution of 'carabeef' in total meat production of India is 26 per cent which accounts for 46.7 per cent of total world's production. The buffalo meat has less cholesterol, more lean: fat ratio and higher content of myoglobins are added advantages over beef. The scope for this resource may well be appreciated. Indian government has placed the export of buffalo meat under OGL (Open General Licence) without any quantitative restrictions (Ministry of Commerce, 1997). Earlier there used to be MEP (Minimum Export Price) which has also been abolished for the export of meat and meat products.

Threats

The major threats to Indian meat industry are:

1. Prevalence of various livestock diseases such as FMD, Rinderpest etc.
2. **Lack of meat breeds:** The livestock is not bred specifically for meat purposes which results in low yield and quality. There is an urgent need to develop high yielding meat breeds for various meat animals especially cattle and buffaloes.
3. The unscrupulous practices of adulteration and unethical meat export leads to rejection of export consignment inturn impede the image of the country.
4. Lack of cold chain systems for transportations of meat and meat products.
5. Lack of quality assurance systems (HACCP, ISO 9000) and Good Manufacturing Practices. Lack of uniform code of ante and post mortem inspections of meat animals.
6. The religious and social taboos against the slaughter of cattle and pig are also a major threat against the development of meat industry in India.
7. There is a need for the promotion and publicity of Indian brands in the international meat market.
8. The rising competition in the world meat trade is also a threat to Indian meat export. Brazil, China and SAARC countries are posing a strong competition in the international market to Indian meat export.

Conclusions

SWOT analysis has given clear and complete picture of Indian meat industry. To augment the meat export, there is a need to realise the strengths, to circumvent the weaknesses/constraints, to grab the opportunities and plug the threats with solutions. It will help the Indian meat industry to keep pace with the galloping progress around the world. This will also help the nation to generate foreign exchange and provides opportunities for the employments.

References

1. Bhasin, N.R. and Kumar, Sushil (1998). Post Seminar recommendations (Round Table 1) of National Seminar on Improvement of Buffaloes for milk, meat, draught and future strategies for processing and marketing of buffalo products (Held at IARI, Pusa, New Delhi from 24-25th June, 1998).
2. FAO (2004) faostat.org 2004.

3. Narain, M.(1998). Agro-food processing and technology scenario and future vision. Processed Food Industry 1(3):17-20.
4. World Bank Report (1996) No. 14522. Livestock Sector Review.
5. www.faostat.com.
6. India Livestock and Products Annual Report Date: 22/09/2010. (USDA Foreign Agricultural Service) prepared by Ritambhara Singh.
7. www.gktoday.in (Indian Economy : Meat and Poultry Industry of India. National Meat and Poultry Processing Board).
8. Recent Developments in the Buffalo Industry of Asia by L.C. Cruz, Philippine Carabao Center, Philippines.
9. Livestock and Poultry: World Markets and Trade from USDA, April 2011.
10. The Meat and Poultry Sector in India (Tiecon 2011).
11. Vision, Strategy and Action Plan for Food Processing Industries In India by RABO India Finance Pvt. Ltd. For MoFPI, 2005.
12. www.exportersindia.com Meat export companies, India.

– *Chapter 2* –

Structure and Chemistry of Animal Tissues

I. Structure of Meat

What is Meat?

Animal tissues suitable for use as food, which includes muscles, bones, connective tissue, fat and vessels. Among all these tissues Skeletal muscles –are of principal interest to the meat industry. Muscle that is attached directly or indirectly to the skeleton is the skeletal muscle. Other muscle tissues are Cardiac muscle – muscle of the heart (Differentiated by the presence of intercalated disks) and Smooth muscle – located in arteries and the lymph system as well as the digestive tractand reproduction systems and are nonstriated in appearance (Figure 2.1). Muscle tissue is primarily muscle then connective tissue (adipose tissue, bone, cartilage, connective tissue proper). Skeletal muscles weigh about 35-65 per cent of carcass wt. and varies in size, form, shape. Abdominal Muscle-long, carpal-short, L.dorsi-34 cm, some muscles may be broad or narrow. There are three types of muscles based on activity – slow/fast/intermediate. Muscle is attached to bone, cartilage or tendon. Meat is postmortem aspects of muscle: Muscles may be striated and non–striated, Voluntary and involuntary. There are more than 600 muscles in animal body.

Muscle Organization

A whole Muscle is made up of Fascicules (Bundle of muscle fibers), which contain Muscle fibers made up of Myofibrils (Figure 2.3). Myofilaments are structural unit of myofibrils and Sarcomere is the structural and functional unit. Each muscle is covered with the connective tissue known as epimysium (Figure 2.6). From inner surface of epimysium, a septum of connective tissue penetrates into muscle to surround the primary and seconday bundles of muscle fibers or fasciculi. This connective tissue is perimysium. It contains major blood vessel and nerves. Muscle fibers or specialized muscle cells are the structural units of the skeletal muscle tissue. Each muscle fiber is surrounded by a connective tissue layer called endomyosin, beneath which is delicate sarcolemma or muscle cell membrane. It transmits nervous signals along the surface of muscle fibre (Figure 2.11).

- **Nerve and Vascular Supply** – Each muscle – at least one artery and vein and nerve fibers from a nerve trunk, these vessels associated with epimysium, enter into the muscle through perimysium and then through endomysium. longitudinally oriented capillaries lying in the endomysium with occasional transverse branches encircling them.
- **Lymph vessels** – also enter and exit the muscle through connective tissue septa nerves fibers – also through connective tissue septa.
- **Nerve fiber:** – interior of muscle – non-myelinated-axon associated Schwann sheath and connective tissue sheath become continuous with the endomysium. The axon endings contact with the muscle fiber at the myoneural junction.
- **Musle spindles:** unique sensory organs function as strain gauges, provide CNS with information about position, movements and tension within a muscle – contain group of muscle fibers and associated nerve endings.
- **Intrafusal fibers:** specialized muscle fiber in the interior of the spindle.
- **Intramuscular fat :** called marbling in meat. Deposited in perimysial connective tissue septa.
- **Intermuscular fat or seem fat:** deposited along the connective tissue septa between individual muscles.

Table 2.1: Characteristics of Types of Muscle Fibers.

Sl.No.	*Characteristics*	*Red Fiber*	*Intermediate Fiber*	*White Fiber*
1.	Colour	Red	Red	White
2.	Myoglobin content	High	High	Low
3.	Fiber diameter	Small	Small-inter mediate	Large
4.	Contraction speed	Slow	Fast	Fast
5.	Mitochondria nos.	High	Intermediate	Low
6.	Mitochondria size	Large	Intermediate	Small
7.	Capillary density	High	Intermediate	Low
8.	Oxidative metabolism	High	Intermediate	Low
9.	Glycolytic metabolism	Low	Intermediate	High
10.	Lipid content	High	Intermediate	Low
11.	Glycogen content	Low	high	High

- **Muscle tendon junction:** ends of myofibrils connect to the tendon fibrils at which noncontractile fibers of each myofibril are attached. Myotendial structure is continuous with tendons which are attached to bones.

☆ **Aponeuroses:** tendinal attachment with bone and myotendial junctions. Some muscles attached by a connective tissue fasciae to skin, ligaments and other muscles.

☆ **Muscle and fiber type:** There are three types of muscle fibers (Table 2.1). Red muscle: higher proportion of red fiber. White muscle - higher proportion of white fiber and Intermediate fiber type.

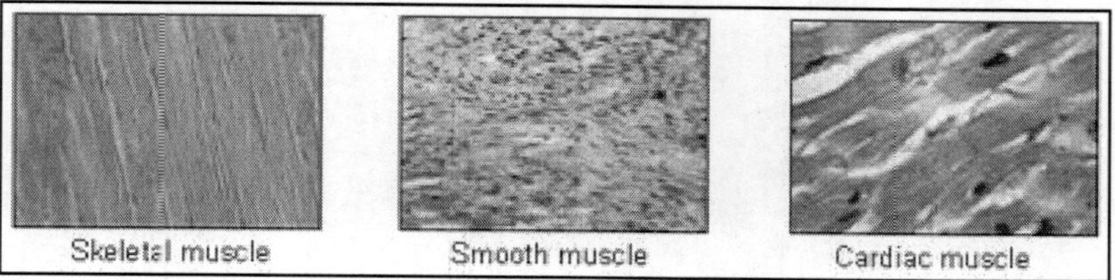

Figure 2.1: Histological Structure of Different Types of Muscles.

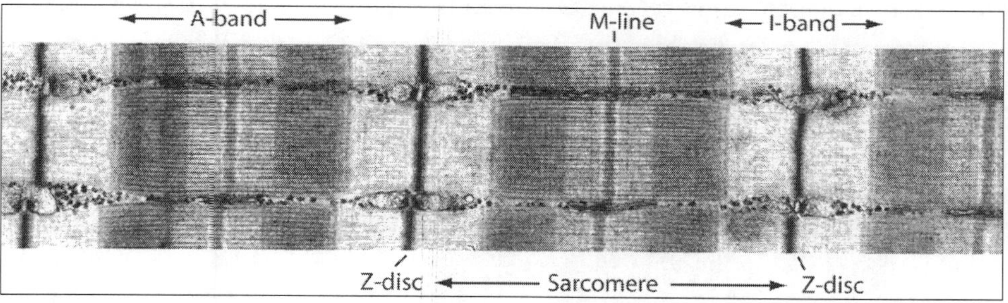

Figure 2.2: Striated Muscle: Striations, Myofilaments.

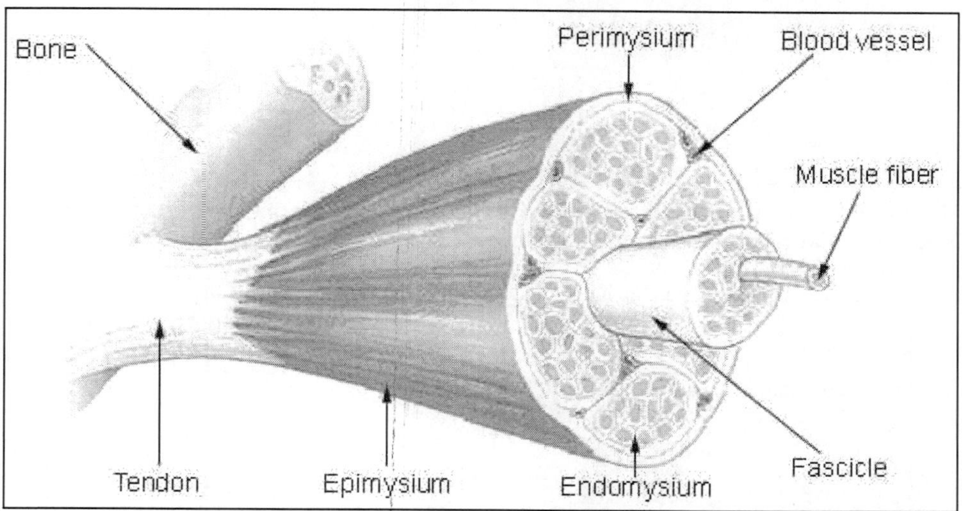

Figure 2.3: Structure of Skeletal Muscle.

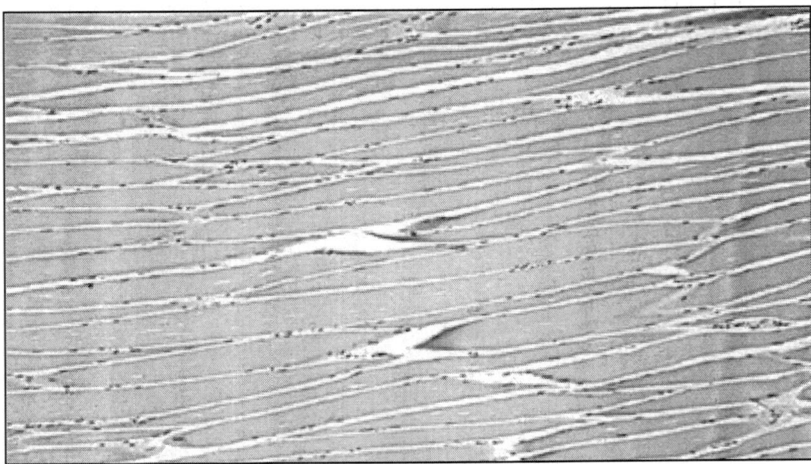

Figure 2.4: Nuclei: Hundreds of Nuclei, Located Peripherally below Sarcolemma.

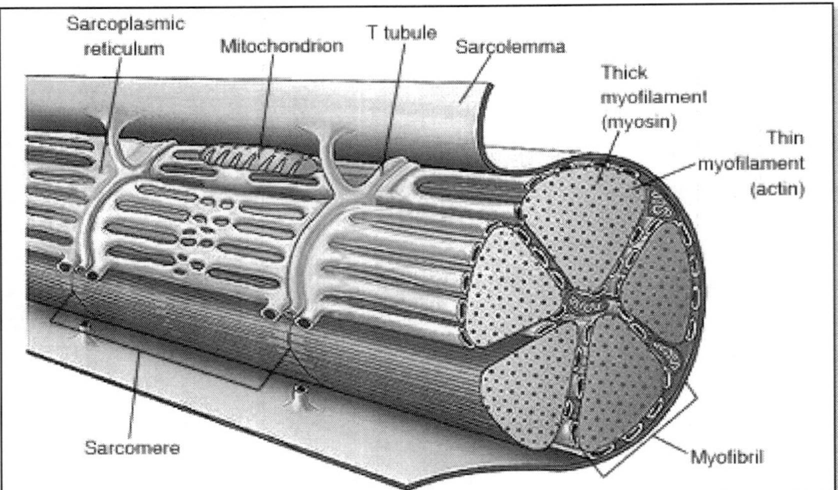

Figure 2.5: Sarcolemma, Sarcoplasmic Reticulum: Transverse tubules or T tubules, longitudinal and fenestrated collar, Invaginations of sarcolemma, Runs transversely through muscle fiber.

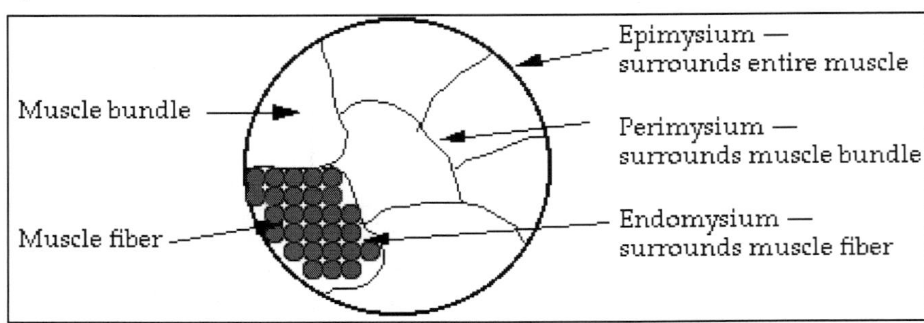

Figure 2.6: Connective Tissues.

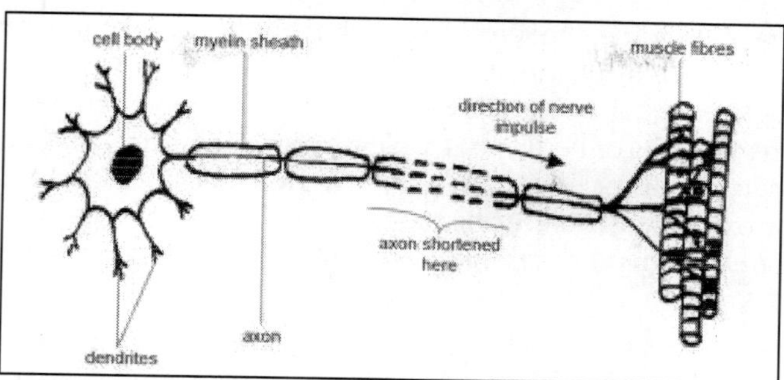

Figure 2.7: Myoneural Junction.

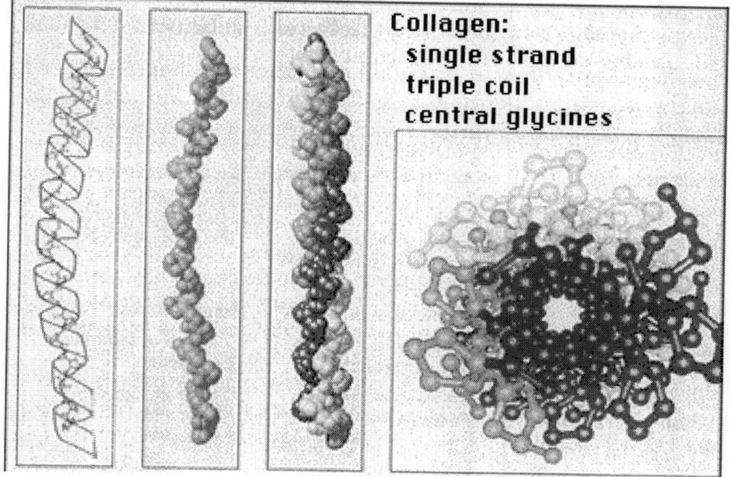

Figure 2.8: Collagen: Single Strand, Triple Coil and Central Glycines.

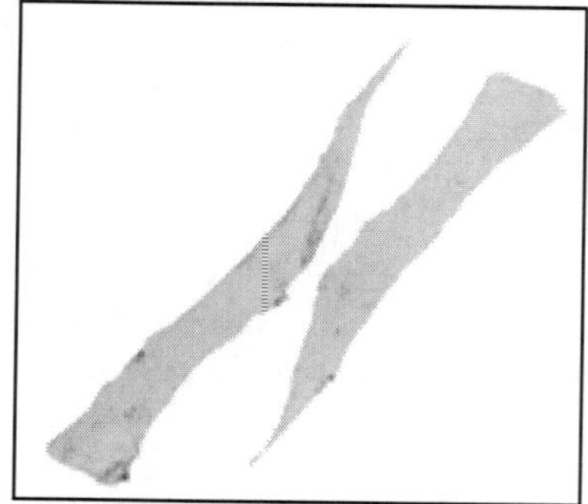

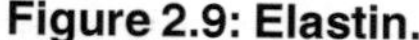

Figure 2.9: Elastin.

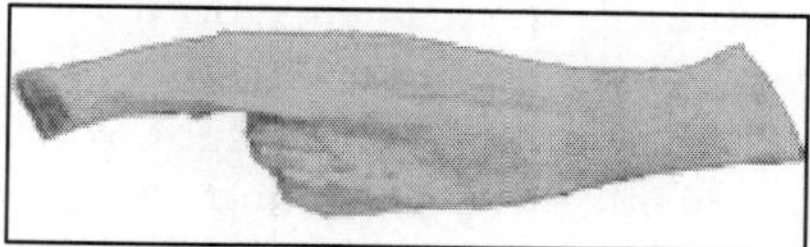

Figure 2.10: Ligamentum Nuchae.

Structure of the Muscle Fibers

Muscle Fibers are also called muscle cells, long, unbranched, thread like cells, taper slightly at both ends; length many centimeters, daim – 10 to 100 µm. Each muscle fiber or cell runs the entire length of the muscle.

A plasma membrane, the sarcolemma, surrounds each muscle fiber (Figure 2.5). The muscle fibers are multi-nucleated (Figure 2.4). The nuclei are located near the surface of the sarcolemma. Muscle fibers are stimulated by motor neurons in specialized regions called synapses or neuromuscular junctions (Figure 2.7). A neurotransmitter chemical, acetylcholine, is released by the neurons into this synaptic region. Acetylcholine excites the muscle fiber and causes the fiber to contract. The contractile filaments or myofilaments are organized into units called myofibrils within each fiber.

The organization of these myofilaments creates light and dark bands, which give skeletal muscle its characteristic, striped or striated appearance (Figures 2.12 and 2.13).

Sarcolemma: Sarco (greek word sarx or sarkos, mean flesh) surffix lemma, mean husk. It is relatively elastic, structure, composition and properties are identical to plasmalemma of other cells along the length of the fiber and around the entire circumference, invaginations of sarcolemma form a network of tubules called transverse tubules (referred to T system or T tubules) (Figure 2.5).

Motor Nerve Endings terminates at the myoneural junction (Figure 2.7). The nerve endings are implanted in small invaginations of the sarcolemma. These structures form a small mound on the surface of the m.f. The entire complex is called motor end plate.

Sarcoplasm: intracellular colloidal substance, organelles are suspended 75-80 per cent water in the sarcoplasm contain lipid droplets, glycogen granules, ribosomes, numerous proteins, NPN compounds, inorganic constituents.

Nuclei: muscle fiber is multinucleated (Figure 2.4), more at tendinous attachment and myoneural junction located at periphery of the fiber beneath the sarcolemma, ellipsoidal in shape, longest axis is oriented parallel to the long axis of the fiber, nuclei of fish skeletal muscle are centrally located.

Myofibrils: an organelle, long thin cylindrical rods, 1-2 μm diam, their long axis parallel to the long axis of the fibre, bathed by the sarcoplasm, extend the entire length of muscle fiber. A muscle fibre with a diameter of 50 μm will have at least 1000 and at many as 2000 myofibrils. Cross section of myofibril- array of dots, two sizes, these are myofilaments – thick and thin filaments arranged parallel to each other, thick and thin overlap at certain places, characteristic banding or striated appearance of the myofibril, bands of each fibril aligned across entire fiber – alternate light and dark areas resulting in striated appearance of muscle fiber. Light band: singly refractive when viewed with polarized light, so isotropic called I-band. Dark band: doubly refractive or anisotropic, A-band, denser. Each myofibril is surrounded by a tubular system, the sarcoplasmic reticulum, which stores the calcium ions that regulate muscle contraction. Rows of mitochondria lay in close proximity to the sarcoplasmic reticulum and myofibrils, ready to supply the ATP needed to fuel the contractile process. Myofibrils are the contractile organelles within each muscle fiber. Each fiber contains many myofibrils, which run the full length of the muscle fiber. Within each myofibril, the thin filaments and the thick filaments are the actual contractile filaments or myofilaments. These myofilaments do not extend the entire length of the muscle fiber, but are arranged in compartments called sarcomeres (Figure 2.13).

The sarcomeres are contractile units that are joined end to end the full length of the muscle fiber. (Functional units) A narrow plate-shaped region called a z disc separates neighboring sarcomeres. During contraction, the length of each sarcomere shortens (Figure 2.15).

Within the sarcomeres, the thin and thick filaments are arranged in parallel, overlapping each other. The thick filaments are about twice the diameter of the thin filaments.

The overlapping filaents create a banding pattern, which makes the muscle cells look striped or striated.

The myofilaments are the contractile elements (proteins) of the muscle fiber. Two main filaments are the thick filaments and the thin filaments. These two filaments are arranged within the sarcomere in an overlapping manner. Interactions between these two filaments cause a contraction by sliding the filaments together, shortening each sarcomere (Figure 2.15). Thin filaments are composed primarily of the protein actin (Figure 2.16). Polymers of actin form the helical backbone of the thin filament. Each actin protein contains an active site which interacts with the myosin head during contraction. Two other proteins are present in the thin filaments, tropomyosin and troponin. These proteins are regulatory proteins, which control the binding of the myosin head to the actin. Thick filaments are composed of a club-shaped protein myosin (Figures 2.18a,b). A third protein, titin, is an elastic filament connecting the thick filaments to the Z discs. Titin helps maintain the position of the thick filaments in the center of the sarcomere following contraction or extension of the fiber.

Sarcomere – unit of myofibril between two adjacent Z-lines.

Functional unit, structural unit.

A band + two half I-band.

H-zone: lighter region in the centre of A-band, M-line: a narrow dense band, bisects the centre of A-band.

Pseudo H zone – low density region on either side of M line in the H-zone.

Myofilaments: thick and thin filaments, Myosin filaments – thick, 14-16 nm diam, 1.5µm length constitute A band, held in transverse and longitudinal register by thin cross bands along their length by cross connections across the centre of the A-band (corresponds to tranverse density characteristics of M-line).

Actin filament: thin filaments, 6-8mm diam extend 1.0µ on either side of Z-line, constitute I-band (Figure 2.16).

H-zone: lighter region of A-band, only myosin, densest area of A-band on either side of the H-zone contain both action and myosin filaments. I-band contain the only thin actin filament is the least dense band.

Cross-section of myofilaments – myosin filaments in the H-zone are oriented in a definite hexagonal pattern, C.S. of A-band where Actin and myosin filaments overlap shows six thin filaments surround each thick filament, gap filament: found when m.f. stretched beyond normal,located at end of myosin filaments, anchor them in position to maintain structural intergrity (Figure 2.15c).

Z-line ultrastructure: longitudinal section:- an actin filament on one side of the z-line lies between two actin filaments on the opposite sides.

The actin filaments do not pass through z-line.

Z-filaments constitute the materials of z-line, connect with actin filaments.

Each actin filament connects to four z-filaments that pass obliquely through the z-line.

Each of the 4 z-filaments then connect with an actin filament in the adjacent sarcomere.

This results in characteristics zig-zag pattern of the z-line (Figure 2.15a).

Sarcoplasmic Reticulum and T tubules: corresponds to the endoplasmic reticulum of other cell types (Figure 2.13a).

A membranous system of tubules and cisternae (flattened reservoirs for Ca^{2+}).

Closely meshed network around each myofibril.

SR and T tubules are two separate and distinct membrane systems.

T tubules are associated with the sarcolemma.

Longitudinal tubules of SR converge in the H- zone SR is intracellular, storage site of Ca^{2+}.

Forming a perforated sheet called fenestrated (window like opening) collar.

At A-I junction the longitudinal tubules converge and join with terminal cisternae a pair of transversely oriented tubular elements.

The longitudinal tubules extend in both directions from the fenestrated collar to the terminal cisternae.

The two terminal cisternae lie parallel to each other – one tubule tranversing the A band the other I-band.

A T tubule runs transversely across the sarcomere at A-I junctions lies between the two terminal cisternae. These three form a structure known as the triad.

Each sarcomere has two triads, one each at A-I band junctions.

SR contribute13 per cent of total fiber volume

Mitochondria

Oblong organelle in sarcoplasm, Power house of cell (Figures 2.13a,b).

Capture energy from carbohydrate, protein and lipid, store and supply energy.

Contain enzymes of oxidative metabolism.

Abundant at the periphery of the fiber near the poles of the nuclei at myoneural junction, also locate between myofibrils, adjacent either to the z-lines, I-band or A-I junction.

Contain 30 per cent of glycoprotein of muscle fiber.

Outer and inner membrane 60A° thickness separatd by a space of 60°A.

Outer chamber : crystae, inner chamber : matrix.

Outer membrane contain enzymes of TCA cycle, fat oxidation, FA elongation and substrate level phosphorylation.

Inner membrane : 3 layers, contain electron transport chain and ATPase.

Lysosomes

Small vesicles in sarcoplasm, number of enzymes capable of digesting cell.

Proteolytic enzymes cathepsins contribute to meat tenderization.

Golgi Complex

in sarcoplasm near nuclei, flatten vesicles – concentration and packaging of cell metabolities.

Smooth Muscle

In walls of arteries, lymph vessels, gastro-intestinal, reproductive tracts.

Vary in size and shape, ellipsoid to triangular and polyhedral shape (Figure 2.1).

Sarcolemma forms membrane to membtane contact bridges with neighbouring fibers.

Mononucleated, centrally located nucleus

SR less developed

Myofilaments are arranged in pairs

Ends of the fibers contain densest aggregation of filaments.

No striations.

Each smoohe muscle fiber is surrounded by a delicate net work of reticular fibers.

Cardiac Muscle

Rhythmic contractility properties of both skeletal and smooth muscle.

Single centrally placed nucleus, Innervated by the ANS, Fibers are branched

Sarcoplasm contain numerous glycogen granules, mitochondria large and numerous.

Myofilaments to myofibrils, of variable size Striated appearance, T tubules larger, occur at z-lines, SR less developed, terminal cisternae absent

Dense lines called intercalated disks transect the fiber at regular intervals, provide a cohesive link between the fibers, facilitate nervous transmission from one fiber to another (Figure 2.1).

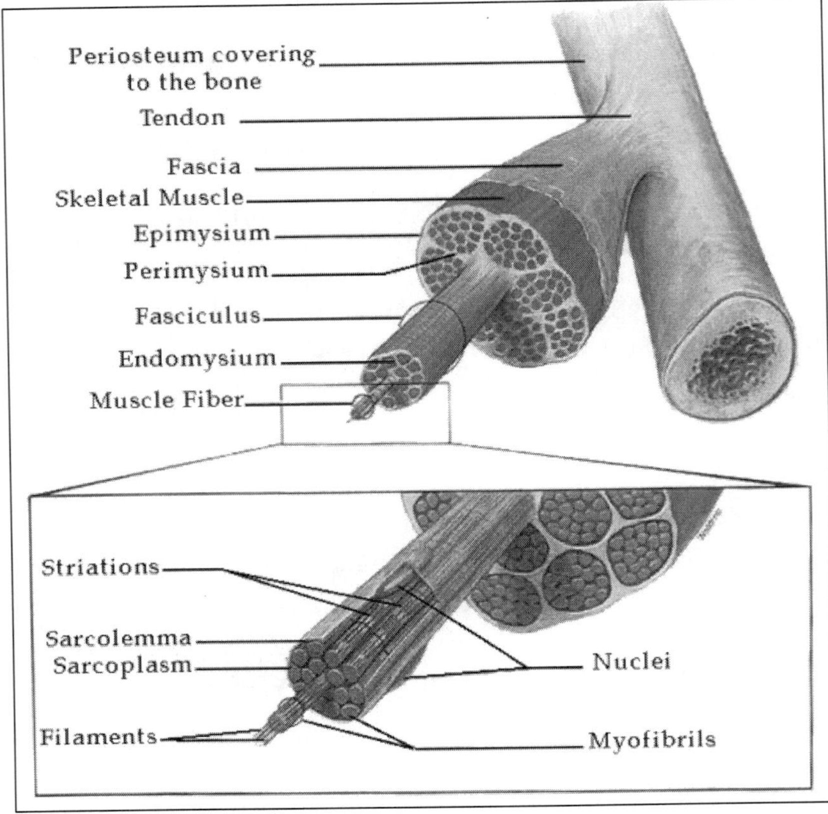

Figure 2.11: Muscle Organization.

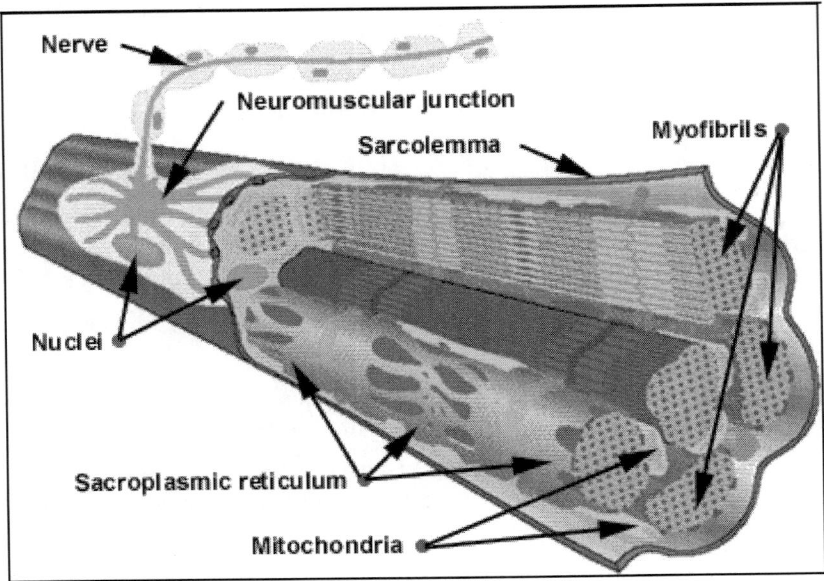

Figure 2.12: Structure of Muscle Fiber.

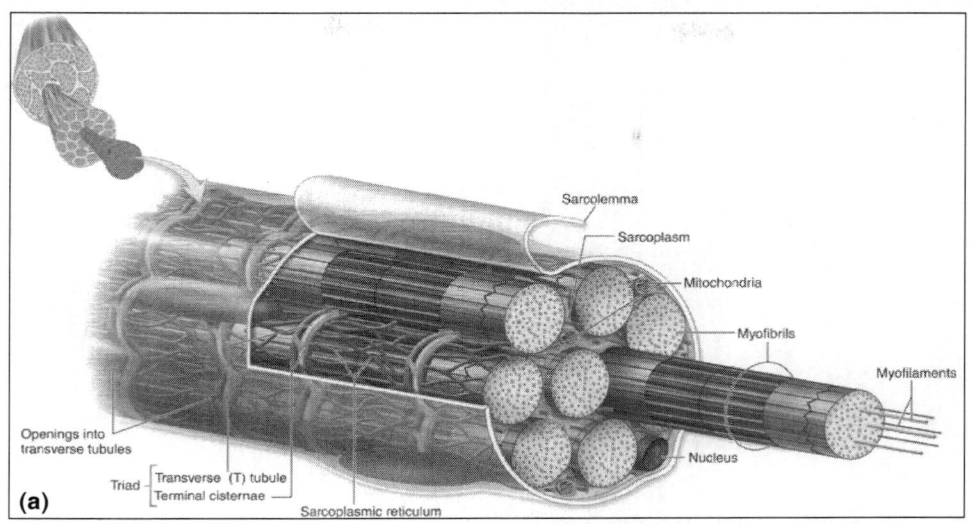

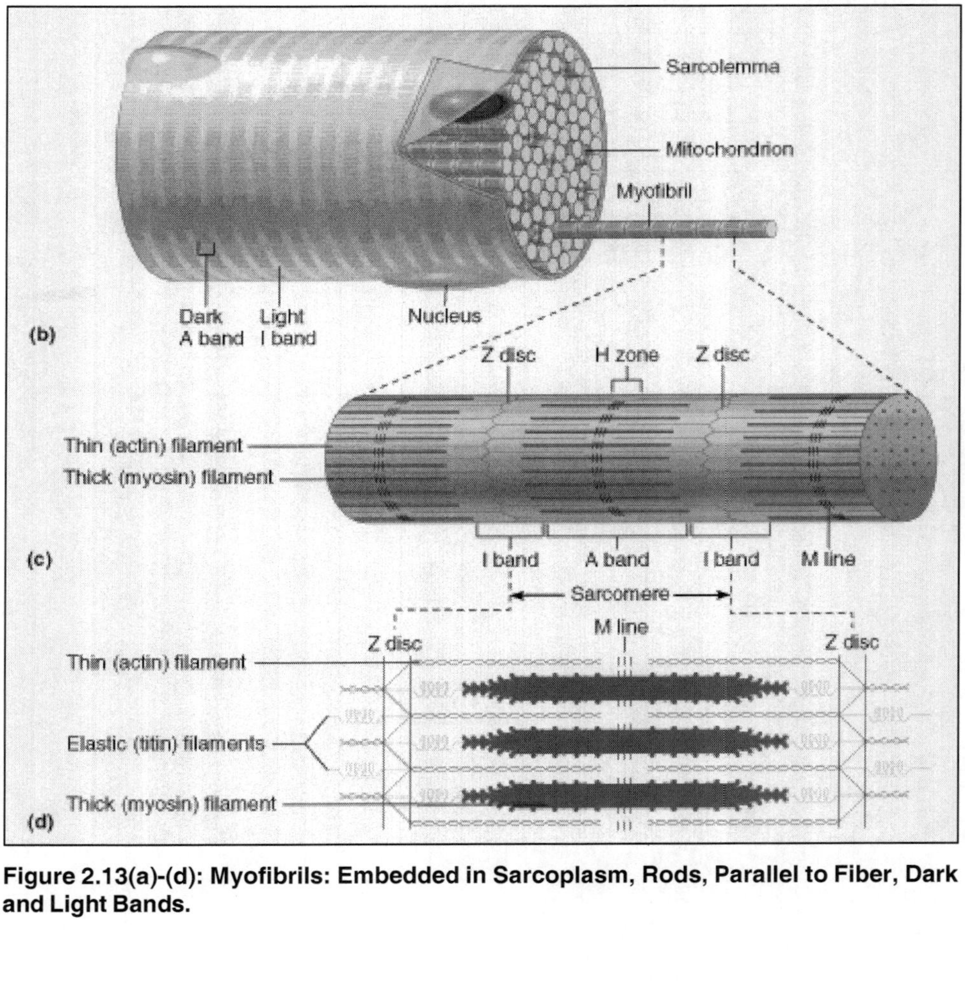

Figure 2.13(a)-(d): Myofibrils: Embedded in Sarcoplasm, Rods, Parallel to Fiber, Dark and Light Bands.

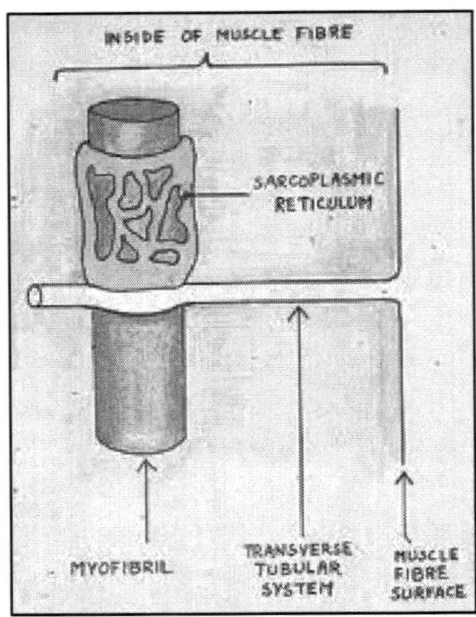

Figure 2.14: Inside of Muscle Fiber.

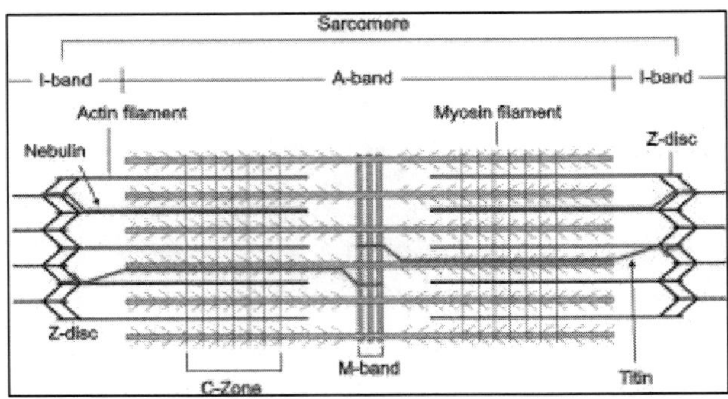

Figure 2.15a

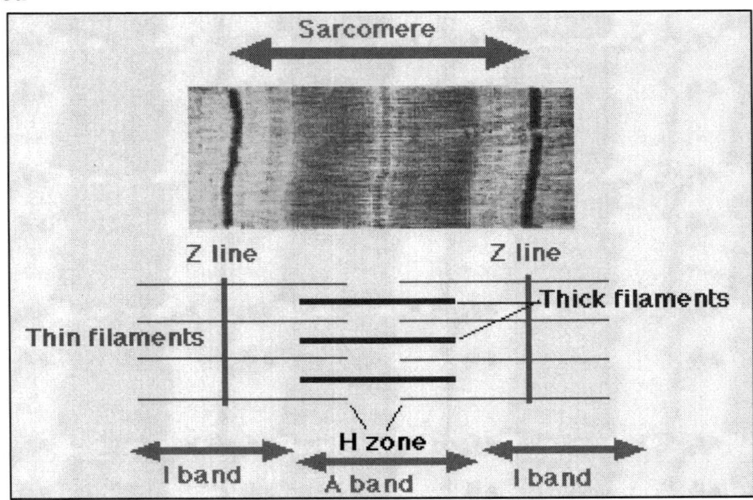

Figure 2.15b

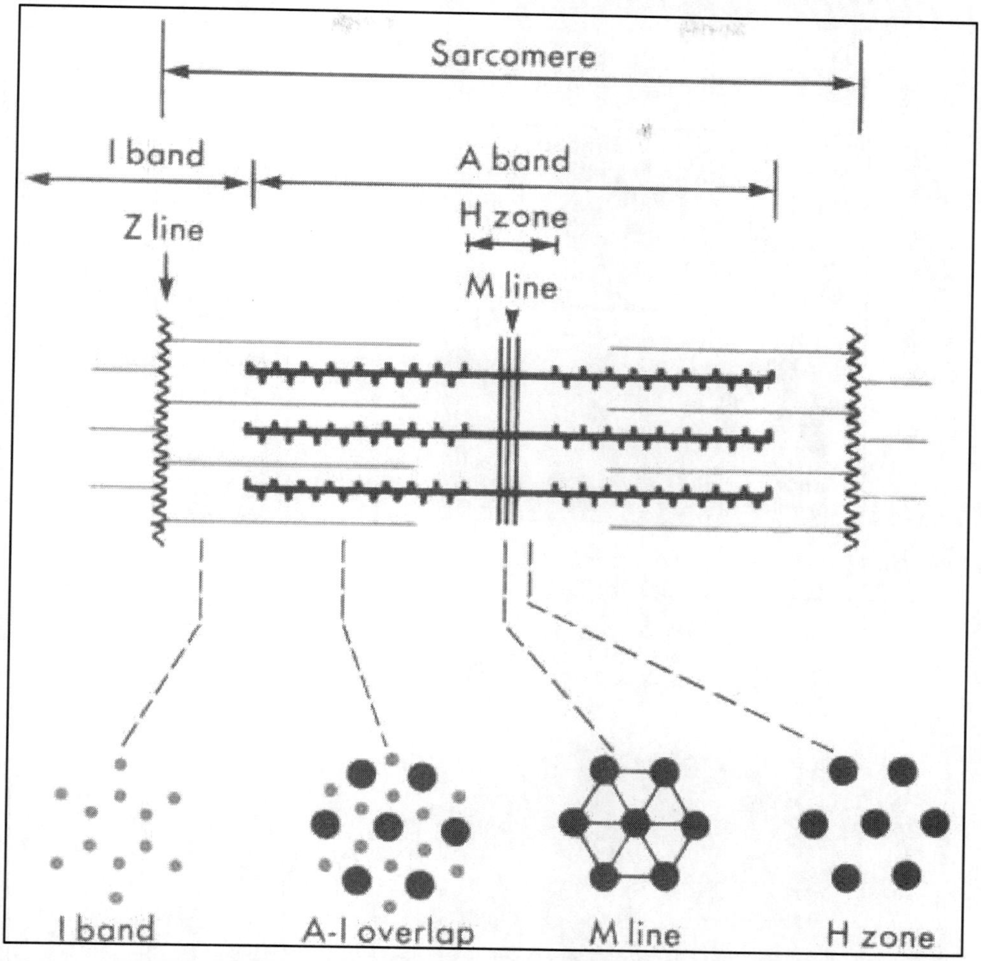

Figure 2.15c: Sarcomere: Between 2 Adjacent Z Disks (Z disc or Z line or Z bodies), Structural Unit.

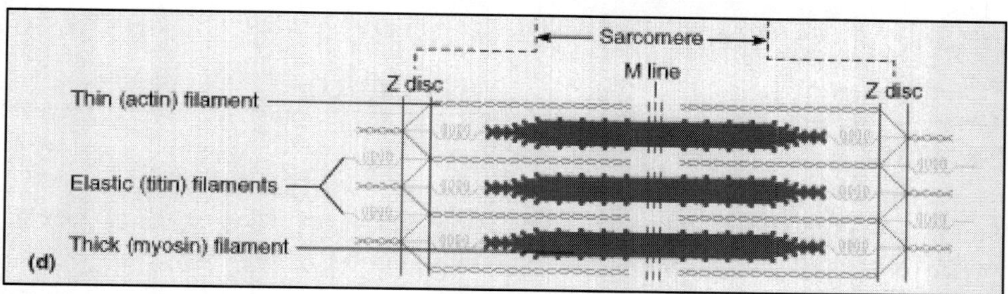

Figure 2.15d

Figures 2.15a-d: Myofilament Systems: Thin Filaments, Myofibrillar Proteins.

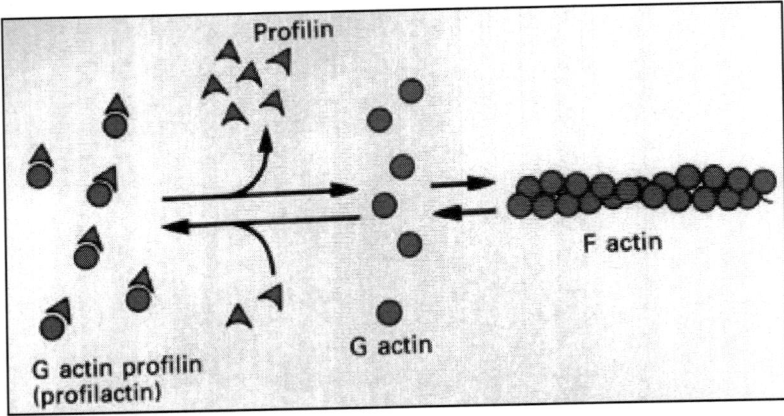

Figure 2.16a

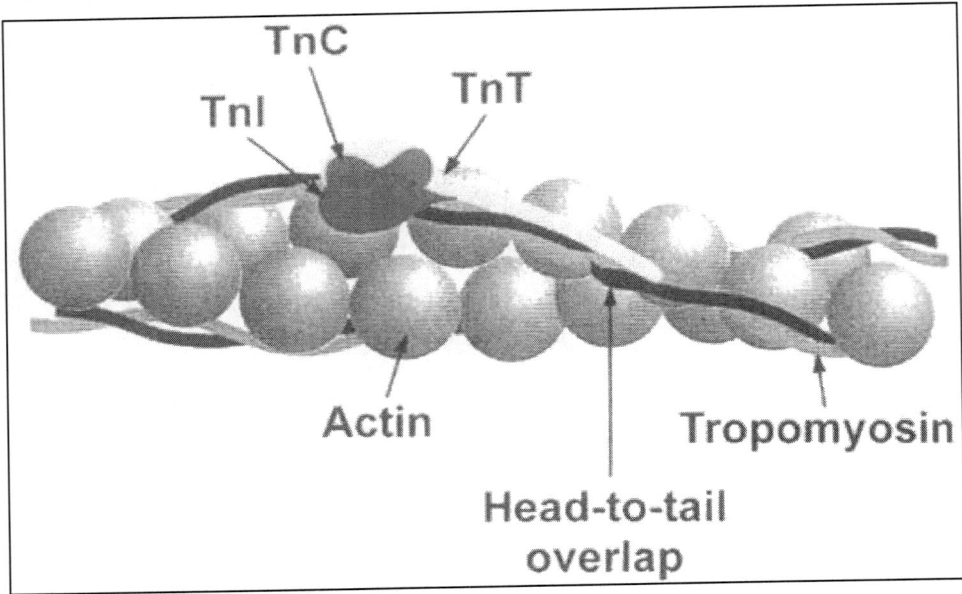

Figure 2.16b

Figures 2.16a-b: Actin: G Actin 40,000 Da, 2 Coils of F Actin String of Pearls Double/ Super Helix.

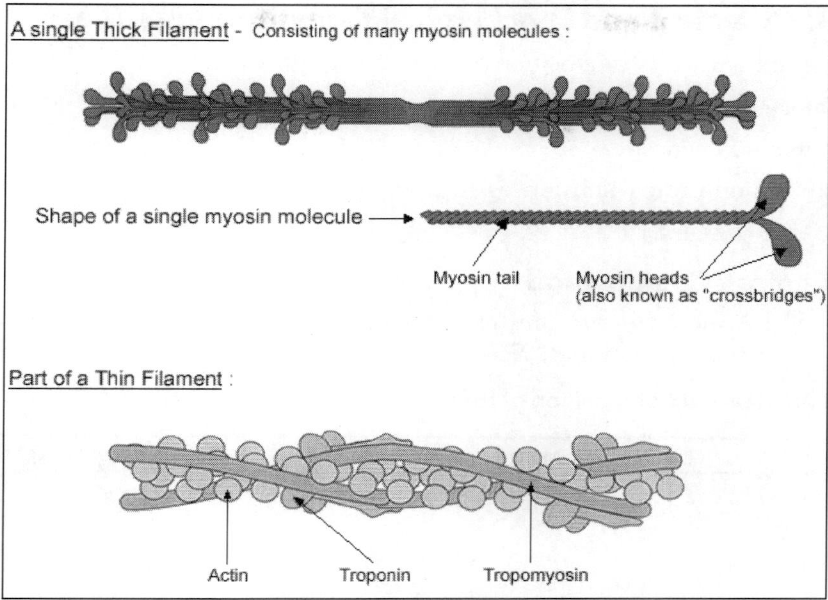

Figure 2.17: Thick Filament: Myosin, Fibrous; Thin Filament.

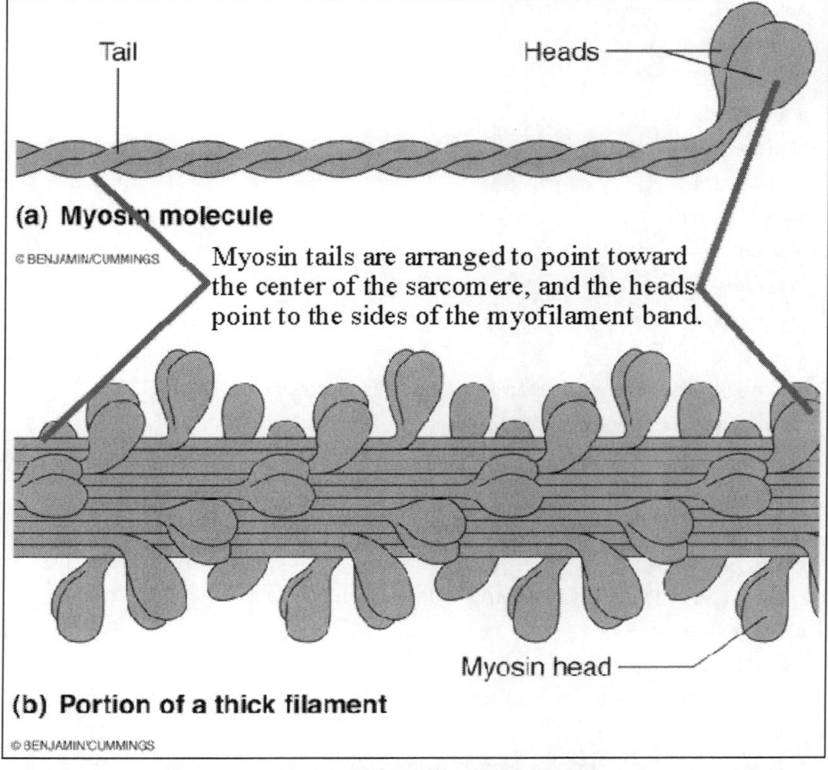

Figure 2.18a-b: Myosin: Rod shaped, 2 Heads, Tail, Neck.

II. Chemical and Biochemical Constitution of Muscle

In broad sense the composition of meat can be approximated to:

Water – 75 per cent

Protein – 19 per cent

Soluble non-protein substances – 3.5 per cent

Fat – 2.5 per cent

1. Chemical Composition

Typical Adult Mammals muscle after Rigor Mortis but before deteriorative changes post-mortem (Lawrie, 1975)

Table 2.2: Chemical Composition of Meat.

Sl.No.	*Component*	*Wet per cent Weight*
1.	Water	75.0
	Protein	19.0
a.	Myofibrillar	11.5
	Myosin (H and L meromyosins and several light chain proteins associated with them	6.5
	Actin	2.5
	Tropomyosin	1.5
	Troponins C, I and T	0.4
	α and β actinins	0.4
	M protein etc	0.2
b.	Sarcoplasmic	5.5
	glyceraldehyde phosphate dehydrogenase	1.2
	Aldolase	0.6
	Creatine kinase	0.5
	Other glycolytic enzymes	2.2
	Myoglobin	0.2
	Haemoglobin and other unspecified extraceliular proteins	0.6
c.	Connective tissue and organelle	2.0
	Collagen	1.0
	Elastin	0.05
	Mitochondrial etc (including cytochrome c and insoluble enzymes)	0.95
3.	Lipid	2.5
	Neutral lipid, phospholipids fatty acids fat-soluble substances	2.5
4.	Carbohydrate	1.2
	Lactic acid	0.90
	Glucose-6 phosphate	0.15
	Glycogen	0.10
	Glucose traces of other glycolytic intermediates	0.05

Contd...

Table 2.2–*Contd...*

Sl.No.	Component	Wet per cent Weight
5.	Miscellaneous soluble Non-protein substances	2.3
a.	Nitrogenous	1.65
	Creatine	0.55
	Inosine monophosphate	0.30
	di-and tri-phosphopyridine	0.30
	Nucleotides	0.10
	Amino acids	0.35
	Carnosine, anserine	0.35
b.	Inorganic	0.65
	Total soluble phosphorus	0.20
	Potassium	0.35
	Sodium	0.05
	Magnesium	0.02
	Calcium, zinc, trace metals	0.23
6.	Vitamins	–
	Various fat and water soluble vitamins quantitatively minute	–

2. Muscle Proteins

Constitutes 16-22 per cent of muscle mass: principal components of solid matter. Broadly divided into:

Sarcoplasmic proteins – soluble in water or dilute salt solutions.

Myofibrillar proteins – soluble in concentrated salt solutions.

Connective tissue and organelle/stromal proteins which are insoluble in conc. salt solution.

Sarcoplasmic proteins (myogen and globulins):

A complex mixture of about 50 components of citric acid cycle and electron transport chain

Mostly enzymes of glycolytic cycle and also include myoglobin and haemoglobin.

Myofibrillar proteins

Myosin – mol wt. 500,000, asymmetric ratio of length to diameter is 100:1

Rich in glutamic and aspartic acids and of dibasic amino acids, highly charged, strong affinity for calcium and magnesium ions.

Built of light (L) and heavy (H) meromyosins.

H-meromyosin contains ATPase and actin-combining properties of myosin, sited on the peripheri of the myosin filaments. The properties depend upon free-SH groups in the molecule.

Tropomyosin: amino acid composition is similar to myosin, a cyclopeptide (a chain of amino acids forming a closed figure).

Actin: exist in two forms: G-actin, F-actin.

G-actin consists of small globular units having a mol. of about 70,000. F-actin: these globular units are aggregated end to end to form a double chain. It is F-actin, which combines with myosin to form actomyosin complex.

Troponin complex promotes the aggregation of tropomyosin, binds calcium and prevents actomyosin formation, three types troponin C, I and T.

α- actinin promotes the lateral association of F-actin.

β- actinin inhibits polymerization of F-actin.

M-line substance – promotes the lateral polymerization of L-meromyosin.

Tropomyosin B- contribute mechanical stability to the muscle filaments. NPN included as amino acids, peptides, creatine, some vitamins, nucleosides etc.

Connective Tissue Proteins

Collagen – highest content of hydroxyproline therefore the hydroxyproline content of muscle is used as a measure of its connective tissue. There is a high proportion of hydroxyl amino acids in collagen and elastin, tryptophan is virtually absent, hydroxylysine is found.

Collagen on heating at > 80°C yield gelatine in boiling, but reticulin does not yield gelatin on boiling.

Elastin is not broken down by heating. It contains a chromophoric residue which gives elastin its characteristic yellow colour and fluorescence. The elastic properties of elastin are due to the presence of two known amino acids – desmosine and isodesmosine at the crosslink areas between adjacent polypeptide chains. The elastin differs from collagen –

By having only 1-6 per cent hydroxyproline

Few polar amino acids

Valine content (18 per cent) is much higher.

3. Intramuscular Fat

Has a considerable content of phospholipids and unsaponifiable constituents *e.g.* cholesterol

Only 3 or 4 fatty acids are present in substantial amount in the fat of meat animals – Oleic, Palmitic and Stearic and four types of glycerides GS3, GS2U, GSU2 and GU3 (S and U represent saturated and unsaturated fatty acids respectively).

The phospholipids consist of phosphoglycerides, plasmalogens and sphingomyelin.

In the phosphoglycerides one of the three hydroxyl groups of glycerol is combined with choline, ethanolamine, serine inositol or glucose. In the plasmalogens the second hydroxyl group of glycerol is esterified with a long-chain fatty aldehyde instead of with fatty acid. In sphingomyelin the amino alcohol sphingosine is bound by an amide link to a fatty acid and by an ester link to Phosphorylcholine, Glycolipids are also present in muscle tissue. Of the total phospholipids in beef muscle

Lecithin – 62 per cent

Cephalin – 30 per cent

Sphingomyclin < 10 per cent

Accompanying the trighycerides are small quantities of substances which are soluble in fat solvents *e.g.* vitamins A, D, E and K and Cholesterol derivatives.

Water: Muscle contains approx. 75 per cent water (range 65-80) by weight. Water is the principal constituent of the extracellular fluid and numerous chemical constituents are dissolved or suspended in it. It serves as the medium for the transport of substances between the vascular bed and muscle fibers.

4. Carbohydrates

Present in small quantities, glycogen is the most abundant carbohydrate in the muscle (0.5 to 1.3 per cent by wt of muscle). The bullk of the remainder of the carbohydrate is comprised of the mucopolysaccharides associated with the connective tissue, glucose and other mono-or disaccharides and the intermediates of the glycolytic metabolism.

5. Inorganic Constituents

Cations and anions of physiological significance – calcium, magnesium, potassium, sodium, iron, phosphorus, sulfur and chlorine. Many of the other inorganic constituents found in the animal body are also present in muscle.

III. Chemistry of Animal Tissues

i) Muscle Proteins

Classification of Muscle proteins

1. Extracellular
   a) Fibrous proteins- i) collagen, ii) elastin, iii) reticulin
   b) Ground substance
   c) Cells- i) fixed cells, ii) wandering cells
2. Intracellular
   a) Sarcoplasmic proteins
   b) Myofibrillar- i) myosin, ii) actin, iii) actomyosin
   c) Regulatory- i) Tropomyosin, ii) Troponin complex, iii) Actinins, iv) M-proteins, v) C- protein
3. Other chemical components:

1. Extracellular Proteins

Extracellular Components:- connective tissue proteins, proteins of interstitial space. insoluble part of extracellular space + insoluble part of sarcolemma- constitute the stroma.

Connective Tissue

Epi-, peri- and endomysium, supporting tissue, extracellular, tendon, ligament bone, blood vessels, skin. Poor quality of meat 30 to 40 per cent by vol in meat, connective tissue proper. It contains (i) **Fibrous protein**: Collagen, reticulin elastin (Extracellular fibers). (ii) ground substance (iii) wander cells, fixed cells.

Extracellular connective tissue: It includes dense connective tissue: dense irregular connective tissue, dense regulat connective tissue (*e.g.* tendons, aponeuroses) and loose connective tissue. The extracelluar fibers include collagen, elastin and reticulin.

(i) Collagen

Most abundant, influence meat tenderness, 20-25 per cent of total protein.

- ✰ Principal structural proteins, amount depend upon exercise of body part, limbs more collagen than back.
- ✰ Is a glycoprotein (galactose and glucose)
- ✰ Glycine is the most abundant a.a. 33 per cent (1/3rd of total amino acids content.
- ✰ Pro 12 per cent and HyP 18 per cent constituteanother 1/3 rd a.a.
- ✰ Hydroxylysine is very low (1 per cent) and alanine 10 per cent.
- ✰ Hyp is a relatively constant component of collagen (13-14 per cent), does not occur in other animal proteins. So chemical assay for quantity of collagen in meat.
- ✰ Tropocollagen structural unit of collagen fibril.
- ✰ Each tropocollagen molecule overlaps its lateral counter part by ¼ of its length, thus straiated appearance of the fibrils.
- ✰ Tropocollagen molecules 2800 A° long 14-15 A° diam with a mol. Wt. of 300,000.
- ✰ Contain three polypeptide chains α, β, γ existing as a left handled triplex with the final collagen chain being the right handed structure.
- ✰ Interlinking bonds in collagen and tropocollagen are formed by the interaction of the OH-group of hexoses and the COOH-group of the polypeptides.
- ✰ Bonds (two linkages), one also involve -NH_2 group of lysine and other an aldehyde intermediate.
- ✰ These two cross linkages are named as
  - (i) Dehydro-hydroxylysinonorleucine (Aldimine)
  - (ii) Hydroxylysino-5-oxo-norleucine (Keto-imine).

  Aldimine crosslinks are formed when the -NH_2 gr. of a lys residue is coverted to an aldehyde which condenses with a OH lys residue in the non-helical region of the tropocollagen.

  Ketoimine cross links – heat and acid stable. Aldimine cross links – heat and acid labile.

These crosslinks result in tensile strength insolubility of collagen. As age advances – tensile strength increase but aldimine and ketoimine decrease as they undergo further reactions producing trifunctional cross-links.

The aldimine cross links react with histidine from adjacent molecule to form histidino-hydroxy lysinonorleucine.

Ketoimine crosslinks react with a hydroxyl lysine-aldehyde from another molecule to form the ring compound hydroxylysyl-pyridinoline.

(ii) Elastin

- ☆ Structural protein of elastic fibers.
- ☆ More resistant to hydrolysis by acids bases and enzymes and to heat denaturation.
- ☆ Fewer polar groups 7 per cent than collagen (34 per cent)
- ☆ Alanine and valine is higher, less HyPro
- ☆ Two unique amino acids *viz.* desmosine and isodesmosine, which are 4-amino 4-carboxy amino acids containing a quarternary pyridinium ring, formed from four lysine residues.
- ☆ High proportions nonpolar a.a. and the cross links of desmosine may be responsible for the insolubility of elastin in most reagents.
- ☆ It is hydrolysed by ficin, papain, bromelin and pancereatic elastase.
- ☆ Two fractions – α and β-elastin, α-contain 17 chains 35 a.a. residues. β – contain 2 chains, 27 a.a. residues.

(iii) Reticulin

- ☆ A mucoprotein
- ☆ Make up finest branched fibers in endomysium
- ☆ Reticulin fibrils are much shorter and finer than collagen, branched and stain black with ammoniacal silver stain.
- ☆ Based on digestion studies of typsin, two types collagenous and non-collagenous fractions
- ☆ 3 forms of collagenous reticulin
  - a) Basement membrane reticulin: protein + carbohydrate + lipid
  - b) Precollagenous reticulin: carbohy only, no lipid
  - c) Stomal reticulins: resistant to peptic digestion.

(b) Ground Substance

- ☆ Occupies the extracellular space
- ☆ A viscous fluid derived from plasma
- ☆ Composed of globular mucoprotein, tropocollagen and tropo-elastin.
- ☆ Impt. mucopolysaccharides are hyaluronic acid, chondroitin sulfates A,B and C keratosulfate, heparitin sulate, heparin.
- ☆ Contain either galactosamine or glucosamine.

(c) Cells: Two Type

i. Fixed cells: fibroblasts, mesenchyme cells, adipose or fat cells.
ii. Wandering cells: mast cells, macrophages, histiocytes, lymph cells, eosinophils, plasma cells – concerned mainly in controlling infection.

2. Intracellur Proteins

Three main groups

(a) Sarcoplasmic proteins
(b) Myofibrillar proteins
(c) Regulatory proteins

(a) Sacoplasmic Proteins

Soluble proteins of the sacoplasm.

Classification: Based on fractional precipitation in ammonium sulfate solution

Myogen

Myoalbumin

Globulin X

Myoglobulin

Mayogen A and B

Based on ultracentrifugation- 4 subclasses

i) Nuclear fraction: nucleoproteins, RNA and DNA lipoproteins.
ii) Mitochondrial fraction: the mitochondria, TCA cycle enzymes, electron transport cahin
iii) Microsomalfraction: microsomes, sarcoplasmic reticulum, the T-system, lysosomes.
iv) Cytoplasmic fraction: enzymes of the glycolytic pathway, glucogenesis, myoglobin, soluble proteins and enzymes of cytrochrome system.

These fractions can be separated by using appropriate centrifugal force and proper buffer system. Each fraction can further be partitioned electrophoretically to characterize individual proteins. 50 to 100 different proteins. They are globular or rod shaped, low viscosity, low mol. wt., constitute 30-35 per cent of total muscle proteins.

(b) Myofrillar Proteins

Myofilamentous – actin, myosin, actomyosin; regulatory

Proteins of the myofilaments: Actin and myosin constitute 75-80 per cent of the protein in the myofibril, remaining 20-25 per cent are regulatory proteins. Myofibrillar proteins: contractile proteins- actin, myosin, actomyosin. proteins of thick and thin filaments + regulatory protein.

Regulatory proteins = tropomyosin, troponin, M-proteins, α-actinin, β-actinin, c-protein.

- ☆ Tropomyosin, troposin and β-actinin are associated with the actin filament.
- ☆ C-protein in myosin filament.
- ☆ α-actinin in z-line.
- ☆ M-proteins- substances of M-line.

Myofibrillar proteins: Myofilaments: actin, myosin – regulatory

i) Myosin

Syn: Myosin-A, L-myosin, myosin -T, β- myosin, Y-protein.

- ☆ 55-60 per cent of myofbrillar proteins 200 to 400 myosin molecules in each thick filament.
- ☆ Myosin molecule length 1.5 μm, diam. 130A°
- ☆ High amount of basic (17 per cent) and acidic(18 per cent) aa, so a highly charged molecule, 38 per cent have polar side groups.
- ☆ Iso-electric pH of myosin is 5.4
- ☆ Myosin molecule is an elongated rod shape with a thickened position at one end.
- ☆ Thickened portion is head region and long rod-like region is the tail region.
- ☆ Between the head and tail region is the neck
- ☆ Double headed *i.e.* bilobed and projects laterally from the long axis.
- ☆ Proteolytic action by trypsin split the molecule near the neck into LMM and HMM
- ☆ LMM is a double or triple stranded α- helical structure.
- ☆ Either side of M-line in H-zone *i.e.* Pseudo H-zone contain only tail poprtion without globular heads.
- ☆ Heads are oriented at an oblique angle on either side of the PseUdo-H zone.
- ☆ The protruding heads (HMM) are functionally active during muscle contraction, each myosin head attaches to a G-actin molecule forming crossbridges of the actomyosin complex.
- ☆ Rest – contraction – relaxation.
- ☆ There are about 400 myosin molecules in each myosin filament.
- ☆ Strong affinity to divalent cations (Ca++, Mg++).
- ☆ HMM carries the ATPase activity and actin binding ability.
- ☆ ATPase activity is stimulated by Ca++ and inhibited by Mg++ ions.
- ☆ Papain splits HMM into HMM S1(anterior globular) and HMM S2 (posterior helical)
- ☆ HMM S1 contain myosin heavy chain (mol.wt.-200,000)
- ☆ Myosin light chain A1 (mol.wt.-18,000) and A2 (mol. Wt. 16000)and myosin – functionally active – i) ATPase activity, ii) forms crossbridges wth actin filament

- ☆ DTNB (5,5-dithiobis 2-nitrobenzoic acid) light chain (mol wt. 25,000
- ☆ DTNB- no ATPase activity

ii) Actin

20-25 per cent of myofibrillar proteins – thin filament 70 µm long 8µm diam.

- ☆ Rich in the amino acid proline.
- ☆ Proline by virtue of its N-H (imino) group contribute to the folding of the polypeptide chains results in a globular (spherical), G-actin of 5.5 nm diam. MW 47,000 linked by a Ca^{2+} or Mg^{2+} bridge.
- ☆ G-actin a monomer of actin.
- ☆ Longitudinal polymerization of G-actin monomers to form F-actin (Fibrous actin)
- ☆ In F-actin, G-actin monomers are linked like the beads on a string of pearls.
- ☆ Two strands of F-actin spirally coiled around one another to form a right handed super helix.
- ☆ The isoelectric pH of actin is 4.7 three forms : α,β,γ actinin
- ☆ In actin 2 per cent acidic amino acids, 13 per cent basic amino acids, 33 per cent polar side chain

Cytoskeletal Proteins (The Cytoskeletal Framework)

Maintenance of the structural frame work within which the contractile proteins function. Different proteins associated with cytoskeletal network are given in Table 2.3.

- ☆ Connectin (titin) high mol. wt., elastic, located at A-I band junction, extrudes as thin filaments on either side of the centre of the myosin filaments through the actin filaments to the Z-disc. Structural component of gap filaments.
- ☆ N-line proteins: runs transversely across the myofibril parallel to the Z-discs, present at 3 locations.
  - i) Close to z-disc
  - ii) Centre of I-band
  - iii) A-I band junction

Protein nebulin, 5 per cent of total myofibrillar proteins, component of N2-lines (centre of I-band) change the configuratin from hexangular lattice at A-I junction to square lattice at the Z-disc, N-line attach to connectin.

Z-disc Proteins

Number of cytoskeletal proteins. α-actinin (previously written) Minor proteins are eu-actinin and filamin, z-protein, z-nin and zeugmatin. Z-disc is surrounded by desmin (skeletin) and vimentin, a peripheral network of intermediate filaments – major structural role in maintaining adjacent myofibrils in lateral register.

- ☆ Synemin: located at periphery of Z-disc. Latticed structures (costameres) run transversely across the sarcomeres on either side of the Z-disc and firmly attached to the myofibrils at the sarcolemma. This consists of protein vinculin.

Table 2.3: Myofibrillar Proteins Associated with the Cytoskeletal Network

Protein	*Location*	*Major functions*
Connectin	Gap filaments	Links myosin to z-disc
Nebulin	N2-lines	Not known
Vinculin	By sarcolemma	Links myofibrils to sarcolemma
α-actinin	z-disc	Links actin to z-disc
Eu-actinin, filamin	z-disc	Links actin to z-disc
Desmin, vimentin	z-disc	Peripheral structure of z-disc
Synemin, z-proteinsz-nin	z-disc	Lattice structure of z-disc

c) Regulatory Proteins

i) Tropomyosin

Syn: Myosin-B, MW 68,000 double helix. two unidentical polypeptide chains. α-tropomyosin (MW 34,000), β -tropomyosin (MW 36,000)

Three types of tropomyosin- α α, α β, β β.

- ☆ 8 to 10 per cent of myofibrillar proteins
- ☆ Highly charged molecule, high content of acidic (28 per cent) and basic (19 per cent) amino acids.
- ☆ Isoelectric pH is 5.1
- ☆ Very low or absence of proline content.
- ☆ Contain two coiled polypeptide chains, attach end to end to one another.
- ☆ Long thin filamentous strands
- ☆ Tropmyosin strands lie alongside each groove of the actin super helix.
- ☆ A single tropomyosin molecule extends the length of 7 G-actin molecules in the actin filament.

ii) Troponin Complex

- ☆ A globular protein
- ☆ High proline content
- ☆ Present in the grooves of the actin filament, lies astride astride the tropomyosin strands.
- ☆ Present near the end of tropomyosin molecules.
- ☆ Present at regular intervals of 38 nm.
- ☆ One molecule of troponin for every 7-8 G-actin molecules along the actin filaments.
- ☆ 3 types Tropponin T, C and I.
- ☆ Troponin T(MW 37,000, isoelerctric point 8.8) binds to tropomyosin and links it to F- actin filaments.

- ☆ Troponin C (MW 18000, isoelectric point 4.1) binds to calcium ions.
- ☆ Troponin I (MW 37000 isoelectric point 5.5) inhibits or prevents the interaction between actin and myosin in relaxed state. Ti binds to Tc and interact directly with actin. Tc binds only to Ti and Tt but does not bind to F-actin or tropomyosis.

iii) Actinins

- ☆ Proline content comparable to actin
- ☆ A globular protein
- ☆ Two types α (MW 102,006) and β (MW 71,000) actinin
- ☆ α-actinin 2-25 per cent of the myofibrillar protein, function as the cementing substance in the Z-filaments, accelerates polymerization of G-actin to F-actin.
- ☆ β-actinin, a globular protein, β1 (MW 37000) and β2 (MW 34,000) two unidentical chains near the z-lines, located at end of actin filaments, regulate the length of actin filament, 1μ in each half sarcomere.
- ☆ γ-actinin (MW 35,000) inhibits the polymerization of G-actin to F- actin.

iv) M-Proteins

- ☆ 30 nm wide M-band in thick filament.
- ☆ 4 per cent of myofibrillar proteins
- ☆ Mol wt. of M-protein is 160,000.
- ☆ Constitute the substance of M-line (M-bridges and M-filaments)
- ☆ M- filaments are paralled to myofibrils and M-bridges run tangent to the myofibrils and interconnect the M-filaments with the myosin molecules.
- ☆ Contain Mα an Mβ proteins in the ratio of 2:3.

v) C-Protein

Associated with actin or myosin and have regulatory functions.

- ☆ Found in myosin filament
- ☆ Single polypeptide chain MW 135-140,000, low α-helical content, high proline.
- ☆ 2-2.5 per cent of the myofibrillar protein
- ☆ Encircle the myosin filament bind the myosin molecules together into the bundle
- ☆ 18 c-protein bands, 43.2 nm apart in each myosin filament
- ☆ 9 bands on each side of H-zone.
- ☆ Control the movement of crossbridges between actin and myosin.

3. Other Chemical Components

a) Water Content

Approx. 75 per cent. water-protein interaction, quality of meat, water dipoles H:O:H two pairs of velence electrons, hydrogen bonding with negatively (Glu and Asp) and positively charged (Lys, Arg, His) amino acids, peptide linkages and with side gr. of amides, (glutamine and asparagine) or tyrosine, amino acids having hydrophobic side chains – leucine alanine, valine repel water.

In muscle water exist in 2 forms.

a) Bound structural or protective form 4-5 per cent firmly held.
b) Free biologically active form

NMR studies – 20 per cent bound water, 15 per cent extracellular 5 per cent intracellular, immobilization of water – sum of polar residues – COOH, NH_2, -OH, SH, NH. Some workers belive carboxyl and amide groups interact strongly, bound water deceases in following order: ionic groups > polar groups > nonpolar groups.

Free water: highly ordered, restricted motional freedom, factors influencing free water.

i) Spatial arrangement of the protein molecules.
ii) Electrostatic forces of the ionic groups
iii) H-bonding
iv) Changes in pH and ionic strength.

WHC – 75 per cent attributed to myofibrillar proteins
20 per cent sarcoplasmic proteins.
10 per cent connective tissue protein

Major share by actomyosin. Myofibrillar proteins responsible for 90-95 per cent variations in WHC of muscle and in emulsifyings property of meat.

b) Ions

Cations- K^+ > Na+ > Mg^{2+} > Ca^{2+} >zn^{2+} >Fe^{2+}. Anions- PO_4^{3-}, Cl^-, HCO_3^-, SO_4^{2-}. other ions are in traces.

Intracellurlar: K^+, PO_4^{3-}, Mg^{2+} (major quantity), Ca^{2+}, Na^+, HCO_3^-, SO_4^{2-} small amounts.

Extracellular: Na^+, Cl^-, HCO_3^- are major ions.

These ions are present in 4 possible forms:

a) Free and mobile form in the aqueous phase
b) Complexed with nonprotein materials
c) Electrostatically bound ions with the charged groups of proteins
d) Strongly bound ions with protein as a structural component.

Small ions (Li^+, Na^+, OH^-, HO_3^+) and multivalent cations Ca^{2+}, Mg^{2+}, Al^{3+}) have strong electrical fields and are structure formers (increase viscosity of water). These ions strongly bind 4 to 6 water molecules adjacent to them. The large monovalent ions (K^+, NH_4^+, CL^-, I^-) have a weak electrical field are structure breakers and reduce the viscosity of water.

c) Glycogen

Glycogen granules are scattered throughout the cell in the sarcoplasm. Some glycogen granules are protein bound, some are free – degraded by muscle phosphorylases. Its metabolic products lactic acid (0.90 per cent) influence meat quality, Glucose 6-phosphate is the next most abundant carbohydrate amounting to about 0.17 per cent of the muscle.

d) Lipids

Are extracellular, deposited as fat globules, major portion deposited in adipose tissue. Small portions exists within muscle cells (intramuscular) as triglycerides, lipoproteins and phospholipids and metabolites such as fatty acids. They are integral part of the cells memberane, mitochondria and sarcoplasmic reticulum. The extracellular lipids are mainly triglycerides varying in composition depending on species, sex and environment. The intracellular lipids are relatively constant within a species.

e) Vitamins

Fat sol. A, D, E and K are low in muscle associated with marbling fat in the intercellular space. They suppress autoxidative changes, guard against rancidity and off-flavour development in meat during storage. Water soluble vitamins are relatively high except vit C. the concentration of different B vitamins in muscles of ruminants falls in the order of: niacin > pantothenic acid > vitamin B_6 > riboflavin (B_2) > thiamine (B_1) > folic acid > biotin > vitamin B_{12}. These vitamins are found in the sarcoplasm; structural components of coenzymes and prosthetic groups and function in the various enzyme systems. The free forms activate the enzymic reactions.

f) Non Protein Nitrogenous Substances

Some are present in sarcoplasm. The major NPN substances are creatine (0.55 per cent), free amino aids (0.35 per cent), peptides (0.30 per cent), nucleotides (0.37 per cent). They constitute 1.5 per cent of the wt of muscles. The nucleotides contribute to the flavour of meat. ADP, AMP and IMP may contribute to the water holding capacity of aged meat due to the presence of PO_4^{3-} groups. NPN also involve in Maillard type reactions (non enzymatic browning reactions) with carbohydrate derivatives and organic acids during cooking and hence impart a characteristic colour and flavour to cooked meat.

ii) Meat Fats

Sources of Meat Fat

From almost every common domestic animal or foul. The greater qualities are provided by beef and pork animals pesser quantities coming form sheep, horse, and poultry.

Killing Fats

In the packing plant fat which are stripped from the animal at the time of slaughter are killing fats.

Cutting Fats

Those trimmed from the animal carcass when it is dicmembered after chilling are known as cutting fats. Two purposes – edible and inedible

Edible

Only from sound healthy non-infection and properly inspected cattle and certified carcasses, rendered pork fat, sheep. This includes swine-lard and edible tallow. The killing fats that may be used for lard are crown fat, caul fat, pate fate, leaf fat, ham facings, ruffle fat, loin and brisket fat, skirt trimmings and pluck trimmings. The crown fat is from rectal end of bung, caul fat from surrounding stomach and intestine, pate fat from upper front of head, leaf fat from abdomen and ruffle fat is mesenteric fat. The cutting fats are back fat, belly, ham, ham trimmings, loin, neck and shoulder, plate, sweet frozen fats and miscellaneous trimming fats. Certain fats from the pork is rendered and termed as "rendered pork fat" include bacon skins and fleshed skins, green bones (other than head), cheek meat trimmings, feet, gullets, skimming from the rendering tank, skin fleshings, sweet pickle fats, tongue trimmings, lips, ears, snouts, head skins, weasands, pancreas, cooked fat and tissue and cooker bottoms'settlings.

Inedible

Large blood vessels, head bones, cured or cooked bones, casings, rancid fats, hearts, kidneys, livers, lungs, skulls and jaws, spleens, stomachs, tails, tonsils, eye-lids, pressings from wet rendered tankage and condemned hogs and parts. The same parts from beef and mutton carcasses also. Also offal and fat from esthetically non-appealing parts are sent to inedible rendering. Other sources are dead or diseased animals like dogs, cats and even horses. Also trimmings and bone from butcher shop and waste fats from hotels and restaurants are sent to inedible rendering.

Production of Fat

Fats are produced by a variety of processes termed rendering. In most cases the fatty tissues are cooked and the fat is relaeased by temperature and cell rupture. In other processes the temp. is kept low and the fat is relased primarily through physical rapture of cells.

Rendering

(i) Wet rendering (ii) dry rendering (Widely Used) (iii) Continuous rendering (not widely used)

(i) Wet Rendering

steam or hot water can be used. The chopped fatty tissues are charged into a steam jacketed vat. Live steam is injected and the rendering tokes place under steam pressure 40 to 60 lbs/sq.in. temp. to hasten the time of cook fatty tissues are disintegrated. After cooking the pressure is slowly released and the mass is settled when water is used – temp not beyond 50°C charge fatty tissues, fat melt., Float on the surface, skim up.

(ii) Dry Rendering

A substantial quantity of lard and almost all the inedible tallows and greases are produced by dry rendering. The fatty tissues are charged into a horizontal steam jacketed cylinder which has a set of internal blades rotating about a central axis and nearly touching the walls. Dry rendering is accomplished under high pressure atmostpheric pressure or sometimes under vacuum. When sufficient water comes out protein coagulates, fat melt, moisture has been cooked out then fat is released from the tissue, the misture is strained or filtereal to remove the cracklings.

(iii) Continous Rendering

Involve grinding the fats, flash heating, centrifuging, comminuting and warming the residue and then spinning out the fat. This method is specially favourable for the production of oleo stock (edible tallow from internal beef fats) and high quality lard. The products are rendered quickly and at low temp. so that they are quite low in free fatty acids, have little colour and a mild flavour. This process is not widely used.

Table 2.4: Trading Specifications a Industrial Standards (Inedible fats are graded for trading purposes Tallows=titre>40°C grease=titre<40°C)

Name of Item	*Titre (Minimum °C)*	*FFA (max per cent)*	*MIU Basis (Per cent)*	*FAC (Max Untreated and Unbleached)*
Edible tallows	41.5 (min)	1 per cent	1 per cent	Color 5
Industrial fancy and/or acidless tallow	41.5 (min)	3 per cent	1 per cent	5 (max)
Tallow Fancy	41.5 (min)	4 per cent	1 per cent	7 (max)
Tallow Choice	41.0 (min)	5 per cent	1 per cent	9
Tallow Prime	40.5 (min)	6 per cent	1 per cent	13
Tallow Special	40.5 (min)	10 per cent	1 per cent	19
Tallow Special No.1	40.5 (min)	15 per cent	2 per cent	33
Tallow Special No. 3	40.5 (min)	20 per cent	2 per cent	37
Tallow Special No. 2	40.0 (min)	35 per cent	2 per cent	No color restriction
Greases choice white	37	4 per cent	1 per cent	11
Greases A white	37 (min)	8 per cent	2 per cent	15
Greases B white	36 (min)	10 per cent	1 per cent	19
Grease Yellow	36 (min)	15 per cent	2 per cent	37
Grease House	37.5	20 per cent	2 per cent	39
Grease Brown	38	50 per cent	2 per cent	No color

Products and Areas of Use of Stearic, Oleic and Mixed Acids for Animal Fat

I. Stearic Acid

1. Candles
2. Ceramics
3. Crayons and chalks
4. Chlorinated products as plasticizers
5. Glues and adhesity
6. Paper sizing
7. Phonograph recorss
8. Sulfonated acids as cmulsifiers
9. Water proofing, cement and metal salts
10. Wire drawing

II. Oleic Acid

1. Asphalt
2. Core oil
3. Hydraulic breek fluid
4. Petroleum demulsifien
5. Soap (liquid sop)

III. Stearic and Oleic

1. Printing inks
2. Polishes
3. Floor waxes
4. Cosmetics and aids
5. Shaving
6. Pharmaceuticals

IV. Stearic and Mixed

1. Mold release powder
2. Resin and plastics
3. Paint and varnishes as flattening agents

V. Stearic, Oleic and Mixed

1. Chemicals, emulsifiers and plasticizers etc.
2. Cutting oil for metals
3. Insulation, linoleum and leather
4. Leather processing
5. Lubricating grease

7. Protective coating I rubber and cloth
8. Rubber (synthetics)
9. Textiles fiber softening

Animal Byproducts and Animal Wastes

Utilization of animal byproducts and animal wastes is extremely vital but this aspect is not yet received due attention in India. Thus there is a colossal loss on this score. Slaughter houses in the country are frenctioning in most primitive conditions. These lacks even ordinary facilities for the timely collection of byproducts from slaughtered stock. Epidemics of deadly diseases, heavy rain and floods dislocating communication are leading to the efficient collection of byproducts from fallen animals. There is a need in the development of transport facilities gradual disappearance of sentiments against handling of carcasses of cattle and buffalo, organisation of collection agencies for theutilisation of animal byproducts and waste in our country. Loss or huge wastage byproducts utilization of byproducts is as follows according for NCOA 1976.

1. **Hides and Skin**: The estimated annual production of hides in the world is of the order of 6 millio tones out of which the score of India is 12 per cent. India stands seconds in the world. in the field of Hide production U.S.A. stand first with 17.5 per cent of world production. The estimated annual production of skin in the world is of the order of 1.3 million tones out of which India accounts for 7.4 per cent and ranks fifth. Two annual production of Hides in India during 1972 was 24,501,000 picese and skin from goat and sheep 49,415,000 pieces. Due to restriction on cow slaughter more than 90 per cent of Hides are obtained from fallen stock. Hides of all dead or fallen animals cannot be claimed as timely faying of dead animals are not available. NCOA: National Commission on Agriculture. In case of skins the wastage due to non collection is neglible. The estimated annual loss of skins due to non-collection form dead stock has been reckoned at 1 or 2 per cent. At present both exports and imports of Hides and skins have declined. Decline in export was largely due to Government restrictive policy on this item. However in view of rarge bovine population there is a scope on increasing export of Hides and skins through timely collection and improvement of their quality. The all India khadi and village industries commission has set up a number of flaying centers in the rural areas through state khadi village industries boards. There is however an urgent need for establishing more flying centers for skilled flaying of fallen animals. Demonstration cum training centers should be established for imparting training in curing, tanning and rational utilization of hides. Cold storage facilities for preserving raw hides and skins may also be provided. Before export compulsory preshipment inspection should be introduced in securing quality in international market. Though there is a decline trend of hides and skin from India leather and leather manufactures have been increasingly exported.

2. **Casings**: There is a great demand in foreign countries for casings produced in India. But now the export of casings has been gradually declined due to lack of international standards of quality because of lack of facilities in slaughter house. So modernization of slaughter houses and provision of a byproducts wing in them are absolutely essential. Adequate water supply in the existing slaughter houses for cleaning the guts properly is very essential. The hygienic conditions of Indian slaughter houses do not meet the minimum requirements prescribed by exporting countries like U.K. and USA and they banned our casings importing to their country from India. In many slaughter houses guts are not removed soon after the slaughter of animals which results in deterioration of quality of guts. The byproducts wing of each slaughter house should have a processing units of guts under hygienic conditions.
3. **Bones**: The collection of bones is only about 40 per cent of the estimated availability in India. Collection of raw bones is very essential for better utilization of these bones; for this Bone purchases depots should be established in blocks. A major portion of the bones collected in India is utilized for the production of crushed bones and bone grits and a small quantity is used for the manufacture of bone meal. There was about 100 bone crushing mills and about 360 bone digestors in the country in the beginning of fifth plan. Most of the mills crush bones with objective of exporting crush bones and bones grits. Bone meal is also being produced for utilization as a fertilizer. State Govt. should set up more bone digesters for manufacture of bone meal and set up factories for production of gelatin glue and Neats foot oil.
4. **Animal Fats**: There is a considerable wastage of animal fats in India due to non collection or delayed collection at present are importing corers of rupees worth of animal fats from other countries. So our Indian big slaughter houses which are being modernized should have a byproducts plant for processing all available fats from fallen animals or slaughtered animals. Since proportion of fallen stock is very much higher in the case of bovines a chain of carcass utilization centre should be set up.
5. **Bristles**: India is one of the few countries which produce high quality bristles mostly from indigenous domesticated pigs and earning a very good foreign exchange. The Indian bristle industry should improve the better use of bristles for making brushes with finish.
6. **Blood**: At present blood is being collected in a few slaughter houses of the country and in most of the S.H. it is wasted due to lack of suitable arrangements for collection. The wastage of blood worked out to 64 per cent, values Rs. 78, 60, 000 in India. So collection of blood from all the S.H. is very important and collection has to be done speedily and without dilution with water.
7. **Goat Hair**: There is a great demand for goat hair in foreign countries. So collection of goat hair is very important 1972-73 74 lakh worth of goat hair exported.

8. **Horns and Hoofs**: The wastage in collection of horns was estimated to 60 per cent and hoofs at about 66 per cent. There is a good demand for export of horns and hoofs. Further processing plants for preparation of gelatin, Neat's foot oil from hoofs and hair is very necessary.
9. **Meat Unfit for Human Consumption**: and Meat received adhered to bones should be properly utilized for meat meal.

Utilization of Fallen Animals

It has been estimated that about 22.8 million carcasses of fallen animals are available annually out of this hardly 53 per cent are being partly utilized and remaining ones are completely wasted. The economic loss for unutilization and underutilization of carcass and defective flaying has been estimated to be about Rs.50 crores/annum. Carcass utilization centers: Well equipped carcass utilization center should be established for better utilization of fallen animals.

Recommendations

1. Improved methods of flaying should be introduced in the slaughter houses. More village flaying centers should be established.
2. Demonstration cum training centers should be established in important places for training people in curing training and rational utilization of hides.
3. A system of compulsory preshipners inspection should be introduced for Hides and Skins meant for export.
4. Cold storage facilitation for preserving raw hides and skins in slaughtered houses and byproducts plant should be improved.
5. Sanitary conditions in slaughter houses and byproduct plant should be improved.
6. The byproducts wing of each plant should have a gut processing unit.
7. For increasing collection of bones, cooperative Bone Collector should be formed.
8. New bone digestors should be set up
9. All pig slaughter house should have a byproducts plant.
10. The pig areas and Bristle merchants should be educated regarding economic importance of bristles and same with goat hair.
11. Blood from small animals should be suitably collected.
12. Export of horns and hooves should be increased.
13. A chain of well equipped carcass utilization centers should be established by the state governments.
14. Meat unfits for human consumption should be converted into meat meal.
15. Modernization of all slaughter houses is very essential to maintain sanitation and hygienic condition of byproducts.

Table 2.5: Characteristics of Representative Animal Fats

	Butter Oil	Neat's Foot Oil	Lard	Tallow	
				Beef	Mutton
Iodine Value	25-42	69-76	53-77	40-48	35-46 (40-45 sometime)
Seponification Number	210-233	190-199	190-202	190-199	192-197
Melting Point	28-35°C	25°F (-4°C)	33-46°C	40-48°C	44-51°C
Density at 20°C		0.912	0.916	0.934 - 0.950	0.934 - 0.948
Viscosity at →	20°C	40°C	50°C	100°C	
Nest foot oil	84	X	X	10	
Lard	X	35	25	X	
Tallow beef	X	X	34	10	
Mutton	7	X	43	19	

- ☆ **Iodine Value:** It is a measure of the unsaturation of fat. It is expressed as the number of grams of iodine observed by 100 gm of fat. The nerve the unsaturated fatty acids present in fat, the more is the iodine value and vice versa.
- ☆ **Saponification number:** It is the number of milligrams of potassium hydroxide (KOH) to saponify 1 gm of fat or oil. It varies inversely with mol.wt. of fat or oil.
- ☆ **Viscosity:** It means the resistance to flow. Viscosity decreases with increasing unsaturation of fat and vice versa.
- ☆ **Titre:** Titre is a measure of temperature developed as a consequence of heat of crystallization during cooling of melted fatty acids of the fat. Measured by °C.
- ☆ **FFA:** Free Fatty Acids.
- ☆ **MIU:** Moisture, insolubles unsaponifiable factors.
- ☆ **FAC:** Fat Analysis Committee colour.

Characteristics and Specifications of Fats

Fats are produced both as edible and inedible grades. The term edible and inedible refer to human consumption. Edible fats may be produced only from the approved portions of the carcasses of clean, sound meat animals, all other fats must be rendered as on inedible grade.

The inedible fats are of many grades. These are graded according to certain physical and chemical characteristics. These are titer, FFA (free fatty acid) contents, MIU (moisture insolubles and unsaponifiables) and FAC (fat analysis committee) color. They are further separated into tallow or grease by the titer test. The titer test is a measure of the temperature developed as a consequence of the heat of crystallization during cooling of melted fatty acids from the fat. Regardless of their source, fat with titer of 40°C (104°F) or higher are called tallows and those with less than 40°C (140°F) are called greases.

Table 2.6: Trading Specifications for Inedible Fats

Fat	*Titer Minimum*		*FFA Maximum (per cent)*	*M.I.U. (per cent)*	*F.A.C. Maximum Untreated and Unbleached*
	°C	*°F*			
Tallows					
Edible	41.5	106.7	1	1	5
Industrial and/or Acidless tallow	41.5	106.7	3	1	5
Fancy	41.5	106.7	4	1	7
Choice	41	105.8	5	1	9
Prime	40.5	104.9	6	1	13 or 11 B
Special	40.5	104.9	10	1	19 or 11 C
No. 1	40.5	104.9	15	2	33
No. 3	40.5	104.9	20	2	37
No. 2	40	104.0	35	2	No colour
Greases					
Choice white	37	98.6	4	1	11
A white	37	98.6	8	2	15
B white	36	96.8	10	1	19 or 11 C
Yellow	36	96.8	15	2	37
House	37.5	99.5	20	2	39
Brown	38	100.4	50	2	No colour

The table shows that the grades within a classification vary widely in FFA (free fatty acid) and colour, the lowest grades having both a very high FFA and a colour so dark it cannot be measured.

Use of Fat

1. Direct use in food gradually decreasing.
2. Used in manufacture of shortening and margarine. The physical properties of tallow are suited for preparation of shortening after eliminating certain flavour defects by a mild hydrogenation.
3. Lard and tallow used for trying purpose are refined and (or deodourized to remove the free fatty acids (FFA) to increase its smoke point. A lard with no FFA will smoke at 220°C (428°F) with 0.2 per cent FFA will reduce the smoke point to 193°C (379°F) and with 0.5 per cent FFA will lower it to 171°C (340°F).
4. Certain internal fats are rendered for oleo stock. This oleo stock is grained (crystallized) at 35°C and then pressed to produce oleo oil and oleo stearin.

These are used in bakery products and confections and a small quality in margarines.

5. The major areas of usage for inedible products are soap, fatty acids, lubricants and animal feeds. The growth of synthetic detergents has seriously disturbed the markets for soup.
6. Long-chain alcohols prepared by reduction of meat fats are useful chemical intermediates. Their sulfate derivatives are marketed extensively as detergents, wetting agents and emulsifying agents.
7. Utilized in animal feeds, especially important in broiler feeds, swine feeds, dog food and cattle feed.
8. The meat fats are composed of 40 to 50 per cent oleic acid, 40-50 per cent stearic and 4-10 per cent polyunsaturated acids. The nitrogen derivatives of these fatty acids *e.g.* amides – used for water proofing and release agents for meat loaves, the polyamines and the hydroxyamines – in liquid detergents.
9. The high mol. wt. esters from meat fat acids – used on plasticizers, lubricating oil additions emulsifiers etc. The esters made with polyhydric alcohols – useful textile sizers and lubricants, water-in-oil emulsifiers, viscosity increasers, pour-point depressants, low-temperature plasticizers, dye solubilizers and detergents. Ethylene oxide addition products are useful in nonsuding detergents and vinyl esters are employed as copolymers in some plastics.
10. The epoxy and dihydroxy compounds from oleic acids – used as plasticizers. Ozonization of oleic acid enables the production of dibasic acid such as suberic and azelaic used in the for, of their polyester and polyamide derivative used as lubricants, plastics and plasticizers.
11. Lard oil, grease oil, horse oil etc are used as industrial cutting oil and in the treatment of leathers and textiles. Lard oil used in microbial cultures for the production of antibiotics.

Processing of Fats

With improved technology and the demands of special as well as general usage, it has become increasingly important to process lard and tallow before utilizing them in foods.

Edible fats may be subjected to hydrogenation, bleaching, deodourization, plasticization, inter-esterification or fractional crystallization. Inedible fats may be subjected to crystallization, hydrogenation, bleaching or fat splitting.

1. Hydrogenation

Unsaturated fats and oils are sometimes hydrogenated to produce harder, higher melting more stable fats. This is accomplished by treatment with hydrogen under some degree of pressure in the presence of a catalyst. Finely divided platinum, palladium or copper chromite may be used but nickel is used most commonly commercially. Only minute quantities of catalyst are required. The hydrogen first dissolves in the catalyst. The unsaturated linkage is then adsorbed on the surface, and hydrogen approaches from inside the metal and becomes attached to the unsaturated carbons. Once saturated, the molecular no longer has an affinity for the catalysis and is released leaving a catalyst site free for another unsaturated molecule. The catalysts may be "poisoned" by substances such as sulfur compounds or carbon monoxide that are adsorbed on the surface of the catalyst and not released.

Tallows are usually so high melting that they are seldom hydrogenated for edible purpose except for a very slight degree. Lards on the other hand are completely hydrogenated to iodine values of five or less.

2. Bleaching

Undesirable colour components may be removed from fats intended for edible purpose by bleaching. Bleaching is common in the processing of tallows and greases for white soaps. Bleaching may be accomplished by adsorption, by chemical action by hydrogenation, by liquid extraction or by heat.

Chemical bleaching: Oxidation by blowing with air, ozone, peroxides, dichromate and acid, permanganate, chlorine and hypochlorite.

Liquid extraction: with propane, it is employed for purifying and bleaching tallow.

Adsorption bleaching: Most widely used, adsorbents used are natural and acid catalyzed clays, activated carbons.

3. Deodourization

Generally, those ingredients of a fat which are responsible for odours and flavours have a low vapour pressure and are removed with difficulty at atmospheric pressures. To minimize heat damage to the fat and to facilitate removal of the odour and flavour components, the fat is stripped at 150°C to 250°C (302°F to 482°F) with a non reactive gas while a good vacuum is applied. Usually dry steam is used as the stripping gas because of its low cost, high specific volume and the ease with which it can be condensed and removed from the system. In addition to the flavour components the free fatty acids in the fats are stripped out and this provides a fat with a high smoke point as well as other desirable properties.

4. Plasticization

Plasticity means the property of acting like a solid and resisting small stresses but yielding instantly and flowing like a liquid when subjected to a stress above certain minimal values. At room temperature meal fats consists of a mass of small crystals in which is enmeshed a quantity of liquid oil. Fats are firmer as the solids content increases. A solids content of 15-20 per cent is usually the most desirable. Lards normally have this content at temperature range of 20°C to 30°C (68° to 86°F). Long plastic rangers are obtained by mixing glycerides of widely differing melting points.

The consistency of a plastic material is influenced by the size of the solid particles and their total volume. A material become firmer as the av. size of the particles decreases and vice-versa. Therefore, a "grainy" lard is softer than a smooth lard. Smooth lard contains many small crystals and this extends the plastic range and gives smooth appearance.

Lard, oleo oil and fat shortenings are plasticized by rapid cooling on a chill roll or in a votator chilling machine. Nearly solidified fats are frequently 'tempered' by holding them at 30°C (86°F) for twenty four hours and then bringing them to 21°C (70°F).

5. Interesterification

It is otherwise called ester interchange. In this process, the fatty acids are re-distributed in glyceride molecule due to rupture and recombination of glyceride ester linkages. The fatty acids are separated from and reunited with glycerol by the action of catalysts such as sodium methoxide resulting removal of saturated fatty acids by crystallization and the remainder of fatty acids are distributed randomly among the glycerides in liquid phase. Ester interchange is used extensively in the processing of meat fats for use in shortening. The solid content in fat is changed and there are modification of crystal habit which provide improved creaming power and ability to incorporate air. This change has made lard a highly desired ingredient for quality shortenings based on meat fats.

6. Fractional Crystallization

It is the separation of solid and liquid portion of the fat based on controlled temperatures. The fats are melted and then are allowed to stand at temperatures controlled such that the more highly saturated trighycerides crystallize out and form crystal aggregates. The fatty masses are pressed, the liquid portions are separated as oil and the solid portions as stearins. Oils made from animal fat by this process are lard oil, oleo oil, tallow oil and grease oil. Oleo oil is used in edible products and other oils in industry as metal cutting oils leather conditioners etc.

Physical Properties of Fats

1. Polymorphic Forms

Triglycerides, diglycerides and monoglycerides all have the property of solidifying in several different crystalline forms *i.e.* they are polymorplic. Each crystal form has its own melting point, heat capacity, crystal structure and solubility. It is agreed that at least three forms exist and these are α' and β. Rapid cooling such as immersion in liquid nitrogen or dry ice acetone, yields the α-forms. Slow cooling or tempering just below the melting point results in the β-form . The β' form may be obtained from the α-form by tempering just above the α-melting point. The melting point of a triglyceride is lowest in the α-form and highest in the β-form *e.g.* Tristearin – 54°C (129°F), β-64.5°C (148°F), β 73°C (163°F). The β-form is the most stable of the three polymorphic forms and the more unstable forms slowly transform to the β-form on standing.

2. Melting Point

The melting point usually given for fats is the open-tube capillary melting point for the most stable polymorphic form (β-form). It should be emphasized that this is not the temperature at which all solid phase changes to an all-liquid phase but is the temperature at which all the solid disappears. The melting point rises with increasing saturation and decreasing chain length *e.g.* Neats foot oil with 79 per cent oleic acid must contain a high percentage of di- and triunsaturated glycerides and has a very low melting point. Butter fat-containing a variety of short-chain fatty acids has a correspondingly low melting point.

3. Viscosity

The property of viscosity is of greatest interest in the design of pumps and piping systems and in selection of the proper temperatures for handling. The viscosity increases with the average chain length of the constituent fatty acids and decrease with increasing instauration.

Table 2.7: Table Viscosities of Simple Saturated Triglycerides

Triglycerides	*Viscosities (70°C, 158°F)*	*Triglycerides*	*Viscosities (70°C, 158°F)*
Triacetin	0.2	Tributyrin	3.0
Tricaproin	5.9	Tricaprylin	8.8
Tricaprin	11.7	Trilaurin	14.6
Trimyristin	17.6	Tripalmitin	20.5
Tristearin	23.4		

4. Specific Heat

Thermal properties are also important in the handling and processing of fats, as well as in the study of the phase changes of such material. These properties vary depending on composition. In an individual fat, they vary with the polymorphic form and the relative amounts of solid and liquid present. At ordinary temperatures the specific heat increases with increasing unsaturation in both liquid and solid states. In the solid state the unstable α-form has a higher specific heat than the stable β-form and the liquid fat has a value which is almost twice that of the solid forms.

5. Heat of Fusion

The unstable α-form has a lower heat of fusion than the stable β-form. As the chain length increases, the heat of fusion becomes greater. The heat absorbed by a sample of a natural fat at temperatures below the melting point but above that of completer solidification is a function of the specific heats of the solid and liquid phases and of the heat of fusion. Such calorimetric data have been used to estimate the relative amounts of solid and liquid in commercial fats.

6. Density

Density is required in the design of apparatus for handling fats. Its most important application is the estimation of the solid-liquid ratio in commercial fats. There are slight differences among the densities of the polymorph modifications *e.g.* tristearin. When suitable dilatometric equipment is used the volume change of a weighed sample of fat may be measured over the temperature range in which the fat melts.

7. Refractive Index

The refractive index of fats and fatty materials is a useful indication of identity and purity. It increases with increasing chain length in fatty acids and esters and may be used to identify fractions obtained in fatty acid ester fractionations. The refractive index also increases with increasing unstauration. This property has been made use of as a control device in the hydrogenation of fats, where a decrease in unstauration causes a corresponding decrease in refractive index. The change in iodine value and refractive index is nearly linear. The refractive index decreases with increasing temperature. For most fats the value for this decrease at temperatures near 40°C (104°F) is given as 0.00038 for 1°C increase in temperature.

8. Solubility

The solubility of fats is important in many areas of processing. Fats in general are completely miscible with non-polar solvents such as petroleum, ether, benzene and some esters. They are virtually insoluble in polar solvents such as water. They may be partially soluble in solvents of intermediate polarity such as alcohol and acetone. The solvents of intermediate polarity are useful in separating the components of a fat mixture *e.g.* the saturated triglycerides (GS3) are only very slightly soluble in cold acetone. Solutions in alcohol of either the fat or a mixture of fat and hydrocarbon solvent will separate into two phases in the cold, leaving the alcohol layer rich in the more polar components of the fat such as fatty acids.

Chemical Reactions at the Easter Linkage of Fats

The ester linkage in fats behaves in much the same fashion as it does in simple esters. It undergoes saponification, alcoholysis, ammonolysis, reduction and hydrazide formation.

1. Saponificaion

Saponification results in the formation of the alkali metal soap and glycerol. Hydrolysis of fats may be accomplished under either acid or alkaline conditions but the energy of activation for acid hydrolysis is greater than that for alkaline hydrolysis.

2. Alcoholysis

This process involves an interchange between the alcohol used and the glycerol in the fat to form the simple esters of the fatty acids making up the fat. This reaction is utilized in a variety of procedures to prepare methyl and other short-chain esters for GLC (Gas-Liquid Chromatography) analysis of the fatty acid composition of various lipids.

3. Ammonolysis

Ammonolysis proceeds with difficulty and is not the method of choice for preparation of the amides which usually result from this reaction. The hydrazides and hydroxamic acids can be prepared from the fatty acids in fats by reaction under suitable condition of the fats with hydrazine hydrate or hydroxylamine.

4. Reduction

Substantial quantities of tallow alcohols are prepared by ester reduction. Reduction is accomplished by sodium and alcohol or by high pressure hydrogenation in the presence of copper chromite. The products are glycerol and long-chain alcohols with the same number of carbon atoms as the fatty acids in the tallow.

5. Interchange

The interchange of the fatty acids in a fat by ester interchange has become important in the use of animal fats in the shortening industry. It is possible by this technique to modify the glyceride composition of a fat.

Chemical Reactions of the Carboxyl Group

The fatty acids of animals fats are capable of undergoing the reactions of organic acids replacing the OH in the carboxyl or complete modification of the carboxyl to form the compounds such as alcohols, Ketones, amines and nitrites.

1. Esters

Easters result from reactions of alcohols with fatty acids or acid chlorides or of alkali metal alcoholates with fatty acids. Simple esters are formed with short chain monohydric alcohols and the waxes are formed by fatty acid reaction with the higer monohydric alcohols such as cetyl and stearyl. The polyhydric alcohols are used to prepare mono-di, or higher polyesters. Esters may be prepared also by alcoholysis of glycerides and by reaction of acids with oxirane compounds.

2. Soaps

The water soluble soaps of sodium and potassium are produced by alkali saponification of fats. Most other soaps are oil soluble and water-soluble salt.

3. Alcohols

Long-chain alcohols are formed by catalytic hydrogenation or by sodium reduction of the ester linkage in a fat.

4. Acid Chlorides

These are usually prepared by reaction of the acid with phosphorus tri-chloride.

5. Amides

Fatty acid amides are formed by passing ammonia into fatty acids and then heating to split out water.

– Chapter 3 –

Muscle Functions and Postmortem Changes: Rigor Mortis, Conversion of Muscle to Meat

Muscle Function

In living muscle, the complete oxidation of carbohydrate to carbon dioxide and water requires oxygen, and it releases a lot of energy. Much of this energy is captured by adding a phosphate group to another molecule that already has two phosphate groups. Thus, adenosine diphosphate (ADP) is converted to adenosine triphosphate (ATP). The ATP molecule carries this energy within the muscle fiber, and it may be released to another biochemical system by cleaving off the added phosphate (ATP ADP + P). Muscle contraction is a primary user of ATP in the living animal, but substantial amounts of ATP are used by the membranes around and within the fibre for maintaining ionic concentration gradients. One molecule of a carbohydrate may be combined with oxygen to add a phosphate group to each of 36 molecules of ADP. In addition to 36 molecules of ATP, this produces carbon dioxide and water. However, if the muscle is without oxygen (anoxic) after slaughter, the most it can normally gain by oxidizing each carbohydrate molecule is two molecules of ATP.

Glycogen is the primary storage carbohydrate in muscle fibers and appears in electron micrographs as single granules or clumps of granules located in the sarcoplasm (cytoplasm) between myofibrils (contractile fibrils) and under the cell membrane. New research using scanning tunnelling microscopy, one of the most powerful types of microscope yet invented, reveals that glycogen granules are ellipsoidal with a laminar structure which suggests they grow from one edge rather than a central point. In longitudinal sections of skeletal muscle, glycogen and its associated enzymes are concentrated at the I bands (one of the transverse bands across the muscle fiber when examined microscopically).

Glycogen is a polysaccharide formed by the linking together of large numbers of glucose units. However, the glycogen from some animal tissues is a proteoglucan (glycoprotein) that may contain other monosaccharides and phosphate ester groups. Straight chains of glycogen are formed by linkages between carbon atoms given numbers 1 and 4, while branch points are formed by 1-6 linkages.

The concentration of glycogen in fetal muscle increases steadily towards the end of gestation and may peak at the time of birth. Pigs have very high muscle glycogen levels at birth but they decline rapidly after birth to reach future adult levels within a week. Glycogenin is a protein that acts as a starting block for the formation of new glycogen.

There is currently a lot of interest in the possibility of post mortem glycogen break-down (glycogenolysis) by pathways other than the normal pathway mentioned above. If appreciable amounts of glycogen may be removed without lactic acid formation, this might account for some of the considerable variability found in post mortem rates of meat acidification or pH decline. About 5 per cent of muscle glycogen may be contained in lysosomes (suicide bags that contain enzymes to destroy damaged parts of the cell) and post mortem glycogenolysis may be a combination of both hydrolysis and phosphorolysis.

After Exsanguination

Once the animal has been exsanguinated, the oxygen within the muscles is rapidly exhausted, and the process of converting muscle to meat really begins.

Glycogenolysis is the enzymatic degradation of glycogen, and is the first step in the release of energy by the oxidation of glucose units (glycolysis). Phosphorylase erodes straight chains (from their non-reducing ends at carbon 4) and attaches a phosphate group to the carbon atom at position 1 as it removes a glucose unit. Phosphorylase erodes straight chains until it comes to the fourth glucose unit preceding a branch point. The three glucose units before the fourth one that carries the branch are removed together, and are added to an adjacent free straight chain so that the 1-6 linkage thus exposed at the branch point may be severed. A second enzyme, debranching enzyme, performs this task. Instead of being released as glucose-1-phosphate, the glucose unit released from a branch point remains as free glucose. Thus, total glycogenolysis liberates glucose-1-phosphate and glucose in a ratio indicating the ratio between the mean length of straight chains and the number of branch points.

While the structure of glycogen and the mechanism of glycogenolysis are important in understanding the conversion of muscles to meat, the remainder of the pathway by which glycogen is anaerobically oxidized to lactate need only be covered in general principle. The most important question to be answered is why lactate is produced under anaerobic conditions, yet hardly at all under aerobic conditions. After a series of steps in the glycolytic pathway, molecules with six carbon atoms derived from the glucose units of glycogen are split to produce two molecules of pyruvate, each with three carbon atoms. All the glycolytic enzymes (except for hexokinase) are concentrated in the I band. If aerobic conditions prevail, pyruvate formed in the cytosol of the muscle fibre now enters a mitochondrion (the metabolic furnace of the cell). After entering a mitochondrion, pyruvate is converted to acetyl-CoA which becomes fused to oxaloacetate to form citrate. The citrate then is oxidized in the well known Krebs' cycle, which is completed by the regeneration of oxaloacetate. Continuous activity of the Krebs' cycle is fuelled by a range of carbohydrates, fatty acids and amino acids, and is the primary system for the aerobic generation of energy. Large numbers of molecules of ATP are produced from ADP by a series of reactions, oxidative phosphorylation, that occur in the mitochondrial membrane.

Under aerobic conditions, the production of two pyruvate molecules from a glucose-1-phosphate molecule results in the reduction of 2NAD+. Thus, somewhere else in the muscle fibre, NADH must be re-oxidized for glycolysis to continue. Aerobically, this occurs as a consequence of mitochondrial Krebs' cycle activity, although NADH and NAD+ do not actually cross the mitochondrial membrane. In anaerobic living muscles and in meat, the Krebs' cycle is halted, and NADH is re-oxidized in the cytosol by lactate dehydrogenase (LDH) during the conversion of pyruvate to lactate. Pyruvate is of no immediate use anaerobically since mitochondrial oxidation has ceased, but its conversion to lactate ensures a continued supply of NAD+ for the continuation of glycogenolysis and anaerobic glycolysis in the cytosol. However, since these events form only the initial stages of complete carbohydrate oxidation, they do not regenerate much ATP. The net gain of ATP is reduced to only two molecules of ATP per molecule of glucose-1-phosphate. Molecules of glucose released from glycogen branch points generate a total net gain of 3ATP.

LDH adds hydrogen to pyruvate to produce lactic acid and exists in a number of isoenzymes separable electrophoretically by their net electrical charge. If LDH-1 is prevalent, it facilitates aerobic metabolism, where possible, since it is inhibited by pyruvate and lactate. LDH-5 is not inhibited by high levels of lactate and pyruvate, and it facilitates anaerobic metabolism. LDH-1 is typical of cardiac muscle while LDH-5 is typical of skeletal muscles, particularly those adapted for anaerobic conditions during contraction. In skeletal muscles, the ratio of LDH-1 to LDH-5 corresponds to the dominant activity pattern of a muscle. For example, muscles capable of sustained activity and which only use aerobic metabolism have high LDH-1. LDH-5 is the dominant isoenzyme in skeletal muscles from slaughter-weight pigs.

The regulation of glycolysis in a muscle fiber of a live animal is integrated with the metabolic state of the fiber and its immediate energy needs. The metabolic state of the fiber is profoundly affected by hormones, particularly adrenaline, and by the extent of recent contractile activity of the fiber. Phosphorylase is particularly important in the conversion of muscle to meat since it may be a primary control site for post mortem glycolysis. Phosphorylase in muscle is most active when it is, itself, phosphorylated (a). When dephosphorylated, it is less active (b). In general terms, therefore, phosphorylase is switched on and off by the addition or removal of its phosphate, with on and off states being relative rather than absolute. The activity of phosphorylase b is dependent on the presence of AMP but the activity of phosphorylase a is not. There are two conflicting requirements that make the mechanism for the activation of phosphorylase rather complex. Firstly, since phosphorylase initiates the release of considerable amounts of chemical energy, there must be safeguards to prevent its uncontrolled activity. In stress-susceptible pigs, for example, the uncontrolled activity of anaerobic glycolysis may lead to excessive heat production and to a level of acidity that may soon prove fatal. The conflicting requirement is that the vast amounts of phosphorylase spread through the muscle mass must be rapidly activated by relatively small amounts of adrenaline. The adrenaline activation of severely frightened animals often is called the "fight or flight" response: neither of these responses is likely to be of much survival value if the anaerobic energy supply to body muscles is delayed.

The conflicting demands for fail-safe but rapid activation are satisfied by two particular features of the activation system. Firstly, the conversion of phosphorylase b to phosphorylase a is inhibited locally in each muscle fibre by high concentrations of ATP and glucose-6-phosphate (an intermediate in the conversion of glycogen to lactate). Thus, if the energy released by phosphorylase is not rapidly consumed, the energy release system shuts down. If the energy is used, however, AMP and phosphate (from ATP ADP + P and from ADP AMP + P) further enhance the activation of phosphorylase. Secondly, to enable the rapid activation of phosphorylase throughout the musculature, the relatively small amounts of adrenaline that arrive at the muscle initiate a series of biochemical changes functioning as an amplifier. A small input leads to a large output. Adrenaline causes adenyl cyclase to increase its formation, from ATP, of cyclic AMP. Then cyclic AMP activates protein kinase. With ATP and magnesium ions present, protein kinase then phosphorylates another enzyme, phosphorylase b kinase b. The active form, phosphorylase b kinase a, in the presence of magnesium ions, finally activates phosphorylase b to phosphorylase a. As a final safety factor, if the supply of inorganic phosphate is inadequate, even phosphorylase a will be relatively inactive but the system will be primed for rapid energy production once muscle contraction is initiated.

When animals require energy anaerobically during normal activity, phosphorylase b kinase is activated by calcium ions released from the sarcoplasmic reticulum - normally the trigger for muscle contraction in living muscle. Glycogen granules are closely related to the sarcoplasmic reticulum and to glycogenolytic enzymes as part of a structural complex. The activation system linking muscle contraction to glycogenolysis is short lived to avoid the continuous use and depletion of glycogen reserves. Glycogen is a rapidly available energy source for both brief muscle activity and the early stages of sustained activity. Phosphorylase activity is curtailed by phosphatase, which dephosphorylates phosphorylase a and phosphorylase b kinase a, when muscle activity ceases or an animal recovers from fright. Many features of the system for activating phosphorylase are shared with the activation system for glycogen synthesis, but the shared features are opposite in effect. Thus, the muscle fibre does not attempt to synthesize new glycogen at the same time that it is breaking it down, and vice versa.

Newborn pigs often have difficulty maintaining their blood glucose levels, and may die of hypoglycaemia after even short periods of starvation. Given that they have high glycogen levels at birth, this is not easy to explain, although stored glycogen may simply be inadequate in amount if milk is not available. Despite an adult predisposition to the excessive accumulation of adipose tissue, newborn pigs have very little adipose tissue so that liberation of free fatty acids is severely limited. Most phosphorylase is in the relatively inactive b form just after birth. In adult pigs, hyperglycaemia readily occurs in response to exercise and adrenaline secretion.

The Fate of Lactate in Living Animals

Meat animals may exhibit a considerable range in their general muscular and cardiovascular fitness. At one extreme, sheep and cattle may roam in search of feed and water for part of the year, coping with adverse conditions much like wild animals. At the other extreme, animals may be reared in close confinement, partly to prevent them wasting feed energy by converting it to muscular work. Pigs that are rarely exercised may have a low oxygen transport capacity whereas regular exercise reduces lactate production in response to a standard test.

In living animals, the lactate produced by contracting muscles is removed by the circulatory system, but first it must travel from the muscle fiber into the interstitial space. Lactate release may be retarded in situations such as exhaustive exercise. A fraction of the lactate leaving a fiber may be in the form of undissociated lactic acid, and this fraction may increase with a rise in external pH. In living animals, blood flow is increased in active muscles (hyperaemia). When hyperaemia occurs as a secondary response to hypoxia, it may be mediated by the release of adenosine (from AMP A + P) into the interstitial fluid between muscle fibers.

On arriving in the liver, lactate may be converted to glucose-6-phosphate, and then stored as glycogen or released as glucose back into the blood. Circulating glucose is available to muscles to be stored as glycogen or used directly as energy for contraction (Cori cycle). After exhaustive exercise, an animal may continue to consume oxygen at an increased rate for some time (oxygen debt). During this recovery period, some lactate may be completely oxidized to release enough energy for the remaining lactate to be converted to glucose (gluconeogenesis) in the liver. When an animal is exsanguinated, the blood can no longer perform its transport function in the Cori cycle, and lactate accumulates in the musculature. There are, however, a number of other possible fates for lactate in living animals.

Heart muscle receives its own blood supply from the coronary artery, straight from the aorta, and cardiac muscle may use circulating lactate as an energy source. The high oxygen concentration in the aorta usually allows complete oxidation of lactate by cardiac muscle. Any lactate remaining in the aorta may not all get pumped to the liver or kidneys to participate in the Cori cycle, because the aorta supplies other major arteries in addition to the hepatic and renal arteries. Much of the circulating lactate may pass through non-contracting muscles that oxidize lactate as an energy substrate, particularly if circulating fatty acids are unavailable. Resting muscles also may take up circulating lactate and reconvert it directly to glycogen, probably via a pathway which is independent of the mitochondrial Krebs' cycle. Finally, also it is possible for all the lactate consumed during an oxygen debt period to be oxidized to CO_2.

Contraction causes an initial drop in muscle fiber pH because of the hydrolysis of ATP, but this may be followed by an increase in pH from the breakdown of creatine phosphate or CP. CP acts as a short term store of energy since it has a phosphate that may be transferred to ADP (CP + ADP ATP + C) by the creatine phosphokinase (CPK). CP is the dominant carrier of energy from mitochondria to myofibrils. CPK and creatine are normally contained within muscle fibers, but may leak into the blood from damaged or diseased fibers. In healthy muscle, creatine is slowly but continuously converted to creatinine. Creatinine is lost in the urine in approximate proportion to the muscle mass of the body. The production of lactate following muscle contraction may cause another drop in pH. The interstitial pH between muscle fibers and the pH at the muscle surface are profoundly affected by overall pH levels in the blood.

Muscle Contraction and Relaxation

Nerves and nature of stimuli: Nervous stimuli in brain or spinal cord transmitted to the muscle via a nerve. Motor nerves – myelinated, nodes of Ranvier. Myelinated nerve fibers have 30-40 fold greater conduction velocities than do unmyelinated fibers.

Resting cell- membrane potential 80-85 mv in nerve and muscle fibers; +ve outside and –ve inside the cell.

Membrane potential is due to:

1. Active transport of ions through the membrane.
2. Selective permeability characteristics of the membrane.
3. Ions composition – intra and extra cellular.

Action Potential

Nerve and muscle fibers exhibit membrane potentials.They are able to transmit an electric impulse, called an action potential, along their membrane surfaces.When an action potential is transferred from a motor nerve to muscle fibers, it initiates muscle contractions.An action potential travels along the membrane surface of the nerve fiber, and is actually a wave of reversing electrical polarization that results from chemical changes in the membrane. Thus it is often referred to as an electrochemical process. The action potential is initiated by a several hundred to several thousandfold increase in the Na^+ ion permeability of the membrane. – cause a rapid rate of diffusion of Na^+ into the cell – reversing the membrane potential. The newly reversed membrane potential reduces the Na^+ permeability to its former low level. The outward flow of K+ continue and reestablish the resting membrane potential. These electrochemical processes can be recorded as electrical depolarization wave. The entire sequence of events in the transmission of an action potential past any point on the nerve fiber requires about 0.5-1 mill seconds.

Myoneural Junction

The stimulus (action potential0 that initiates muscle contraction is transferred from the nerve fiber to the muscle fiber at the myoneural or neuromuscular junction.At this junction the motor nerve branches into several terminal endings that are implanted in small invigilation of the sarcolemma. The combined structures of the myoneural junction form a small mound on the surface of the muscle fiber, called the motor end plate. When the action potential arrives at the motor end plate, it causes a chemical transmitter, acetylcholine (stored in small vesicles in the terminal nerve branches) to be released.

- ☆ Sarcolemma become more permeable to Na^+ ions.
- ☆ Its polarity reverses – Action Potential propagated.
- ☆ Acetyl choline (Ach) destroyed by cholinesterase, abundantly found in myoneural junction, so Ach acts for short time.

Action Potential (AP) in Muscle

Duration of AP 5-10 milliseconds in muscle fiber as compared to 0.5-1milliseconds in nerve fibers. AP begins at myoneural junctions, progress longitudinally in both directions along the sarcolemma and stimulates the entire length of the fiber. The AP enters the interior of the fiber along the T tubules and at the triad, is transferred to the SR that sorrounds each myofibril.

Contraction of Skeletal Muscle

Involves actin, myosin, tropomyosin and troponin. Resting muscle: Ca^{2+} ion conc. 10^{-7} moles/lit. in sarcoplasmic fluid, total Ca^{2+} conc. is 10^{-4} moles/lit. in muscle. Mg-ATP complex serves as a plasticizer, inhibits crossbridges formation by myosin and actin. Action potential – release bound Ca^{2+} ions to sarcoplasmic fluid – free Ca^{2+} ions conc. increases– initiate contraction mechanism. It requires 10 to 100 times (10^{-6} to 10^{-5} moles/lit) more Ca^{2+} ions to initate a contraction.

Ca^{2+} ions released – bound by troponin complex – myosin become free to form cross bridge – actin filaments are pulled toward centre of the sarcomere – actomyosin complex formed - decrease sarcomere length. Width of A-band does not change I-band and H-zonc width decrease.

$$\text{Energy ATP} \xrightarrow[\substack{\uparrow \text{ ATPase} \\ \text{Free } Ca^{2+} \text{ ions}}]{\text{Myosin}} \text{ADP} + \text{Pi}$$

The cross bridges convert the chemical energy to mechanical energy and initiate filament sliding, thus generation a contractile force.

Relaxation of Skeletal Muscle

It is re-establishment of resting state.

- ☆ Decrease in muscle tension.
- ☆ Re-polarization of action potential
- ☆ Membrane potential to its resting value.
- ☆ Free Ca^{2+} bound to tubule of SR
- ☆ Transferred to terminal cisternae of the triads for storage.
- ☆ Troponin molecules release the Ca^{2+} ions, thus inhibits the formation of cross-bridge (at Ca^{2+} ions conc. of 10^{-7} moles/lit or less)

- ☆ Cacium pump mechanism helps in accumulating Ca^{2+} in SR, energy for this is from ATP hydrolysis by an enzyme which is activated by increase in free Ca^{2+} ions.

Source of Energy for Muscle Function

1. Muscle glycogen → 1 glucose-1-phosphate
2. 1 molecule of glucose-1-phosphate → 2 pyruvic acid
   Net = 3 ATP (-1 ATP, +4 ATP)
3. 2 pyruvic acid → aerobic → TCA cycle → $6CO_2$
   Products of fat and protein degradation → aerobic
   20 H → aerobic → mitochondria → 30 ATP
4. 2 pyruvic acid → Anaerobic → 2 lactic acid
5. Glycolysis → 4H → Anaerobic → 2 lactic acid
6. Glycolysis → 4H → aerobic → cytochrome chain → 4ATP
   Blood supply → $6O_2$ → cytochrome chain – mitochondria → 12 H_2O
   ↓ ↓
   4ATP 30 ATP

Thus, when a single glucose molecule, derived from glycogen is degraded to CO_2 and H_2O, 37 ADP molecules are converted to 37 ATP molecules.

Developments in Post-mortem Changes in Meat Influencing its Quality

Slaughter of food animal is followed by a series of physical and chemical changes over a period of several hours or even days resulting in the conversion of muscle to meat. After slaughtering there is immediate loss of oxygen supply to the muscle due to exsanguination. As the stored oxygen in myoglobin gets depleted, there is inhibition of aerobic pathway through citrate cycle as well as cytochrome system. The store of creatine phosphate used for rephosphorylation of ADP to ATP gets soon exhausted. Energy metabolism is then shifted to anaerobic pathway resulting in the breakdown of glycogen to lactic acid. This process continues till all the glycogen stored in the muscle is exhausted. This resynthesis of ATP by anaerobic pathway is not enough to maintain the required ATP level and as it depletes. There is formation of actomyosin resulting in the onset of rigor mortis. The important changes that take place during post-mortem period are as follows:

A. Chemical Post-mortem Changes

1. Loss of homeostasis
2. Post-mortem glycolysis and pH decline
3. Rigor mortis
4. Loss of protective mechanisms
5. Degradation due to proteolytic enzymes

6. Loss of structural integrity
7. Other chemical changes

B. Physical Post-mortem Changes

1. Change in colour
2. Change in water binding capacity

A. Chemical Post-mortem Changes

1. Loss of Homeostasis

Maintenance of a physiologically balanced internal environment is termed as homeostasis. This homeostatic regulation gives an organism the ability to survive under many different and sometimes adverse environmental conditions, including extreme variation in temperature, oxygen deficiency, and psychological stress. The homeostatic mechanism is presided over by the nervous system and the endocrine glands. These two system serves as communication and triggering mechanisms that co-ordinate adjustments in the function of various organs during period of stress. This mechanism ceases within 4-6 minutes after bleeding. In the absence of blood supply, there is loss of body heat and temperature starts declining. The concept of homeostasis becomes very important during conversion of muscle to meat for two reasons:

a) Many of the reactions and changes that occur during the conversion are a direct result of attempts to maintain living functions.
b) Conditions in the immediate pre slaughter environment are stressful and may alter post-mortem changes and affect meat quality.

2. Post-mortem Glycolysis and pH Decline

One of the most serious consequences of circulatory collapse is the interruption of the oxygen supply of the muscles. As the stored oxygen supply becomes depleted after exsanguination, the aerobic cycle through the TCA cycle and the electron transport chain stops functioning. Energy metabolism is then shifted to anaerobic pathway, in much the same fashion as when oxygen debt develops in the living muscle tissue during period of heavy exercise.

$$\text{Glycogen} \xrightarrow{\text{Anaerobic conditions}} \text{Lactic acid} + 2\ \text{ATP}$$

Lactic acid is produced by anaerobic metabolism in the living animal is transported from the muscles to the liver, where it is resynthesized into glucose and glycogen, or to the heart, where it is metabolized to carbon dioxide and water. Since circulatory system is no longer available to the exsanguinated animal, lactic acid remains in muscle tissue and increases in concentration as metabolism proceeds. It continues to accumulate until nearly all the original glycogen stored in muscle is depleted, or until tissue pH becomes so low that the enzymes of glycolysis become inactive.

This lowering of muscle pH is the most significant post-mortem changes. In most species, a gradual decline continues from approximately pH 7 in the living muscle during first few hours (5-6 hrs) and then there is little drop in the next 15-20 hrs, giving an ultimate pH in the range of 5.5-5.7. The rate of pH decline is enhanced at high environmental temperature. A low ultimate pH is desired to have a check on the proliferating micro-organisms during storage.

Development of acidic conditions in the muscle, before natural body heat and heat of continuing metabolism have been dissipated through carcass chilling, causes denaturation of muscle proteins. The proteins in some species are more sensitive to this type of denaturation than are those of others. For example, fish muscle proteins are more labile than most mammalian muscle and are denatured at lower temperature and higher pH. Denaturation of proteins causes a loss of protein solubility, loss of water and protein binding capacity, and loss in intensity of muscle pigment coloration. All these changes are undesirable, whether the muscle is going to be used as fresh meat or subjected to further processing.

Muscles that have very rapid and extensive pH decline will be pale and have very low water holding capacity, the latter of which causes cut surfaces to appear wet. In severe cases, fluid will actually drip from the surface of the meat. On the other hand, muscles that maintain a high pH during conversion of muscle to meat may be very dark in colour, and very dry on the exposed cut surface, because naturally occurring water is tightly bound to proteins.

Normally, the pH in the muscle decreases from 7.0 upon slaughter to approximately 5.3 to 5.8 (Smulders, Toldra, Flores, and Prieto, 1992). In extreme cases, this decline can take only 1 h. The typical decline for pork is in the range of 6 to 12 h, and beef usually completes its pH decline in 18 to 40 h (Smulders et al., 1992). Howard and Lawrie (1956) suggested that the rate of pH decline has an inverse relationship to tenderness. As the pH drops, it nears the iso-electric point. At this point, all of the negatively and positively charged amino acid side chains equal, which causes the maximal attraction between the two. This attraction holds the filaments closely together and does not allow any water to get in, greatly reducing the water holding capacity (Smulders et al., 1992). Because pork experiences a quicker pH decline than other species, it is more likely to experience elevated temperatures during the onset phase of rigor, which can be detrimental to the myoglobin pigment. This causes the myoglobin structure to be "open" and scatter light, creating a pale colored product (Lawrie, 1998). When pork is not able to hold water, it loses colour and firmness. This condition is described as pale, soft, and exudative (PSE). Quickly lowering the temperature post-mortem will decrease the velocity of these chemical and biochemical reactions, therefore decreasing the rate of pH decline (Lawrie, 1998). Blast chilling will help with the reduction of this type of reaction (Meisinger, 1999). Offer (1991) reported that the effect of chilling on PSE conditions is strongly dependent on the rate of pH decline. Meisinger (1999) suggested chilling pork to muscle temperatures of less than 10°C in 12 h, and 2 to 4°C in 24 h to reduce the occurrence of P SE.

3. Rigor Mortis

It refers to the stiffening of muscles after death and is another important post-mortem change in the process of conversion of muscle to meat. Stiffening observed in rigor mortis is due to formation of permanent cross-bridges in muscle between actin and myosin filaments. During the period immediately following exsanguination, muscle is quite extensible. At this time, only very few actomyosin bridges are present to prevent extension by a force. The period of time during which the muscle is relatively extensible and elastic is called the delay phase of rigor mortis. Stores of creatine phosphate are used for phosphorylation of ADP becomes insufficient to maintain the tissue in a relaxed state. Then, glycogen stores are used for further phosphorylation of ADP. Actomyosin bridges begin to form, and the muscle gradually becomes less extensible under an externally applied force. The onset phase of rigor mortis begins when the muscles begin to lose extensibility, and this phase lasts until the completion of rigor mortis.

ATP complexed with Mg^{2+} is required for a muscle to be maintained in the relaxed state. As ATP is depleted from the muscle, permanent cross- bridges begin to form. As these cross-bridges form the muscles contract, shortening sarcomere lengths and tension increases. In the absence of ATP, the actomyosin bonds can't be broken because the Ca pump (SRATPase) has run out of fuel (ATP); consequently, tension is at its maximum. During PM storage tension decreases, but it never returns to prerigor levels. The decrease in tension with time, PM is glibly described as the "resolution" of rigor mortis. This is misnomer because the actomyosin bonds of rigor mortis are not broken during post-mortem storage as implied by the term "resolution" of rigor. Thus, the decrease in tension is due to events other than breaking actomyosin bonds. Proteolytic degradation of specific myofibrillar proteins results in dissolution of Z disk, loss of ultra structural integrity, and decreases tension. Rigor shortening differs from normal contraction because more cross bridges are formed. During normal contraction, cross-bridges form at only about 20 per cent of the possible binding sites, but in rigor, nearly all binding sites in the area of overlap between actin and myosin filaments contain cross-bridges.

Rigor mortis and pH decline are closely correlated because both are related to energy metabolism of glycogen. In muscle with abbreviated pH decline, onset and completion of rigor mortis are rapid because the initial energy supply is limited. In the case of rapid early pH decline, onset and completion of rigor also are rapid because energy supplies are rapidly metabolized, or low pH conditions curtail important chemical reactions in energy generation. The intermediate pH decline curve is associated with a longer time of rigor mortis development than either of the two extremes.

4. Loss of Protective Mechanisms

In healthy living animals, muscles is protected from the invasion of micro-organism by a series of defenses, the first line of which is the tissue that cover the body and surround many of the internal organs. The lymphatic system and circulating WBC are available to destroy organism that enter the body. During PM period, body defense mechanism stops operating and membrane properties are altered. With increasing time post-mortem, all homeostatic mechanisms are eventually lost. Nervous control from the central system is lost within 4-6 minutes after exsanguination So, during conversion to meat, muscle is quite susceptible to invading micro-organisms. Except for low pH, most of the other PM changes favour bacterial growth. Hence, utmost handling precautions are necessary to prevent contamination of meat.

The structurally important sites of enzyme actions by calpains and lysosomal enzymes (including cathepsins B, D, L) during conditioning can be summarized as below:

a) CASF (Calpains)

1. Troponin T (above pH 6)
2. Z lines (desmin)
3. Connectin, "gap filaments"
4. M-line proteins and tropomyosin

b) Lysosomal Enzymes (including cathepsins B, D and L)

1. Troponin T and I (below pH 6) and C-protein: relatively rapidly)
2. Myosin (heavy and light chains), actin, tropomyosin, alpha actinin, nebulin and titin ("gap filaments"): relatively slowly above pH 5 or below 35°C
3. Cross-links of non-helical telopeptides of collagen
4. Mucopolysaccharides of ground substance

5. Degradation due to Proteolytic Changes

Several enzyme systems present in skeletal muscle have been implicated as being responsible for post-mortem proteolytic degradation of myofibrillar proteins. These systems include the calpains, the multicatalytic proteinase complex (both of which are present in the Sarcoplasm) and the cathepsins, present only in lysosomes of muscle fibers. The autolytic lysosomal enzymes called cathepsins which remain inactive in a living muscle tissue, are activated as the muscle pH declines. These enzymes initiate the degradation of muscle protein structure. In fact, catheptic enzymes are capable of breaking down even collagenous connective tissue of the muscle and cause tenderisation of meat during aging. The improvement in tenderness during PM storage is due almost entirely to proteolytic degradation of myofibrillar proteins. Obviously, degradation of collagen would improve meat tenderness, especially if intermolecular cross-linkages were degraded. However, PM proteolysis of collagen is minimal, and intermolecular cross-linkages are not degraded. The small amount of proteolytic degradation of collagen that does occur appears to takes place only during the early PM period.

6. Loss of Structural Integrity

PM alterations of membrane properties initiate the degradation of muscular proteins. There is progressive disruption of myofibrillar structure. The resolution of rigor mortis is known to occur due to disintegration of Z-line structure and complete loss of Z disks may occur due to proteolytic degradation of proteins associated with the disk, notably desmin and possibly titin. A rapid decline in muscle pH also causes denaturation of collagenous connective tissue.

7. Other Chemical Changes

By the time ultimate pH has been reached, ATP has been broken down to inosinic acid, inorganic phosphate and ammonia. Although some degradation of inosinic acid to phosphate, ribose and hypoxanthine will have occurred at this stage, the latter process is substantially a function of time, temperature and pH after tha attainment of the ultimate pH (Solevev, 1952; lee and Webster, 1963). According to Howard, lee and Webster (1960), conditioning is organoleptically at an optimum when the hypoxanthine level has reached 1.5-2.0 micromoles/g. this is attained after 10-13 days at 0°C, 4-5 days at 10°C, 30-40 hr at 20 °C and 10-11 hr at 30°C (Lee and Webster,1963). It has been shown that inosinic acid (or inosine and inorganic phosphate) when heated with a glycoprotein containing alanine and glucose (also isolated from the water soluble extracts of beef) produces a basic meat flavour and odour (Batzer, Santoro and Landmann, 1962). The breakdown of protein and fat during conditioning also contributes to flavour by producing hydrogen sulphide, ammonia, acetaldehyde, acetone and diacetyl (Yueh and Strong, 1960); but prolonged conditioning, e.g. 40-80 days at 0°C is associated with loss of flavour (Hoagland, and Powick, 1917). Apart from the increase in free amino acids arising from proteolysis, their concentration is also augmented by the breakdown of various peptides. During conditioning, e.g. the dipeptides carnosine and anserine are progressively hydrolyzed to beta-alanine and histidine (Bouton *et al.*, 1958. the accumulation of free amino acids, and of soluble carbohydrates, such as glucose (by the action of alpha-amylase on glycogen; Sharp, 1958), glucose 6-phosphate (one of the intermediaries in the glycolytic pathway), ribose (from nucleotide breakdown) and the other sugars in traces, is potentially undesirable. Although conditioning enhances the water holding capacity of proteins to some extent, the loss due to denaturation changes and to post-mortem pH fall predominates, and meat exudes fluid post-mortem.

B. Physical Post-Mortem Changes

1. Changes in Colour

In living animals, muscles with sufficient oxygen have bright red appearances. In PM muscle, as oxygen is used in metabolism, the colour becomes dark purplish red. When fresh meat is cut, the exposed surface has this dark red apperances immediately after cutting, but, on exposure to atmosphere for a few minutes, the myoglobin becomes oxygenated and changes to a brighter red colour. If the muscle has been subjected to severe denaturation, colour intensity will be reduced to a pale red.

2. Changes in Water Holding Capacity

Water accounts for 65-80 per cent of total muscle mass. Much of the water in muscle cells is tightly bound to various proteins. If the proteins are not denatured, they continue to bind water during conversion of muscle to meat, and to a great extent, even during cooking. This retained water contributes to juiciness and palatability of meat as a food.

Changes occur in WHC, during conversion of muscle to meat, depend on the rate and extent of pH drop and on the amount of protein denaturation. When the pH of post-mortem muscle remains very high, the water binding properties of meat are similar to those of living muscle. When the pH drops rapidly during the early PM period, it results in low WHC.

Ageing of Meat

Postmortem aging is a process that occurs naturally in all muscle tissues, whether vacuum packaged or in the form of carcasses or wholesale cuts. In the conversion of muscle to meat, natural enzymes found in muscles, break down specific proteins into smaller molecules i.e. polypeptides, peptides and amino acids. This breaking or fragmentation of these protein stands, called myofibrils, by natural enzymes results in improved tenderness of the muscles during postmortem aging. Tenderization occurs at relatively rapid rate until 3 to 7 days postmortem, and then the rate of increased tenderness diminishes with time. Practically speaking, the increased in tenderness of different cuts after 7 to 10 days relatively small, compared with the increase during the first 7 to 10 days postmortem. Although extensive proteolysis causing increased tenderness, but the protein of connective tissue are not normally changed in this way during conditioning. There is no increase in water soluble hydroxyproline-containing derivatives, even after storage of sterile, fresh meat for one year at 37°C. However there is evidence for the operation of lysosomal enzymes which can attack the cross links in the non-helical telopeptide region of collagen. It has been found that collagenolytic cathepsins from bovine spleen cleaved the non-helical telopeptide region of native tropocollagen between the lysine-derived cross-links and the triple helix of the main body of the molecule.

Three types of endogenous enzymes present in meat- calpains, the multicatalytic proteinases complex (present in sarcoplasm) and the cathepsins (present in lysosome). The multicatalytic proteinases complex does not cause post mortem proteolysis of any myofibrillar proteins that place a role in improvement in meat tenderness. However, activity of calpains (calcium activated sarcoplasmic factors; CASF) and cathepsins (B, D and L) depends on pH of the muscle fibers.

Calpains are located in the sarcoplasm of muscle fibers. As calpains are known as calcium activated sarcoplasmic factor, their activity mainly depend on intracellular calcium ion concentration. There are two major calpains: millimolar (mM) calpain and micromolar (μM) calpain. Millimolar and micromolar calpain so called as requires a high (0.3M) and low (0.005M) concentration of free calcium for their activation, respectively. The high concentration of calcium is rarely present in muscle tissues until injected from externally. This precludes the activity of mM calpains. So, micromolar (μM) calpains have major function in tenderizing of pre-rigor meat as both the calpains have optimal activity at higher pH (6.6 to 6.8). Post rigor meat pH varies in the range of 5.4 to 5.8. Both the calpains are acts on following muscle fiber proteins:

1. Troponin T (above pH 6)
2. Z-line proteins (desmin)

3. Connectin (gap filaments)
4. M-line protein and tropomyosin.

Though various cathepsins are identified in the lysosomes of muscle fiber only cathepsins B, D and L have major activity on tissues. These enzymes are best act at acidic pH (5.2>pH). It is believed that these enzymes are act on actin and myosin so producing a more tender product. Cathepsins act on following myofibrillar proteins.

1. Troponin T degradation
2. Cross links of non-helical telopeptide of collagen
3. Mucopolysaccharides of ground substances
4. Actin and myosin, but at pH below 5.0, and at a temperature of 35°C

Types of Postmortem Ageing

Two types of postmortem aging processes are practiced commercially- dry and wet aging.

Dry Ageing

It is the traditional process of placing entire carcass or whole sale cut without covering or packing in a refrigerated room for 21 days to 28 days at 0-2 °C and 80-85 per cent relative humidity (RH), with an air velocity of 0.5 to 2.5 m/sec. All three conditions though varying widely in commercial practice, are extremely important in the proper postmortem aging of carcasses, as well as beef ribs and loins. Too much RH will allow excessive microbial growth, whereas too little will cause excessive shrinkage. Eighty five percent RH is a happy medium in slowing microbial growth and moisture loss. Tenderness development can be accelerated by aging at higher temperature; however, increased microbial growth becomes a serious problem at higher temperature. Air velocity is essential because it acts as a medium for moisture removal from the refrigerated area. Insufficient air velocity will allow excessive moisture to condense on the product, and as a result, off-flavours and aromas, as well as spoilage, will occur. Too high an air velocity, on the other hand, will result in excessive surface drying, with resulting weight and trim losses. The main disadvantages of dry aging with the cost associated with these weight and trim losses.

Wet Ageing

It is the aging of meat in vacuum bags usually the middle meats under refrigerated conditions of 0-2°C. Obviously, humidity and air velocity are not necessary requirements for the proper wet aging. Because most meat is vacuum packaged at the site of carcass fabrication, wet aging is the predominant method of postmortem aging today. The aging process continues when a primal or sub primal cut has been placed in vacuum package. By the time the cut reaches the retail store, at least 7-10 days have normally elapsed following slaughter, during holding at the packing plant for carcass chilling and fabrication, inventory storage, shipping to the retail warehouse, and subsequent shipping to the retail store level. Therefore, the time associated with the rapid tenderization and that associated with product movement to the retail store are similar. However, additional aging time is generally beneficial.

Dry and wet aging both result in a similar degree of palatability of meats, however, there can be distinct flavour differences. Meat from vacuum aged cuts has a more bloody or serumy and metallic flavour, whereas meat from dry aging has more brown-roasted flavour.

Factors Affecting Ageing

Aging rate and time are postmortem variables affecting tenderness. Different rate of aging means some carcasses and/cuts tenderize very early, while other tenderize gradually. In fact, some meats does not tenderize appreciably, regardless of aging time. Muscles that are moderately high to high in connective tissue generally are not very tender after adequate aging because the connective tissue is not fragmented sufficiently during aging. Widely differed amounts of time for postmortem aging occur in commercial practice, due primarily to the time that vacuum packed cuts are held in inventory prior to being processed into retail cuts for sale. Aging beyond 18 days results in little benefit to enhanced palatability, and may even be detrimental in terms of increased flavour changes. Specific muscles and quality grades are also considered important variables in postmortem aging. The tender loin is the tenderest muscle in the carcass, and interestingly requires little postmortem aging. The loin muscle, a relatively tender muscle, because of high fragmentation and small quantities of connective tissue, has a similar pattern of postmortem aging as the eye of the round, a less tender muscle of low fragmentation and more quantities of connective tissues. Steaks from different USDA quality grades, although differing in tenderness within and between grades, have a similar pattern of aging. That is beef cuts from USDA Choice will age very similarly to beef cuts from USDA Select.

While postmortem aging can have a profound effect on improving palatability, breeding, feeding, processing and preparation all play an important role in final consumer's satisfaction. When carcasses are suspended by obturator foramen proved to be most effective because it causes the tenderness of biceps femoris, semimembranosus and *L. dorsi* more than double by processing lamb carcasses in a standing rather than a vertical position. Processing conditions such as pre-rigor prompt chilling (cold shortening), pre-rigor freezing (thaw rigor) and even freeze drying (woody) are subjected to increase of toughness of meat. Cooking often can be the most profound factor in determining meat tenderness. Cooking makes connective tissue tenderer by converting collagen to gelatin, it coagulates and tends to toughen the proteins of the myofibril. Prolong cooking times and relatively low temperatures are thus justified for meat which has much connective tissue and conversely. The tenderizing effects of prolong cooking is additional to that of ageing. Cooking method like microwave heating preferentially increases the solubilization of collagen. Ionizing radiation at sterilizing doses or above causes changes in the meat proteins which increase tenderness. This is due to changes in the collagen molecule, for the shrink temperature of isolated collagen decreases from 61 °C to 47 °C with 5 Mrad and to 27 °C with 40 Mrad.

Influence of Electrical Stimulation on Post-mortem Aging

The electric stimulation accelerates natural tenderization process by increasing the proteolytic enzyme activity at the high temperature and damage to the micro-structure of muscles during vigorous contraction. The acceleration of post mortem glycolysis is achieved by a concomitantly high rate of ATP breakdown following application of high voltage current, reflects marked activation of the contractile actomyosin ATP-ase by release Ca^{++} ions. These also enhance the titre of phophorylase A, which is an additional factor increase of tenderness. Generally, buffalo carcasses need to be stimulated either before or immediately after dressing and splitting into sides, preferably within 1 hour of slaughter, using 600 volt (15 to 25 pps) for 1.5 to 2.0 min. Sheep or lamb carcasses require immediate electrical stimulation, as their sensitivity of electrical falls off more quickly than buffalo or beef carcasses. Electrical stimulation is generally employed within 30 min of slaughtering of animals. Further it has also been observed that a high voltage current (1000 volts) is desirable for this animal carcass as current flows to stimulate the whole musculature.

References

Lawrie, R.A. Meat science. Second Edition. Pergamon Press. Oxford, New York.

Forrest, J.C., Aberle, E.D., Hedrick, H.B., Judge, M.D. and Merkel, R.A. Principles of Meat Science. W.H. Freeman and Company. San Francisco.

J.W. Savell*, S.L. Mueller, B.E. Baird, The Chilling of the Carcass, Meat Science Section, Department of Animal Science, Texas A and M University, College Station, TX, 77843-2471, USA

http://www.meat-us.com/quality.php?page=1

– Chapter 4 –

Effect of Transport on Meat Quality: Its Veterinary and Clinical Importance

I. Effect of Transport on Meat Quality: Its Veterinary and Clinical Importance

Transportation of Animals

Production of good quality of meat not only related to hygiene of meat processing plant but also depends on how they are shifted from farm to the plant. To ensure high standards of welfare for transported animals, they should be treated in a humane and require well-maintained vehicles.Vehicular transport of animals to slaughter is slowly gaining ground in the poorer countries in place of the on-the-hoof method. This is quite evident with sheep, goats and pigs because of difficulties of herding numerous small stock on-the-trotters to slaughter, a practice which also subjects the animals to stress, exhaustion, weight losses and lower quality carcasses. Road transport featuring special trucks is probably the cheaper, commoner and more convenient means of conveying animals because it affords more direct links with production and marketing centres than does rail or air. A few precautions are worthwhile in road transporting small ruminants to slaughter: (a) the trucks must be specially designed or conveniently modified to convey the stock; (b) they should allow ample ventilation and lighting; (c) if open trucks are used, the top should be covered with a tarpaulin or canvas material to protect the animals from rain and sunshine; (d) they should have easy loading and unloading mechanisms to prevent injuries, and above all; and finally (e) they must provide for maximum comfort of the animals. In loading the trucks, the animals should be kept away from a state of excitement. Rushing them in with force or with violent beatings must be avoided: heavy whips often cause bruises which ruin the quality of the meat. A moderate size flock must be transported at a time. Overloading and overcrowding should not take place: animals get bruised, suffocate or become exhausted when this happens, and over long distances they may lose weight.

Sheep and goats may be trucked together, but should not be mixed with cattle especially the bulky, long-horned type which is apt to squeeze and trample upon them or cause them injuries. When trucking is routine and over long distances clearly defined routes must be followed, these being provided with resting stops for feeding and watering. On arrival at the slaughter holding ground, they must be discharged, with patience, avoiding all cruelty. Immediately upon unloading, the animals should be stored out: the sick and fatigued to be placed in special pens and the normal animals in the kraal. It is necessary to lift and carry the sheep or goat, one hand must be placed under the jaw with the other at the hock. They should not be lifted by grasping the skin or hair as this causes surface bruising. To catch them, a leg must be grabbed first. The trucks in which the animals are conveyed should be washed and disinfected after the discharge, but if this is not possible, they should be swept thoroughly and sprinkled with sawdust.

Essential to see that meat animals are properly loaded, unloaded, laired without any discomfort, injury and disease to them to produce wholesome meat

Transportation of Livestock

Detailed regulations of humane transport of animals in most countries

Following are prohibited:

- ✰ Exposure to inclement weather
- ✰ Transport of injured birds
- ✰ Use of unsuitable receptacles
- ✰ Mixed consignments
- ✰ Long confinement in crates are prohibited.

General provisions for road and rail vehicles, receptacles, separation of animals, cleansing and disinfection, floor and ramps of vehicle, nonslippery, vehicles partitions, ventilation, rigid sides and coverings

Overcrowding is forbidden, supply food and water every 12h., minimum floor space- 335 cm^2 for pigs, 213 cm^2 for sheep, 271 cm^2 for calves.

Loss of Weight during Transport

Species	*Loss of Wt.*	
	Live Wt. (kg)	*Carcass Wt. (kg)*
Pigs 24h transport	2.2 to 5.4	–
Sheep 24h lairage	0.9 to 1.8	–
24h transport	3.6	–

Contd...

Contd...

Species	*Loss of Wt.*	
	Live Wt. (kg)	*Carcass Wt. (kg)*
Calf of 149.6 kg live wt.		–
In 1st day travel	4.0	–
In 2nd day travel	1.8	–
Bullock 609.6kg live wt.		–
In 1st day travel	30.0-40.0	–
In 2nd day travel	5.0-7.0	–
Bacon pig per day journey	–	0.9
Pigs, over exertion, excitement during transit	–	6.7 per cent wt. of liver
Cattle 161 km journey	–	1.48
402-482 km	–	2.10

Increase wt. loss when increase temp. and decrease R.H.,

In pigs sprayed with cold water- pigs traveled 80 km wt. loss reduced by 50 per cent.

Affections Induced by Transport

1. Transit (Shipping) fever without food, long journey, cold weather. *Myxovirus, Pasteurella hemolytica, P. multocida, Mycoplasma, Chlamydia.*
2. Transit tetany: cows with adv. Pregnancy, warmer months associated with hypocalcaemia.
3. Salmonellosis- calves, lambs precipitated by lack of food, water and by chilling.
4. Miscellaneous conditions: heat shock, indigestion, abortion, post-parturient disorder, ketosis, foot diseases, enterotoxaemia, mastitis, gastric ulcer etc.

Stress

Many stressors- loading, unloading, detention in lairage, handling up to point of slaughter, physical trauma, sound, light, humidity, cold, wind, excitement

Two main reactions when exposed to stresses

i. Alarm or Emergency Reaction

- ☆ Increased activity of sympathetic nervous system supplying to involuntary muscles, secreting glands and the heart.
- ☆ Outpouring of catecholamines, noradrenaline and adrenaline.
- ☆ Increase heart rate, constriction peripheral blood vessel, increase blood pr, dialation of bronchi, cessation of digestion, mobilization of liver glycogen, increase blood sugar.

ii. General Adaptation Syndrome

Longer lasting- ACTH released, production hydrocortisone, cortisone, decrease carbohydrate metabolism, increase protein metabolism, amino acids converted to glycogen in liver. Fat mobilized, metabolized to ketone bodies. Overall result high blood glucose level and ketosis, adrenal hypertrophy, eosinopenia, lymphopenia, polynucleosis, increased susceptibility to disease.

Changes in Meat Quality

1. Decrease glycogen level, less lactic acid, higher pH, poor keeping quality of meat. PSE meat, DFD meat.
2. Bruising : causes are–Rough handling, vehicle design defects, presence of horns, temp. of animal, stunning box design, mixing of animals, transport condition, breed etc.

Downgrading of carcass, quantitative loss, this depends upon time and extent of bruising.

A Bruise Dated by Appearance

Red and hemorrhagic	0-10h
Dark coloured	24h
Watery consistency	24-38h
Rusty orange colour and soapy to the touch	3+ days

By Bilirubin Test

Based upon formation of bilirubin from hemoglobin in the area of bruise

Bruised meat +	no reaction upto	50h
Foucher's reagent	light blue	60-72h
	Dark green	4-5 days

Age of bruise - electrical conductivity increases

Transport Mortality

Result of suffocation feeding heavy meal before journey, inadequate ventilation, summer season, distant journey.

Tranquilizers can reduce aggression and stress - dose rate and inj. technique impt., may cause loss of meat due to tissue reaction – gelatinous infiltration, hemorrhage, necrotic muscle changes, residual effect in meat.

II. Pre Slaughter and Post Slaughter Loss

Introduction

Food shortage is not only due to failure to produce enough amount per capita. It is aggravated when the product is affected by inadequate knowledge of production, poor handling, processing and preservation, storage leading to low quality and spoilage. Post harvest loss and illness from contaminated food is cause of reduced economic productivity (FAO, 1983).Foods of animal origin are the most liable to loss because suffer from slight defect to meet the desired quality, are ideal environment for microbial contamination, are perishable and result to spoilage. Meat from the huge number of livestock plays a crucial role in food security. Issue of meat quality, safety and post slaughter loss should be seriously considered. Meat quality can be summarised in to product and process oriented, user-oriented and quality control. Meat safety and post slaughter meat losses are accounted, when the product endanger public health-pathogens, when shelf life is reduced due to spoilage organisms. Presumed poor meat quality, safety and post slaughter loss is related to: Husbandry practices, meat quality assurance systems, animal welfare issues. In view of this, pre- and post-slaughter losses of meat aspects are discussed below:

Loss in Tenderness of Meat

Meat from the hindquarters is made up of much larger muscle groups, with less cartilage and connective tissue and is therefore more tender. Meat with the fat deposited within the steak to create a 'marbled' appearance has always been regarded as tenderer than steaks where the fat is in a layer around the outside. Both stress before slaughter in particular, and lack of aging of the meat has more to do with toughness than most other factors, including marbling. There is a complex interplay between pasture species effects, protein intake, calcium status, stress before and at killing, breed, the age of the animal, and how the meat is treated after slaughter. The best meat cuts on an animal can be made tough by stress, and an older animal can have relatively tender meat if it is docile, handled and slaughtered without it becoming stressed, and the meat aged correctly. The message for the person killing beasts for the home freezer is that a quiet and humane kill gives superior meat; for the hunter, an animal ambushed and killed cleanly and instantly will have superior meat to that chased by dogs or not killed cleanly. The message for the consumer is that the more you pay, the more likely the meat is to be tender. Any expensive cut that is not tender may have been stressed before slaughter. For cheap cuts, we must resort to pounding it with a tenderizing hammer, marinating it with ginger, or cooking it long and slow.

Loss during Transportation of Livestock

It is essential to see that meat animals are properly loaded, unloaded, laired without any discomfort, injury and disease to them to produce wholesome meat. Regulations of humane transport of animals in most countries prohibit: exposure to inclement weather, transport of injured birds, use of unsuitable receptacles, mixed consignments, long confinement in crates. General provisions for road and rail vehicles, receptacles, separation of animals, cleansing and disinfection, floor and ramps of vehicle nonslippery, vehicles partitions, ventilation, rigid sides and coverings are required. Overcrowding is forbidden. Supply food and water every 12h.and minimum floor space- 335 cm^2 for pigs, 213 cm^2 for sheep, 271 cm^2 for calves should be provided. There is loss of weight of animals during transport. The information in tabular form is already given above.

Affections Induced by Transport

1. Transit (Shipping) fever without food, long journey, cold weather. Myxovirus, *Pasteurella hemolytica, P. multocida*, Mycoplasma, Chlamydia.
2. Transit tetany: cows with adv. Pregnancy, warmer months associated with hypocalcaemia.
3. Salmonellosis: calves, lambs precipitated by lack of food, water and by chilling.
4. Miscellaneous conditions: heat shock, indigestion, abortion, post-parturient disorder, ketosis, foot diseases, enterotoxaemia, mastitis, gastric ulcer etc.

Preslaughter Care of Animals Resting in Lairages

1. Preslaughter rest: importance, inadequate rest- ultimate P^H affected, Penetration of putrefactive bacteria from intestine, these are causes of bone taint in cattle, ham taint in pigs
2. Rail gaps of proper wide- otherwise head of animal strangled
3. Isolation of horned animals, females in estrus, spray of water on pigs
4. Supply ample drinking water, decrease bacterial load in intestine, easy removal of hide or pelt, effective electrical stunning
   - Withhold food prior to slaughter: better bleeding, easier to dress, brighter appearance of meat, pigs fed before slaughter (milk, sugar), loss of carcass weight from 7 per cent to 3 per cent and of live wt. from 30 per cent to 8 per cent.

Loss in Meat Quality (PSE and DFD Meat)

Colour is important qualities attribute that Influence consumer acceptance of many food products. Consumer will often reject products in which the colour varies from the expected normal appearance. Colour is often used to determine Economical value of food. Off colour is associated with a lack of product wholesomeness. Because of emphasis consumer place on colour it is critical that meat should be produced of normal colour. So as to insure attractive and high quality meat products for consumers. (Williams W.D. 1992).

Pale, Soft and Exudative (PSE) Meat

Meat PSE meat is a result of accelerated post mortem glycolysis which results in a rapid post mortem decline in pH while the carcass temperature is still high.(Fercot 1995, Barbut 1996,Mcee and Sam 1997) PSE meat is pale in colour and soft in touch.

Dark, Firm and Dry (DFD) Meat: When an animal in physical exhausted state at the time of slaughter, the extent of post mortem glycolysis is very limited resulting in higher ultimate pH than normal. This results in very dark, firm and dry meat.

III. Ante-mortem Factors Affecting Meat Quality

1. Influence of Genetics Meat Breeding

Tenderness of loin steaks – particular sire colour and firmness ratings of beef – breed of dam.

2. Influence of Blood Characteristics

More tender and finer grain meat producing animals have:

i. Lower alkaline-to-acid phosphatase ratio, oxaloacetate to pyruvic transaminase ratio, oxaloacetic transaminase and amylase activity.
ii. Lower total and free cholesterol level.
iii. Higher level of phosphomonoesterase-1 activity
iv. Blood serum calcium and tenderness – significant correlation.

3. Influence of Sex

Castration males results in fatter carcasses Bulls and rams produce

- ☆ Heavier carcasses
- ☆ Larger L.dorsi muscle area
- ☆ Less external and internal fat
- ☆ Higher conformation scores

Hormonal status of the animal serum testosterone level higher in bulls and rams than steers and weathers- Marbling and more tender meat, in increase stress more intramuscular connective tissue in males. More UFA in ram fat than wether, lower flavour scores for meat – heavy ram lambs. Differences in tenderness, juiciness and flavour in chops from boars, barrows, gilts, ovariectomized gilts.

Biological value of meat from yearling bulls is higher than that from steers. Undesirable flavours in entire males of pig, goat and sheep – adrenal hypertrophy and C_{19} – 16steroids, 5-α- androst-16-ene-3-one-bore taint, 4-methyl fatty acids and 2-pentyl pyridine-objectionable flavour of mutton.

4. Influence of Age and Maturity

Juiciness and tenderness ↓ scores ↑ age inter-and intermolecular cross links of stromal ↓ proteins. Solubility of collagen, Age ≤ cooking loss, Age ≤ tenderness

5. Influence of Nutrition

High plane of nutrition in cattle-desirable quality and palatability characteristics of beef pasture + concentrates in lamb – carcass quality higher than only pasture. High energy rations in cattle – high quality meat. Highest level of digestible energy – marbling and carcass grade ↑ higher. Forage fed steers – less fat, higher UFA than grain fed. Arolled barley diet to lamb – fat c ↑ SFA than oats Diet 72 per cent or more corn in rams – fat c PUFA. Feeding UFA to mature sheep – objectionable flavour. Related to (i) V-dodeca-lactone (ii) Volatile carbonyl compounds.

Under Nutrition

1. Nutritional stress secretion of adrenaline, 17-hydroxycortico-sterone and 11-deoxycorticosterone. Adrenaline effect.

(i) K^+ from muscle to blood

(ii) Glycogen catabalism lactic acid by stimulating phosphorylase a nad converting phosphorylase b to phosphorylase a.

2. Lower grade of carcass, yield of valuable cuts retards growth of individual muscles. Loss of fat and protein and a gain in proportion of water in meat.
3. Reduction in flesh volume, loss of fat, shrinkage of the muscle fibers.
4. Composition - ↑ water, Cl^-, Na^+, extracellular protein and decrease in K^+, P^{5+} and intracellur protein.
5. Adversely affect meat tenderness
6. ↓ BV, NPU, PER.

Supplementing diet with carotene and lysine (i) improve colour, flavour, tenderness, nutritive value, (ii) decrease Hypro, increase Try.

6. Influence of Hormone

Inj. Epinephrine 24 hrs pre slaughter control PSE, produce DFD meat, no adverse effect on palatability. Oral feeding of adrenaline - ↑ ultimate pH ≤ and β adrenergic block agents – ↑ block symp. Nerve slow decrease PM pH. Diethylstilboestrol (DES) administration to cattle and sheep - growth performance, feed efficiency deposition of more protein, water less fat in meat. Combination of testosterone and diethylsilboestrol or thyroxine - ↑ growth rate in heifers, ↑ growth rate, feed efficiency and grade of lambs.

Influence of Antemortem Treatments

Proteolytic enzymes – papain, bromelin, ficin, trypsin, trypsin, chymotrypsin, pepsin, pancreatin, certain microbial enzymes. Inj. Papain – tenderization of meat β-aminopropionitrile – utility grade live steers affected metabolism of collagen either by solubilization by blocking collagen synthesis at the tropocollagen stage or by interference in inter and intra molecular formulation of cross links.

Pre-slaughter Inj. of Ions

Mg^{2+} ions – prolonged onset of rigor mortis ↓ rate pH fall and ATP breakdown. Ca^{2+} ions – opposite effect. $Cacl_2$ alone or in combination with epinephrim – lower pH value, accelerate rigor dev. – increase muscle toughness. Pyrophosphate - ↑ aerobic glycolysis extensive catabolism of ATP.

Climatological Condition

High temperature - ↑ PM glycolysis, ↑ PSE sudden change from warm to cold weather – In pigs rapid ↓ muscle glycogen and ATP break down.

Pre slaughter exercise: depletion of glycogen, high ultimate pH high WHC, dark colour of meat.

Periodic AM Electric Shock

In swine improve the structure, colour and tenderness of meat. In general, pre slaughter treatments effect glycogen content, rate of rigor, rate of glycolysis, ulitimate pH. If pH<5.8 at 1h P.M. → PSE meat, pH>6.2 at 24h P.M. → DFD meat. Such meats not suitable for dry sausage and cured ham (fresh).

– Chapter 5 –

PSE and DFD in Meat Quality

I. Effect of DFD and PSE Conditions on Sensory Quality of Meat and Meat Products

Introduction

Sensory evaluation is of the simplest analytical tool for monitoring quality control at all stages of food product development starting from the inspection of incoming raw material to surveillance of their finished product. The sensory evaluation is defined as a scientific discipline used to evoke, measure analyze and interpret result of those characteristics of foods and material as they are procured by the sense of sight, smell, taste, touch and hearing. The definition makes clear that sensory evaluation encompasses all the senses and not the taste testing alone. Sensory evaluation takes into account several different discipline knowledge of food science and technology and it emphasizes the behavioral bases of perception.

Meat

Meat is defined as those tissue which are suitable for use as food, nearly every species of animal can be used as meat, the majority of meat can be used by humans come from domestic animals and aquatic organism.

Properties of Fresh Meat

1. Water Holding Capacity

It is defined as the ability of meat to retain its water during application of external forces such as cutting, heating, grading, or pressing. Many of the physical properties of meat (including the colour, texture and firmness raw meat and the juiciness and tenderness of cooked meat) are partially dependant on water holding capacity. The water holding capacity of muscle tissue has a direct effect on the shrinkage of meat during storage. When the tissue have poor water holding properties, the loss of moisture and consequently the loss of weight during storage is great.

Pale Soft Exudative (PSE) pork has a high percentage of free water that accumulates on the surface of meat soon after the cuts are packaged. This condition is the most serious problem associated with PSE pork when it is merchandised on a fresh meat basis. The formation of PSE muscle is characterized by a fast pH fall within 1/2 -3 hr. to a final pH from 5.0 to 5.6.

2. Color

The most important contribution to meat colour are the pigments. The pigments in meat consist largely of two proteins; haemoglobin, the pigment of blood and myoglobin the pigment of muscle. Myoglobin quantity varies with species, age, sex, muscle and physical activity. The following list shows the most typical colour of meat from various species;

- ✰ Beef: bright, cherry to dark red
- ✰ Fish: gray, white to dark red
- ✰ Horse: dark red
- ✰ Lamb and Mutton: light red to brick red
- ✰ Pork: grayish pink
- ✰ Poultry: Gray white to dull red
- ✰ Veal: brownish pink

The reaction of pigments with any of several materials can result in colour changes in meat. Upon cutting, grinding or expose to air, the pigment in meat undergo colour changes due to their reaction with oxygen. If only small quantities of oxygen are present, such as in partial vacuum or a sealed semipermeable package; the iron portion of pigment becomes oxidized and changes to a brown colour. In this oxidized state the pigment is called metmyoglobin. The prevention of metmyoglobin formation is an important requirement for fresh meat merchandising. Meat dicolouration by metmyoglobin formation can occur during several phases of meat processing. When a product is permitted to remain in contact with flat surfaces, such as pans or tables, the oxygen may drop to a level that favour the development of the brown colour. In other instances, the meat may be wrapped in a paper that only permits the passage of small quantities of oxygen to the surface of the meat. When meat is allowed to come in full contact with the air, the reduced pigments will react with molecular oxygen and form a relatively stable pigment called oxymyoglobin. This pigment is responsible for the bright red colour that consumers expects in fresh meat. The bright red colour on the surface depends on the availability of oxygen in the superficial layers of the tissues. Fresh meat wrapping materials are designed to provide an abundant amount of oxygen at the muscle surface. Clean film are available that have high oxygen and low water permeability. Cellophane, polyvinyl chloride and polyethylene provide the oxygen transmission rate that is necessary for the retention of a red meat color.

The paleness of PSE pork is believed to be the result of a high proportion of free water in tissue, compounded by the direct effect of the low pH on the pigments. The free water in PSE tissue probably influences colour because it is located between the muscle cells rather within them. Tissue containing a great amount of extracellular water have many reflecting surfaces that totally reflect light, but have only a limited light absorption capability. The colour intensity is therefore greatly reduced. The pigments of PSE muscle might also appear light in colour because of a possible denaturation during the early postmortem period, or because of a direct effect postmortem period, or because of a direct effect on the low pH on the light reflecting properties of the pigments.

In dark cutting meat, the high water binding capacity maintains an unusually large proportion of water as intracellular water. Because of this, white light reflections between the cells are minimized. In addition, colour absorption is enhanced. Dark cutting tissue also has a high rate of oxygen-using enzymes actually, due to its pH. This reduces the proportion of pigment in red oxygenated state. Discoloration of meat may occur as a result of myoglobin distruction due to bacterial growth. A discolouration, in the form of a darkening of the meat, may also occur after cuts have been exposed to the air for a long time because the cut surfaces is drying out. As the drying progresses the pigment become concentrated the color became a deeper red.

3. Structure, Firmness and Texture

Physical properties of fresh meat, such as structure, firmness and texture are difficult to measure objectively. These factors are usually evaluated by consumers with their visual, tactile and gustatory senses.

Meat tenderness is one of major palatability factor that must be maintained or improved in most of the meat producing species. Meat tenderness is affected greatly by the age of animal. Meat from the carcasses of relatively young animals is tenderer than that from older animals. Marbling or the interspersing of fat within the lean, has often been discussed as factor associated with tenderness in meat has a major influence on the consumer when meat is purchased at retail. Most consumers have a concept of the proper appearance of meat from any given species, and any significant deviation from that color will be discriminated against. They might associate darker than normal color with dryness, toughness, or even with an off flavour. Quality evolutions can also be made using mechanical shearing or penetration devices of fat in muscle to quantitative marbling and spectrophotometers or colorimeter for evaluating color. The ultimate in quality evaluation is the case of a trained taste panel or a consumer panel, but even these methods are not without substantial error. Some variations in quality assessment obviously stems from the variation in preferences among the panel members. If during the course of carcass chilling, muscle firmness is compared to that of the carcass of a freshly slaughtered animals, there are noticeable differences. The change is said to result from the carcass "Setting up" during chilling. This increased firmness develops from the loss of extensibility that accompanies, the completion of rigor mortis; and the solidification of fat within and surrounding muscles. The degree of water holding capacity or both or with the rate of postmortem change is observable because of large scale effects on firmness, structure and texture.

Those muscle with an extremely high proportion of bound water are firm, have a light structure and a dry or sticky texture. Conversely, tissue with poor water binding ability are soft, have a loose structure and a wet or grainy texture.

Intramuscular fat contributes to the firmness of refrigerated meat. The solidification of fat that occur during chilling increase its firmness. Thus, fat has an important merchandising influence. It helps retail cuts, such as steaks and chops, retain a uniform thickness and characteristic shape during handling and storage. The amount of connective tissue in muscle affects the texture of meat such as the biceps femoris or semitendinosus of the rear leg, tend to appear coarse in texture. On the other hand, a muscle such as the infrequently used psoas major, loin appear fine in texture. Most meat cutting method incorporate the objective of separating tender from less tender cuts so that maximum palatability is realized and the usefulness of each cut is not limited by a large internal variation in connective tissue or tenderness. A coarse texture is sometimes apparent in muscle from older animals. Although the amount of connective tissue doesn't increase with advantage its prominence and strength become greater.

The texture and consistency of meat render it highly susceptible to the absorption of volatile material. Aromatic compounds from other foods, such as apple or onions are readily absorbed by meat tissue consequently off flavour may occur when meat is stored in the presence of such products.

pH

The accumulation of lactic acid in the postmortem period can have an adverse effect on meat quality. The development of acidic conditions in the muscle before the natural body heat and the heat of the continuing metabolism have been dissipated through carcass chilling, cause denaturation of muscle protein. The amount of denaturation depends upon have high a temperature and low a level of pH is reached. Temperature appears to play a icy role in denaturation, since muscle can attain a fairly low pH after it has been thoroughly chilled without excessive denaturation occurring. The proteins in some species are more sensitive to this type of denaturation than are the proteins of others. Denaturation of the protein causes a loss of protein solubility, loss of water holding capacity and a loss in the intensity of muscles pigment coloration. These changes are all undesirable whether the muscle is going to be utilized as fresh meat or be subjected to further processing. Muscle which have a very rapid and extensive pH decline will be pale in color and have a very low water holding capacity, that will give a cut surface a very pale appearance. In several cases fluid will actually drop from the surface of muscle. On the other hand muscle that maintain a high pH during the conversion of muscle to meat will tend to be very dark in color and very dry on the exposed cut surface because the occurring water is tightly bound to the proteins.

Pale Soft Exudative (PSE) Meat

Meat of a pale, soft and exudative nature is a serious problem in the meat industry. The incidence of the PSE problem in commercial turkey flocks range from 5 to30 per cent. Pale soft and exudative pork is causing considerable economic loss to the meat industry due to its poor color and low water holding capacity. The fast glycolysis and rapid pH decline in PSE muscle early post mortem, combined with high pre-rigor temperature cause partial protein denaturation, in particular of the myosin and sarcoplasmic proteins causes of the development of PSE pork have been breeding extensively focusing on genetics of breeding pigs, pre-slaughter stress and slow chilling of pre rigor muscle.

A study was conducted by Banon et all in 1997 on effects of the PSE defects of fresh hams on quality and yield of the final cured products have been discussed. Experiments were conducted with refrigerated and frozen PSE and normal fresh hams. Effects on composition colour, intramuscular fat content, proteolysis index, white participate formation and sensory quality were assessed. In general, only a minority of consumers could differentiate ham made from PSE meat from those made with normal meat. The differences between hams made from PSE and normal meat are significantly decreased by prior freezing. Although the PSE defects had only a limited effect on consumer acceptability of the final product processing yield was lower for hams made from PSE meat.

Barbut, S. in 1997 found the occurrence of Pale Soft Exudative meat in mature turkey hens. Color distribution of mature turkey hen breast meat was evaluated during the year in 7 commercial flocks to assess the occurrence of PSE problem. Evaluation was done on the processing have 24 hr. postmortem. In addition, 10 selected flocks were analyzed for pH, water holding capacity and texture. The pH ranged from 5.68 to 6.64. WHC ranged from 7 to 102 per cent. Increase in strength for the cooked samples ranged from 3 to 54N. Correlation between color and WHC indicated the potential use of a fast colour measurements to indentify PSE meat. Breast muscle sample with <*e" 52 exhibited poor WHC. When this value was used as a cut off point for identifying was 5 per cent and the highest was 40 per cent.

Sorhium in 1997 studied the effects of modified atmosphere storage on color, bacteriological quality and drip loss were investigated containing low level of residual O_2 for 21 days at 3°C. Compared with normal pork loins before packaging, the PSE loins were lighter and less red. After MA storage with CO_2 and low level of residual O_2. Normal and PSE pork were equally susceptible to discoloration surface color of both PSE and normal pork was highly affected by the conc. of residual O_2 in the atmosphere.

Dugan, M.E.R *et al.*, in 1997 studied Ca infusion through the vasculature of meat has been reported to accelerate meat tenderization. However in pork a rapid influx of Ca into muscle cell results in development of PSE meat which is less tender than normal meat. Effect of infusion of solution containing various conc. of a Ca chelator or Ca salt on pork quality were studied. Results showed that osmotic shock gave rise to an PSE-like condition, regardless of type of infusate. Unlike PSE which generally produces tougher meat, infusion of either $CaCl_2$ or EDTA solutions resulted in tenderization. The infusion process also resulted in an acceleration of glycolysis increased drip loss and decreased shear values.

Barbut in 1997 stated the occurrence of PSE problem in broiler chicken breast meat was monitored 700 birds. A rapid method of color measurement was used in the plant to assess the color of skinless pectoralis muscle at 24 hr post mortem. In addition 10 selected samples from each flock were further evaluated for pH, water holding cap and most of the physical measurements were observed, suggesting that a rapid color measurement method could be used to recognize PSE meat or identify flocks with a high occurence of PSE. Breast muscle sample with <*>49 showed water holding capacity, which inducted that these samples would be classified as PSE meat. Using this criterion it was shown that the occurrence of PSE ranged from 0 to 28 per cent. However the precise cut off point for PSE muscle should be determined by each processor depending on final product requirements.

Arnau, J in 1995 studied the changes in moisture content, pH, NaCl, nitrate and nitrite in different zones of normal and PSE dry cured hams during processing were evaluated. No differences in pH was found between PSE and normal hams. PSE hams contained more moisture and NaCl than normal hams in certain muscle zones. In most zones, pH increased during processing.

Petronic, L in 1993 made a study on appearance and color of cooked ham in foil made of PSE muscle with the addition of skin hydrolysates and blood plasma. Results showed that processing PSE meat by the modified process with increased mechanical treatment and addition of skin hydrolysates or blood plasma gave good appearance and colour characteristics. Processing PSE meat by the conventional method gave poor color and appearance.

Scenic, D. in 1991 studied the PSE defects of pork, is discussed with reference to: incidence of the defect, the relation of PSE to the porcine stress syndrome; breed differences in susceptibility to PSE, the physiological basis of PSE, selection against PSE in breeding survive and the halothane taste for susceptibility to PSE.

Dark, Firm, Dry (DFD) Meat

Garrido, M. in 1994 several objective methods for estimating pork quality were studied: internal light scattering (FOP) electrical conductivity (ELC), pH, color, water holding capacity, soluble protiens, pigment content, intra muscular fat and moisture. Most of measurements were significantly different between normal PSE and DFD quality categories.

Rohschinkenherstellung, Guerreso *et al.,* in 1991, studies were conducted on a total of 160799 hams 6 slaughter house to assess the effects of various parameters on losses of raw cured ham. Of the hams studied 12.55 per cent showed DFD and 44.22 per cent showed PSE. Incidence of PSE and DFD differed considerably between slaughter houses; this may be due to differences in pre-slaughter method. PSE includes was highest in the hottest part of year DFD incidence varied seasonally, but without any clear relation to ambient temp. losses were significantly correlated with incidence of DFD. Delayed or slow cooling increased microbial counts on the hams, but had little effect on losses. Total count detected significantly between slaughter houses. Hygiene status of the transport vehicle was not closely correlated with losses.

Shakelford, S.D. in 1994 studied the effect of biological type of cattle on the incidence of the DFD condition in longissimus muscle. It is concluded that there is genetic variation in the incidence of the DFD condition, however genetic variation was small relative to environment variations.

Vanderzant, C. in 1983 studied the effect of addition of glucose, citrate and citrate-lactic acid on microbiological and sensory characteristics of steaks from normal and DFD beef carcasses displayed in polyvinyl chloride film and in vacuum package.

Mojto, J. *et al.*, in 1994 indicated that ketobion preparation has been successfully used to treat energy metabolism disorders in cattle. The efficacy of using ketobion for prevention of DFD defect in beef was examined. Meat sample were examined for pH at 48 hr. postmortem and for color, free water content, shear force and cooking losses. Administration of ketobion did not prevent a steep fall in glycogen content, occurring during preslaughter housing. High terminal pH value were found in experimental and control meat indicating DFD defects. Other quality characteristic value were also within the range associated with DFD. It is concluded that ketobion is not effective in preventing DFD in slaughter bulls.

Bartos, L *et al.*, in 1993 studied a method for prevention of dark cutting (DFD) in beef, based on recognition of social relationships between of bulls was tested on 2234 bulls slaughtered under commercial conditions. When the influence of time between loading the animals and slaughter was eliminated statistically bulls of socially stabilized group showed the lowest pH24 values, whereas those of the stabilized group whether they are stabilized group whether they were slaughtered immediately after transport or during the following day. In contrast, in bulls from the socially instable groups, the pH24 value increased substantially after overnight lairage at the abattoir. In conclusion for longer transport, bulls from loss housing with stable social relationships should be used. It is necessary to keep the same social groups from loading to slaughter, strictly avoiding any mixing of strange bulls. Bulls from tethered stalls should be transported and slaughtered within as a short time after regrouping as possible.

References

1. John C. Forrest, Elton D.Aberle, Harold B. Hedrick, Max D. Judge, Robert A.Merkel. 1995; Principles of Meat Sciences W.H. Freeman and Company. San Francisco.
2. D.J.A. Cole and R.A. Lawrie, 1975, Meat Proceeding of the twenty-First Easter School in Agriculture Science, University of Nottinghan.
3. Maynard A. Amerine, Rose Maric Pangborn, Edward B.Roessler, 1965 Principles of Sensory Evaluation of Food. Academic Press New York and London.
4. Ralston Lawrie 1992, Developments in Meat Science-2. Applied Science Publishers. London and New Jersey.
5. Frank Gerrard, 1964. Meat Technology, A Practical textbook for Student and Butcher. Leonard Hill: London.

List of Abstracts Consulted

1. Banon, S.; Granados, M.V.; Alvarez, D., Garrido, M.D. PSE effect on cured ham in FSTA Vol. 30 (1998) No.2
2. Barbut, S. Occurrence of Pale Soft exudative meat in mature turkey hens. In FSTA Vol. 29 (1997) No.8.
3. Sorheim, O.; Erlandsen T.; Nissen, H.; Lea P.; Hoyun, T. Effects of Modified atmosphere storage on color and microbiological shelf life of PSE Pork. In FSTA Vol. 30 (1998) No.1.
4. Dugan, M.E.R.; Aalhus, J.L.; Murray, A.C.; Latsen, I.L.; best D.R. Development of PSE pork in halothane –ve pigs through postmortem infusion. In FSTA Vol.29 (1997) No.12.
5. Barbut, S. Problem of PSE Meat in broiler Chicken. In FSTA Vol.30 (1998) No.3.
6. Arnau, J.' Guerrero, L., Casadanont, G., Gou. P. Physical and Chemical changes in different zones of normal and PSE dry curred ham during processing. In FSTA Vol. 27 (1995) No.4.
7. Petronic, L.; Okanovic, D.; Popov-Raljic, J.; Funic, D. appearance and color of cooked ham in foil made of PSE muscles with the addition of skin hydrolystes and blood plasma. In FSTA Vol. 26 (1994) No.7.
8. Sencic, D. Problems with PSE pork. In FSTA Vol.24 (1992) No.2.
9. Garrido, M.D.; Pedauye, J.; Banon, S.; Laencina, J. objective assessment of pork quality FSTA Vol. 26 (1994) No. 7.
10. Rohscurkenherstellung, Rohstoff-Qualitatskontrolle als Massnahme zur Minderung der Verluste. Guerrero, l.; Arnau, J.; Garriga, M., Manufacture of raw ham. Ram material quality control as a measure for maximization of losses. In FSTA Vol. (1992) No.2.
11. Effect Shakelford, S.D.; Koohinaraie, M.; Wheeler, T.L.; Cundiff, L.V.; Dikeman, m.E. Effect of biological type of cattle on the incidence of the DFD condition in longissimus muscles. FSTA Vol.26 (1994) No.7.
12. Vanderzant (c), Chesser (LK), Savell (JW), Garclner (FA) and Smith (GC). Effect of addition of glucose citrate and citrate-lactic acid on microbiological and sensory characterstics of steak from normal and DFD beef carcasses displayed in polyvinyl chloride film and in vacuum packages. In J. of Food Tech. Vol. 19, No.203, Sept. 1984
13. Mojto J.; Palanska, O.; Benusk. N.; Szakacsova, D: Testing of the glucoplastic preparation ketabcon used for prevention of DFD meat occurrence in slaughter bulls. In FSTA Vol. 27 (1995) No.5.
14. Bartos, L.; Franc, C.; Rehak, D.; Stipkova. A practical method to prevent dark cutting (DFD) in beef. In FSTA Vol. 25 (1993) No.7

II. Constraint in Using PSE and DFD Meat in Product Development

Introduction

Colour is important qualities attribute that Influence consumer acceptance of many food products. Consumer will often reject products in which the colour varies from the expected normal appearance. Colour is often used to determine economical value of food. Off colour is associated with a lack of product wholesome- ness. Because of emphasis consumer place on colour it is critical that meat should be produced of normal colour so as to insure attractive and high quality meat products for consumers. (Williams W.D. 1992).

Pale, Soft and Exudative (PSE) Meat

PSE meat is a result of accelerated post mortem glycolysis which results in a rapid post mortem decline in pH while the carcass temperature is still high.(Fercot 1995, Barbut 1996,Mcee and Sam 1997) PSE meat is pale in colour and soft in touch.

Dark, Firm and Dry (DFD) Meat

When an animal is physical exhausated state at the time of slaughter, the extent of post mortem glycolysis is very limited resulting in higher ultimate pH than normal. This results in very dark, firm and dry meat.

Factors resulting in Development of PSE and DFD Meat Conditions

1. Stress Prior to Slaughter

Meat scientists have divided meat animals in 2 categories.

a) Stress Susceptible

b) Stress Resistant

Stress resistant animals are able to maintain normal temperature and homeostasis in their muscles in spite of severe stress like fatigue, excitement, exercise, fasting, fighting etc. However they may accomplish this at the expense of muscle glycogen store. Glycogen deficiency usually occurs when animal survives stress and when these animals are slaughtered before given sufficient time to replenish their muscle glycogen level. Muscle glycogen deficiency in these animals cause slow rate and limited extent of glycolysis after death. The resultant high pH will minimize the change in colour. The muscle reflects less total light due to minimum structural change and gives dark colour. Tissue of this type is also dry and shows DFD condition.

Stress susceptible animals have usually high temperature, rapid glycolysis and early onset of post mortem rigor mortis in their muscles and the muscles become pale, soft and exudative.

2. Growing Environment

It exerts important influence on the properties of meat. Among animals which are stress susceptible, the long term mild stress caused by some growing environment (such as close confinement, hard or slippery floors, chronic diseases, fluctuating temperature etc.) probably exhausts their ability to resist the severe stress. Stress is also experienced during marketing. Survey shows that confinement reared pigs are more susceptible to stress than those reared in the natural environment. Animals reared in careful experimental environment are more susceptible to PSE condition after slaughter. Stress resistant animals are capable of adjusting to certain level of discomfort in the rearing environment and consequently retain high level of stress resistance. So stressors imposed during marketing do not cause serious carcass defects in these animals.

3. Breeds

Certain breeds are particularly susceptible to stress due to endocrinological imbalance induced by selection for leanness and enhanced growth rate *e.g.* the Danish Landrace and Pie train in Europe and the Poland China in USA appears to be prone to rapid post mortem glycolysis and the production of PSE meat.

4. Diet

The influence of diet on the physical properties of meat is of minor importance as long as there are no serious nutritional deficiencies. However it should be noted that the growth pattern of body tissues can be changed by controlling dietary energy, thus affecting the composition of meat. If pigs were started on the high level of nutrients and then switched to a low level, they produce carcass with more muscles and less fat and vice versa. Different nutrients of food have different effect on growth and development of muscles. Proteins act as building blocks and important in growth and maintenance of muscles. Fat are more concentrated source of energy. Certain fatty acids are essential for growth. Carbohydrates are energy source to the animals. Energy in muscles is stored as glycogen which will determine the ultimate pH of meat.

5. Pre Slaughter Handling

Conditions prior to slaughter have a marked effect on meat quality.

a) Holding of animals in stockyard prior to slaughter provides opportunity for resting and feeding.This interval can influence the level of energy stored in muscles (Ngoka *et al.*, 1982). Starchy feeds and sugars specially will restore the muscle glycogen level thus permitting the development of normal pH.

b) Immobilization of animal Although it is not free from stress but it probably reduces stress responses. The properties and composition of meat is influenced by the type and effectiveness of the immobilization process. The severity of this process is usually expressed in the muscle by the degree of muscle glycogen depletion. Stunning has been reported to minimize perimortem struggling that decreases the utilization of glycogen resulting in a higher muscle pH early post mortem. There is delay in the rate of colour development due to stunning.

c) Anaesthetization of animal prior to slaughter cause delay in the development of rigor mortis and delay in the breakdown of phosphocreatine and ATP so there will be delayed glycolysis and pH of meat remain high for longer time after slaughter and this will lead to DFD meat condition. (Froning *et al.*, 1978)

d) When animals are exposed to low temperature prior to slaughter, meat will exhibit DFD condition. As such animals either don't or have limited struggle prior to slaughter as most of glycogen is utilized for maintenance of body temperature.

Effect of PSE and DFD Meat Conditions on different Properties of Meat

PSE and DFD meat differ in different properties of normal meat. These differences are well notable and make them different from normal meat. Some important properties are as follows:

1. Colour

Major pigment responsible for meat colour is myoglobin, hemoglobin from trapped blood and other heme pigment like cytocrome gives minor contribution. Myoglobin is a conjugate protein consisting of a globin apoprotin and heme. The central iron of heme group has six coordinating sites. Four with nitrogen atoms of the protoporphyrin ring. One with imidazole group of a histidine in the globin portion and sixth complexes with any atom which has an electron pair to donate. The molecules functionality and perceived colour is determined by the ligand at the sixth site and the redox state of iron. The purple red colour of freshly cut meat is due to deoxy myoglobin (Iron is in ferrous state). Desirable bright red pigment is oxymyoglobin and is formed by oxygenation of iron, which is in ferrous state. Undesirable brown coloured metmyoglobin is formed by oxidation of iron to ferric form and water is complexed at the sixth site.

Some normal colour of meat from various species is:

- ☆ Beef: Bright Cherry Red,
- ☆ Fish: Gray White to Dark Red,
- ☆ Horse: Dark Red,
- ☆ Lamb and Mutton: Light Red to Brick Red,
- ☆ Pork: Grayish Pink,
- ☆ Poultry: Gray White to Dull Red

PSE and DFD both conditions have abnormal color. Abnormal colour in PSE and DFD condition is partially the result of an unusual water binding capacity and its influence on light reflection. The paleness of PSE is believed to be the result of high proportion free water. This free water is extra cellular and has many reflecting surfaces that totally reflects light and have only limited light absorption capability. Total pigment myoglobin, Fe concentration were significantly lower in PSE meat as compared to normal meat. At lower pH there is denaturation of sarcoplasmic proteins resulting in greater scattering of light so gives paler colour. (Fletcher D.L. 1995). DFD meat has higher WHC so there is large proportion of water as intracellular water because of this white light reflection between the cells is minimized and colour absorption is enhanced. So DFD meat is more red than normal.

2. pH

Normal pH of meat is due to the anaerobic glycolysis of muscle glycogen which leads to accumulation of lactic acid. Normal pH of meat is 5.1 to 5.8. In PSE meat there is rapid decline of muscle pH as a result of accelerated post mortem glycolysis while the carcass temperature is still high. pH of PSE muscle is below 5.4 and temperature is 36-40°C. DFD meat has pH value greater than the normal because of delayed or reduced glycolysis.

3. Water Holding Capacity (WHC)

It may be defined as ability of meat to retain in water during application of external forces such as cutting, heating, grinding or pressure. Water in muscles is held by capillary forces between thick and thin filaments *i.e.* thick filament of myosin and thin filament of actin/tropomyosin. Water exists in muscle in two forms 'Bound' and 'free' form. Diminution of in vivo WHC is manifested by exudation of fluids known as 'Weep' in uncooked meat which has not been frozen. 'Drip' in thawed uncooked meat and as 'Shrink' in cooked meat. In PSE meat there is rapid decline in pH and the ultimate pH is lower resulting in denaturation of sarcoplasmic and myofibrillar proteins and myosin. Denaturation of myosin results in shrinkage of myosin head drawing the thick and thin filaments closely together. This shrinkage in addition to myofilaments shrinkage at low ultimate pH results in more fluid expulsion between fibers and fiber bundles *i.e.* in PSE condition there is decline in WHC. In DFD condition the pH of post mortem muscle remains high so there will be no denaturation of proteins and there naturally occurring water is tightly bound to the protein. The water binding capacities of DFD meat is higher than normal meat.WHC can be determined by expressible moisture and cook loss. Expressible moisture involves using force to express water from the meat. Water bond by protein is not expressed from meat. So, increase in expressible moisture indicates greater proportion of the water that holds more loosely thus indicating lower water holding capability. PSE meat has higher cook looses and higher expressible moisture value than normal meat so have lower WHC.

4. Emulsification Capacity

The emulsification capacity is one of the primary factors which determine the utility of food products. Emulsion is defined as a mixture of two immiscible liquids one of which is dispersed in the form of small droplets or globules in the other liquid in which these droplets are dissolved is called continuous phase. Meat emulsion is a 2-Phase system in which dispersed phase consisting of either liquid or solid fat particles and continuous phase being water containing dissolved or suspended salts and proteins. Solubilised protein acts as emulsifier agents. The solubility of emulsion depends upon the emulsifier agent which is soluble protein in case of meat emulsion.

In PSE meat, there is denaturation of protein, solubility of protein are decreased, so the emulsifying capacity of PSE meat is lower than normal and emulsifying capacity of DFD meat is higher than normal.

Disadvantages/Limitations of Using PSE or DFD Meat in Manufacturing different Meat Products

1. Cook Loses/Lower Yield

PSE meat has higher shear value and lower taste panel score for tenderness.PSE meat result in lower yield and increased post cooking labour. During cooking PSE meat there is increase in purge in the cook-in bags which results in a product with increased yield losses during cooking, poor meat binding and dry soft texture.

2. Shelf Life

Meat is a highly perishable food. Shelf life of meat and meat products depends upon the microbial load they carry. Microbial contamination can take place from the contaminants present in air, water, soil, contamination from floor, handlers hands processing equipments; animals may themselves carry micro-organism from various disease conditions. There are different intrinsic and extrinsic factors which will determine the growth of microorganisms. Bacterial growth is generally favoured by near natural pH. The normal ultimate pH favours the growth of molds, yeast and acidophilic bacteria. Meat with lower pH values have markedly reduced microbial growth as compared to normal pH. At lower pH bacteria have longer lag phase and slower rate of growth which results in lower bacterial density. On the other hand DFD meats with higher pH have shorter lag phase time and growth of microorganism is high, so shelf life of DFD meat is low. (Allen *et al.*, 1997)

3. Palatablity and Visual Acceptance

After 5-6 hrs PSE meat starts to develop a gray-greenish cast so their acceptance decreases sharply. This is because of greater instability of myoglobin as myoglobin had a rapid rate of auto-oxidation, greater heat instability of both met and oxy form. PSE meat develops rancidity at a faster rate when stored at low temperature for longer period.

4. Texture

Texture properties, tenderness and juiciness are very important in consumer quality perception. PSE muscles are less desirable for production of pasteurized canned hams and emulsified products, as PSE ham are found to shrink significantly more than normal. PSE muscles are lower in juiciness, tenderness, flavour and is dry soft in texture. DFD ham has higher moisture content and is softer, pastier, more crumbly and adhesive than normal.

How to Use PSE or DFD Meat in Meat Products

PSE meat is either mixed with normal meat or meat products requiring low WHC can be prepared from it. Attributes such as firmness, high WHC, tenderness, juiciness makes DFD meat very acceptable to processing. In order to avoid excessive paleness and exudation PSE meat must be chilled rapidly. DFD meat can be consumed or processed to comminuted and heated meat products.

Conclusions

Care and all precautions should be taken by the producer to prevent the production of DFD or PSE meat. Specially stress factors should be taken into account. Propagation of stress resistant breeds should be carried out. The norms of transportation of animals as per regulations and animal welfare issues must be followed. Adequate resting period should be provided to the animal prior to slaughter. Rough handling of the meat animals during slaughter must be avoided. Post-slaughter care of meat and meat products during chilling, ageing, freezing, packaging including various processing techniques for development of meat products should be meticulously followed to prevent pre- and post-slaughter loss of meat.

References

Allen C.D. *et al.* (1997) :The relationship of broiler breast meat colour and pH to shelf life and odour development.Poul.Science 76, 1042-1046.

Allen C.D. *et al.* (1998): The relationship of broiler breast colour to meat colour and shelf life. Poul. Science 77, 361-366.

Barbut S. 1996: Estimates and detection of the PSE problem in young turkey breast meat. Canadian J.of Animal Sci. 76 455-457.

Barbut S. 1997a: Occurrence of PSE meat in mature turkey hens. British Poul. Sci. 38, 355-358.

Bendall J.R. *et al.*, 1988: A review of relationship of Ph with physical aspects of pork quality. Meat Sci. 24, 85-126.

Ferket P.R. 1995: PSE breast meat in turkey. Turkeys 43, 19-21.

Fletcher D.L 1995: Relationship of breast meat colour variation to muscle pH and texture. Poul. Sci. 74 (suppl. 1) 120.

Froning G.W. *et al.*, 1978: The effect of preslaughter temp., stress, struggle and anesthetization on colour and textural characteristics of turkey muscles.Poul. Sci. 57, 630-633.

Forrest *et al*: Principals of meat science.

Fernandez X. *et al.*, 1994: Effect of high P.M. temp. on the development of PSE pork quality. Interaction with ultimate pH. Meat sci. 37, 133-147.

Fox J.D. *et al.*, 1980: Physical, Chemical, Sensory and Microbiological properties and shelf life of PSE and normal pork chops. J. Food Sci. 45, 786-790.

Gree G.G. *et al.*, 1988: Effects of pork meat quality on bacterial growth and retail case life. Meat Sci. 24, 61-71.

Guerrero L. *et al.*, 1999: The influence of meat pH on mechanical and sensory textural properties of cured ham. Meat Sci. 52, 267-273.

Kannan G. *et al.*, 1997: Effect of crating and transport on stress and meat quality characteristics in broiler. Poul. Sci. 76, 523-529.

Lawrie R.A.: Meat Science.

McCurdy R.D. *et al.*, 1996: Seasonal effect on PSE occurrence in young turkey breast meat. Food Res. International 29, 363-366.

Mckee S.R. *et al.*, 1998: Rigor mortis development at elevated temp. induce PSE meat characteristics. Poul. Sci. 77, 169-174.

Mugler W.D. 1972: Factors affecting poultry meat colour. A Review. World Poul. Sci. J. 28 (4), 400-406.

Newton K.G. *et al.*, 1981: The microbiology of DFD fresh meat. A review. Meat Sci. 5, 223-232.

Ngoka D.A. *et al.*, 1982: Effect of sex, age, preslaughter factors and holding conditions on quality characteristics and chemical composition of turkey breast meat. Poul. Sci. 76, 523-529.

Owen C.M. *et al.*, 2000: The characterization and incidence of PSE turkey meat in commercial plant. Poul. Sci. 79, 553-558.

Poultry Meat Science edited by R.I. Richardson and G.C. Mead.

Rey C.R. et.al 1976: Microbiology of pale, dark and normal pork. J. of Food Sci. 41, 111-116.

Sosniciki A.A. 1993: PSE in turkey. Meat Focus Int. Feb. pp. 75-78.

Santos C. et.al 1994: Incidence of different pork quality categories in a Portuguese slaughter house. A survey. Meat Sci. 38, 279-287.

Stabursvik E. et.al 1984: Myosin denaturation in PSE porcine muscle tissue as studied by differential scanning calorimetery. J. of the Sci. of Food and Agri. 35,240-244.

Swatland H.J. 1987: Fiber optic specterophotometery of colour intensity problems in raw and cooked turkey breast. Poul. Sci. 66, 679-682.

Tarrant P.V. 1989: Animal behaviour and environment in dark cutting condition in beef. A review. Ir. J. Food Sci. and Tech. 13, 1-9.

VanHoof J. 1979.: Influence of anti and peri mortem factors on biochemical and physical characteristics of turkey breast muscle. Vet. Q. 1, 29-36.

Williams W.D.1992: Origin and impact of colour on consumer preference for food. Poul. Sci. 71, 744-746.

Woelfel R.L. et.al 2001: Marination performance of pale broiler breast meat. Poul. Sci. 80,1519-1522.

– Chapter 6 –

Composition, Essential Nutrients in Meat and Poultry Meat

I. Chemical and Biochemical Constitution of Muscle

In broad sense the composition of meat can be approximated to:

- ☆ Water – 75 per cent
- ☆ Protein – 19 per cent
- ☆ Soluble non-protein substances – 3.5 per cent
- ☆ Fat – 2.5 per cent

1. Chemical Composition

Chemical Composition of Typical Adult Mammals muscle after Rigor Mortis but before deteriorative changes post-mortem (Lawrie, 1975)

Table 6.1: Chemical Composition of Meat

Sl.No.	*Component*	*Wet per cent Weight*
1.	Water	75.0
	Protein	19.0
A	Myofibrillar	11.5
	Myosin (H and L meromyosins and several light chain proteins associated with them	6.5
	Actin	2.5
	Tropomyosin	1.5
	Troponins C, I and T	0.4
	α and β actinins	0.4
	M protein etc	0.2

Contd...

Table 6.1–*Contd...*

Sl.No.	*Component*	*Wet per cent Weight*
B	Sarcoplasmic	5.5
	glyceraldehyde phosphate dehydrogenase	1.2
	Aldolase	0.6
	Creatine kinase	0.5
	Other glycolytic enzymes	2.2
	Myoglobin	0.2
	Haemoglobin and other unspecified extraceliular proteins	0.6
C	Connective tissue and organelle	2.0
	Collagen	1.0
	Elastin	0.05
	Mitochondrial etc (including cytochrome c and insoluble enzymes)	0.95
3.	Lipid	2.5
	Neutral lipid, phospholipids fatty acids fat-soluble substances	2.5
4.	Carbohydrate	1.2
	Lactic acid	0.90
	Glucose-6 phosphate	0.15
	Glycogen	0.10
	Glucose traces of other glycolytic intermediates	0.05
5.	Miscellaneous soluble Non-protein substances	2.3
a	Nitrogenous	1.65
	Creatine	0.55
	Inosine monophosphate	0.30
	di-and tri-phosphopyridine	0.30
	Nucleotides	0.10
	Amino acids	0.35
	Carnosine, anserine	0.35
b	Inorganic	0.65
	Total soluble phosphorus	0.20
	Potassium	0.35
	Sodium	0.05
	Magnesium	0.02
	Calcium, zinc, trace metals	0.23
6.	Vitamins	–
	Various fat and water soluble vitamins quantitatively minute	–

2. Muscle Proteins

Constitutes 16-22 per cent of muscle mass: principal components of solid matter. Broadly divided into:

Sarcoplasmic proteins – soluble in water or dilute salt solutions.

Myofibrillar proteins – soluble in concentrated salt solutions.

Connective tissue and organelle/stromal proteins which are insoluble in conc. salt solution.

Sarcoplasmic Proteins (Myogen and Globulins)

A complex mixture of about 50 components of citric acid cycle and electron transport chain

Mostly enzymes of glycolytic cycle and also include myoglobin and haemoglobin.

Myofibrillar Proteins

Myosin – mol wt. 500,000, asymmetric ratio of length to diameter is 100:1

Rich in glutamic and aspartic acids and of dibasic amino acids, highly charged, strong affinity for calcium and magnesium ions.

Built of light (L) and heavy (H) meromyosins.

H-meromyosin contains ATPase and actin-combining properties of myosin, sited on the peripheri of the myosin filaments. The properties depend upon free-SH groups in the molecule.

Tropomyosin: amino acid composition is similar to myosin, a cyclopeptide (a chain of amino acids forming a closed figure).

Actin: exist in two forms: G-actin, F-actin.

G-actin consists of small globular units having a mol. of about 70,000. F-actin: these globular units are aggregated end to end to form a double chain. It is F-actin, which combines with myosin to form actomyosin complex.

Troponin complex promotes the aggregation of tropomyosin, binds calcium and prevents actomyosin formation, three types troponin C, I and T.

α- actinin promotes the lateral association of F-actin.

β- actinin inhibits polymerization of F-actin.

M-line substance – promotes the lateral polymerization of L-meromyosin.

Tropomyosin B- contribute mechanical stability to the muscle filaments. NPN included as amino acids, peptides, creatine, some vitamins, nucleosides etc.

Collagen – highest content of hydroxyproline therefore the hydroxyproline content of muscle is used as a measure of its connective tissue. There is a high proportion of hydroxyl amino acids in collagen and elastin, tryptophan is virtually absent, hydroxylysine is found.

Collagen on heating at > 80°C yield gelatine in boiling, but reticulin does not yield gelatin on boiling.

Elastin is not broken down by heating. It contains a chromophoric residue which gives elastin its characteristic yellow colour and fluorescence. The elastic properties of elastin are due to the presence of two known amino acids – desmosine and isodesmosine at the crosslink areas between adjacent polypeptide chains. The elastin differs from collagen –

By having only 1-6 per cent hydroxyproline

Few polar amino acids

Valine content (18 per cent) is much higher.

3. Intramuscular Fat

Has a considerable content of phospholipids and unsaponifiable constituents *e.g.* cholesterol.

Only 3 or 4 fatty acids are present in substantial amount in the fat of meat animals – Oleic, Palmitic and Stearic and four types of glycerides GS3, GS2U, GSU2 and GU3 (S and U represent saturated and unsaturated fatty acids respectively).

The phospholipids consist of phosphoglycerides, plasmalogens and sphingomyelin.

In the phosphoglycerides one of the three hydroxyl groups of glycerol is combined with choline, ethanolamine, serine inositol or glucose. In the plasmalogens the second hydroxyl group of glycerol is esterified with a long-chain fatty aldehyde instead of with fatty acid. In sphingomyelin the amino alcohol sphingosine is bound by an amide link to a fatty acid and by an ester link to Phosphorylcholine, Glycolipids are also present in muscle tissue. Of the total phospholipids in beef muscle

Lecithin – 62 per cent

Cephalin – 30 per cent

Sphingomyelin $<$ 10 per cent

Accompanying the trighycerides are small quantities of substances which are soluble in fat solvents *e.g.* vitamins A, D, E and K and Cholesterol derivatives.

Water: Muscle contains approx. 75 per cent water (range 65-80) by weight. Water is the principal constituent of the extracellular fluid and numerous chemical constituents are dissolved or suspended in it. It serves as the medium for the transport of substances between the vascular bed and muscle fibers.

4. Carbohydrates

Present in small quantities, glycogen is the most abundant carbohydrate in the muscle (0.5 to 1.3 per cent by wt of muscle). The bullk of the remainder of the carbohydrate is comprised of the mucopolysaccharides associated with the connective tissue, glucose and other mono-or disaccharides and the intermediates of the glycolytic metabolism.

5. Inorganic Constituents

Cations and anions of physiological significance – calcium, magnesium, potassium, sodium, iron, phosphorus, sulfur and chlorine. Many of the other inorganic constituents found in the animal body are also present in muscle.

Composition of Meat

The composition of muscle obtained from different animal species is relatively constant in terms of protein, fat, mineral and water content, regardless of the degree of fatness of the animal.

The Proximate Composition and Energy Value of Meat

Fresh Muscle and Organ Meats

The average values for the proximate composition and energy value of the edible portion of fresh meat cuts is as follows:

- ✰ Protein – 17 per cent
- ✰ Fat – 20 per cent
- ✰ Moisture – 62 per cent
- ✰ Ash – 1 per cent
- ✰ Calories – 250/100 gm

} Medium cut with covering fat layer of ½ inch thick

Lean muscle meat may have the following average proximate composition values:

- ✰ Protein – 20 per cent
- ✰ Fat – 9 per cent
- ✰ Moisture –70 per cent
- ✰ Ash – 1 per cent
- ✰ Calories – 160/100 gm

Fresh muscle meats contains essentially no carbohydrate (less than 1 per cent) and no fiber or indigestible carbohydrate. Several of the organ meats however contain small amounts of glycogen and glucose (upto 4 per cent).

The degree of finish (fatness) affects values for proximate composition, meat from lean animals generally has higher protein and moisture content, whereas fat or very fat meats have lower values for protein and moisture alongwith substantially greater fat content.

The proximate composition and energy values of fresh organ meats differ significantly from the values observed for fresh muscle meats. With the exception of sweet breads (beef pancreas and beef thymus) and tongue fat level are generally lower and moisture levels are higher with some increase in ash levels. Thus the organ meats provide levels of protein similar to those of fresh muscle cuts with substantially fewer calories per unit of wt.

Composition of Poultry Meat

Please refer Part II "Poultry and Fish Products Technology" of the book.

II. Nutritive value of Fresh Meat

Nutritive value of meat is attributed to its protein, fats, carbohydrates, vitamins and minerals. Though meat does provide calories from the proteins, fats and carbohydrates that are present, its more vital contributions to the diet are derived from the high quality and quantity of its proteins, the available supply of B-vitamins and certain minerals and the presence of essential fatty acids.

Proteins

The largest proportion of total muscle proteins are those of the myofibrils. The sarcoplasmic proteins consisting of muscle enzymes and myoglobin make up the next largest fraction. This is followed in abundance by the connective tissue proteins consisting largely of collagen and some elastin. Raw muscle contains approx. 18-22 per cent protein. This content varies inversely with the amount of fat present. Meat products generally supply a major portion of the recommended dietary allowance (RDA) of protein. The RDA for an adult man is 56 gms per day. Large amounts of protein cannot be stored in the body, so it is essential that protein be consumed everyday. A normal sized serving of cooked meat is 100 gms and its protein content is 25-30 per cent *i.e.* it furnishes 25-30 gms of protein or about 45-55 per cent of the RDA.

In addition to its protein contents skeletal meat provides a high quality protein with a high biological value, a high quality protein is one that contains all of the essential amino acids in amounts that are equivalent to the requirements of the human body, is highly digestible and is easily absorbable. Amino acids are basic building blocks of protein. Essential amino acids are those that cannot be synthesized by the body in amounts sufficient to meet its requirements. Adult human beings need 8 EAA. These are phenylalanine, valine, tryptophan, threonine, methionine, leucine, isoleucine and lysine. The high amounts of non-essential amino acids glycine, proline and hydroxyproline in collagen are responsible for its lower biological value.

In addition to proteins, meat also contain some non protein nitrogenous compounds, such as the free amino acids, simple peptides, amines, amides and creatine. They are a potential source of nitrogen that can be used for amino acid and protein synthesis.

Lipids

The lipids content of meat is generally the most variable content. The amount of lipid depends upon the cut of meat and the amount of fat that is left after cutting and trimming. The lipid contents that are important from a nutritional stand point are the triglycerides, phospholipids, cholesterol and fat soluble vitamins. The caloric value of lipids in meat is derived from the fatty acids in triglycerides and phospholipids. The fatty acids constituting the triglycerides of meat are relatively saturated, when compared to the vegetable fats. In meat fat the most abundant fatty acid is unsaturated oleic acid, with one double bond. The other fatty acids that are present in high proportions are saturated palmitic and stearic acids. The consumption of saturated fat and cholesterol is linked to the cardiovascular diseases. But several studies indicate that high caloric intake is related to obstity and in turn, obesity, stress and relative inactivity are factors which are directly related to the occurrence of cardiovascular diseases.

Meat fats contain variable quantities of cholesterol. Cholesterol content of lean muscle is 65-75 mg/100g, kidney 400mg/100g and liver is 430mg/100g. Eventhough blood cholesterol values rise following the ingestion of cholesterol in foods, it should be pointed out that the body is capable of synthesizing more cholesterol than is normally ingested. Therefore, the cholesterol controversy is still unresolved.

Meat fats contain ample quantities of the fatty acids that are essential in the diet of humans. Since the daily need of these essential fatty acids is relatively small, the RDA is easily met from intramuscular fat. The fatty acids that are known to be essential are linoleic and arachidonic.

Carbohydrates

Carbohydrates constitute less than 1 per cent of the weight of meat; most of which is present in the form of glycogen and lactic acid. Since the liver is the principal storage site of glycogen most of the carbohydrate in the animal body is present in the liver. Thus most meats are poor source of carbohydrate.

Minerals

Meat is generally a good source of all minerals except for calcium. Most of the calcium in the body is present in bones and teeth. The minerals in meat are associated with the lean tissues.

Meat is essentially a good source of iron, a nutrient that is essential for maintaining good health. Iron is required for the synthesis of haemoglobin myoglobin and certain enzymes. Since little iron is stored in the body a regular intake of dietary iron is important and meat provides it is a form that is easily absorbed.

Vitamins

Excellent source of water soluble B-complex group but a poor source of water soluble vitamin C. The fat soluble vitamin A, D, E and K are found primarily in the body fat. All of the B-complex vitamins are present in the meat; but the amine, riboflavin and niacin are present in the highest quantities. Pork contains higher levels of B-complex vitamins than beef, veal, lamb, fish or poultry. In fact the lean portion of pork is 8-10 times higher in thiamine than other meats as well as being slightly higher in riboflavin, pyridoxine, pantothenic acid and biotin content. Pork contains approx. the same amount of niacin and slightly less vitamin B_{12} than other meats.

Table 6.2: Composition of Lean Muscle Tissue of Meat Animals (per cent)

Species	*Water*	*Protein*	*Lipid*	*Ash*	*Kcal/100g*
Buffalo	76-78	18-22	1-2	1-1.5	
Beef	70-73	20-22	4.8	1.0	118
Chicken	73-75	20-23	4.7	1.0	
Lamb	73	20	5-6	1.4	
Pork	68-70	19-20	9-11	1.4	
Chevon	74.2	21.4	3.6	1.1	

Source: Fennema, O.R – (1985) Food Chemistry Marcel Dekker, New York.

Table 6.3: Nutritive Value of 100g Meat/Chicken

	Moisture (g)	*Protein (g)*	*Fat (g)*	*Ash (g)*	*Calories (Kcal)*	*Cholesterol mg per cent*
Raw meat	71	21	3	1.03	150	75
Cooked meat	57	30	7	1.21	210	110
Raw chicken	74	23	1.70	1	115	45
Cooked chicken	64	31	4.2	1	170	70

Table 6.4: Comparative Nutritive Value of different Meats (per 100g)

Nutrients	*Chicken*	*Mutton*	*Pork*	*Fish*	*Milk*	*Soya bean*
Energy (Kcal)	163	194	200	160	117	375
Protein (g)	19	18	18.5	17	4.3	35
Fat (g)	4.6	13.30	15	6.15	5.5	18
Cholesterol (mg per cent)	35	71	62	55	14	–
Iron (mg)	2.6	2.5	2.2	2.0	0.2	0.2
Vitamin A (IU)	730	500	500	700	160	–

Table 6.5: Amino Acid Composition of Meat Proteins (g/100g)

Amino Acids	*Beef*	*Chicken*	*Lamb*	*Pork*
Arginine	13.7	12.8	12.7	12.2
Cystine	2.6	2.6	2.7	2.6
Histidine	7.5	6.2	6.7	8.9
Isoleucine	10.4	9.5	9.7	9.2
Leucine	16.3	15.4	15.0	14.5
Lysine	18.5	18.4	20.3	19.7
Methionine	5.5	4.9	5.3	5.6
Phenylalanine	9.1	9.2	8.0	7.9
Threonine	9.4	8.5	9.7	8.9
Tryptophan	2.6	2.3	2.7	2.3
Tyrosine	7.8	7.2	7.3	7.6
Valine	10.7	9.8	10.0	9.9

Source: Paul, A.A., Southgate D.A.T. and Russel J (1980). First supplement to Mc Cance and Widdowson. The composition of foods HMSO, London.

Protein Quality Parameters Biological Value (BV)

B.V. of a protein is the fraction of the nitrogen retained in the body for growth and maintenance. It is determined by nitrogen balance expermiments:

$$BV = \frac{1N - UN - FN}{1N - FN}$$

where,

1N: Nitrogen intake
UN: Urinary nitrogen
FN: Faecal nitrogen out put.

Net Protein Utilisation (NPU)

It is the ratio of nitrogen retained and total protein nitrogen intake. NPU is influenced by biological value and digestibility of the protein:

Table 6.6: Net Protein Utilisation of Protein Foods

	BV	*NPU*	*Digestibility*
Meat	0.75	80	94-97
Human milk	1.0	–	–
Wheat protein	0.50	52	–
Egg	–	100	94-97
milk	–	–	94-97

Table 6.7: Fatty Acids Composition of Fat (per cent)

F.A.	*Mutton*	*Beef*	*Pork*	*Chicken*
14:0	2.0	2.5	1.5	1.3
14:1	0.5	0.5	0.5	0.2
15:0	0.5	0.5	–	–
16:0	21.0	24.5	24.0	23.2
16:1	3.0	3.1	3.5	6.5
17:0	1.0	1.0	0.5	0.3
18:0	28.0	18.5	14.0	6.4
18:1	37.0	40.0	43.0	41.6
18:2	4.0	5.0	9.5	18.9
18:3	–	0.5	1.0	1.3
20:0	0.5	0.5	0.5	–
20:1	0.5	0.5	1.0	–
P/S ratio	0.07	0.11	0.25	0.64
Iodine value	42.6	48.7	60.3	78.3

Source: Rossell J.B. (1992). In the chemistry of meat based foods (eds DE Johnston, M.K. Knight and D.A. Ledward). Royal society of Chemistry, London.

III. Health Benefits of Eating Meat

There are innumerable health benefits of eating meat, to say, for example, it serves as a fabulous source of high quality proteins, which a single vegetarian food is not able to provide. It contains all the essential amino acids that the body requires. The red meat contains very high quantities of iron, when compared with plant origin foods. 100 grams of Liver contains 6000 mcgm of iron as against 325 mcgm in 100-gram carrots. Read further to explore information about the advantages of eating meat.

The phosphorus content present in meat gets much more easily absorbed than that present in cereals and legumes. This is owing to the fact that cereals and legumes contain phosphorus, usually in the form of phytic acid that must be hydrolyzed before absorption. Meat also serves as the main source for the intake of vitamin B_{12}. Though meat is rich in nutrients, but, there are certain things that meat lacks in. It doesn't contain any kind of fiber, which helps to keep your digestive system in order. Also it is very high in saturated fats, thus it is recommended to eat meat, but in moderate quantities.

Preserved meats like ham, bacon, salami etc should be avoided, as they are very high in terms of fats, salts, nitrites and nitrates that are often held responsible for causing cancer. It is recommended to eat not more than 60-75 grams of meat per day and not more than thrice a week.

Rabbit

Farm-raised rabbit is a lean, slightly sweet meat with a closely textured flesh that has virtually no fat and is very high in protein. Rabbit is an alternative to chicken, with the additional advantage that it is commonly raised without the use of hormones or steroids. Rabbit meat contains calories 136, protein 20.05, fat 5.55, cholesterol 57.

Table 6.8: Nutritional Information Comparison of Ostrich Meat

Species	*Description*	*Protein per cent*	*Fat Grams*	*Calories*	*Iron (mg)*	*Cholesterol (mg)*
Ostrich	Cut Composite	26.9	3.0	142	3.2	83
Chicken	Whole (no skin)	28.9	7.4	190	1.2	89
Turkey	Whole (no skin)	29.3	5.0	170	1.8	76
Beef	Retail Composite	29.9	9.3	211	3.0	86
Pork	Retail Composite	29.3	9.7	212	1.1	86
Veal	Retail Composite	31.9	6.6	196	1.1	118
Duck	Meat Only	23.5	11.2	201	2.7	89
Deer	Meat Only	30.2	3.2	158	4.5	112

Table 6.9: All Measurements taken from 100 gram Servings

	Protein	*Cholesterol*	*Saturated Fats*	*Total Fat*	*Calories*	*%Calories from Fat*
Fish	22.9g	47mg	.104g	.81g	105	6.9 per cent
Chicken	31.0g	85mg	1.0g	3.5g	165	19.5 per cent
Pork	29.3g	86mg	3.4g	9.7g	212	41 per cent
Beef	25.9g	88mg	8.5g	21.5 g	305	63.6 per cent
Beefalo	30.7g	58mg	2.7g	6.3g	188	30.3 per cent

All figures taken from the USDA Nutrient Database for standard release 11 (September 1996).

Notes

1. Finfish, cod, Pacific, cooked, dry heat (NDB #15192)
2. Chicken, broilers or fryers, breast, meat only, cooked, roasted (NDB #05064)
3. Pork, fresh, composite of trimmed retail cuts (leg, loin, and shoulder), seperable lean only, cooked (NDB #10093)
4. Beef, composite of trimmed retail cuts, seperable lean and fat, trimmed to 1/4" fat, all grades, cooked (NDB #13004)
5. Beefalo, composite of cuts, cooked, roasted (NDB #17153)

Table 6.10: What is the Relationship of the Calories, Fats and Cholesterol in Ostrich, Chicken, Turkey, Beef, and Pork?

3 oz Portion of:	*Calories*	*FatGrams*	*Cholesterol mg.*
Ostrich	96.9	1.7	58.0
Chicken	140.0	3.0	73.0
Turkey	135.0	3.0	59.0
Beef (ground)	230.0	16.0	74.0
Beef (steak)	240.0	15.0	77.0
Pork	275.0	19.0	84.0

Farming of nutritious and tasty Japanese quails is becoming a popular business. Considered to be more profitable, many entrepreneurs are switching over from poultry farming to this business.

With an initial investment of about Rs 2,000, anyone can start a small quail unit in one's own household.

A PTI report has quoted the Indian Council of Agricultural Research's (ICAR) findings as saying that the Japanese quails being comparatively free from disease problems could be taken up even by small farmers with low financial resources.

Dressed quail meat fetches a higher market price ranging from Rs 90-110 a kg, compared to Rs 60-80 for chicken meat.

Because of the advantages of profit and lesser disease problems, quail farming introduced as part of the rural uplift schemes have caught up in many states. Still its availability in major urban markets, like Delhi, is erratic for want of organised production and supply arrangements.

ICAR, the central organisation for all research and development activities inagricultural crops, animal husbandry, poultry and fisheries, has entrusted quail development to the Central Avian Research Institute (CARI) near Bareilly in Uttar Pradesh.

CARI has come out with new lines of quails that have more body weight, complete white feathers and bigger egg yield than the traditional yellowish speckled quails introduced originally from Japan. CARI has developed simple breeding and management practices which are also inexpensive.

The quail egg, though slightly smaller than the chicken egg, has higher protein and other nutritive contents. Because of the erratic demand-supply position, quail eggs are better available in the market in pickled form. Each bird yields more than 300 eggs in a year.

From a small 6-10 gm body weight in a day-old chick, the quail can grow to a 175-220 gm bird within five to six weeks. The quail meat is reputed to be very tasty, tender and delicious with low calorific and cholesterol value.

Quail meat has a definite game flavour and is recommended in thediet of children, expectant women and convalescent patients.

The female quail chicks achieve maturity in seven to eight weeks and starts egg laying. The incubation period of quail eggs is only about 17 days. This is very advantageous to the quail farmers.

The ICAR has started supplying seed birds of quails to the animal husbandry departments of states. The departments, in turn, are supplying them to farmers on a subsidized rate. The CARI has also arrangements for training small farmers intending to take up farming of Japanese quails.

IV. Nutritive Value of Different Types of Meats

Food is one of the foundations of human life and the consumption of meat in the human diet date back to the time when *Homo sapiens* first appeared on the earth. Since ancient times, meat consumption has been a factor differentiating the society and creating a measure of social position. Cultural and religious considerations have always played a significant role in the preparation and consumption of meat products. A product regarded as a delicacy in one Cultural group can be considered as inedible in another one. Every human has grown up only after consuming nutrient of animal origin because as babies in uterus, we receive all nutrient of animal origin. It has also been shown that modern disease such as obesity, cancer, diabetes and coronary heart disease were absent in the Paleolithic men who had a high dependence on animal foods rather than on plant foods.

Nutritive Value of Meat

Numerous studies have been conducted to seek out the nutritional benefits from the meat and meat products. The quality and quantity of different compositional attributes of meat depend upon various factors such as the species, age, diet, cut-up-part of the carcass etc. of animal.

Protein

Muscle food is a good concentrated source of nutrients and can make a valuable concentration to the overcome nutrition problems. The protein content of meat products ranges between 21-25 per cent proteins. Meat proteins have high biological value and consist of all the indispensable/essential amino acids (EAA). Essential amino acids cannot be synthesized by the body, it should always be available in diet for adults these are eight for adults and ten for childern include arginine and histidine also. Beef has more of leucine, lysine and valine than pork and lamb. The content of these EAA increases with age and varies with the type of muscle. In comparison all plant protein are lacking atleast one of these amino acids called as limiting amino acid. Meat protein and it contain all essential amino acids. Taurine is a an essential amino acid for the new borns. Human requirements for protein have been thoroughly investigated over the years (FAO/WHO 1985) and are currently estimated to be 55 g per day for adult man and 45 g for woman. (There is a higher requirement in various disease states and conditions of stress). The protein requirement varies with the age, children requirement is much higher than the adults.

The quality of dietary protein can be measured in various ways (FAD/WHO 1991) but basically it is the ratio of the available amino acids in the food or diet compared with needs. In the earlier literature this was expressed on a percentage scale but with the adoption of the S.I. system of nomenclature it is expressed as a ratio. Thus a ratio of 1.0 (100 per cent) means that the amino acids available from the dietary proteins are in the exact proportions needed to satisfy human needs; a ratio of 0.5 means that the amount of one (or more) of the essential amino acids present is only half of that required. If one essential amino acid is completely absent (a circumstance that can occur only experimentally with isolated proteins since any food, let alone a whole diet, consists of a mixture of many proteins) the protein quality would be zero. The qualities of proteins from animal sources are greatly superior to those from plant sources. Many animal sources have Net Protein Utilization, NPU, (a measure of the usefulness of the protein to the body) around 0.75 while that of many, but not all plant foods is 0.5-0.6.

Lipids

Lipids (fats) are found at three sites in the animal body viz; under the skin (Subcutaneous fat) and around the organs (visceral fat), in between the muscle bundles (intermuscular fat), fat within the muscle structure (intra muscular or structural fats).

The fat content of meat varies from 2-25 per cent depending upon the species and cut-up-portion. This adipose tissue is composed largely of phospholipids, triglycerides contained in proteinaceous cells with relative little water.

For the modern meat consumer taste and nutritional value are two important quality attributes of the meat. Tendency is to get leaner meat but fact is that the fat contributes to the eating quality of meat. Fat also influence the tenderness and flavour. The proportions in which each of the fatty acids is present determine the fatty acid profile of a food.

The predominant saturated fatty acids in meat are stearic acid (C18 :0) and palmitic (C16:0). In general saturated fats are known as 'bad fat' as they tend to raise the blood cholesterol and cause atherosclerosis however, studies have shown that stearic acid does not raise the blood lipids and these acids make 35 per cent of sheep/ goat fat. Myristic acid (C14:0), which is most atherogenic fatty acid is found only in minor quantities (1-2 per cent) in meat. Meat contains mixture of unsaturated fatty acid, polyunsaturated fatty acids and monounsaturated fatty acids. Approximately 40 per cent of the total fats in meat are MUFA, which is considered to be neutral to blood cholesterol level. The principal MUFA in meat is Oleic acid (Cis 18:1 n-9), which is alos found in olive oil. Amongst PUFA, omega-3 and omega 6, meat supplies 18 per cent and 17 per cent respectively. Moreover meat is good source of essential fatty acids such as linoleic and linolenic acids. Studies conducted by GISSI-Prevenzione Investigators (1999) showed that one gram of eicosapentaenoic acid and docosahexanoic acid daily reduced coronary heart disease death by 25 per cent. Meat and fish are the only significant source of very long chain n-3 PUFA in the diet. PUFA also have anti-inflammatory and anti tumergenic properties. Long chain n-3 PUFA are absent in vegetarian diets as plants cannot produce these long chain PUFAs. Next important thing is ratio of n-3 and n-6 in diet which should be less than 4. Now a days, with the modification of diets of animals and processing manipulations various health oriented meat products are available which has desired ratio.

Meats are considered as best dietary source of Conjugated Linoleic acid (CLA) which help in reduction in tumor forming cells, reduces atherosclerosis. It also delays the onset of diabetes and reduces adiposity. Different isomers of CLA are responsible for different biological effects.

Trans Fats raises LDL cholesterol and decrease HDL cholesterol. Main trans fatty acid is Vaccenic acid (t-11) 48 per cent of t-18:1 isomers. So it is recommended to avoid the large intake of trans fats. It is present both milk and meat of ruminants which accounts for 5 per cent only whereas their level is as high as upto 48 per cent of the junk foods available in the market.

The most recent nutrient intake goals published as a result of a joint WHO/FAO expert consultation (WHO,2003) are based on the widespread consensus that a "balanced diet" has preventive effects on chronic non-deficiency diseases, *e.g.* obesity, type 2 diabetes, cancer and cardiovascular diseases. These guidelines include the following targets for fat intake: total dietary fat, 15–30 per cent of energy (En per cent); saturated fatty acids (SFA), <10 En per cent; *n* À 6 polyunsaturated fatty acids (*n* À 6 PUFA), 5–8 En per cent; *n* À 3 polyunsaturated fatty acids (*n* À 3 PUFA), 1–2 En per cent; *trans*-fatty acids, <1En per cent. The target for monounsaturated fatty acids (MUFA) is calculated as follows: MUFA = total fat À (SFA + PUFA + *trans*-fatty acids).

Table 6.11: Relative Proportion of Types of Fatty Acids and Other Lipids

Cooked Meat	*Percentage of Total Fat*			
	SFA	*MUFA*	*PUFA*	*Other Lipids*
Beef	38.2	42.1	3.4	16.3
Pork	35.4	44.7	7.5	12.4
Lamb	35.7	43.8	6.5	14.0
Veal	28.0	35.7	9.0	27.3
Chicken	27.5	35.9	22.8	13.8
Tuna Fish	28.5	35.9	22.8	13.8
Salmon Fish	16.2	27.1	39.2	17.5

Vitamins

Meat and meat products are important sources of all the B-complex vitamins including thiamin, riboflavin, niacin, biotin, vitamins B_6 and B_{12}, pantothenic acid and folacin. The last two are especially abundant in liver, which, together with certain other organs is rich in vitamin A and supplies appreciable amounts of vitamins D, E and K. The amount of vitamins depends on the method of processing. Thiamine is a required as part of co-enzyme that convert carbohydrate and fat in to fuel. it also promote normal appetite and normal nervous functional. A typical serving of red meat will supply daily requirement of thiamine. Offal like kidney and liver are good source of riboflavin. Folic acid intake at level of >400µg/day is recommended for pregnant women. Meat is richest source of niacin. Niacin helps to supply energy to body by converting fats and carbohydrates to fuel. Liver and kidney are rich source of pantothenic acid. Vitamin B_6 is a co-factor for several cellular enzymes. Reactions including those related to amino acid metabolism and inter-conversion reactions.

Vitamin A is essential for growth and development of cells and tissues. In its active form, retinoic acid, it controls the regular differentiation as a ligand for retinoic acid receptors and is involved in the integration of cell formations. Vitamin A plays a substantial role especially in the respiratory epithelium and the lung. Vitamin a deficiency lead to diseases of respiratory tract and repeated respiratory infections can be influenced therapeutically by vitamin A supplementation.

Vitamin B_{12} is exclusively of animal origin as it is a product of bacterial fermentation, which occurs in intestine of ruminant animal. This important vitamin is required to produce red blood cells and act as a cofactor for many enzymatic reactions. Its deficiency causes the megaloblastic anemia, neuropathy, and gastrointestinal system. Vegetarians are at a risk of its deficiency because it is of animal origin exclusively. A 100 gram intake of meat everyday will supply all the daily requirement of this vitamin.

Vitamin B_6 and B_{12} are cofactor for enzyme reaction that reduces homocystine level by catabolizing homocystine to cystine. Research shows that deficiency of these two vitamins will raise homocystine levels, which is a risk factor for cardiovascular disease.

Vitamin D is essential for skeletal development and severe deficiency leads to rickets in children osteomalacia in adults. Severe insufficiency causes increased bone losses and fracture. sunlight exposure is main source of vitamin D. However there are certain subgroups in the population who are at the risk of vitamin D deficiency so they have to depend on sunlight and diet, and these subgroups include infants toddler pregnant and lactating women and those has less sunlight exposures. Meat and meat products contain sufficient 25-hydroxychole calciferol, which is 5 times biologically active than cholecalceferol. Thus meat is recognized as a rich source of vitamin D.

Minerals

Meat is very good source of minerals. Almost all the minerals necessary for the growth of the human body and other physiological functions are available in meat except Calcium which is more available in the bones can be extracted out in meat soups etc. The mineral content increases on cooking of meat.

Iron

Iron supports oxidative metabolism. It is essential for gas exchange a tissues and cellular level through the hemoglobin oxygenation in red cells and myoglobin in skeletal muscles. Moreover iron-containing enzymes are involved in cellular energy metabolism and in host defense responses. These various roles are due to biological catalytic activity of iron. Iron deficiency is most common and widespread nutritional disorder due to its biological losses such as cyclical monthly bleeding of fertilized women, excessive infestation with blood filled parasite Depending on the composition of individual diet the bio-availability can differ 5 to 10 fold. The different bioavailability depends on presence or absence of different ligands (phytates from cereal products, tannins from coffee and tea and oxalates from vegetables.), which block their absorption by forming complexes with iron and zinc. A vegetable diet consists of rice, beans and corn is having poor iron bioavailability. Meat is recognozed as a chief food source of of haem iron.Human body readily absorbes the haem iron.Meat also influence the availabilty of non haem iron present in other foods. This effect is known as magic factor.

Selenium

Selenium is often considered as belonging to the group of antioxidant nutrient. Since it is incorporated in to enzyme glutathione peroxidase, which act as a cellular protector against free radical oxidative damage and protective against degenerative disease. Supplemental may reduce the incidence and mortality from cancer. But its role as an anti cancer agent is still a topic under study. It also has a great role if boosting the immune system. Meats has been reported to be highly bioavailable for selenoprotein synthesis. Broccoli and beef were produced in a manner that resulted in high concentrations of selenium in the edible portions however it is easy to take 300g of meat in the diet than 300g of broccoli.

Zinc

Zinc is primarily found in animal products such as meat, shellfish and dairy products. Beef, liver and liver-based products are particularly rich in zinc. A vegetarian diet contains a lot of phytate, which inhibits zinc absorption due to binding with Phytate Zinc is an important co-enzyme for more than 80 enzyme systems and it plays a role in immune function, protein synthesis, wound healing, DNA synthesis and cell division. Zinc also supports normal growth and development during pregnancy, childhood, and adolescence and is required for proper sense of taste and smell. Meat counteracts the phytate-zinc bond so that the body can absorb zinc.

Energy

The amount of energy provided by meat is variable. Meat contains virtually no carbohydrate, and is principally composed of protein (which provides 17 kJ/4 kcal of energy per gram). Meat also contains fat in varying amounts (providing 37 kJ/9 kcal of energy per gram).The more fat that meat contains, the higher will be the energy content.

Meat-Based Bioactive Compounds

Chemical found as natural component of the other ingestible form that have been determined to be beneficial to the human body in preventing or treating one or more diseases and improving physiological performance are known as nutraceuticals.in addition to these compounds several bioactive compound are present in meat. Feeding conditions of animals can affect the content of bioactive components.

Biogenic amines are naturally formed from bacterial decarboxylation of amino acids. They improve gut health and cognitive performance. Nucleotides found in organ meats which enhances the general immune function. Glutathione is a tripeptide, which has major role in meat factor beneficial in absorption of non haem iron.

Conjugated Linoleic Acid

The CLA content is affected by several factors such as breed, age and fat composition. Beef fat contain 8 mg of CLA per gram of fat. CLA isomer in the meat is octadeca-c9 which have anticarcinogenic activity, antioxidative and immonomodulative property. Recent study has shown that intake of CLA may reduce the risk of colorectal cancer. CLA may also play a role in the control of obesity, reduction of risk of diabetes and has a role in bone metabolism.

Histidyl Peptides

Carnosine and anserine are antioxidant and composed of alanine and histidine and found most abundant in meat. The concentration of carnosne in meat range from 500mg/kg of chicken thigh to 2700mg/kg of pork shoulder. On the other hand, anserine is the especially abundant in chicken muscle. They can chelate transition metal like copper. These peptide also inhibit the ageing related to the oxidative stress. Recent study demonstrated the bioavalibilty of carnosine by determining its concentration in the human plasma after ingestion of beef.

L-Carnitine

L-carnitine, β hydroxyl-γ-trimethyl amino butyric acid is biosynthesized in human body, mainly in liver and kidney. It transport long chain fatty acid across the inner mitochondrial, where they are processed by beta –oxidation to produce biological energy. It also helps in energy production in muscle at the time of hard exercise. It is abundant in beef (1300 mg/kg of the thigh). It also help the body to absorb the calcium to improve skeletal strength and chromium picolinate to help build lean muscle. Recent studies have shown that l-carnitine blocked apoptosis and prevented skeletal muscle myopathy in heart failure. Most of carnitine are made from a byproduct of corned beef.

Lipoic Acid

Lipoic acid has antioxidant properties and has beneficial in diabetes and in prevention of cataract development in animal models and cell lines. Organ meats contain higher quantities of lipoic acid than muscle meat.

Choline is an essential nutrient required for the development of Central Nervous System, homocysteine metabolism and plays a role in immune system, fat metabolism and improves atheletic performance. Liver is one of the richest source of choline.

These bioactive compounds are used for developing novel functional meat products.

Concerns

The concerns about public health is the different meat borne diseases parasitic diseases Measly beef (*Cysticercus bovis*), *Measly pork* (*Cysticercus cellulosae*), ascariasis etc. The recent outbreaks of Bovine Spongiform Encephalopathy (BSE) in cattle and Avian Influenza in chicken with the suspicion that it might be transmitted to human beings through affected meat. In addition there is concern, about the presence in meat of pesticides, residues of hormones and growth promoters used to increase yields, increase blood pressure due to sodium in meat products. Therefore, there should be stringent implication of laws for the proper Ante mortem and post mortem examination of animals and maintenance of proper hygienic practices such as Good Hygienic Practices (GHP), Good Manufacturing Practices (GMP) and Hazard Analysis Critical Control Points (HACCP) so that the end product is safe and nutritious.

Conclusions

Attitudes and mindset of the consumers are the outcome of a clear philosophy of living and determine the demand of goods and service. The word 'Meat' is contradiction in India as it has a great sociocultural importance like "maha prasad"(Grand Blessing) to the food of "satan" (Devil) provoking 'lust and passion' thus hindering spiritual progress in life.

There has been considerable emotive debate over the last two decade on the importance of meat in the diet of modern man. Early dismissive arguments have been challenged with the recent research and information. A serious rethinking is required for an holistic approach of diet and lifestyle.

Busy and sedentary life style, lesser physical activity, erratic dietary practices like junk food intake has lead to serious health related problems like CHD and CRC. Vegetarians lobby has been blaming red meat as a sole reason behind these fatal

Table 6.12: Meat Composition of different Species of Animals

Nutrients	*Lamb*	*Pork*	*Beef*	*Chicken*	*Quail*	*Duck*	*Turkey*	*Buffalo*	*Rabbit*	*Chevon*	*RDA/day*
Moisture (per cent)	71.50	71.95	71.60	74.00	71.50	58.00	60.00	70.00	70.00	70.84	2.7 - 3.7 L
Protein (per cent)	19.50	20.22	20.94	18.50	20.50	20.00	19.50	23.70	21.00	20.60	50 g
Fat (per cent)	7.00	6.75	6.33	6.00	5.50	19.80	18.00	6.30	8.00	7.25	65 g
Ash (per cent)	1.50	1.04	1.03	0.80	1.20	0.50	1.00	1.00	1.00	1.10	–
Calorie per 100g	145.00	147.00	147.00	125.00	125.00	300.00	270.00	188.00	160.00	109.00	2400 Calorie
Minerals (mg/100 gm)											
Na	75.00	70.00	65.00	46.00	–	–	–	–	40.00	64.48	2400 mg
K	295.00	285.00	355.00	248.00	–	–	–	–	300.00	350.00	4700 mg
Mg	15.00	18.00	18.00	29.00	26.00	15.00	22.00	–	–	19.70	400 mg
Fe	1.20	2.30	2.80	0.70	3.05	2.70	1.80	–	1.50	4.37	12 mg
Ca	10.00	9.00	11.00	5.80	19.00	11.00	15.00	–	20.00	11.00	1000 mg
P	147.00	175.00	171.00	407.00	151.00	139.00	178.00	–	350.00	155.50	1000 mg
Vitamins (mg/100gm)											
Thiamine	0.15	0.76	0.06	0.07	0.15	0.20	0.06	–	0.10	0.10	1.5 mg
Riboflavin	0.20	0.18	0.13	0.38	0.50	0.21	0.16	–	0.05	0.56	1.7 mg
Niacin	4.70	4.10	3.60	5.60	6.00	3.90	4.10	–	13.00	3.60	20 g
Pantothenic Acid	0.50	0.60	0.40	0.91	1.10	0.95	0.81	–	0.80	–	10 mg
Biotin	0.003	0.004	0.003	–	–	–	–	–	–	–	300 μg
Folic Acid	0.003	0.003	0.01	0.006	–	0.013	8.00	–	–	–	400 μg
Vitamin B_6	0.40	0.50	0.30	0.35	0.52	0.19	0.41	–	0.45	–	2 mg

diseases. But a serious rethinking is needed. Balanced diet with a sufficient quantity of animal proteins, meat should be consumed along with vegetables and fruits to live longer with a sound health.

V. Meat and Health: Benefits and Concerns

Food is one of the foundations of human life and the consumption of meat in the human diet date back to the time when *Homo sapiens* first appeared on the earth. Since ancient times, meat consumption has been a factor differentiating the society and creating a measure of social position. Cultural and religious considerations have always played a significant role in the preparation and consumption of meat products. A product regarded as a delicacy in one cultural group can be considered as inedible in another one. Every human has grown up only after consuming nutrient of animal origin, as babies in uterus; we receive all nutrient of animal origin. It has also been shown that modern disease such as obesity, cancer, diabetes and coronary heart disease were absent in the Paleolithic men who had a high dependence on animal foods rather than on plant foods.

Concerns

The major concerns include microbial contaminants, parasitic infestations, presence of pesticides, hormones, growth promoters and drug residues in meat and their products which may lead to various health hazards. The parasitic diseases including Measly beef (*Cysticercus bovis*), Measly pork (*Cysticercus cellulosae*), ascariasis etc are very important. The recent outbreaks of Bovine Spongiform Encephalopathy (BSE) in cattle and Avian Influenza in chicken with the suspicion that it might be transmitted to human beings through affected meat. The major concerns in relation to meat quality are listed below:

Microbial Contaminants

Among food borne pathogens, *Salmonella* and *Campylobacter* are the most serious. These two pathogens are causing as many as 4 million illness and 4000 deaths per year in USA. Epidemiological data in India is still unclear. The most common clinical manifestation is that of acute gastro-enteritis with a short and shelf limiting clinical course. *Escherichia coli* (VTEC; *E. coli* 0157:H7) is an indicator organism showing the unhygienic practices followed during meat processing. It is associated with infant diarrhoea, hemorrhagic colitis, thrombotic-thrombolytic purpura, and haemolytic uremic syndrome in human.

Other important pathogenic bacteria associated with food safety issue is *Listeria* and coagulase positive *Staphylococcus*. Listeriosis can occur in healthy adults and children, however, the most vulnerable groups include pregnant women, infants, elderly and immunocompromised persons. The common symptoms include involvement of central nervous system, pneumonia endocarditis, localized abscess, skin lesions or conjunctivitis with high mortality rate, whereas *S. aureus* is responsible for a variety of pyogenic skin diseases in man.

Microbial toxins *e.g.* mycotoxin Aflatoxin B_1 the most important mycotoxin may cause mutagenic, carcinogenic, teratogenic or hepatotoxic effect.

Pesticide Residues

Among all residues, pesticides receiving most interest worldwide in recent years due to its wide spread use in meat and poultry production systems, their persistence in environment, and varying toxicity. The acute and malicious consumption involving higher dose results in death whereas, chronic insidious intake lead to elevated cancer risk and disruption of body's reproductive, immune, endocrine, and nervous system. The carcinogenicity of organochlorine (OC) pesticides such as DDT is well known. DDT and its metabolites inhibited gap-junctional intracellular communication. Pesticides can suppress immune system,

Drug Residues

The exposure of veterinary drug residues to the consumers is very common through injectables or feed ingredients to the food animals. The overuse of antimicrobials such as tetracyclines, sulfonamides, amino glycosides, β-lactam derivatives etc. in animal production or their residues in food system pose potential allergic reactions in sensitized individuals, but sub therapeutic and therapeutic levels may perturb human gut micro flora. Immuno-depression and phototoxicity may also occur in animals and human beings. Therefore, the requisite withdrawal period is necessary for the food animals are being sent to the slaughter house.

Similarly, uses of hormonal compound as growth promoter, beta-adrenergic agonist (clenbuterol, salbuterol, cimeterol)in meat production system known to have strong carcinogenic effects and are banned from use for food producing animals.

Heavy Metals Residues

The health implications from heavy metals lead to kidney damage, cardiovascular diseases, induction of hypertension, growth inhibition, interference in haeme synthesis, irreversible changes in brain and nerve cells and also some of these residues are known to be carcinogenic in nature. The pulmonary and nervous systems and skins are the main target organs of arsenic contamination. Cadmium associated with kidney damage and Lead considered being associated with learning deficits in children. Copper and zinc are essential micronutrients but in higher amount may impact metallic taste to the product resulting unacceptability of the product.

Chapter 7

General Quality Characterization and Evaluation of Meat and Meat Products

I. Discolouration Problem in Meat and its Prevention

Introduction

Color is the single most important factor of meat products that influences consumer buying decision and affects their perception of the freshness of the product. Knowing the factors that affect color is important to understanding problems when they occur. Everyone dealing with meat products should have a working knowledge of the color.

What is Discolouration?

Discoloration usually is due to the presence of metmyoglobin, which contributes brown or grayish-brown color to fresh and processed meat. The brown color is detectable when approximately 60 per cent of myoglobin is in metmyoglobin form. Metmyoglobin formation is accelerated by conditions that cause denaturation of the protein portion of myoglobin, and by oxidation under conditions of low oxygen tension. Factors causing denaturation of the protein portion of myoglobin include heat, salts, ultraviolet light, low pH, and surface dehydration. Oxygen tension is increased at meat surfaces by low temperatures, as in refrigerated storage, because oxygen-using enzymes surviving in meat are suppressed.

Discolouration due to Microbial Changes

1. Green Discolouration

Bacteria causing green discoloration in raw meat include *S. putrefaciens* and *Proteus vulgaris*, and *Lactobacillus* and *Leuconostoc sp*.

2. Pink Discolouration

In processed and vacuum-packaged meats -pink discoloration of microbial origin in cooked meat product can be due to psychrotrophic *Clostridia*. In addition to the pink discoloration, a strong hydrogen sulphide odor is produced. The combined offensive odor and internal pinkness results in product rejection.

3. Orange and Yellow Pigmentation

This is mainly due to *Flavobacterium*.

4. Black Spots

This is mainly reported due to meat spoilage by mold- *Cladosporium herbarum*.

5. White Spots

This is due to molds such as *Sporotricus* and *Geotrichus*.

6. Red to Orange Pigmentations

This is due to bacteria such as *Serratia* (red), *Halococcus* (red to orange) and *Halobacterium* (pink, red and orange)

Prevention

1. Control of the relative humidity in chill rooms, *i.e.* by reducing the water activity can reduce bacterial spoilage.
2. A reduced oxygen partial pressure in the vicinity of stored meat is of value in curtailing spoilage, as is increased partial pressure of carbon dioxide.
3. In recent years attempts have been made to counter the adverse action of spoilage bacteria by the use of irradiation, mainly with gamma rays. Using a dose of about 0.1 Mrad immediately before shipping, the storage life of carcass under refrigeration has been prolonged and Salmonellae eliminated.
4. Proper controls for cooking.
5. Proper layout of the production facility to separate raw meat processing areas from cooking, chilling, storing and packaging areas can virtually eliminate the risk of recontamination by microorganisms.

Pale Soft Exudative (PSE) Meat

PSE in pigs is caused by severe, short-term stress just prior to slaughter, for example during off-loading, handling, holding in pens and stunning. Here the animal is subjected to severe anxiety and fright caused by manhandling, fighting in the pens and bad stunning techniques. All this may result in biochemical processes in the muscle in particular in rapid breakdown of muscle glycogen and the meat becoming very pale with pronounced acidity (pH values of 5.4-5.6 immediately after slaughter) and poor flavour. This type of meat is difficult to use or cannot be used at all by butchers or meat processors and is wasted in extreme cases.

Prevention

Allowing pigs to rest for one hour prior to slaughter and quiet handling will considerably reduce the risk of PSE.

Dark Firm and Dry (DFD) Meat

This condition can be found in carcasses of cattle or sheep and sometimes pigs and turkeys soon after slaughter. The carcass meat is darker and drier than normal and has a much firmer texture. The muscle glycogen has been used up during the period of handling, transport and pre-slaughter and as a result, after slaughter, there is little lactic acid production, which results in DFD meat. This meat is of inferior quality as the less pronounced taste and the dark colour is less acceptable to the consumer and has a shorter shelf life due to the abnormally high pH-value of the meat (6.4-6.8). DFD meat means that the carcass was from an animal that was stressed, injured or diseased before being slaughtered.

Prevention

Animals should be given minimum period rest before slaughter as per the species requirements. Pre-slaughter stress to the food animals should be avoided.

Discouration due to pH

If meat is very dark, it will have a high pH, likewise, if meat is very light, it will have a low pH. The pH of boneless-skinless broiler breast meat is determined by how much glycogen is in the breast muscle prior to slaughter and how rapidly the remaining glycogen is converted to lactic acid after slaughter. Fletcher (1995) reported that there was considerable variation of pH among breast meat fillets collected from commercial processing facilities. He also noted that there was a direct correlation between the color of the breast fillets and the pH of the meat.

Prevention

Pre-slaughter stress should be avoided and proper rest should be given.

Discouration due to Temperature

The Canadian Meat Packers Council recommends that internal meat temperatures should not exceed 39° F or 4° C, and other studies have suggested that the optimal storage temperature for meat is just below the freezing point. Psychrotrophic bacteria are capable of multiplying in refrigerated atmospheres between 26° F to 41° F (-3° C to 5° C) and grow at optimal rates at 68° F to 86° F (20° C to 30° C), but their growth can be restrained by keeping meat at 29° F or -1° C, which is also cold enough to prevent the growth of food-borne pathogens. The density of the meat prevents it from freezing at these temperatures, and though bacteria can grow at -3° C or colder, they grow much more slowly at cold temperatures. Even small increases of a degree or two can result in an enormous increase in bacterial growth.

For example, raising the temperature from -1.5° C to 2° C can cut the shelf life of meat in half. Bacteria on meat that is kept at 41° F or 5° C grows at twice the rate of bacteria on meat kept at 33.8° F or 1° C, and at 50° F or 10° C the rate of bacterial growth is triple. Temperature has an even more profound effect on the spoilage rate of meat. Beef at 5° C spoiled three times faster, and beef at 10° C spoiled five times faster, than beef stored at 0° C. High meat surface temperatures not only encourage psychrotrophic bacteria to grow exponentially, accelerating the rate of discoloration and spoilage, but also provide ideal conditions for the growth of food borne pathogens such as Salmonella.

Prevention

1. Shelf life can be lengthened by controlling the temperature of the meat and by improving sanitation as the meat is being processed.
2. While moving the meat to coolers overnight where they can be stored at 1° C will extend the shelf life of the meat to 5 days, this may not be worth the added labor costs and loss of refrigeration cooler space

Iridescence in Processed Meat Products

Iridescence is a common problem in sliced roast beef and ham products. The iridescence of meat products is produced by a combination of the angle of incidence of the light on the muscle fibers and the wetness of the surface. If the fibers are pulled slightly out of alignment during slicing, the light strikes the fiber at an angle scattering light which appears as the rainbow or greenish color on the surface of the meat.

Prevention

Addition of phosphate seems to exacerbate the problem by increasing the amount of water that is retained by the product.

Freezer Burn

Freezer burn is a condition that occurs when frozen food has been damaged by dehydration and oxidation, due to air reaching the food. It is generally induced by substandard (non-airtight) packaging. It appears as grayish-brown leathery spots on frozen food, and occurs when air reaches the food's surface and dries out the product. This can happen when food is not securely wrapped in air-tight packaging. Color changes result from chemical changes in the food's pigment. Although undesirable, freezer burn does not make the food unsafe. It merely causes dry spots in foods.

The condition is primarily caused by sublimation. Water evaporates at all temperatures, even from what appears to be solid ice. In meats, air can cause fats to oxidize. This process occurs even if the package has never been opened, due to the tendency for all molecules, especially water, to escape solids via vapor pressure. Fluctuations in temperature within a freezer also contribute to the onset of freezer burn because such fluctuations set up temperature gradients within the solid food and air in the freezer, which create additional physical motivation for water molecules to move from their original positions.

Prevention

1. It is possible to slow down freezer burn by filling plastic containers with water (leaving room for expansion) and leaving them open in the freezer to help maintain humidity.
2. Proper packaging can also help delay freezer burn because small, air-tight packaging allows local homeostasis of humidity, and, to a lesser degree, temperature.
3. Meats stored in a manual defrost freezer will last longer than those stored in automatic defrost freezers. That is because the temperature of a manual defrost freezer remains closer to 0 °F/-18 °C while the temperature of automatic defrost freezers fluctuates.

Discouration due to Carbon Monoxide

Carbon monoxide combines with natural pigments in meat to produce a dark red color in raw and cooked meat. Small amounts of the gas may come from dry ice, or carbon dioxide freezer tunnels used in hamburger production and it will affect color. Carbon monoxide, which has a greater affinity for myoglobin than oxygen, binds almost irreversibly to the raw color pigment. Research has shown that if CO is used in modified atmosphere packages a dark red color develops and it remains after cooking.

Prevention

Avoid use of CO for packaging. Safe gas like Nitrogen can be used.

Drying Out

Drying of the meat surface affects the way that light is reflected and absorbed. The drier the meat surface, the greater the reduction in reflected light. During drying, the concentration of meat pigment increases at the surface and produces a darkening effect. Drying out also leads to increased brown pigment formation. This darkening, due to dehydration, can often be seen on the cut surface of the topside on sides of chilled beef.

Two-Toned (Pale and 'Dark') Meat

In two-toned meat there are undesirable gradations in meat colour within a cut, with the deep meat tissue being paler than the normal red meat closer to the surface. Pale coloured meat will discolour more quickly than normal-coloured meat in the presence of oxygen because of the effect on its enzyme system and the faster progression of the metmyoglobin reaction. The two-tone effect is sometimes evident in beef (particularly heavy carcasses), but is not seen in small stock carcasses to any extent because of their more even chilling rate. The paleness causes a ring effect in the meat, sometimes called a **'heat ring** and is due to the comparatively slow cooling of the deep meat compared to that of the surface meat. The undesirable paleness leading to two toning is due to denaturation of meat proteins at relatively high temperatures (30-40°C) and acidity resulting from the natural development of lactic acid during the early stages of rigor mortis (acid production is also faster at higher temperatures). The paleness normally occurs in the deep muscle where slower chilling conditions are experienced.

Prevention

1. Electrical stimulation tends to even up the colour, making it more uniform, and lighter.
2. Fast chilling of hot, heavy beef sides after slaughter gives more evenly coloured meat, and firmer muscles. It also minimizes the subsequent unsightly weep (drip) in display or vacuum packs that might lead to customer complaints.

Browning

Browning of meat stored in a vacuum package indicates that there is too much oxygen in the pack. This occurs fastest at moderate (1 per cent) level. If there are poor seals, punctures, or poor air evacuation at the time of packing and sealing, the meat will turn brown during storage. The oxygen permeability of the films used for vacuum packing is also very important and is a matter to which the packer should pay close attention.

Prevention

1. To prevent oxygen from gaining access to the meat surface, care is needed to ensure that the appropriate degree of impermeability is chosen.
2. Meat should be packed and sealed as quickly as possible after boning or cutting the carcass, provided that the carcase deep muscle temperature is adequately reduced.
3. Efficient refrigeration during chilling, holding, transportation, storage, preparation and display; and proper hygiene, packaging and selection of meat.

References

1. http://books.google.co.in/books?id=NHN25jAMwo8C and pg=PA83 and dq=Flavobacterium-yellow+pigments+in+meat
2. http://books.google.co.in/books?id=KPi6XkazZYIC and pg=PA346 and dq=Flavobacterium-yellow+pigments+in+meat
3. http://www.google.co.in/url?sa=t and source=web and cd=1 and ved=0CBYQFjAA and url=http%3A%2F%2Fen.engormix.com%2FMA-poultry-industry%2Fnews%2Fbreast-meat-low-can
4. http://www.google.co.in/url?sa=t and source=web and cd=1 and ved=0CBYQFjAA and url=http%3A%2F%2Fen.wikipedia.org%2Fwiki%2FFreezer_burn

5. http://www.google.co.in/url?sa=t and source=web and cd=2 and ved=0CCIQFjAB and url=http%3A%2F%2Fwww.promolux.com%2Fenglish%2Fretail_meat_color.

6. http://www.google.co.in/url?sa=t and source=web and cd=4 and ved=0CDIQFjAD and url=http%3A%2F%2Fonlinelibrary.wiley.com

7. http://www.google.co.in/url?sa=t and source=web and cd=9 and ved=0CEkQFjAI and url=http%3A%2F%2Fanimalrange.montana.edu%2Fcourses%2Fmeat%2Fmeat_color.

II. Fat Oxidation Problems

The reaction of unsaturated components of fats with oxygen is one of the most important reactions in lipid chemistry. This reaction is responsible for the development of odours and flavours of rancidity and reversion. Oxidation takes place with oxygen in the air under the influence of heat, light, high energy radiation and various prooxidant catalysts. Oxidation also takes place with peracids hydrogen peroxides, ozone, nitrite acid, permanganate chronic acid and many other agents.

Among the many reactions with oxygen, auto-oxidation is one of the most important and has received a great amount of attention. It was earlier observed that when fats and oils became rancid peroxides were developed to a varying degree. Careful study revealed that these were primarily hydroperoxides (00Ḣ) and are found on the carbon atom adjacent to a double bonded carbon atom in a fatty molecule. It has been generally agreed that canto-oxidation proceeds by a free radical chain machinery. The imitation reaction is believed to be one in which oxygen reacts first at the double bond to form a biracial.

The biradical thus formed then combines with the hydrogen of methylenic group adjacent to a double bond in another molecular to yield two/radicals:

These radicals continue the chain reaction, which leads to formation of α-methylenic hydroperoxides.

The auto-oxidation process may be represented most simply by the following equations:

$$R\bullet + O_2 \longrightarrow ROO\bullet$$

$$ROO\bullet + RH \longrightarrow ROOH + R\bullet$$

Where RH = USFA etc. the reactions which form ROO• and ROOH tend to be self-perpetuating and are termed the propagating steps of auto-oxidation. The terminating steps results in insert products and determine the length of the reaction chain.

The hydrperoxides formed are composed of methylene-interrupted polyenes for the most part are on a carbon atom to or conjugated double bond system. There is abstraction of a hydrogen from the methyl group between two double bonds. A resonance hybrid results, in which the bonding tendencies favour a shifting of the double bonds to the more stable conjugated system, leaving the terminal carbon from one of the initial double bonds with the unpaired electron, thus providing site at which the oxygenation takes place. A similar explanation can be made for the formation of the 8,9,10 and 11 hydroperoxidooleates when oleic acid or its esters undergo auto-oxidation.

The positional shift of the double bonds during hydroperoxidation is generally accompanied by geometric isomerization of the double bond. The double bonds is oleic acid are cis but those in hydroperoxidooleates are predominately trans in configuration.

The hydroperoxides are quite stable at low temperatures but are readily decomposed at temperatures above. 80°C. the decomposition products found in auto-oxidized fats are many and complex. The most commonly found products are the shorter chain aldehydes resulting from scission and the acids from further oxidation of the carbonyl formed. This further oxidation to acid and the scission of hydroperoxides is favoured by the presence of certain pro-oxidant metals such as iron, copper, cobalt manganese etc. these multivalent metals through electron transfer act as peroxide decomposer and acetate the rate of auto-oxidation by producing an increased no. of radicals for reaction in the auto-oxidizing fat system.

Anti-oxidants

Anti-oxidants that delay or prevent rancidity of fats caused by oxidation react with the chain-carrying free radicals to form inert products in one of the termination steps. Peroxy radicals ROO probably predominate in this termination step since hydrocarbon free radicals react very readily with molecular O_2. Anti-oxidants are substances capable of slowing the rate of oxidation in anti-oxidizable materials.

Features of an Anti-oxidants

- ✰ Effective at low conc.
- ✰ No undesirable characteristics to the system in which it is used,
- ✰ Convenient and safe to handle
- ✰ Low in cost.

Mode of Action

Antioxidants may terminate oxidative chain reactions by (1) donating an electron to a peroxy radical ROO· (2) donating a hydrogen atom to a peroxy radical (3) adding to a peroxy radical before or after being partially oxidized. (4) possibly involve hydrocarbon radicals instead of peroxy radicals.

The antioxidants used in food fats have the ability to survive baking or frying operations and provide improved keeping quality *e.g.* Gum guaiac, gamma-tocopherol have carry through effect during processing.

Nordihydro guaiacetic acid, n-propyl gallate = limited carry through Butylated hydroxyanisole (BHA) – best carry through – is a mixture of the isomers 3-t-butyl 4-mothoxypheol and 2-t-butyl-4 methoxy phenol.

Butylated hydroxyl toluene (BHT) – second only to BHA, carry through – 2, 6 – t-butyl-4methoxyphenol. A combination of antioxidants is frequently used in food fats. Numerous combinations of BHA, BHT, n-propyl gallate, and citric acid are available commercially BHT was found to synergize with propyl gallate to produce the best all-round antioxidant. The mixture of BHA and BHT produced the best carry through stability in lard, particular when high temperatures were used. Antioxidants combinations which include propyl gallate are generally used in fats subjected to long storage period.

Disadvantage: Propyl gallate reacts with soluble iron to form blue and black discoloration so economic loss in fatty foods, use of metal scavengers, such as citric acid prevent these discolourations.

Ascorbic acid, citric acid: act as synergists with phenol-antioxidants – chelate metals, such as copper and iron that catalyze auto-oxidation of fats. Trace metals promote the first oxidative changes *e.g.* Reverted, tallowy, beany, metallic etc. Phosphoric Acid: reacts with fatty peroxides to form dark phosphorus containing polymeric precipitates.

Spices: can also act as free radical acceptors to retard the off-flavour. Radiation induced auto-oxidation of methyl linoleate – best antioxidants are tocopherol and BHT.

Auto-oxidation

Auto-oxidation *i.e.* lipid oxidation in muscle food is one of the major degradative processer responsible for loss in quality. Auto-oxidation leads to formation of short chain aldehydes, ketones, fatty acids and some polymers, all of which are believed to contribute the oxidized flavour in meat. The important lipids involved – oleic, linoleic, linolenic; rate of oxidation; degree of unsaturation of fatty acid.

Mechanism

Free radical chain mechanism, simple pathways reactions given earlier. When two double bonds are separated by one or more methylene groups, the UFA is unconjugated; when they are adjacent and separated by one single bond the unsaturation is called conjugated.

$-CH = CH - CH_2 - CH = CH -$ Unconjugated

$CH_2 - CH = CH - CH = CH$- Conjugated

The conjugated form is the more stable configuration and the reaction is irreversible – strong characteristic of U-V absorption and basis for spectrophotometric determination of unsaturated Fatty Acids.

- ☆ (OOH) hydroperoxides are stable at low temp., readily decomposed above 80°C (176°F) – decomposed products are short chain aldehydes, acids from further oxidation of carbonyls. Scission of OOH – by peroxidants catalysts Fe, Co.
- ☆ Formation of Malonaldelyde in Auto-oxidation reaction, is a three carbon dialdehyde.

Unsaturated FA are mostly found in phospholipids, so phospholipids are important in rancidity in meat. Phosphotidyl ethanolamine (PE) exerts a more pro-oxidants effects than phosphotidyl choline (PC).

Warmed Over Flavour (WOF) in Meat

- This is oxidized flavour of meat.
- Phospholipids (PL) the major contributor in turkey, chicken, beef, lamb
- Total lipids important role in pork.
- PL readily oxidized due to high UFA
- Both Mb and Fe++ accelerate the oxdn. Of PE
- Turkey most susceptible to WOF followed by chicken pork, beef and mutton in decreasing order.
- Red muscle more susceptible WOF than white muscle.

III. Taste and Olfaction

Sensation of Taste

The word "taste" means not only sensory response to soluble materials in the mouth but also aesthetic appreciation. Hollingrowth and Poffenberger (1917) noted that the words for the other senses are also employed figuratively, "odorous" for something reprehensible, "vision" for something impersonal and intuitive "touch" for an expression of sympathy or pity and "warmth" or "chill" for a depth of emotion. "Taste" is reserved for judgements involving harmony, especial fitness, critical capacity or quality in general.

From the view point of the food processor and food scientist, the sense of taste commands interest because of its role in food recognition, selection and acceptance in addition to its pleasurable aspects.

Taste or some aspects of it, is very important for lower animals life in the ocean, the chemical senses functions as warning and as feeding mechanisms. Moncrieff (1951) devotes an entire chapter to chemicals sensibility in sea animals, insects, birds, reptiles and non- human mammals. Apparently as land animal developed, taste became secondary to smell. The importance of taste in rats has been stressed by Harlow (1932) who showed that complete removal of the olfactory bulbs did not result in any dietary deficiencies whereas presumably removal of the taste buds would. For man, both taste and smell contribute to the enjoyment of food.

Aristotle defined taste as one of the five senses. According to Boring (1942), the various forms of papillae are considered to be the organs of taste. Taste is initiated by contact of an aqueous solution of a chemical with the taste buds on the surface of the tongue and the adjacent regions of the mouth and throat. In this, taste, differs from smell, which reacts primarily to chemicals in gases.

Experimentally, the taste sense can be demonstrated by plugging the nose and keeping the taste-temperature of the test-substance at body temperature. Dilute taste-substances affect the tongue whereas stronger solutions elicit sensations of pain and sharpness in all parts of the mouth including the tongue.

The sense of taste has been approached from three directions: behavioural, electro-physiological and molecular (Beidler,1952). Behavioural responses constitute the main volume of studies made to date and have provided useful information on palatability. Increasing numbers of electrophysiological studies have yielded results of great utility in elucidating the nature of the gustatory process. Molecular approaches are still in their infancy.

The salivary glands are important in tasting particularly in dissolving or diluting tasteful substances and carrying them to the receptors. Saliva also buffers acids and helps control temperature by means of the relatively high specific heat content of the water component (Beidler, 1962). Saliva is secreted by three pairs of glands the parotid, submaxillary and sublingual reinforced by numerous small buccal glands. In the parotid saliva is wartery, and has a high digestive power, whereas the secretions from the other glands are more viscous and higher in mucin. The rather high potassium content has been suggested as a sensitizer of taste receptions. Thiocyanate ion, which is present in relatively high concentration in saliva, has been shown by Ehrenberg and Guttes (1949) to raise the threshold for sweet and decrease that for bitter. Chewing stimulates salivary secretions as do stimuli brought about by the thought, sight or odour of food. Chouncey and Shannon (1959) indicated that the rate of salivary secretion was a liner function of the log of the of the bolus volume of the masticating stimuli. More work is needed on the enzyme functions and the effect of the composition of the saliva on taste responses. Human salt thresholds have been found to reflect the state of adaptation to salivary sodium (MC Burney and Pfaffman, 1963). Bartoshuk *et al.* (1964) demonstrated that the tongue could be adapted to various concentration of sodium chloride. Adapting solutions became tasteless; solutions weaker than the adapting concentration tasted sour or bitter and stronger solutions were sweet or salty.

The tongue itself probably facilitates tasting by its muscular movements which bring the taste materials into contact with the taste buds. The movement of the tongue also constantly disturbs concentration gradients near the receptors and thus tends to prevent adaptation to a given stimulus intensity.

I. Anatomy

According to Boring (1942) the raised portions to tongue, the papillae were selected as the organs of taste. In 1803 Charles Bell demonstrated that the tongue was insensitive to taste in the regions where there were no papilla; gustatory sensibility was confined mainly to the tip and edges and was absent in the middle of tongue.

Four kinds of papillae are found on the human tongue: foliate, circumvallate fungiform, and filliform. Filliform papillae evenly distributed on the anterior two thirds of the tongue, are the most numerous but have no taste buds. Fungiform papillae, large and round and mushroom like in appearance (0.8-1.0 mm in diameter and 1.0-1.5 mm high) are greater in number at the tip and sides of the tongue. They are scattered over the anterior two thirds of the tongue. It is estimated that they number 150 to 400. The foliate papillae on the posterior third of the tongue (in folds on the sides) are not well developed in man and have little functions. The circumvallate papillae form a V-shape on the back of the tongue. There are usually 6 to 15 of these are present. They are large, 2mm high 1-1.5mm in diameter and 1-1.5mm deep) and easily visible. The name arises from their shape-a small mound sorrounded by a ditch. With age the number of papillae varies, becoming less in number and more restricted in distribution.

In adults, the taste buds containing the receptors are located mainly in depressions or moats of the papillae except for the fungiform type, but in children they may also be found in the chicks. A few are found on the larynx and pharynx. Besides the taste buds in the papillae, there are a few in the mucosa of the soft palate and in children on the sides and even roof of the mouth. Henning (1924) suggested that taste buds occur even in the nose. The taste buds of the fungiform papillae occur on their upper surface whereas those of the foliate and circumvallate papillae occur on their grooves. According to Beidler (1962) the taste stimulus is apparently "carried down into the grooves by convection forces exerted by the contraction and expansion of the grooves due to the dynamics of the musculature of the tongue". According to Heiderich (1906), the number of taste buds per papille in the human varies from 33 to 508 averaging about 250.

The taste buds also called "taste beakers" or "taste onions". The term taste beaker arose from their resemblance in form to a modern brandy snifter, the taste onion term refer to the spindle shaped cells bulging out at the root and coming together at the taste pore, very much like the petals of a bud. Each bud contains a number of taste cells 5 to 18 together with other cells, which may be immature taste cells. Human taste buds are about 0.07mm long and 0.05mm wide at their widest diameter. Within the taste buds are sustentacular cells and gustatory cells (or a mixture of the two in a transitional state from one to the other) arranged to enclose a small chamber *i.e.* grouped together into a budlike structure.

Murray and Murray (1960) found only one type of gustatory cell in the taste buds of rhesus and cynomolgus monkeys. Beidler (1960, 1961a) reported that the cells had a relatively brief life. From each receptor cell a fine hair was believed to project into the chamber and above its inner surface. Since these have not been observed with electron microscopy, Beidder (1961b, 1962) believes they were artifacts, noting, however, that the apical processes of many of the cells of the taste bud bear numerous microvilli each of which is about 2μ long and 0.12μ wide and extends into the taste pore. The microvilli could facilitate rapid absorption of the taste substances.

The taste bud is innervated by myelinated nerve fibers, arising from the subepithelial plexus which wind around the taste cells and terminated in knoblike projections on the cell. About two nerves innervate each taste bud of a fungiform papilla. For example, the intact tympani of the cat contained 1955 sensory and motor axons and that of the dog 3347 of these respectively 1157 and 2205 were sensory axons. The majority of the sensory and motor axons. The majority of the sensory and motor axons in these cases are myelinated.

For gustation according to Erickson (1958) there is chain of three stages of neurons from the periphery to the cortex. The first order neurons originate in the tongue and terminate in the second-order neurons presumably terminate in the thalamus on the third-order neurons which end on the neurons in the cerebral cortex. Krarup (1959) indicated that in all cases the taste filers from the anterior part of the tongue have the following course: lingual nerve chorda tympani, facial nerve and intermedius of Wrisberg.

Cutting the nerve connections results in degeneration of the whole bud. The unusual properly of the end organs of the taste is that the nerve fibers regenerate and new taste buds are formed from epithelial tissue. Beidler (1962) noted that human sensory nerve induces epithelial cells to form taste cells.

The anterior two thirds of the tongue and the filliform and fungiform papillae are innervated by a portion of the nervus intermedius division of the seventh cranial (facial) nerve. These taste fibers branch away from the lingual nerve to become a part of the chorda tympani nerve; which then passes through the middle ear and enters the brain stem as a part of the seventh cranial nerve. The posterior third of the tongue and the foliate and the cercumvallate papillae are innervated by the glossopharyngeal (ninth cranial) nerve. In some individuals taste sensations may be conveyed almost completely by the seventh cranial nerve. Halpern (1959) reported that chemical stimulation of the anterior portion of the tongue yielded the same overall response functions in both the chorda tympani nerve and medulla oblogata. Posterior tongue stimulation with quinine hydrochloride gave large bulbar response than did sodium chloride stimulations. The vagus nerve may receive a few taste fibers from the epiglottis and pharynx. The nerve pathways for taste have also been determined from intracranical division of isolated cranial nerves in humans. The trigeminal nerve (fifth cranial) is not involved since its cutting does not affect taste. Cutting of the sensory portion, nervus intermedius of the facial nerve, so as to control facial too, results in complete and permanent abolition of taste sensation from the anterior two thirds of the tongue.

In the brain the region of the cortex of the operculum, insula and supratemporal planes of the temporal lobe are involved in taste but there is no special primary cortical receiving zone with exclusive gustatory functions. The medulla oblongata and the thalamus are also involved.

There are only four basis tastes, but that these four, at least appears to be distinct from each other. In general, sweet and salt are best tasted at the tip of the tongue. Bitter is best tasted at the back of the tongue. Therefore many substances do not taste bitter until swallowed. The sour taste is best appreciated along the edge of the tongue.

II. Classification of Taste

Odours were confused with taste in the earlier studies. Henning's classical taste prism is given below:

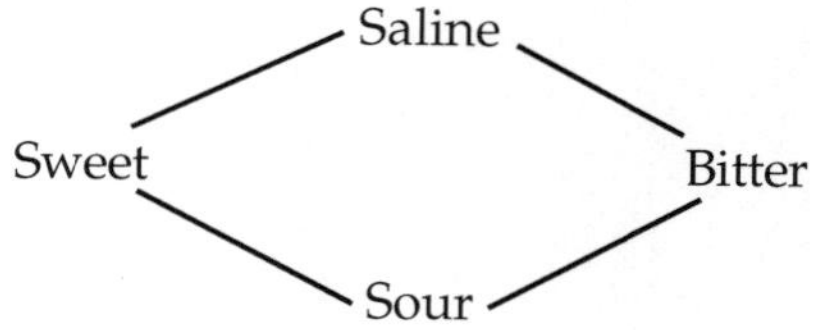

Other tastes have been postulated particularly alkaline and metallic. Probably these sensations are more tactile than taste or at least fusions of taste and touch and possibly of smell. A mixture of conc. solutions of salt and sugar will approximate the alkaline taste. Sour and salt together stimulate the metallic taste.

III. Four Tastes

The number of distinct tastes is very large but many believe they are only combination of four basic tastes. Skramlick (1921) reported that inorganic salt solutions with multiple taste *i.e.* sweet, salty, sour and bitter could be duplicated by suitable mixtures of sucrose, sodium chloride, tartaric acid and quinine. The proportions of the match changed with concentration and varied with the individual.

Wenger *et al.* (1956) gave the following summary of data in favour of four primary taste modalities.

1. Introspective evidence: the ability of normal individuals when deprived of sense of smell to describe their gustatory sensations in terms of these four qualities.
2. Differential distribution of taste qualities on the surface of the tongue. This seems to indicate different sensory systems.
3. Differential effects of narcotics.
4. Fibers sensitives to certain tastes.
5. Interactions of tastes to change each other's threshold. A subliminal concentration of acid on one side of the tongue becomes intensively acid-tasting when other side is coated with a subliminal concentration of sucrose.

In summary, on the basis of recent electrophysiological data, there seems to be the little physiological ordering of chemoreceptors into four catagories and there are unspecific responses where single peripheral gustatory units respond to a variety of compounds. The afferent neural code apparently depends on some sort of patterning of input and this provides a basis for taste discrimination. According to Erickson (1958) discrimination would depend on the relative amounts of activity in several parallel afferent fibers. From a behavioural stand point, however, the four modality classification still appears useful.

The Basic Tastes

Sour

Along with saltiness, sour is considered to be a primitive taste and is a true taste since we can taste concentrations lower than those which affect the common chemical sense. Not all acids are sour: amino acids are often sweet, and picric acid is very bitter. The apparently sour taste of carbon dioxide may be an artifact representing no gustatory sensations.

Table 7.1: Taste Threshold for Selected Acids

	Medium	
Acid	*N*	*per cent*
Hydrochloric	0.0009	0.0033
Nitric	0.0011	0.0069
Sulfuric	0.001	0.0049
Formic	0.0018	0.0083
Acetic	0.0018	0.0108
Butyric	0.0020	0.0176
Oxalic	0.0026	0.0117
Succinic	0.0032	0.0189
Lactic	0.0016	0.0144
Malic	0.0012	0.00905
Tartaric	0.0012	0.00905
Citric	0.0023	0.0152

Source: Pfaffman (1959a).

The reaction time to acid was given as 0.536 sec. by Kiesow (1903) and as 0.3315 sec by Vintschgau and Honigschmied (1877a). Such differences are to be expected with variations in the volumes and concentrations used, the specific portions of the tongue exposed, the temp of the solution and individual variability. The order of intensity of common organic acids is usually given as tartaric, citric, malic, hydrochloric, lactic and acetic but this is subject to various variables. Richards (1898) – weak acids have a lower hydrogen ion concentration and taste less sour. Acetic acid is more sour than hydrochloric acid at the same pH but at the same molar concentration the stimulus is the reverse. Near- threshold equinormal solution of organic and inorganic acids taste equally sour.

Barath and Vandorfy (1926) – The threshold for weak organic acids is about pH 3.7 to 3.9 where as for strong organic acid it is about 3.4 – 3.5. Clendenning (1940a,b,c) claimed that it is possible to raise the pH wit sodium salts and not change the acid taste.

According to Richard's theory the reaction of hydrogen ions at the receptor surface causes the sour taste, and as hydrogen ions are used up more appear from the dissociation of acid. This would indicate that repeated tasting of sub-threshold concentrations of an acid should produce a sour taste. Sugar may enhance or depress sourness. The taste of sourness depends on the pH of the saliva, neural response, speed at which the acid penetrated the cells.

Salty

The saline test is typified by sodium chloride. The chlorides, bromides, iodides, nitrate and sulfates of potassium and lithium are also salty, but usually give a mixed taste. Potassium chloride is salty and bitter. The particular taste depends not only on the salt employed but on its concentration. It can also be shown that it is the ions that give the taste. The anion series of sodium salts is SO_4>Cl > Br > I > HCO_3 > NO_3. Hahn *et al.* (1938) concluded that human threshold for a just perceptible salty taste are about equimolar for all sodium salts.

Table 7.2: Threshold Values for Selected Salts

Substances	*Medium*	
	M	*Per cent*
Lithium chloride	0.025	0.106
Ammonium chloride	0.004	0.021
Sodium chloride	0.03	0.175
Potassium chloride	0.017	0.127
Magnesium chloride	0.015	0.143
Calcium chloride	0.01	0.111
Sodium fluoride	0.005	0.021
Sodium bromide	0.024	0.247
Sodium iodide	0.028	0.420

The saltiness of different salts was found to be additive (Hahn and Ulbrich, 1948). The saline taste of mixtures of various chlorides is reported to have synergistic effect. There is evidence that the degree of saline taste is proportional to molecular weight. The cation strength for chlorides has been variously reported. The generally accepted order is NH_4 > K> Ca> Na > Li> Mg. In electrophysiological study the order of response for carnivorses is NH_4 > Ca > Sr > K > Mg > Na > Li and for rats it is Li > Na > NH_4 > Ca >K >Sr >Mg. Note that sodium is much more effective for rodents than for carnivores, whereas potassium is relatively ineffective for both.

Sweet

The sweet taste is produced by a variety of nonionized aliphatic hydroxyl compounds particularly alcohols, glycols, sugar and sugars derivatives. Electrolytes such as beryllium and some lead salts are sweet and many α- amino acids are also sweet but β and gamma-amino acids are not sweet. β-Glucose derivatives are more bitter than α-glucose derivatives but both are sweet. Saccharin is the best known sweetening agent, being 200 to 700 times as sweet as sucrose. Other sweet substances are dulcin, cyclamate, and 4-alkoxy-3-amino-nitrobenzenes. Dulcin (n p-ethoxyphenyl urea) is over 300 times as sweet as sucrose at low concentration. Many glycols are sweet, erythritol is more than twice as sweet as sucrose. The lower homologs of halogenated hydrocarbons are usually sweet and increasing the no of halogen atoms in the molecule tends to increase the sweetness. Most amides are bitter, but the introduction of groups such as halogen, phenyl or hydroxyl tends to give a sweet taste. A few aldelydes and ketones are sweet. Many esters are sweet, but some are bitter or produce burning sensation. Esters of low mol. wt. alcohols and increasing the molecular weight tends to increase the sweetness. Furane derivatives and nitriles are often sweet. The n-propyl derivative of 4- alkoxy-3-amino nitrobenzene is about 5000 times as sweet as sucrose and is also toxic.

Table 7.3: Threshold for Selected Sweet Compounds

Substances	Median	
	M	Per cent
Sucrose	0.017	0.582
Glucose	0.08	1.442
Saccharin (N)	0.000023	0.00047
Beryllium chlorides	0.0003	0.0024
Sodium hydroxide	0.008	0.0320

The sweetness of a sugar is related in part, to its solubility. The reaction time for sucrose is 0.446 sec. according to (Kiesow 1903) It has been noted that the amount of sugar appears to be related to the blood sugar level. The tasters with blood sugar at a normal level found 30 per cent sucrose sickeningly sweet whereas tasters with blood sugar at one half the normal level found that the same concentration lasted very good. Stress may influence acceptability by changing palatability.

Bitter

The typical bitter stimuli are alkaloids such as quinine, caffeine and strychnine. The bitter taste is often associated with compounds harmful to man. Several electrolytes (magnesium and ammonium salts) are bitter. Salts of cesium or rubidium are bitter, as are iodide salts. Nitro- compounds such as picric acid are often bitter and the bitterness increase as the number of nitro groups increase. Kancko (1939) and Berg (1953) - the L-isomers of the α-amino acids are generally bitter to man. In man, the amino group may obliterate the taste of a bitter substance. If there are enough amino groups to make the compound distinctly. alkaline, the taste is bitter. Most amides are bitter. Glucosides, benzamide and the substituted benzamides are usually bitter. As some aldehydes, ketones, esters, nitriles, isocyananides, urethans, N,N′ hydrazine dicarboxylic acids and substituted benzenes and naphthoisotriazines.

Some compounds are first bitter and then sweet eg. O-benzoylbenzoiac acid, p-aminoazobenzene sulfonic acid, L-leucyl-D-tryptophan and phenolphthalein. Tetrachloroethyl ether and 2,3-dicholoro-hexane are bitter and slightly sweet. Hexenylglycerin is slightly bitter and sweet. Sodium ethyl sulfonate is bitterish and later slightly sweet. Phenyl urea C_6H_5-$NHCONH_2$ is bitter but p-tolylurea p-$CH_3C_6H_4NHCONH_2$ is sweet. Glycol CH_2OH CH_2OH is sweet but phenylglycol C_6H_5 $CHOH$ CH_2OH is bitter.

It is generally considered that bitterness is a taste sensation which can be evoked by the lowest concentrations. Tannins occur frequently in foods imparting bitterness and astringency.

The mechanism of human sensitivity to the bitter taste is not as well understood as that to the other tastes. In fact, tasters often find considerable difficulty in identifying dilute bitter solutions, confusing them with other tastes, particularly sour solutions.

Interaction of Tastes

Although threshold tastes of individual tastes are of interest we seldom encounter this problem in practice. Foods contain two or three or probably all the basic taste. Heymans (1899) showed that the presence of increasing amounts of another taste raised its threshold. Hahn and Ulbrich (1948) observed a reduction in saccharin thresholds by adding to the taste solution subliminal concentration of quinine sulfate, sodium chloride and hydrochloric acid. Hambloch and Puschel (1928) showed that the effect of one taste on another dependent on their relative concentrations. If one component is present in a very much high concentration than other its taste tends to predominate. Bujas (1934) – at low sugar levels, the salt sensibility is increased, higher sugar levels had a reverse effect. Hahn *et al.* (1938) –Previous exposure to a specific salt raised the threshold for that salt but not for the others. Fabian and Blum (1943) studied the competitive and compensatory action that sub-threshold levels of one taste had on supra-threshold levels of another when the two were mixed together. Following observations were mode.

1. Sub-threshold levels of sodium chloride reduced the sourness of acetic, hydrochloric and citric acids moderately and of lactic, malic and tartaric acids markedly.
2. Sodium chloride increased the sweetness of sugars in the order maltose, lactose, fructose, glucose and sucrose.
3. Hydrochloric acid did not influence the taste of sodium chloride. All other acids increased the salty taste.
4. Acids did not influence the sweetness of glucose except hydrochloric and acetic which reduced its sweetness. The sweetness of sucrose was increased by lactic, malic, citric, and tartaric acids, but remained unchanged with HCl and acetic acid.
5. Sugars reduced the salty and sour testes.

Quinine hydrochloride was shown to reduce sweetness Kaman at al.(1961) summarized their results as follows:

1. Caffeine did not affect saltiness and vice versa.
2. Caffeine did not affect sweetness but sucrose depressed bitterness.
3. Caffeine enhanced the effect of salt and vice versa.
4. Salt decreased sweetness but the opposite effect was not found.
5. Salt did not have a monotonic effect on sourness but citric acid increased saltiness.
6. Sucrose decreased sourness but citric acid enhanced sweetness.

Taste Theories

Beidler (1952) suggested that any theory of taste must account for the following:

1. The taste receptors respond rapidly to a chemical stimulus.
2. All substances tasted must be in a liquid soluble form.
3. A variety of substances stimulate the taste receptors.
4. The threshold concentrations for stimulation are not large.
5. Many taste substances are non-physiological *i.e.* they do not result in any rapid deterioration of the receptor cells; this is true of 0.1 M sodium chloride 10 mM strychnine and acids with a pH down to about 2.5.
6. The taste receptor rapidly elicits a steady level of response with a magnitude that is a function of the concentration of the applied substances.
7. The response to many substances remains constant over a long period of adaptation.
8. Receptor stimulation must be followed by electrical depolarization of the nerve membrane and possibly preceded by depolarization of the end organ itself.
9. A water rinse rapidly reduces the taste response.
10. The receptors are the site of the chemical specificity.
11. There are genetic variations in taste ability

To these he added (1962).

1. The taste receptors response of the rat to sodium chloride is almost independent of temperature between 20° and 30° C and of pH between 3 to 11.
2. The presence of saliva is not necessary.
3. Different species reveal different cationic series of taste receptor excitability.

Warfield (1954) – Searched for a molecular factor related to taste. He proposed a **"taste couple" –a proton and a neighbouring unshared electron pair**. This is tentative, needs detail explanation.

Lasareff (1922) - Considered that each receptor was responsive to a single taste, the applied stimulus caused decomposition of a material in the cell. This produced ions which stimulated the nerve endings.

Enzyme Theory

Baradi and Bourne (1953) hypothesized that enzyme activity in the vicinity of nerve fibers produces ionic changes which induce the formation of nerve impulses. The taste substance would inhibit enzymes in some sites, leaving enzymes in other sites unaffected, thereby producing a change in the pattern of impulses reaching the brain. Different tastes could thus be distinguished. However, the enzyme theory would seem to deny the association of gustatory nerve fibers with specific taste sensations. The main criticism is that the magnitude of taste response is fairly independent of temperature whereas enzyme reactions are very dependent on temperature. Although enzymes may not be involved in the initial reaction of the stimulus with the receptor, enzymatic processes are most certainly involved in overall maintenance of the integrity of the receptors.

Beidler's Theory

Beidler (1954) believes that taste sensation is dependent on:

1. The particular types of chemoreceptor that are activated.
2. The magnitude of their response.
3. The pattern of the nerve discharge over each taste nerve fiber.

The different peripheral innervations of the fungiform, foliate and circumvallate papillae suggest that there may be different spatial representations of the taste of chemical compounds on this basis alone (Halpern, 1959). Erickson (1958) believed that first –and second –order neurons did not differ significantly in patterns of sensitivity to chemical stimulation. The distinction between tastes might be due to the number of impulses resulting from discharge, the fibers stimulated and the pattern in time of the discharge.

Another possible theory is that taste substances participate in an adsorption process possibly with proteins at the surface of the receptor. This result in a rapid depolarization of the receptor surface which spreads to the attached nerve fiber and excites it.

Other Theories

Frings (1951, 54) taste spectrum concept- The determining factor in taste quality is thought to depend on;

1. The simulative effectiveness of the substances.
2. The penetration or adsorption of the compound by the receptors. The population of the receptors is variably sensitive to stimulation. with sweet least stimulating, then salt bitter and sour. The receptors are differently susceptible to penetration or adsorption.

Beidler (1961a) favours a biophysical rather than a biochemical explanation of the taste mechanism. Beidler (1962) showed that the number of potential sites on the microvillus of the taste cells is adequate to account for the various types of taste.

IV. Taste Qualities

The four fundamental taste qualities give variable sensations of pleasantness and unpleasantness, depending on concentration. Engel (1928) noted that the pleasantness of sucrose increased as the concentration increased and at a rather high concentration, it decreased slightly. Solutions of sodium chloride, tartaric acid and quinine sulphate increased in pleasantness over a small range of increasing concentration, and then gave an unpleasant sensation. In mixtures of tastes, however pleasantness or unpleasantness is less predictable. If one taste is at or near the threshold and the other very strong, the lesser will not be perceived even by the most sensitive subjects. Likewise, in practices we reduce the strong sensation of one taste with another: salt on melons to reduce the sweet taste, sugar in tea to mollify the bitter taste, sugar in lemonade to ameliorate the sour taste etc. Thus although one taste may modify another, it does not neutralize it.

Contrast phenomenon is also easy to demonstrate with taste. For example, salt on one side of the tongue will cause distilled water on the other side to taste sweet or insipid. Application of salt to one side of the tongue and only a subliminal concentration of sucrose to the other, causes the latter to the easily recognised or sweet or even very sweet. A sugar solution on one side will enhance the saltiness reaction on the other. Salt also sensitizes to salt, bitter has little tendency to contrast with the other tastes.

Bartoshuk *et al.* (1964) showed that subjects adapted to sodium chloride reported weaker sodium chloride solutions tasted sour or bitter and stronger solutions sweety or salty. The taste of water and weak sodium chloride solutions thus depends on prior adaptation. The tongue is normally adapted to saliva which in man contains relatively low concentrations of salt. Thus it is near the lower limit of the adapting level at which it is one reason why water usually tastes flat or nearly tasteless. Bartoshuk *et al.* (1964) attributes the sour-bitter taste of water, after adaptation to sodium chloride to a gustatory after image.

V. Relative Intensity

Lewis (1948) constructed psychological scales of taste intensity. This suggested comparisons of the taste intensity of the different tastes. Beebe Centes and Waddell (1948) used two subjects who could match relative strength of solutions of quinine sulphate, tartaric acid or sodium chloride against 1 per cent sources. In cross-qualitative matching, there was considerable variability. The concentration that matched 1 per cent sucrose was called a "gust". The gust values of compounds at various concentrations is given below:

Table 7.4: Guest Values of Various Compounds

Gust	Sucrose[a]	Quinine Sulfate[a]	Tartaric Acid[a]	Sod. Chloride[a]
1	1.00	0.00020	0.0085	0.30
1-8	1.62	0.00043	0.0142	0.46
3-2	2.76	0.00087	0.0234	0.70
5-6	4.68	0.00174	0.0389	1.15
10.0	8.32	0.00339	0.0661	2.00
18.0	15.50	0.00646	0.118	3.80
32.0	28.80	0.0120	0.209	7.41
56.0	56.20	0.0224	0.407	15.90
100.0	115.00	0.0417	0.794	34.70

a: Concentration in grams per 100cc.

Quinine sulphate alone was predominantly unpleasant at a concentration of 0.0011 per cent which was only 5 gusts, whereas commercial ale had a bitterness of 28.2 gusts. Note that the addition of 5 per cent sucrose raised the sweetness of coffee by only 2.2 gusts but reduced the bitterness by 18.5 gusts. Therefore, it was concluded that sweetness had no advantage over sourness or bitterness in determining acceptability.

Gridgeman (1958) was able to get comparison of relative intensity of sucrose, sodium chloride, citric acid and quinine hydrochloride. His comparison of 1:14:220:2300 is similar to that of Beebe centre even though they used different methods.

VI. Reaction Time

The reaction time to taste *i.e.* the interval between initial stimulations of the receptors and the report of a reaction, was estimated at 0.02-0.06 sec. in electro-physiological studies (Pffafman, 1955). Compared to oral response reaction-times of 0.307 sec. for salt, 0.446 sec. for sweet, 0.536 sec for sour and 1.082 sec. for bitter. Taste has the slowest reaction time as compared other senses such as vision, hearing and touch. The faster the reaction the shorter the persistence. The over-all response depends somewhat on concentration and the stimulus: for sodium chloride 0.370 to 1.007 sec. for citric acid 0.480 to 1.32 sec. the minimum is about 0.25 sec. However Beidler (1953), Pfaffman(1955) and Nejad (1961) reported that the response latency to sodium chloride decreased as the concentration increased.

Bujas and Ostojecic (1939) showed that taste intensity increased rapidly after a sapid solution was applied to tongue. then more slowly and finally showed no further increase. For salty and bitter, the concentration did not influence the maximum intensity attained. For sweet the time to reach max. increased with conc. However, the beginning of a sensation is quicker at higher concentration. The time required to establish a sensation was greatest with bitter and least with salty.

VII. Effect of Disease

Disease and accident may result in ageusia, hypogeusia or parageusia (loss of, decreased or altered taste sensations). These may be temporary or permanent and uni- or bilateral.

The relation of disease to tasting ability has been studied by some workers. They noted that irradiating the side of the tongue of a patient with cobalt source or X rays reduced taste sensitivity to all taste except sour. Recovery took about 2 months. In many individuals the lesions of the fifth cranial nerve reduce or cause a temporary loss of taste sensitivity from the front of the tongue. Taste sensitivity returns after a short or longer period.

In cases of diabetes, a sweet taste may be experienced in the absence of stimuli on the tongue. A bitter taste was reported in the case of jaundice. Bartley (1958) found a tingles and metallic taste at the tip of the tongue within a few seconds of intravenous injections of nicotinic acid. Patients with adrenal insufficiency exhibit increased sensitivity to salt, sweet, bitter and sour tastes. There was a greater sensitivity in patients with cystic fibrosis.

After prolonged vit A depletion, rats showed a decrease in degree of rejection of quinine sulphate solutions. The rejection of sodium chloride increased towards the end of the depletion period.

Sensitivity to citric acid increased with increased ascorbic acid deprivation, sugar in the blood (diabetic or added) reduced sensitivity to sweetness. In pregnant women, citric acid thresholds were also low.

VIII. Taste Thresholds

Measurement of thresholds is the most common procedure for studying the psychologises of taste. The absolute threshold, S_0 or better the absolute limen t_0 is the minimum detectable concentration. The limen is not a sharply defined stimulus increment since subjects vary in sensitivity, the limen can only defined as a statistical measure. The absolute or sensitivity limen is usually set as the stimulus magnitude at which the subject can identify a difference in taste in half of his attempt in a paired test.

The 'recognition' threshold is the concentration at which the specific taste can first be recognized and is higher than the sensitivity threshold concentration.

A. Effect of Sleep and Hunger

Lack of sleep upto 72 hrs did not affect the thresholds to salt and sweet, but lack of sleep for 48 and 72 hrs raised the sour threshold significantly. In studies on hunger by Yensen (1959) sensitivity to the four basic taste qualities was greatest at 11:30 AM. There was a significant decrease in sensitivity for about 1 hour after a meal, followed by an increase in 3 or 4 hrs. The decrease of sensitivity appeared to be related to the caloric value of the meal. Depletion of body salt content increased the sensitivity to salt but did not affect the other taste threshold. Loss of body water caused a decrease in sensitivity to salt but did not affect the sour threshold.

B. Age

The new born apparently have little taste differentiation until about 35 to 40 days. However, response to saltiness has been demonstration in 2 days old children. Ritcher and Campbell (1940a) found a much higher sweet threshold in a 52 to 85 yr group than in a 15 to 19 yr. group. There is decline in taste senstivitity for the basic taste in people having more than 60 yrs. of age. This may be due to degenerative changes in the taste receptors. It has been found that women has higher sensitivity than men for sweet and salty but less for sour and no difference between the sexes for bitterness.

C. Smoking

Smoking may affect taste preferences via the taste mechanism. Krut *et al.* (1961) found no differences between smokers and non-smokers in their thresholds for sweet, sour, or salty but the mean threshold for bitter was significantly ($P<0.001$) higher for smoker. The decrease in sensitivity was progressive with age and thus appears to be the result of prolonged addiction. It was suggested that the nicotine and other alkaloids in cigarette smoke fatigue the mechanisms for perception of bitter. In studies by Sinnot and Rauth (1937), sugar and thresholds were higher among smokers than non-smokers.

D. Other Factors

Henning (1921) reported that taste sensitivity to sucrose was not affected by chronic alcoholism, excessive smoking, badly infected gums, marked tooth decay, mild head colds, hay fever or allergy. Water unless specially purified has a taste (Anderson 1959). Very sensitive persons frequently note a taste or flavour in distilled water. These impurities could influence the results of threshold tests.

IX. Effect of Temperature

The influence of temperature on taste is not uniform. Optimum have been reported of 35-50°C for sucrose and hydrochloric acid, 18-35°C for saltiness and 10°C presumably at or near its threshold concentration. Increasing temperature appears to increase the response to sweet and decrease it to salty and bitter. The effect of temperature requires control of the area stimulated and the rate at which the liquid passes over the tongue.

X. Effect of Taste Medium

Skramlik (1926) noted that the intensity of taste was greater in aqueous media. Crocker (1945) speculated that the physical state of a food influenced taste by partially controlling the quantity of sapid matter reaching the taste receptors in a given time. He further theorized that the viscosity of fluid thickened with algin, gum tragacanth, flaxseed or other source of mucillaginous material interferes with diffusion of soluble substances to the receptors. According to Tritton (1939), pectin depresses free hydrogen ions, thereby reducing apparent sources in food products. The taste thresholds for sucrose, sodium chloride, caffeine and tartaric acid were lower in water solutions than in tomato juice and custard each prepared as liquid, gels and foams (Mackey and Valassi, 1956). Mackey (1958) observed that the tastes of caffeine, quinine and saccharin were more easily detected in water than in mineral oil and theorized that the lipid inhibited the solubility of the taste compounds in saliva. Simon (1962) indicated that, at thresholds concentrations, sensitivity to sodium chloride was lower in agar solutions than in pure water. Conversely at a level of 0.5 per cent sodium chloride, ability to detect differences in saltiness was greater in the ager than in water solutions. Pangborn (1963) observed that on a weight basis, fructose was sweeter than sucrose in water, but the reverse was true when both sugars were compared in pear nectars at various levels of citric acid.

XI. Taste and Chemical Configuration

Taste responses are related to chemical specificity. For example, there are taste difference between o-, m-, and p- tolylurea. The compounds p-anisonitrile is sweet whereas p-ethoxybenzonitrile is bitter. The sterioisomers sorbitol and dulcitol are not equally sweet. Kaneko (1938) found that D-tyrosine compounds were sweet and the L-compounds bitter or disagreeable. The taste was related not to the optical rotation but to the stereo structure. The D-configurations of leucine, isoleucine, valine, histidine, tryptophan and asparagine were sweet, whereas the L-forms were not. Ferguson and

Lawrence (1958) found that isomaltose (6-α-D-glucopyranosyl-D-glucose) was sweet whereas its anomer, gentiobiose (6-β-D-glucopyranosyl-D-glucose) was bitter. Application of enzyme inhibitors, sodum azide, potassium fluoride, sodium iodoacetate and sodium cyanide modified the sweet taste. α-galactose is reported to be sweeter than β-galactose, but β-fructose is sweeter than α-fructose. 5 out of 8 observers found L-mannose less sweet than D-mannose, and L-glucose not sweet but slightly salty. Pangborn and Gee (1961) noted that the α-configuration of galactose was significantly sweeter than the β-forms whereas the reverse was true for fructose and lactose. Steinhardt *et al.* (1962) observed that the α-anomer of D-mannose was sweet whereas β-anomer was bitter. Shallenberger (1963) proposed that the sweetness of sugars is influenced by hydrogen bonding. When hydroxyl groups, which elicit sweet taste, are hydrogen bonded, the ability of the compounds to cause a sweet taste appears restricted. Besides, the other parameters such as resonance energy, vibratory hydrogen, solubility and rate of diffusion into taste bud receptor sites, may also be related to sweetness.

The Sense of Olfaction

Smell is a primitive sense-more primitive than vision and more complex than taste. The sense of smell is more highly developed than the sense of taste. The olfactory organ can detect dilutions of alcohol 24,000 times greater than those required to stimulate the organ of taste. The distribution of olfactory nerve endings in the nose are related directly to the animals position on the evolutionary scale; man's receptor area is restricted to a small portion of the olfactory mucosa, whereas dogs possess highly convoluted turbines which greatly increase the olfactory area.

Importance of Odour

The food industry is particularly cognizant of the importance of odours in the acceptance of various food products since odours can attract or repeal consumers.

Definition: Sagarin (1954) –

Phenomenological Definition – "Odour is the property of substance or substances that is perceived, in the human and higher vertebrates, by inhalation in the nasal or oral cavity that makes an impression upon the olfactory area of the body; and that during and as a result of such inhalation is distinct from seeing, hearing, tasting or feeling and does not cause or result in choking, irritation, cooling, warmth, drying, wetting, or other functions foreign to the olfactory area."

Physiological Definition: Sensations perceived from response of the olfactory nerve or first

Cranial nerve.

Henning believed that all odours would find a place on the surface of the Henning's smell prism.

Schutz (1964)- Identified nine odour factors

1. Fragrant (methyl salicylate)
2. Burnt (guaiacol)

Table 7.5: Odour Classification

Sl.No.	Linnaeus (1752)	Haller (1763)	Zwaardemaker (1895)		Henning (1916)	
			Type	Example	Type	Example
1.	Aromatic	–	Aromatic	Camphor Citral	Spicy	Clove Anisaldelyde
2.	Fragnant	–	Fragnant (balsamic)	Vanillin	Flowers Fragrant	Heliotrope coumarin
3.	Ambrosiac	Sweet or Ambrosiac	Ambrosiac	Musk	Resinous	Pinene Turpentine
4.	Alliaceous	–	Alliaceous	Onion mercaptan	–	–
5.	Hircine	–	Hircine (caprylic)	Strong cheese caprylic acid	–	–
6.	Foul	Stencher	Foul (repulsive)	Some Night shades Bed bug	Putrid (foul)	Hydrogen Sulfide Mercapton
7.	Nauseous	–	Nauseous (faetid)	Faeces skatol	–	–
8.	–	Intermediate	Ethereal	Fruit Acetic acid Amyl ether	Fruit Ethereal	Fruit citral
9.	–	–	Empyreumatic (burned)	Phenol pyridine	–	–

Source: Boring (1942).

3. Goaty or sulfurous (ethyl disulfide)
4. Etherish (1- propanol)
5. Sweet (vanillin)
6. Rancid (butyric acid)
7. Oily (heptanol)
8. Metallic (hexanol)
9. Spicy (benzaldehyde)

Chemical Specificity

Odour is frequently found in compounds containing hydrogen, carbon, nitrogen, oxygen, and sulfur. Some compounds of halogens and of phosphorus, arsenic, selenium, boron, antimony and silicon are also odourous. A chemical entity which confers odour on an otherwise odourless compound is called an osmophoric group. Among the strong osmophores are phosphorus, arsenic, sulfur, selenium, chlorine and bromine. Also good osmophores are carbonyls, esters, amines, imines, and lactones. Henning (1924) believed that spicy odours had the osmophoric group in the para position, flowery odour in the meta position, resinous odours in a position within the ring, burnt odours with a smooth ring, foul odours with a fragmentary ring and fruity odours with a forked ring. Odour intensity increases with increase in the mol. wt. of the chemical compound. The polarity and form of the molecules also seem to influence odour. When isomerism is created by a double bond, the odour of the cis- and trans-isomers is very distinct. The quality and intensity of odour are influenced by the position of the double bond in the molecule, the distribution of electrons, resonance or induction of the molecule and the kind of group adjacent to the osmophore. In general molecules with greater adsorption capacity are more odours.

Anatomy of Olfactory Region

In man, the two nasal cavities are separated by a smooth median septum. The lateral walls of the cavities have a series of folds, approximately horizontal, varying from two to six. The lower folds extends over most of the length of the nasal cavity. The two above this, called conchae are smaller and protrude into the cavities to provide three channels, the inferior, median and superior meatus. Meatus is confluent with a large common meatus, which communicates with the olfactory cleft above the superior concha and the septum. These spaces are all connected by very narrow passages with the posterior naris (choana) and with the pharynx. The upper and lower nasal passage are mere slits nowhere wider than 1-2 mm.

The deeper part of the cavity contains a pseudo-stratified columnar epithelium containing ciliated walls whose cilia beat toward the choana. The cavity also contains many alveolo- tubular glands with mucous cells. The chonchae are very vascular and their edges are erectile and capable of enlargement through reflex excitation.

Only the inner surface of the superior concha and the adjacent outward face of the septum are innervated by the olfactory nerve –about 2.5 cm^2 or 500-625mm^2 in man (max 750mm^2). The olfactory regions contains basal cells sustentacular (supporting) cells, and sensory (olfactory) cells. It is estimated that man has 10 to 20 million such receptors: 100 million for the rabbit. The olfactory epithelium as well as the rest of the nasal surface is also innervated by bare nerve fibers from the trigeminal nerve.

The sensory cells are bipolar neurons with oval shaped cell bodies. The olfactory rod or dendrite extends from the peripheral part of the cell body, ending in a rounded enlargement, the olfactory vesicle. Very thin hair like projections protrude from the vesicle into the mucous. They appear to be 1-2μ long and 0.1μ wide, but a fine process may extend to 100μ and this increase their total surface enormously. Beidler (1961b) noted that the nuclei of the receptors are situated at different depths in the olfactory mucosa, with olfactory rods, 20-90μ long extending to the surface. He and others have suggested that these differences in receptor morphology may be related to differential sensitivity to odours and might be a basis for odour quality determinations. The whole region is covered with secretion from numerous branched alveolotubular glands which contain both mucous and serous cells. The proximal part of the body of the sensory cells tapers down to a fine process which continues as the olfactory nerve fiber and finally terminates in the olfactory bulb.

This chart emphasizes the following aspects:

1. The prospective odourous material must be volatile.
2. The odour laden air must reach the olfactory receptors.
3. Differences in diffusion rates may be a factor in stimulation.
4. The odour must dissolve in aqueous mucous and then diffuse through it.

Neural Mechanisms

Ogasawara (1954) found no discontinuity between the sensory endings in the mucosa and the cell bodies in the bulb. This is at variance with most result, although it is recognized that the connection are very intimate. The fine unmyelinated proximate ends of the olfactory cells are the axons which enter the olfactory bulb. Here the sensory is both the receiver and conductor, *i.e.* a primary neuron. These nerve fibers end in a series of intricate basketlike terminations called glomeruli. These they synapse with the large mitral and the tufted cells. Axons from both types form the olfactory tract which then passes along the base of the frontal lobe. The arrangement in the olfactory bulb of cells and axons provides a convergence of pathways and a return route back to the glomerulus by way of collaterals. Hence there is a sort of closed of reverberating system a " feed batch" and this may partially account for the great sensitivity of the sense of smell. As Ottoson (1963) says " the structural arrangement of the synaptic connection between primary and secondary neurons in separate units represented by the glomeruli may serve an important function in olfactory discrimination. It was suggested that there is a concentration of fibers from functionally similar receptors onto particular glomeruli" However much more evidence is needed on the nature of the " feed back" system.

The olfactory membranes develops a slow, negative, purely, monophasic potential when stimulated by odourous material. A wave like oscillation of 25-30 cycles per second (cps) is a particularly striking features of the olfactory bulb. Olfactory stimulation initiates long or short bursts of activity. The activity seems to arise peripherally rather than within the neuronal network inside the bulb. The mechanism is not yet completely understood.

Olfactory Abnormalities

- ☆ Cryptosmia = obstruction in nasal passage
- ☆ Anosmia = temporary or permanent loss of smelling capacity.
- ☆ Hemianosmia or hyperosmia = excessive response.
- ☆ Merosmia = loss of only certain odours.
- ☆ Heterosmia or in parosmia = false odours perceived
- ☆ Autosmia = odour sensation in the absence of odour stimuli
- ☆ Cacosmia = persistent perception of unpleasant odours.

The above conditions are due to accident in disease, endocrine disorders, congenital and inherited, vitamin A deficiency (rats).

Thresholds

The apparent olfactory threshold for the most powerful odours are about 10,000 times lower than the lowest taste threshold. The variation of threshold of olfactory are due to purity of compounds, external variables (duration and rate of flow of inspired air, prolonged noise, humid/dry conditions, methods of presentation of samples; effect of hunger and chemicals, individual variation (physiological state of the nose, age, hormonal imbalance, occupational effect)

Table 7.6: Recognition Threshold Concentrations of Various Odourous Materials

Substance	*Boiling Point (°C)*	*Mg/lit of Air*
Ethyl ether	35	5.833
Carbon tetrachloride	76.7	4.533
Chloroform	62	3.300
Ethyl acetate	77.4	0.686
Amyl alcohol	137.8	0.225
Nitrobenzene	209.4	0.146
Ethyl mercaptan	37.0	0.046
Methyl salicyllate	222.2	0.100
Pyridine	115.2	0.032
Amyl acetate	148	0.039
Valeric acid	186.4	0.029
Methyl isothiocyanate	119	0.015
Butyric acid	162.3	0.009
Isobutyl mercaptan	88	0.008
Allyl isothiocyanate	151	0.008
Propyl mercaptan	67	0.006
Phehyl isocyanide	165	0.002
Amyl thioehter	95-98	0.001

Source: Allison and Katz (1919)

Table 7.7: Corrected Threshold Concentration from International Critical Tables

Compound	*Nature of Odour*	*Threshold (mg/litre)*
Methyl salicylate	Winter green	0.100
Amyl acetate	Banana oil	0.039
n-Butyric acid	Perspiration	0.009
Benzene	Kerosene-like	0.0088
Safrol	Sassafras	0.005
Ethyl acetate	Fruity	0.0036[a]

Contd...

Table 7.7–*Contd...*

Compound	*Nature of Odour*	*Threshold (mg/litre)*
Pyridine	burned	0.00074[a]
Hydrogen sulfide	Rotten eggs	0.00018
n-Butyl sulfide	Foul, sulfurous	0.00009
Coumarin	New mown hay	0.00002
Citral	Lemon	0.000003
Ethyl mercaptan	Decayed cabbage	0.00000066[a]
Trinitro-tert-butyl xylene	Musk	0.000000075

a: Detection threshold not recognition threshold.

Source: Wenger *et al.* (1956).

Theories of Olfaction

Three main theories have been proposed

1. Direct radiation from the odour
2. Chemical activity as part of reception
3. A radiation mechanism in the olfactory region

The first theory seems impossible since odours travel with the wind and are not transmitted through solids or reflected from mirrors. The others are discussed below.

Any theory for odour must explain a wide variety of conditions. Among these are: need for volatiles, solubility of odourous material in the watery mucous and in the fatty or lipoid ends of the olfactory cells, and some idea of the chemical reactions in the cells. Volatility and solubility in fat solvents seem most important. Moncrieff (1951) suggested the following requirement for any theory of odour:

1. All normal people can smell
2. Anosmia occurs in people with obstructed nasal passage, brain lesions or injured olfactory nerve.
3. The possibility of preferential must be considered.
4. Some substances are odourous others not.
5. We can smell at a distance.
6. Substance with different chemical compositions may have similar odours.
7. Substances with similar compositions usually have similar odours.
8. High mol.wt. substances usually are nonodourous.
9. The quality and strength of the odour may change on dilution.
10. The sense of smell fatigues rapidly.
11. Fatigue for one odour has little effect on perception of dissimilar odours, but interferes with the perception of similar odours.
12. Odours can cancel each other out.

13. Odours travels downwind.
14. Many animals have keener senses of smell than man.

A. Adsorption

Moncrieff (1954 b, 57b) and Davies and Taylor (1957) noted that the olfactory membrane adsorbed odourous material. These was a correlation between the odours of two materials and their relative adsorbance on inorganic adsorbents. Davies and Taylor (1957,1959) showed that olfactory thresholds depended on the adsorption energy of the odourous molecules passing from air to the lipid-aqueous olfactory membranes and on the dislocation of the membrane which is caused by these adsorbed molecules (depends on the shape, size, and flexibility of the odourous molecules). In other words, their basic concept is that odour molecules initiate the nerve impulse by causing localized changes in the cell membrane. Davies (1962) further elaborated this theory, noting that as the olfactory substances penetrates the olfactory nerve cells, a small region of the wall is dislocated. This dislocations allows potassium and sodium ions to move across the membrane, thus initiating the nerve impulse.

B. Physio-chemical

Mullins (1955 b) and Timmermans (1954) considered that olfaction is related to two molecular parameters. **Cohesive energy density** (defined as the energy of vaporization of liquid per unit volume) and **molecular shape** Mullins (1955 a, b) suggested that the olfactory membrane is formed of macromolecular cylinders arranged in a regular hexagonal pattern with pores at the junctions between any three cylinders. Such a membrane should show considerable specificity in terms of interaction between the walls of the pores and the molecules in contact with the membrane Molecular wt., **vapour pressure, lipoid solubility, thermodynamic activity** and other physical parameters have a correlation with the olfactory effectiveness of some compounds, but not of all.

C. Enzyme

Lauffer (1954) believed that adsorption of the **stimulant on the enzyme surfaces of the sensory cell might be a factor**. Kistiakowsky (1950) and Baradi and Bourne (1951a, b) assumed that odourous compounds inhibit the activity of one or more of the enzyme systems in the olfactory regions. This selective inhibition alters the relative concentration of various compounds at the receptors and thus initiates neural response. **Alkaline phosphatase** found in the olfactory and gustatory epithelia was inhibited by vanillin, coffee oil and aniseed, esterase was inhibited by quinine.

D. Absorption

Beck and Miles (1942) revived the old concept that the infrared absorption of a compound was related to its odour. Stereoisomers with identical infrared absorption spectra and differences in odour are known. Not all substances that absorb radiation in the infrared region possess an odour and the theory, therefore, still remains unproven. Ottoson (1956) obtained no odour if the olfactory membrane was covered with a plastic membrane that transmitted infrared radiation within the range supposedly involved. It seems established that **odourant particles must come into direct contact with the olfactory receptors.** Dyson (1928 a, b, 1937) was convinced that the **atomic vibrations within the molecule stimulated the nerve endings directly** . Raman shifts of 1400 to 3400 units were believed to account for all distinctive odours But this was latter challenged by Hallan (1954) and Thompson (1957).

E. Physiological

Adrian (1948) concluded that olfaction is a **"patterned" sense of restricted repertoire**. Different loci of impingement of odourous particles on receptor cells, varying rates of nervous discharge and variable latencies all provide **pattern differentiation**. Different receptors may come into operation at different times according to their chemical affinities and their position on the olfactory surface.

IV. Aroma and Flavour of Meat

Introduction

The flavour of meat is of great academic, as well as practical importance but we are still unable to completely understand this important sensory quality of muscle foods. Flavour is a complex sensation. It involves odour, taste, texture, temperature and pH. Physiologically the perception of flavour involves the detection of four basic sensations *viz.* salty, sweet, sour and bitter by the nerve endings on the surface of the tongue. Aroma is detected when numerous volatile materials stimulate the nerve endings in the lining of nasal passages. Thus the sensations of aroma and flavour are a combination of gustatory (taste) and olfactory (smell) stimulation. Odour probably involves chemical reactions between the molecules and the nerve endings in the taste cells, interpretation of the sensation again being made in the brain. Odour and taste are most difficult to define objectively. The evaluation of odour and taste still depends mainly on taste panel.

Fresh raw meat usually has a very slight odour. The flavour and aroma are more pronounced on cooking the meat. The meaty flavour and the aroma stimulate the flow of saliva and gastric juices, thus aiding in the process of digestion. The odour and taste of cooked meat arise from water or fat soluble precursors and by the liberation of volatile substances, pre-existent in the meat. Precursor studies have shown that proteins per se contribute little to meat flavour, but that amino acids such as cysteine, methionine, phenylalanine, valine, leucine, tryptophan and reducing sugars are important meat flavour precursors. Carbonyl compounds produced due to oxidation of fatty acids are potent flavour contributors. Fat may also act as a storage depot for odoriferous compounds that are released on heating. The volatiles derived from fat may be responsible for the characteristic differences associated with the flavour of beef, pork and lamb. Approximately, more that 600 compounds have been identified in the volatiles derived from beef which are broadly classified as hydrocarbons, aldehydes, ketones, alcohols, acids, esters, ethers, lactones, aromatics, "S" compounds and "N" compounds. Inosine monophosphate (IMP) and hypoxanthines enhance the flavour or aroma. These are the breakdown products of Adenosine triphosphate (ATP). It is obvious that muscle with large energy stores would have a more pronounced flavour, *e.g.* strong flavour of game animals. Besides there are many types of undesirable flavours of meat encountered in different conditions are summarized in Table 7.1.

The factors affecting the meat flavour and aroma are broadly divided into preslaughter and post slaughter factors.

A. Pre slaughter Factors

1. **Species:** Among various pre slaughter factors, species of the animal from which the meat is derived plays an important role in determining its flavour. Perhaps this is due to variation in the muscle composition and flavour precursor substances present. There is not much difference in the flavour of cooked beef, lamb and pork when only lean meat is used, but when fatty tissues of different species of animals are cooked, different types of odours are evolved. The volatile carbonyls from heated pork fat include octanal, undecanal, hepta 2:4 dienal and nona-2:4 dienal (Hornstein et al, 1963). Deca-2:4dienal present appreciably in beef and pork fat whereas it is absent in lamb fat and 4-Methyl octanoic acid is responsible for the odour of mutton and goat flesh. MacLeod (1984) identified two S-containing compounds *viz.* bis-mercaptomethylsulphide and 1,2,3,5,6 pentathiopome (Lenthionine) from aroma volatile of cooked mutton. Some of the amino acids also act as essential precursors of meat flavours. The most important are cysteine, methionine, phenylalanine, tryptophan, leucine and valine.
2. **Breed:** The odour and taste of meat are affected by breed in sheep and cattle (Jacobson et al, 1962, Bryce-Jones et al, 1963). It has been observed that the flavour quality of lean obtained from Hereford, Angus, Shorthorn and Brahman breed is different. The intensity of flavour is more in beef breeds when compared to the dairy breeds.
3. **Sex:** It is well known fact that meat obtained from male animals whether bull, ram or boar always possesses an unpleasant odour characteristics of the male. The sex odour is more prominent in pigs are compared to cattle and sheep. The substance responsible for "boar taint" is identified 5-α androst-16-en-3-one from the adipose tissue of the entire boar.
4. **Age:** The intensity of flavour starts increasing with the advancement of age. Perhaps due to the change in their metabolic processes. Veal is much milder in flavour than beef. It has been observed that calves up to six months age does not exhibit the typical beef flavour which is quite conspicuous when they grow over 12 months and near 18 months age. In sheep at 12 months age flavoursome meat is produced. Once the animals reach their maturity age, flavour intensity in their meat remain almost stationary.
5. **Nutrition:** Beef animals fattened on crops sprayed with dieldrin may require a taint of this chemical. Similarly animals reared on pastures containing certain weeds (rag weed) impart a skatole taint to the flesh. Lambs receiving clover emitted a strong flavour through their fat and lean when compared to those raised on rye grass. Rape in forage gives the meat a nauseating flavour, oats a pungent note and vetch an intense meaty flavour when the

Table 7.8: Some Undesirable Flavours of Meat–Their Reasons and Remedial Measures

Sl.No.	*Type of Flavour*	*Reason (s) of Such Flavour*	*How to Prevent it*
1.	Boar Taint	5-Androst-16-ene-3-one in adipose tissue of entire boar	Castration
2.	Skatole Taint	Rag weeds in pasture	Remove weeds from pasture
3.	Nauseating flavour	Rape in forages	Avoid these plants in forages
4.	Pungent note	Oats in forages	– do –
5.	Intense meaty flavour	Vetch in forages	– do –
6.	Burnt, faecal oily and rubbery flavour of pork	Administration of diethylstilboesterol and methyl testosterone	Avoid such drugs for growth promotion of pork type pigs
7.	Fishyness in pork bacon	Feeding of fish meal and cod liver oil	Discontinue such feed at least six weeks before slaughter
8.	Turnipy odour	Feeding of turnip	Six weeks before slaughter do not feed turnip
9.	Rancid odour and soapy taste	Feeding of fermenting beet to sheep	Avoid beet feeding to sheep
10.	"Pig" odour of lamb	Intensive feeding of fish meal, soybean meal and barley to lambs	Maintain proper nutritional level of such ingredient in feed
11.	Musty taint in poultry meat	Chloroanisoles released by the micro-organisms from wood preservatives in deep litter	Wood savings used for deep litter should be checked before using
12.	Drug odours in meat	Intake of drugs such as linseed oil, turpentine, carbolic acid, ether, chloroform, asafoetida, spirits, ammonia, aniseed, chlorine vapour, tar, DDT	Avoid contaminated feed and water with such drugs
13.	Gammy or aged aroma	Meat stored unfrozen for some time	Proper refrigeration of meat should be done
14.	Sulfury flavour	Prolonged braising of beef cuts	Recommended cooking methods should be followed
15.	"Canned meat" flavour	Severe heat process during canning	Proper time and temperature schedule should be followed
16.	"Catty" odour	Hydrogen sulphide from meat proteins react with mesityl oxide from tin lacquers	Avoid temperature abuse. Use good can material.

Contd...

Table 7.8–*Contd...*

Sl.No.	*Type of Flavour*	*Reason (s) of Such Flavour*	*How to Prevent it*
17.	Putrid odours	Protein decomposition	Maintain proper storage temperature and time
18.	Sour or tainted odours	Microbial growth	– do –
19.	Rancid odours (tallowy, cheesy, acrylic, fishy, oily)	Prolonged storage under unfavourable conditions	– do –
20.	"Bone Taint"	Insufficient cooking of deep seated meat/lymph nodes having reservoir of micro-organisms	Hygienic production of meat and sufficient chilling of the carcasses
21.	Cabbage odour	Methanediol produced by proteins in sliced bacon	Strict hygienic measures to manufacture bacon
22.	Oily aroma of pork	Increased levels of trans, trans 2,4 decadienal	Avoid feeding of formaldehyde treated feed containing a high percentage of unsaturated fatty acids
23.	Sweet aroma and flavour of beef and mutton	Increased amounts of cis-6-V-dodecenolactone	
24.	Sharp odour	Feeding of lucernae, white clover, sweet glycerine plants	Do not feed these fodder/plants to the meat animals
25.	Strong meat odour/flavour	Feeding of perennial rye grass, panic grass, kikuya grass	

sheep are raised on lucern or phalaris pastures. Use of growth promoting substances like diethyl stilbosterol and methyl testosterone can produce undesirable flavour in pork meat leading to off-flavour which can be described as burnt, faecal, oily and rubbery. If animals consume wild onion, meat produced from it will have undesirable odour. Fishiness in pork or bacon can be avoided if the feeding of fish meal is discontinued six weeks (safer period four months) prior to slaughter. Turnipy odour develops, if cattle is fed on turnip. A rancid odour and soapy taste may develops, if cattle is fed on turnip. A rancid odour and soapy taste may develop in sheep fed on fermenting beat. Intensively fed lambs with diets containing fish meal, soybean meal and barley, possess a 'pig' odour in their flesh.

6. **Stress:** Biochemical condition of a given muscle influenced by stress factors have been observed to influence the meat flavour due to the depletion of glycogen reserve in muscles causing higher ultimate pH. The higher the ultimate pH of muscle tissue, the lower is the flavour. Perhaps, this is due to swollen structure of meat tissue which interferes with the access to the palate of the odoriferous substances.
7. **Rearing system:** Meat from conventionally raised chicken has a more characteristics flavour than meat from the chicken raised in germ free environment. "Musty taint" in poultry meat may be caused by choloroanisoles released by the micro-organisms from the wood preservatives in certain types of savings used in deep litter.
8. **Drug Administration:** the odour of drug persists longest in the thickest parts of the carcass. Drugs which may effect meat adversely are linseed oil, turpentine oil, carbolic acid, ether, asafoetida, chloroform, aromatic spirits of ammonia, aniseed etc. Abnormal odour may occasionally occur due to inspiration of air containing the vapour of chlorine or carbolic acid used in cleansing of transport vehicles. The drinking of water impregnated with tar many render the flesh unmarketable. DDT may accumulate in fat as a result of spraying or by the animal consuming contaminated feeds.

B. Post Slaughter Factors

1. **Location of Muscle:** Beef *Longissimus dorsi* has apparently a better flavour than *Semitendinosus*. The flavour of skirt or diaphragm is more than psoas muscle (Doty and Pierce, 1961; Howard and Lawrie, 1956).
2. **Biochemical condition of muscle:** In general the higher the ultimate pH, the lower is the flavour, because the consequently swollen structures interfere with access to the palate of the odoriferous substances. The flavour score decreased from 5.5 to 4 when the ultimate pH increased from 5.7 to 6.5 (Bouton et al, 1957). In case of cured meat, especially bacon of relatively high ultimate pH appears less salt to the palate than that of low pH, even when the salt content is the same (Ingram, 1949).
3. **Ageing:** There is increase in the meat flavour during ageing. This may be related to the progressive breakdown of nucleotides producing IMP, ADP,

inosine, ribose and hypoxanthine. The increase in the concentration of hypoxanthine parallels the organoleptic changes during ageing. Changes in the free fatty acids during ageing no doubt contribute the flavour alterations observed. High temperature condition of meat, especially when meat held at 49°C, causes undesirable flavour due to greater risk of bacterial growth. True beef flavour is fully developed after about 8 days ageing at 32 to 35°F, as the beef becomes more tender during ageing. Meat stored unfrozen for sometime develops a gammy or aged aroma.

4. **Cooking Methods:** The aroma of cooked meat is affected by the cooking method, the kind of meat and the precooking treatments. Weir (1960) stated that lamb leg roasts cooked to an interior temperature of 65°C (149°F), have an aroma and taste more distinctive of lamb than similar roasts cooked to an interior temperature of 75°C (167°F). Braised beef cuts cooked to 90°C (194°F) internal temperature, are considered to have a more desirable flavour than similar cuts held at this temperature, are considered to have a more desirable flavour than similar cuts held at this temperature for an additional hour. The additional holding period results in an increase in the "sulfury" flavour component. Broiled lamb has a predominant animal flavour and a greasy mouth coating effect and after taste. The distinctive flavour of cooked cured meat is due mainly to the ingredients used in the curing process. Cured meat may be smoked which contributes an additional flavour components. The "canned meat" flavour associated with canned meat is due to the severe heat process. On heating, hydrogen sulphide liberated from meat proteins can react with mesityl oxide (from tin lacquers) to give various compounds including 4-Methyl, 4- mercapto-penta-2-one, which produces most offensive "catty" odour (Aylward et al, 1967). Pressure cooking of meat has somewhat better flavour due to high temperature attained in the depth of the meat. The odour and taste of beef roasts cooked to an internal temperature of 82 °C in an oven at 177 °C are generally lower than grills from the same animal cooked to the same internal temperature over ½ hour in an oven at 288 °C (Howard, 1956; Howard and Lawrie, 1956; Bouton *et al*, 1957, 1958). This is due to the effect of prolonged cooking.

5. **Storage Conditions:** Flavour changes occur after extended period of storage due to chemical breakdown of certain meat constituents due to protein denaturation, fat oxidation, deamination and decarboxylation of amino acids, proteolysis, escape of volatile materials, oxidation of certain components and microbial growth. Some flavours changes occur during storage are considered desirable and others are undesirable. The ageing of meat results desirable flavour changes that are appreciated by many consumers. Such changes include the formation of AMP and IMP and the production of some flavour compounds by microbes, particularly by yeasts and in long term ageing by moulds. Undesirable flavour can develop during storage *e.g.* rancidity of fat. The formation of carbonyls, particularly low molecular weight volatile aldehydes, is directly responsible for the rancid flavour and sharp aroma. The end products of microbial growth can produce

undesirable flavour *e.g.* bone sour. Prolonged storage under unfavourable conditions may cause the development of putrid odours from protein decomposition "sour" or "tainted" odours from the microbial growth and rancid odours are described as tallowy for beef, muttony for mutton and stable, cheesy, acrylic, fishy or oily for pork. A faint odour of diacetyl is frequently observed in frozen meat stored at -10°C. High temperature of storage produces putrid off odour through the breakdown of proteins as in pre-packaged bacon stored at 20°C (Cavett, 1962) or "bone taint" in those deep seated portion of the carcasses which are insufficiently cooled and having reservoir of micro-organism in the lymph nodes (Nottingham, 1960). Free fatty acids produced by microbial action accelerate the development of oxidative rancidity in intra muscular fat (Lea, 1939; Watts, 1954). Meat, especially meat fat which has been in refrigerated storage for more than a week become unmarketable due to taints absorbed from extraneous sources such as diesel oil and fruits. Activated charcoal, placed in cold store, frequently reabsorbed the taint from the meat (Macara, 1947). The phospholipids of meat fat are most unstable and may play a major role in flavour deterioration (Younathan and Watts, 1969). The separated cephalin fraction of both beef and pork intramuscular fats produce fishy odours (Hornstein *et al*, 1961). When meat is stored after cooking, a distinctive stale, warmed over odour develops. This may be due to myoglobin catalyzed fat oxidation after cooking (Reineccius, 1979).

6. **Processing methods:** The commercial processes such as dehydration, freeze drying and irradiation may cause flavour changes. Dehydrated and freeze dried meat is susceptible to oxidative rancidity resulting mealy and paint like odours. In the absence of oxygen, bitter tastes develop because of Maillard type reactions. Irradiation causes both immediate and storage changes in the odour and taste of meat. The production of hydrogen sulphide, mercaptans, carbonyls and aldehydes especially in beef (Huber *et al*, 1953), is largely responsible for the off flavour of irradiated meat. In this context within package odour scavengers (*e.g.* activated charcoal), the addition of protective compounds such as ascorbic acid and irradiation at temperature far below the freezing point have been used with some success. On storage, the irradiated meat develops stale and bitter flavours which may be due to the meat's proteolytic enzymes producing free tyrosines.
7. **Microbial Cultures:** In previous years systematic attempts have been made to introduce micro-organisms deliberately in order to produce particular desirable flavour. Niven *et al.* (1958) have proposed the use of *Pediococcus cerevisiae* as a sausage starter culture. McLean and Sulzabacher (1959) had demonstrated that the addition of a species of *Pseudomonas* to meat curing brine significantly altered its flavour.

Conclusions

The basic information as discussed above regarding the aroma and flavour of meat, are very much helpful to understand the different reasons why there is development of some desirable and undesirable flavours of meat at different storage and processing conditions. Besides, this gives guidelines how to prevent the undesirable flavours, at the same time to enhance the desirable flavours of meat. Since, the commercial viability and consumer demand depend upon flavours in meat, the most important eating quality parameter, further research is required to develop and enhance the desirable flavour of meat according to the need of different classes of people in a community and prevent the unacceptable off flavours of meat.

References

Alward, F., Coleman, G. and Haisman, D.R. (1967) Chem. Ind. 1563

Bouton, P.E., Howard,A. and Lawrie, R.A. (1957). Spec report Fd Invest Bd. London No. 66

Bouton, P.E., Howard,A. and Lawrie, R.A. (1958). Spec report Fd Invest Bd. London No. 67

Bryce-Jones, K, Houston, T.W. and Harries, J.M. (1963). J Sci. Food Agric. 14:637

Cavett, J.J. (1962). J Appl. Bact. 25 :282

Doty, D.M. and Pierce, J.C. (1961). US Deptt. Agric. Tech. Bull No. 1231

Hornstein, I., Crowe, P.F. and Heimberg, M.J. (1961) Food Res. 26:581

Hornstein, I., Crowe, P.F. and Sulzabacher, W.L. (1960). J Agric. Food Chem. 8, 65

Hornstein, I., Crowe, P.F. and Sulzabacher, W.L. (1963). Nature, London 199, 1252

Howard, A. (1956). C.S.I.R.O. Food Res. Quart., 16: 26

Howard, A. and Lawrie, R.A. (1956). Spec. Report. Fd. Invest. Bd., London. No. 63

Huber, W., Braach, A. and Wely, A. (1953) Food Tech. 7:109

Ingram, M. (1949) Food Manuf. 24:292

Jacobson, M., Weller, M., Galgon, M.W. and Ruphew, E.W. (1962). Factors in the flavour and tenderness of lamb, beef and pork. Washington Agric. Exp. Sta.

Lee, C.H. (1939). Rancidity in edible fats. Chemical Publishing Co. New York

Macara, T.J.R. (1947). Mod. Refrig. 50:63

MacLeod (1984). Cited by Lawrie, R.A. in Meat Sci. 4th Ed. 1985 pp 201, Pergamon press

McLean, R.A. and Sulzabacher, W.L. (1959). Appl. Microbiol. 7:81

Niven, C.F., Deibal, R.H. and Wilson, C.D. (1958). Amer. Meat Inst. Found. Cir. No. 41

Notingham, P.M. (1960). J Sci. Food. Agric. 11:436

Reineccius, G.A. (1979). Off-flavours in meat and fish- A Review. J Food Sci. 44(1):12-21

Watts, B.M. (1954). Adv. Food Res. 5:1

Weir, C.E. (1960). The science of meat and meat products. Ed. Amer. Meat Inst. Found pp 212. Reinhold Publ. Co., New York

Younathan, M.T. and Watts, B.M. (1960). Food Res. 25:538

V. Physical and Chemical Tests Related to Sensory Properties of Food

I. Colour and Appearance

The colour data can be accumulated for two purposes: (1) the identification and characterization of a food type and the permissible colour variation before the type is downgraded and (2) the effect of perceived colour on its appreciation by consumers. A very good instrumental measurements are available for the visual characteristics of food. Mossel (1950) reviewed the sensory properties of food and spectrophotometer analysis properties of their colour. Scofield (1954) pointed out that the difficulties in improving the colour grading systems originate in a lack of fundamental knowledge effectively. He listed four points which are applicable to most problems in foods: (1) the difficulty in relating what is normally seen with what the spectrophotometer measures (2) the mental processes by which colour matches are made (3) the visual spacing of standards on an empirical basis without underlying theory and (4) the metal correlation for depth. Nothing has been done to improve the correlation between the grade and what the user sees (making and Little, 1962).

Definition of Colour

Physically colour is a characteristic of light, measurable in terms of intensity (radiant energy) and wave length. It arises from the presence of light in greater intensities at some wave lengths than at others. Physiologically it is further limited to the band of the spectrum from 380 to 770 mμ, since the human eye is practically insensible to the wave lengths of radiant energy. Thus the phenomenon of colour is said to be psychophysical and is defined as consisting of the characteristics of light. Light being that aspect of radiant energy of which a human observer is aware through the stimulation of the retina arise from the stimulation of the retina of the eye.

Visual inspection of food items has occasionally given erroneous results because the light source did not emit sufficient radiant energy at the eritical wave lengths. To correct this situation three standard illuminates have been established by the international commission of illumination. These are: Illuminant A – incandescent lamp (28540K), Illuminate B – moon sunlight (50000K) and Illuminant C – cloudy day light (68000K) whereas 0K = degrees Kelvin.

A. Spectrophotometry

The colour of any object may be defined comprehensively by measuring the amount of reflection of light from the surface of the object at each wave length in the visible range of approx. 380 to 770 mμ. This determination may be made by the use of a spectrophotometer. Instruments are:

1. Hardy (General Electric) or the backman spectrophotometer – which use a prison
2. Bansch and Lomb Spectronic 20 – which uses a grating for isolating the spectral bands

B. Tristimulus Colourimetery and the Standard Observed

C. Munsel Colour System

The munsel system is based on the use of 3 or 4 colour discs, each of which has been carefully calibrated in term of the three notations of hue (red, green etc.) value (lightness or darkness) and chroma (strength of the colour). This method is most satisfactory when used with a disc colorimeter.

D. Hunter Colour and Colour Difference Meter

It is a tristimulus photoelectric colourimeter. Advantage over spectrophotometric curve method economic rapid method.

E. Abridged Methods

This method involves the extraction of the colour from the product by the use of one or more solvents and the measurements of that extract in a spectrophotometer in terms of present transmittance of light at a specific wave length. The greater the intensity of the pigment the lower the percent transmittance.

F. Kubelka–Munk Concept

The Kubelka-Munk concept has been defined by K/S = kc where K = light absorbed; S = light scattered; C = concentration of colourant and K = a constant. The K/S is related to reflectance's at a given wavelength by $K/S = (1\text{-}R)^2/2\,R$. where R = the reflectance of an infinitely thick samples. A knowledge of the K and S values enables one to predict whether the color of a particular sample should be measured by reflectance or transmittance. This approach also shows promise for measuring the internal colour and quality characteristics of foods without destroying the sample.

II. Taste and Flavour

1. Refractometry –
2. Polarimetry – to establish the configuration of optically active compounds whose anomers may vary in taste intensity
3. Spectrophotometric measurements of the ultra-violet absorbing materials in hydrocarbon extracts.
4. Total titrable acidity of food products correlates more closely with sourness than does pH because of the various natural buffering agents in foods. With canned fruit products a common index of palatability is the sugar/acid ratio or Brix-acid ratio which is determined by percent total soluble solids by weight. Percent total titrable acidity by weight eg. The sugar-acid ratio that correlated with optimum consumer acceptance was 38/39 for caned apricots, 75/85 for canned cling peaches 138/170 for canned Bartlett pears; 65/75 for canned freestone peaches.
5. Objective measure of flavour (odour) – mass spectroscopy, infrared and Raman spectroscopy. Fractional distillation enzyme techniques, chromatography. Stewart (1963) There is no doubt that some important components contributing to the aroma of foods have been isolated and

identified but what is not being done is to establish which of the compounds isolated are responsible for what sensory properties.

6. Gas liquid chromatrography (GLC) – Sensitively of the instrument to very small amounts of volatile material.
7. Andersson and Danielson (1961) – good correlation of fish rancidity with the peroxide value or with the malonaldehyde content test (TBA test).
8. Insecticides/pesticides residues – correlated with reduced palatability.
9. Sweetness can be determined by very satisfactorily by the use of hydrometers or refractometers in relatively pure solutions of syrup in terms of degrees Brix or to a commercially satisfactory extent
10. Sourness can be measured: by pH meter, total titrable acid.
11. Saltiness can be estimated by chloride determination or more rapidly by sodium determine with the use of a flame photometer (Brown *et al.*, 1952).
12. Odour or olfaction – chromatographic separation and spectrophotometer charting (infrared or ultraviolet spectrophotometry)

III. Texture or Kinesthetics

Meats

1. Tenderness measured by sensory panel and shear strength measurements by Warner-Bratzler shear press.
2. Household food grinder and modified Christel Texturemeter in measuring beef texture.
3. Kramer shear instrument. No chemical tests appear to yield sufficiently high correlations with sensory measurements of tenderness or fibrousness.
4. Strain gage denture tenderometers for foods: Canco tenderometer

Other Foods

1. Shortometer – shortening quality of lards oil.
2. Soluble protein viscosity and degree of cell disruption were useful in predicting sensory quality of fish.
3. Viscometers – oils, cream etc.
4. Texturometer
5. Puncturemeter
6. Succulometer
7. Fibrometers

Physical Chemical Methods

In the absence of adequate devices for measuring directly kinesthetic properties, empirical, physical-chemical tests have been devised and used successfully. Some of these are highly accurate, particularly when the details of the methods are adhered to rigidly.

Table 7.9: Relation of Kinesthetic Characteristics to Physical Methods of Application of Force

Firmness	*Compression*	*Pressure Tester, Shear-Press*
Yielding quality	Compression	Pressure tester, shear-press, ball compressor
Juiciness	Compression (Juice extraction)	Puncture-tester, succulometer, shear press moisture test
Chewiness	Shear pressure	Tenderometer texture meter, shear press, sq. gr., solids
Fibrousness	Cutting comminuting	Fibrometer shear-press fiber analysis
Grittiness	–	Comminution, elution, sedimentation
Mealiness	–	Starch or gum analysis
Stickiness	Tensile, strength	Jelly strength, pectin and or gum analysis

Source: Kramer and Twigg: Quality control for the food industry pp. 85.

1. Moisture content: (i) AOAC method: vacuum oven – drying 6 hrs.
2. Toluene distillation and Brown – Duvel methods involve the distillation of water from a sample mixed with toluene or oil, time reqd is < 1 hr.
3. Barbender moisture tester.
4. Cenco moisture balance
5. Electronic moisture tester – steinlite Model No. 300
6. Nuclear magnetic resonance

2. Alcohol Insoluble Solids

Consists of extraction of the sample with 70 to 80 per cent alcohol. The filtered, washed and dried residue is a measure of the alcohol–insoluble starches, cellulose, fiber pectins and proteins which account for the chewiness and mealiness of the products. The method is particularly suitable for vegetables.

3. Fiber

AOAC method rapid methods by Bonney at FDA – suitable for canned green and wax beans asparagus.

4. Grit

Sand particles in food product. National canners Assoc. 1941 Dried Fruit Assoc. 1950

5. Density

Nrine floatation or froth floatation equipments suitable for peas and lima beans.

IV. General Quality

The number of physic-chemical methods is so great that only a few representative examples can be mentioned. Weight, size, moisture content, alcohol-insoluble solids fiber content, density, colour, acidity, sugar concentration, pH, salt, tannins, volatile reducing, substances, peroxide value, non-protein nitrogen and phosphor-18-tungstic acid-positive material are all the basis of one or more procedures which attempt to relate food quality to an objective measurement. Objective methods have been given or determining contamination of foods by biological agents such as insects, rodents, bacteria, molds and yeasts.

Chapter 8

Meat Microbiology

I. Microbiological Quality of Meat Products

Food security is a global issue, where livestock products (principally meat, fish, milk and eggs) are generally regarded as high risk commodity in respect of pathogen contents, natural toxins and other possible contaminants and adulterants. These products have been major global causes of food borne disease in humans and are also prone to microbiological growth and spoilage. Consequently, monitoring the safety and quality of these products remains a primary concern. Recognizing this, the World Health Organization (WHO) developed its Global Strategy for Food Safety (Adak *et al.*, 2005). Microbiological analysis is an established tool in controlling the safety and quality of foods. Recent advances in preventative and risk-based approaches to food safety control have reinforced the role of microbiological testing of foods in food safety management. WHO emphasizes that "where a food represents an actual or potential health hazard, microbiological examination should be made and microbiological specifications, wherever appropriate, should be established for the foods".

Microbiological Testing

Foods may contain a variety of microorganisms, many of which are harmless. Even those that can cause illness can be present in foods at low levels and if this food is consumed, illness is unlikely. In addition, some foods, such as fermented foods like cheese and yoghurt, contain beneficial microorganisms.

In fact, tissues from healthy animal are sterile. The possible sources of these bacteria are likely to come from the skin and intestinal tract of the animal from which the meat is obtained. Other potential sources of microbial contaminations are the equipments used for each operation that is performed until the final product is eaten, the clothing and hands of personnel and the physical facilities are all implicated. Retail cut could also result in greater microbial load because of the large amount of exposed surface area, more readily available water, nutrient and greater oxygen penetration available. External contamination of meat is a constant possibility from the moment of bleeding unit consumption. Among the factors that affect microbial growth in meat are intrinsic properties (physical and chemical properties of meat) and extrinsic environmental factors; however the factors having the greatest influence on the growth of microorganisms in meat and meat products are the storage temperatures, moisture and oxygen availability.

As such, when deciding on the type of analysis to perform it is important to understand the food and how it is produced.

Some of the factors influencing the choice of test include:

- Type of ingredients in the finished product
- Status of ingredients (*i.e.* cooked vs raw)
- Type of cooking/processing undertaken
- Level of handling after cooking or processing
- Presence of preservatives, including acids and salt
- Presence and type of packaging
- Distribution and storage of finished product

Most common tests performed on ready-to-eat foods and their relevance to different types of product and ingredients is as follows:

Aerobic Plate Counts

There are many different types of aerobic plate counts like total mesophillic aerobes, psychrophillic, lipolytics and proteolytic etc., However the most commonly used test is Standard plate count (or total plate count or total viable count) that provides a general indication of the microbiological quality of a food. A standard plate count will not differentiate between the natural microflora of a food, spoilage microorganisms, organisms added to fermented foods or pathogenic microorganism. It can not be used to predict the safety of the product and will be influenced by the storage conditions of the product. Depending on the product, a high standard plate count may indicate that the product may have been prepared unhygienically or stored inappropriately. While assessing standard plate count results, the processing and/or ingredients present in the foods needs to be considered along with a knowledge of the processing conditions. Care should be taken when assessing a single result as series of results over time generally provide a better understanding. Individual survey reports will justify the undertaking (or not) of a standard plate count test.

Indicator Organisms

Coliform Bacteria (*Escherichia, Enterobacter, Klebsiella*)

These are of a great importance to food microbiology. Coliform bacteria are important microbiological sanitary indicators, which emphasizes hygiene in processing and handling of products. In some cases, it highlights various heat treatments (pasteurization type) applied to meat products.

Escherichia coli

E. coli is an organism that is part of the normal microflora of the intestinal tract of humans and warm-blooded animals. Contaminated food and water are the major sources by which the bacteria are spread. *Escherichia coli* is commonly used as surrogate indicator, its presence in food generally indicate direct and indirect fecal contamination. As such, their presence in foods can be an indication of poor hygiene and sanitation or inadequate heat treatment. Ideally *E. coli* should not be detected and as such a level of < 3 per gram (the limit of the Most Probable Number test) has been given as the satisfactory criteria for this organism. Levels exceeding 100 per gram are unacceptable and indicate a level of contamination which may have introduced pathogens or that pathogens, if present in the food prior to processing, may have survived.

Enterobacteriaceae

The family *Enterobacteriaceae* includes many bacteria that are found in the human or animal intestinal tract, including human pathogens such as *Salmonella* and *Shigella*. They can also be found in soil, vegetable matter and marine environments. The group includes both pathogenic and non-pathogenic bacteria. *Enterobacteriaceae* are useful indicators of hygiene and of post-processing contamination of heat processed foods. Their presence in high numbers($>10^4$ per gram) in ready-to-eat foods indicates that an unacceptable level of contamination has occurred or there has been under processing (*e.g.* inadequate cooking). As they can be found in raw foods, testing for *Enterobacteriaceae* is not applicable to fresh fruits and vegetables or foods containing these.

Pathogens

Coagulase Positive Staphylococci (CPS)

Staphylococcus aureus can be routinely isolated from humans and associated environments. As such, the presence of coagulase positive staphylococci (a subgroup of *S. aureus*), is an indication of human contact. Some CPS strains produce a toxin which can cause food poisoning. Even minimal handling of foods can result in coagulase positive staphylococci being present in foods at low levels. This is unlikely to be a food safety concern provided the food is either consumed immediately or stored under temperature control. In raw or fermented foods, coagulase positive staphylococci are likely to be outgrown or inhibited by the naturally occurring microorganisms. In fully cooked foods that support the growth of coagulase-positive staphylococci, the absence of competing microorganisms may provide the opportunity for growth and toxin production. Coagulase-positive staphylococci appear to be of greatest concern in products such as custard or cream-filled pastries, mayonnaise-based salads and processed meats. Unsatisfactory levels of coagulase-positive staphylococci indicate that time/temperature abuse of a food is likely to have occurred following improper handling during food preparation. A test for enterotoxin, SET, may be appropriate where levels of coagulase-positive staphylococci exceed 10^3 cfu per gram or where poor handling practices are suspected but it is likely that viable organisms may no longer be present in significant numbers. Levels of greater than or equal to 10^4 cfu are considered as potentially hazardous as foods with this level of contamination may result in food borne illness if consumed.

Clostridium perfringens

C. perfringens can be isolated from a variety of environments and foods. As the spores of *C. perfringens* can survive cooking, it is of most concern in cooked foods that have been temperature abused as this provides the opportunity for spores to germinate and grow. Potential temperature abuse scenarios include:

- ✰ Holding cooked foods at warm temperatures for extended periods of time, and
- ✰ Cooling foods too slowly.

C. perfringens is of particular concern for cooked meats (large joints or rolled meats), gravy and meat and vegetable dishes such as stews and pies. *C. perfringens* can be present in herbs and spices and where these are added after cooking low levels of *C. perfringens* may be detected. As *C. perfringens* can be present in a variety of foods, their detection at low levels in foods with raw components is not unexpected.

Bacillus cereus

B. cereus can be detected in many raw foods of plant origin and in raw milk. As with C. perfringens, their spores will survive cooking, and poor temperature control after cooking may result in germination of the spores and subsequent growth. B. cereus is of greatest concern in plant or cereal based ready-to-eat foods and cream based sauces. Ready-to-eat foods containing raw components may contain low levels of B. cereus.

Vibrio parahaemolyticus

V. parahaemolyticus is present in the marine environment and is of relevance to foods containing seafood. It is common for raw seafood to contain low levels of V. parahaemolyticus and this would not be an indication of poor food processing practices.

Effective cooking of seafood will destroy V. parahaemolyticus and their presence in cooked food may be an indication of post-cooking contamination or insufficient heat treatment.

Salmonella

Salmonella species are enteric bacteria and can be found in the intestinal tract of animals, including birds. As such, Salmonella can frequently be isolated from raw foods of animal origin. Environmental contamination can also result in Salmonella being present in a wide variety of foods, although generally at lower numbers. Their presence in ready-to-eat foods may be a result of undercooking, poor handling practices and cross contamination. Salmonella can occasionally be isolated from fresh fruit and vegetables, and these may be a source of contamination when included in ready-to-eat food. Foods should be free of Salmonella as consumption of food containing this pathogen may result in food borne illness.

Campylobacter

Campylobacter can be found in the intestinal tract of wild and domesticated animals. They can be found in raw meats and poultry and have been known to be present on eggs and in raw milk and untreated water. In ready-to-eat foods the presence of Campylobacter may be an indication of undercooking or cross contamination due to poor hygiene practices, especially poor handling of raw and cooked animal products. *Campylobacter* should not be present in ready-to-eat foods as consumption of food containing this pathogen may result in food borne illness.

Listeria monocytogenes

L. monocytogenes is widely distributed in the environment and can be isolated from a wide variety of foods. As such it can be expected to be present in ready-to-eat foods that contain raw ingredients. Moreover, this organism is able to multiply slowly at 4°C. The shelf life of the foods varies enormously. Certain foods – such as soft ripened cheese, vacuum packed pâté, and sliced meats – have a long shelf life under refrigeration, and the presence of *L. monocytogenes* at any level may be of significance due to its potential for growth during storage. The use of an enrichment procedure, in addition to enumeration, should therefore be considered to ensure that the organism is absent from the product. The risk posed by L. monocytogenes is dependent on the food and how long it is stored. Foods in which all components have been cooked in the final food preparation, or have received some other listericidal treatment, should be Listeria free. Additionally, the detection of *L. monocytogenes* in foods which have been prepared specifically for 'at risk' population groups such as the elderly, immunocompromised and infants should be considered as potentially hazardous. Foods with a long shelf life stored under refrigeration should have no *L. monocytogenes* detected in 25g.

Yeasts and Molds

Yeasts and molds are widely distributed in environment and can enter the foods through inadequately sanitized equipment or as airborne contaminants. They become predominant on foods when conditions for bacterial growth are less favourable *e.g.*, low pH, high salt, high sugar etc. Their counts are used as a part of microbiological standards of various dairy products specially fermented ones.

Indian Regulations

- ☆ **Essential Commodities Act, 1955** of Government of India, aim at regulating sanitary and hygienic conditions at all levels of supply chain and lay down sanitary and hygienic conditions of premises, surrounding environment and personnel. A number of quality control orders issued under Essential Commodities Act, 1955 such as Fruit Product Order (FPO), 1955; Meat Food Products Order (MFPO), 1973,and Milk and Milk Product Order (MMPO), 1992.

- **Bureau of Indian Standards (BIS)** is engaged in formulating the standards for a number of food items including the foods of animals origin. Limits of microbiological parameters for processed food products are specified in respective Indian Standards. As far as microbiological criteria are concerned Indian Standards are elaborate. BIS has formulated standards on test methods for detection and enumeration of pathogenic microorganisms in food and specifications for ingredients used in media for microbiological work.

Microbiological standards defined under Prevention of Food Adulteration Act, 1956 (Appendix B: Definitions and Standards of quality)

Meat and Meat Products

(Corned beef, luncheon meat, cooked ham, chopped meat, Canned chicken, canned mutton and goat meat)

- Total plate count 1000/gram maximum
- *E. coli* Absent in 25 gram
- *Samonella* Absent in 25 gram
- *Staphylococcus aureus* Absent in 25 gram
- *Clostridium perfringens* and *Clostirdium botulinum* Absent in 25 gm

Forzen Mutton, Goat, Beef and Buffalo Meat

- Total plate count 10000/gram maximum
- *E. coli* 100/gram maximum
- *Samonella* Absent in 25 gram
- *Staphylococcus aureus* 100/gram maximum
- *Clostridium perfringens* and *Clostridium Botulinum* 30/gm max
- *Listeria monocytogenes* Absent in 25 gram
- Yeast and mould count 1000/gram maximum

Continued progress on the part of regulators and industry to improve food safety are dependent on local, state, and central agencies' ability to conduct epidemiologic and laboratory investigations that identify the offending agents and link them with specific foods and this should be put in place. Fresh meats to be used for consumption purposes should be adequately cooked before use and the relevant agencies should ensure and enforce strict compliance of the recommended food standards as regards the production and sales of processed and packaged meat products.

References

Adak GK, Meakins SM, Yip H, Lopman BA, O'Brien SJ. Disease risks from foods, England and Wales, 1996-2000. Emerging Infectious Diseases, 2005 March [*cited* 2009 August 18]. Available from http://www.cdc.gov/ncidod/EID/vol11no03/04-0191.htm

Clarence SY, Obinna CN, Shalom NC. 2009. Assessment of bacteriological quality of ready to eat food (Meat pie) in Benin City metropolis, Nigeria. *Afr. J. Microb. Res.* 3(6): 390-395

Filimon M. N. et. al, 2010, Microorganisms, Qualitative Indicators for Meat Products Scientific Papers: *Animal Science and Biotechnologies* 43 (2): 346-349.

Subcommittee on Microbiological Criteria, Committee on Food Protection, National Research Council 1985: An Evaluation of the Role of Microbiological Criteria for Foods and Food Ingredients.

James M. Jay.2000 (Ed) *Modern Food Microbiology*. Aspen Publishers, Inc. Gaithersburg, Maryland

Okonko I.O. *et al.*, 2010. Assessment of bacteriological quality of fresh meats sold in Calabar metropolis, Nigeria: *EJEAFCHE*, 9 (1), [89-100]

Rao VA, Thulasi G, Ruban SW. 2009. Meat quality characteristics of non-descript buffalos as affected by age and sex. *World Applied Science Journal*,; 1058-1065.

V N Bachhil, Malik S V S and Singh D K 2004. Microbiological specifications and Food safety in *Sherikar AT, Bachhil V N and Thepliyal D C 2004 (Eds.) Textbook of Elements of Veterinary Public Health*, ICAR New Delhi. 259-284.

II. Microbial and Other Deteriorative Changes in Meat and their Identification

- Bleeding, circulatory failure, defense mechanism lost
- Physical, chemical and microbial processes
- Handling processing and storage conditions
- Deteriorative changes include; caused by microorganisms (bacteria, moulds, yeasts) insects, endogenous enzyms (naturally present in meat tissue) exogenous enzymes (secreted by microorganisms) chemical reactions (Oxidative rancidity), physical effects (freezer burn, exudation or drip, light fading and discolouration)
- Major cause is microbiological contamination and
- So preservation methods aimed at activity minimizing microbial contamination retarding microbial growth and activity.

Sources of Microbial Contamination

- Unsterile knives used for sticking
- Hide, feet, manure, dirt, viscera.
- Equipments in each operation
- Clothing and hands of personnel
- Water supply
- Air-borne organisms in chilling, aging, storage room

Microorganisms in Meat

Fungi (Moulds yeasts) and bacteria growth phase (lag, log or exponential, stationary, death)

- ☆ Type and nos. microbes impt.
- ☆ Factors affecting microbial growth
- ☆ Intrinsic factors – moisture, pH, O-R potential,nutrients
- ☆ Extrinsic factors – temp., RH, O_2, physical form of meat (wholesale cut, retail cut)
- ☆ Factors having greatest influence are – storage temp, moisture, O_2 availability

Assessing Microbial Number, Growth, Activity in Meat Nos. of Methods

1. Total plate count
2. Indicator and dye reduction test

Deteriorative changes in meat: Spoilage – decomposition and putrefaction

Chemical changes: degradation of protein, lipids, carbohydrates, other complex molecules into simpler ones by the action of endogenous enzymes in meat.

Aerobic: proteins to peptides, amino acids.

Anaerobic: proteins to sulfur containing compounds, ammonia – so abnoxius odour.

Bacterial lipases: triglycerides to glycerol, fatty acids, phospholipids to nitrogenous bases and phosphorus.

Extensive lipolysis can accelerate lipid oxidation. Bacteria change carbohydrates to alcohol and organic acids (lactic acid).

Physical Changes

Aerobic Spoilage

Slime formation, undesirable lipolytic changes.

Oxidizing compounds by bacteria cause formation of MMb from Mb or MbO_2 "greening" in sausages, surface colourations by pigmented bacteria and yeast.

Lipolytic bacteria and yeast:- oxidative rancidity, undesirable odour, flavours.

Moulds cause "whiskers" – creamy, black or green colour mould colonies, moulds cause lipolysis, enhance oxidative rancidity.

Aerobic spoilage occur in surface of meat. Anaerobic spoilage occur in the interior of meat. Caused by facultative and anaerobic bacteria.

Souring: due to accumulation of organic acid. Proteolysis without putrefaction.

Taint: Undesirable odour, flavour.

Round Sour/Ham Sour, Bone Sour

Putrid odour surrounding bones caused by anaerobic bacteria present in the lymph modes, bone joints if chill room temp. inadequate for rapid dissipation of body heat, growth of anaerobes.

Bacteria – fresh meat

Moulds – cured and smoked meat.

Caused by Insects

Country cured ham. Processed pork cuts "Skipper" a leaping larvae, ladder, beetle, cheese or ham mite, blow flies.

Hole formation, discolouration, weight loss.

USDA approved – methyl bromide fumigation.

Food poisoning and infections:

Botulism – toxins by *Clostridium botulinum* in canned meat, fish

Staphylococcal enterotoxin produced by *Staplylocccus aureus;*custard, pastries, cooked ham, tounge, poultry.

Clost. perfringens food poisoning – toxins by the organism (cooked meat, poultry, fish held in non-refrigerated temperature for long time.)

Salmonellosis (food infection) – Insufficiently cooked meat, poultry, egg, dairy products Trichinosis infection by *Trichinella spiralis*– insufficiently cooked pork and products.

Chapter 9

Factors Affecting Quality of Meat

I. Factors Affecting Quality of Fresh Meat

Introduction

Fresh meat eating quality and consistency is an important component of meat production systems. It is generally understood that production of meat must be tied to the production of a product that consumers find visually appealing, that they will continually purchase and that consistently delivers an acceptable eating experience. Therefore, meat quality encompasses the visual appearance and eating quality. Both of these quality factors can be influenced by pre-slaughter and post-slaughter production factors.

Fresh meat can be referred as a product which has undergone imminent post-mortem changes following slaughter but has not been subjected to any processing.

Quality is defined by consumers according to their own personal preferences and goals. Definitions of quality thus differ between the different stages of the supply chain and, as a result, consumer needs are not always met efficiently. We will approach our definition of quality by presenting first the consumer perspective and then the producer perspective. Quality in a market is the result of the interplay of demand and supply.

Some of the quality factors are given below:

Smell

Another quality factor is smell. The product should have a normal smell. This will be different for each of the species (*i.e.* beef, pork, chicken), but should vary only slightly within the species. Any rancid or strange smelling meat should be avoided.

Firmness

Meat should appear firm rather than soft. When handling the retail package, it should be firm, but not tough. It should give under pressure, but not actually be soft.

Visual Identification

The visual identification of quality meat is based on color, marbling and water-holding capacity. Marbling is small streaks of fat that are found within the muscle and can be seen in the meat cut. Marbling has a beneficial effect on juiciness and flavour of meat. Meat should have a normal color that is uniform throughout the entire cut. Beef, lamb, and pork should also have marbling throughout the meat.

Table 9.1: The Relationship between Species of Origination of Muscle Foods, Fresh Meat Colour, Myoglobin Content, and Major Factors Influencing Quality of Meat

Species of Origin of Muscle Food	*Animal Age*	*Myoglobin Content, mg/g*	*Visual Color*	*Major Factors influencing Quality Listed in Decreasing Order of Importance within a Species*
Beef	12 days 3 years >10 years	0.70 4.60 16 to 20	Brownish pink, Bright, cherry red to dark red	Tenderness, Juiciness and flavour
Lamb	Young	2.50	Light red to red	Flavour, Juiciness and Tenderness
Poultry dark meat	8 weeks 26 weeks (female) 26 weeks (male)	0.40 1.12 1.50	Dull red	Flavour Juiciness Tenderness
Fish dark meat	–	5.3 to 24.4	Dull red, dark red	Flavour, Juiciness and Texture
Pork	5 months	0.30	Grayish pink	Flavour Juiciness Tenderness

Juiciness

Juiciness depends on the amount of water retained in a cooked meat product. Juiciness increases flavour, helps soften meat - making it easier to chew, and stimulates saliva production in the mouth. Water retention and lipid content determine juiciness. Marbling and fat around edges helps hold in water. Water losses are from evaporation and drip losses. Meat aging can increase water retention and therefore increases juiciness.

Tenderness

Has been linked to several factors, such as the animal's age, sex or the muscle location. One important way to tenderize meat is by aging. Carcasses are aged by holding them at refrigeration temperatures for extended periods of time after slaughter and initial chilling.

Flavour

Flavour and aroma are intertwined to create the sensation the consumer has during eating. These perceptions rely on the smell through the nose and on the sensations of salty, sweet, sour and bitter on the tongue. Meat flavour is affected by type of species, diet, cooking method and method of preservation (*e.g.* smoked or cured)

Factors Affecting Quality of Fresh Meat

There are mainly two type of factors:

1. Pre-slaughter
2. Post-slaughter

Both of them are extremely important in the overall effort to control and improve the quality of the fresh meat, and are discussed as follows:

Preslaughter Factors

1. Stress

The term stress is a general expression referring to physiological adjustments, such as changes in heart rate, respiration rate, body temperature, and blood pressure. That occur during the exposure of the animal to adverse conditions, such conditions are called *stressors*, occur when the environment becomes uncomfortable or hazardous to the animal.The nature of the changes depends upon the duration and severity of stress and level of the animal's stress resistance at the time of death. Animals may be characterized as *stress susceptible* or *stress resistant.* Stress susceptible animals have unusually high temperatures,rapid glycolysis(pH drop) and early post mortem onset of rigor mortis in their muscles.

The muscles usually become pale, soft, moist or exudative after a normal 18 to 24 hr chilling. The PSE condition is associated with lowered processing yields,increased cooking losses and reduced juiciness. A dark, firm, dry muscle condition also can be produced in meat from animals with a degree of stress susceptibility, if they have survived a stress of sufficient duration to deplete their glycogen reserves. Stress resistant animals are able to maintain their normal temperature and homeostatic conditions in muscles, but they accomplish this at the expense of glycogen, so slower glycolysis and resultant high pH leading to *dark firm dry* muscle condition.

2. Genetic Effects

As meat quality is affected by the lipid, muscle fiber and connective tissue components within an animal, it is not surprising that animal genetics can play a major role in meat quality. It has long been understood that the unique genetic code for each animal regulates the production of proteins and that genetic variation exists within meat animal species for important meat quality attributes. Meat quality traits are generally recognized as being moderate to highly heritable. Livestock producers therefore could make important improvements in the acceptability of muscle as food by selecting breeding animals whose close relatives had muscles with normal color, moderate firmness, optimum or minimal intramuscular fat, and low resistance to shearing force (high degree of tenderness).

3. Age

Animal aging is accompanied by darkening of muscle color due to increasing myoglobin concentration. High myoglobin muscles are desirable when used in processed meats for their contribution to product color, but otherwise, dark color is useful only as a guide to animal age. As the age increase tenderness decreases. But during rapid phase of growth tenderness increase with time because rapid development of muscle fiber size "dilutes" existing connective tissue. Thus market weight beef animals (12 to 18 months of age) often have more tender meat than growing calves (6 months of age).toughening is evident at about 30 months of age. Meat flavour intensity increases with age, the likely cause of this flavour change is increased concentration of nucleotides in muscle. which degrade to inosinic acid and hypoxanthine postmortem.

4. Muscle Location

Muscles that are free to shorten during rigor mortis onset often lack tenderness. Degree of tension placed on the individual muscles by the skeleton and temperature. Some differences in tenderness among muscles result from different quantities of connective tissue.

5. Sex

Meat quality varies among sexes largely due to the levels of circulating hormones. Unacceptable meat quality is associated with intact males. An objectionable onion like odor known as *sex odor* is often found in pork, which represents most serious sex-associated quality problem. It is usually because of the degradation of a metabolite of testosterone (5-α- androst -16ene-3one).

6. Diet

As long as there are no serious nutritional deficiencies, the influence of diet on the physical properties of muscle is of minor importance. However, any feeding practice in the immediate ante-mortem period which alters the quantity of glycogen stored in muscles can influence the ultimate physical properties of meat. Starchy feeds and sugar will restore depleted muscle glycogen level, permitting a normal postmortem pH. But it is advisable to withhold feed for 24 hrs prior to slaughtering order to facilitate the process of evisceration and minimize the chances for microbial contamination of the carcass from the gastrointestinal tract. High forage diets produce some undesirable meat flavour compounds.

7. Pre-slaughter Handling

Procedures necessary to convert the tissues of living animals into edible food are necessarily stressful. Animals are exposed to a combination of environmental stimuli. The several steps involved in marketing process may include sorting, loading onto trucks, transport(this is the most stressful, it is during transit that most death losses and tissue bruises occur), weighing, driving, water spraying and immobilization. The severity of effects of these treatments depend on the climate, equipment used, personnel etc. Undesirable effects include carcass bruising, dark cutting meat, and PSE meat.

8. Immobilization Method

Immobilization of meat animals, except those slaughtered for kosher meat, is accomplished by carbon di-oxide, electric shock and captive bolt (or projectile) immobilization. These processes reduce stress responses compared to exsanguination without immobilization. But overall effectiveness is dependent on careful design and operation of equipment used. Most systems are designed to cause animals to be rendered unconscious without stopping action of the heart, so that it can aid the bleeding process."Deep stunning" systems stops heart action but also minimize reflex struggling, which can produce hemorrhage in muscle tissue. Immobilization should be followed, as quickly as possible, by rapid bleeding to prevent animals from regaining consciousness, and to release blood pressure. Unless bleeding is accomplished within few seconds of immobilization, the meat may exhibit a condition known as *blood splash,* which consists of blood spots (petechial hemorrhages) that can be removed. These problems can be minimized by use of proper voltage and correct placement of electrodes.

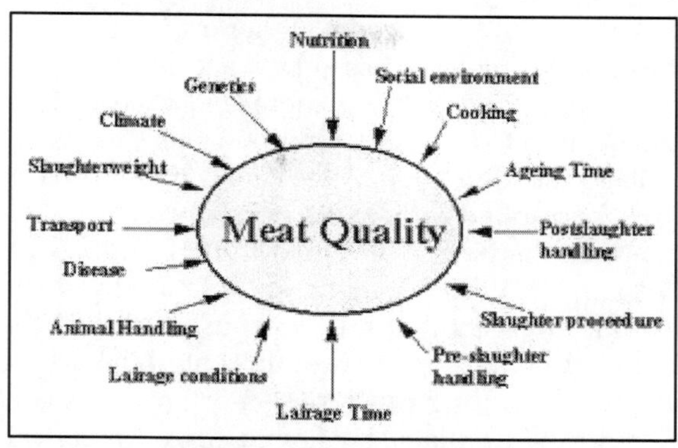

Post-slaughter Factors

1. Temperature

Temperature at which freshly slaughtered animal carcasses are stored may bring about distinct changes in rate of chemical reactions occurring in muscle tissue. Temperature differences of 10°C may cause rates of these reactions to change by a factor of three or more. It is desirable to reduce muscle temperature after death as quickly as possible, to minimize protein denaturation and to inhibit growth of microorganisms. But one needs to avoid extremely rapid reduction as it may cause undesirable consequences. Two conditions, known as *thaw rigor and cold shortening*have been recognized resulting from low temperatures in muscles before onset of rigor mortis. Thaw rigor is a severe type of rigor mortis that develops when muscle that was frozen pre-rigor is thawed. Cold shortening develops when muscle is chilled below 15°C-16°C before onset of rigor mortis. Complete disappearance of I band is seen in cold-shortened muscle. Beef and lamb are most susceptible. Contraction is caused by sudden release of Ca^2z into the sarcoplasm and may cause a physical shortening of 80 per cent of original length, accompanied by release of large quantities of meat juices and severe toughening. Severe shortening and early onset of rigor mortis may be induced by maintaining muscle at relatively high temperature (up to 50°C), thus *Heat Rigor* is produced, which is a result of of a rapid depletion of ATP stores. Consequently, there appears to be an optimum temperature at which muscle should be held during the onset of rigor mortis to minimize shortening, toughening and other undesirable effects of the rigor process.

2. Electrical Stimulation

The use of electrical pulses to use up energy reserves in meat is called electrical stimulation. Savell *et al.* (1978) showed that by applying electrical stimulation to beef carcasses, cold-induced toughening was reduced. They showed that electrically stimulated beef carcasses had accelerated post-mortem pH decline and longer sarcomeres that resulted in more tender meat. High or low voltage electrical stimulation can be used to reduce variation in beef quality. The major differences between low-voltage and high-voltage electrical stimulation is that low-voltage electrical stimulation must be applied early in the post-mortem process and results in more gentle muscle contractions when compared to high-voltage electrical stimulation. Additionally, with high-voltage electrical stimulation there can be some tearing at the molecular level in muscles that are rigorously worked that provides additional tenderness improvements. Electrically stimulated carcasses also have brighter cherry red color at shorter chilling times post-mortem. As rigor proceeds at a more rapid rate in electrically stimulated beef carcasses, ultimate pH is obtained more rapidly and post-mortem physiological changes stabilize sooner. It has shown that electrically stimulated beef carcasses have brighter cherry-red color and higher amounts of marbling. Carcasses with low levels of external fat, usually less than 0.64 cm, chill rapidly and the resultant Longissimus muscle may appear darker red along the exterior rim of the meat and be lighter in color in the center. This condition is called heat ring, but it is actually a result of pH differences in the muscle due to a more rapid chilling of the exterior surface of the cut compared to the center. The exterior surface will have a higher pH that is a result of rapid chilling in lean carcasses. At cold temperatures, glycolysis proceeds at a reduced rate until it eventually is halted. In rapidly chilled muscle, glycolysis halts when there is still substrate, glucose, available for further pH decline, but the system to convert glucose to lactic acid is not functioning. Therefore, ultimate pH is higher. In the center of the muscle, rigor mortis continues at a more normal rate and glycolysis is not limited due to cold temperatures. The ultimate pH is lower. Electrical stimulation reduces or eliminates this effect by forcing the muscles to work and use up ATP reserves, rigor mortis proceeds at a more rapid rate and ultimate pH is more closely reached before chilling can inhibit glycolysis and rigor mortis development. Electrical stimulation has not commonly been applied to pork. As pork has more problems with rapid rates of post-mortem pH decline due to short-term excitement, electrical stimulation traditionally has induced higher levels of PSE.

Future Trends

Quality as a meat industry issue will continue. Providing consumers with high quality, consistent product is a key to the success of the meat industry as with any food entity. Today's consumers demand consistency and quality and their demands are met by other segments of the meat industry. Those livestock/meat producers who can ensure consistent quality will be the viable players of the future. To ensure consistency and quality, links between the production segments of the livestock industry that have genetic verification of animals and that then manage these animals to maximize their genetic propensity will be producers of the future. The slaughter and manufacturing segments of the meat industry will have control points within their production segments to assure meat quality and will control the end product from slaughter to the final package for the consumer. Technological advances to improve meat quality will be viewed as interventions to help control consistency and quality. A fully integrated meat production system that assures quality will have economic benefit and returns.

References

http://ag.ansc.purdue.edu/meat_quality/mqf_other_factors.html

http://en.engormix.com

Fletcher, D. L. 1997. Quality of Poultry Meat: Texture and Color. Proceedings Georgia International Poultry Course, Athens, GA.

Harold B. Hedrick, Elton D Aberle, John C Forrest, Max D Judge, Robert A. Merkel 1993. "Principles Of Meat Science". Kendall/Hunt Publishing Company. 4050 Westmark Drive P.O. Box 1840 Dubuque, Iowa 52004-1840.

Kerry J, Kerry J and Ledward D (2000) Meat Processing Improving Quality (chapter-2,3 page no.3-56) Woodhead Publishing Limited ISBN 1 85573 583 0 England.

Lawless, H. 1991. The sense of smell in food quality and sensory evaluation. *J. Food Quality 14:*33-60.

II. Factors Affecting Quality and Composition of Meat and Meat Products

Meat quality is normally defined by the compositional quality (lean to fat ratio) and the palatability factors such as visual appearance, smell, firmness, juiciness, tenderness, and flavour. The nutritional quality of meat is objective yet "eating" quality, as perceived by the consumer, is highly subjective.

Some of the quality factors are given below:

Visual Identification

The visual identification of quality meat is based on colour, marbling and water holding capacity. Marbling is small streaks of fat that are found within the muscle and can be seen in the meat cut. Marbling has a beneficial effect on juiciness and flavour of meat. Meat should have a normal colour that is uniform throughout the entire cut. Beef, lamb, and pork should also have marbling throughout the meat.

Smell

Another quality factor is smell. The product should have a normal smell. This will be different for each of the species (*i.e.* beef, pork, chicken), but should vary only slightly within the species. Any rancid or strange smelling meat should be avoided.

Firmness

Meat should appear firm rather than soft. When handling the retail package, it should be firm, but not tough. It should give under pressure, but not actually be soft.

Juiciness

Juiciness depends on the amount of water retained in a cooked meat product. Juiciness increases flavour, helps soften meat - making it easier to chew, and stimulates saliva production in the mouth. Water retention and lipid content determine juiciness. Marbling and fat around edges helps hold in water. Water losses are from evaporation and drip losses. Meat aging can increase water retention and therefore increases juiciness.

Tenderness

Has been linked to several factors, such as the animal's age, sex or the muscle location. One important way to tenderize meat is by aging. Carcasses are aged by holding them at refrigeration temperatures for extended periods of time after slaughter and initial chilling.

Flavour

Flavour and aroma are intertwined to create the sensation the consumer has during eating. These perceptions rely on the smell through the nose and on the sensations of salty, sweet, sour and bitter on the tongue. Meat flavour is affected by type of species, diet, cooking method and method of preservation (*e.g.* smoked or cured)

Factors Influencing Composition of Meat

1. **Heredity** : animals of different breeds grow and develop in characteristic manners and produce carcasses with distinctive characteristics peculiar to the breed. In meat animals *phenotypic variation*: the outward visible expression of the hereditary constitution of an individual are due to heredity, environment or interaction of both. Heredity provides the necessary potential for growth and development, and the environment will tend to maximize or minimize the realization of this potential.
2. **Physiological age**: all animals within a species or a breed grow at different at different chronological age. Physiological age refers to the stage of development of an animal that can be described by identifiable stages of body development or function, such as body height and weight, body composition, or onset of puberty. So animals may attain these stages of physiological age at different chronological ages and being described as early or late maturing.
3. **Nutrition**: although heredity dictates the maximum amount of growth and development, nutrition along with environmental factors,governs actual rate of growth and extent to which development is attained. It is possible to control the rate at which different tissues and parts of the body grow and develop by altering the nutritional level of animals at critical limits. But if under nutrition occurs at early postnatal growth period, subsequent feeding at high nutritional levels lead to a greater increase in fat than in muscles. Highest efficiency in converting feed energy into body wt. gain is achieved when animals are fed *ad libitum.*
4. **Hormones and hormone like materials**: hormones are substances secreted into body fluids by ductless endocrine glands or other tissues such as the intestinal tract. They act as regulators of chemical reactions involved with

growth of tissues and other physiological processes. Combinations of these hormones are involved in the growth process, and their interactive effects results in "normal" carcass composition *e.g.* Growth hormone or somatotropin produces lean tissue growth. Hormones of adrenal medulla like epinephrine and norepinephrine assist Immobilization of glycogen to provide energy and influence muscle protein as well. They activate β *receptors.* Some hormone like substances known as β-adrenergic agonists are effective repartitioning agents : they shift available nutrients away from fat deposition and towards muscle accretion. The hormones of the testes (androgens) and ovaries (estrogens and progesterone) play an important role in growth and development of body. Androgens stimulate growth in muscles by increasing protein synthesis, accompanied by decreased fat deposition. Estrogens are effective in promoting deposition of body fat. Synthetic progesterone is effective in increasing carcass leanness by stimulating muscle growth and suppressing fat deposition.

5. **Environment**: environmental conditions under which animals are reared may have marked influence on growth rate, and even on body composition. Any environmental conditions that require body heat generation or dissipation reduce efficiency of growth.

Changes in carcass composition result from such energy partitioning, depending on the growth stage of the animal and the tissue priority for nutrients prevalent at the time.

Factors Affecting Quality of Meat

There are mainly two type of factors:

1. Ante-mortem
2. Post-mortem

Both of them are extremely important in the overall effort to control and improve the quality of the meat, and are discussed as follows:

Ante-mortem Factors

Stress

- The term stress is a general expression referring to physiological adjustments, such as changes in heart rate, respiration rate, body temperature, and blood pressure. That occur during the exposure of the animal to adverse conditions, such conditions are called *stressors,* occur when the environment becomes uncomfortable or hazardous to the animal.
- The nature of the changes depends upon the duration and severity of stress and level of the animal's stress resistance at the time of death.
- Animals may be characterized as *stress susceptible* or *stress resistant*
- Stress susceptible animals have unusually high temperatures,rapid glycolysis (ph drop) and early post mortem onset of rigor mortis in their muscles.

- ✰ The muscles usually become pale, soft, moist or exudative after a normal 18 to 24 hr chilling. The PSE condition is associated with lowered processing yields,increased cooking losses and reduced juiciness.
- ✰ A dark, firm, dry muscle condition also can be produced in meat from animals with a degree of stress susceptibility,if they have survived a stress of sufficient duration to deplete their glycogen reserves.
- ✰ Stress resistant animals are able to maintain their normal temperature and homeostatic conditions in muscles, but they accomplish this at the expense of glycogen, so slower glycolysis and resultant high pH leading to *dark firm dry* muscle condition.

Heredity

- ✰ Physical properties of muscle(meat quality) are at least moderately heritable.
- ✰ Livestock producers therefore could make important improvements in the acceptability of muscle as food by selecting breeding animals whose close relatives had muscles with normal color, moderate firmness, optimum or minimal intramuscular fat, and low resistance to shearing force (high degree of tenderness.

Age

- ✰ Animal aging is accompanied by darkening of muscle color due to increasing myoglobin concentration. High myoglobin muscles are desirable when used in processed meats for their contribution to product color, but otherwise, dark color is useful only as a guide to animal age.
- ✰ As the age increase tenderness decreases.
- ✰ But during rapid phase of growth tenderness increase with time because rapid development of muscle fiber size "dilutes" existing connective tissue.
- ✰ Thus market weight beef animals (12 to 18 months of age) often have more tender meat than growing calves (6 months of age).toughening is evident at about 30 months of age.
- ✰ Meat flavour intensity increases with age, the likely cause of this flavour change is increased concentration of nucleotides in muscle, which degrade to inosinic acid and hypoxanthine postmortem.

Muscle Location

- ✰ Muscles that are free to shorten during rigor mortis onset often lack tenderness.
- ✰ Degree of tension placed on the individual muscles by the skeleton and temperature
- ✰ Some differences in tenderness among muscles result from different quantities of connective tissue.

Sex

- ✰ Meat quality varies among sexes largely due to the levels of circulating hormones.

- Unacceptable meat quality is associated with intact males.
- An objectionable onion like odor known as *sex odor* is often found in pork, which represents most serious sex-associated quality problem. It is usually because of the degradation of a metabolite of testosterone (5-α- androst -16-ene-3one).

Diet

- As long as there are no serious nutritional deficiencies, the influence of diet on the physical properties of muscle is of minor importance.
- However, any feeding practice in the immediate ante-mortem period which alters the quantity of glycogen stored in muscles can influence the ultimate physical properties of meat.
- Starchy feeds and sugar will restore depleted muscle glycogen level, permitting a normal postmortem pH.
- But it is advisable to withhold feed for 24 hrs prior to slaughtering order to facilitate the process of evisceration and minimize the chances for microbial contamination of the carcass from the gastrointestinal tract.
- High forage diets produce some undesirable meat flavour compounds.

Preslaughter Handling

- Procedures necessary to convert the tissues of living animals into edible food are necessarily stressful.
- Animals are exposed to a combination of environmental stimuli. The several steps involved in marketing process may include sorting, loading onto trucks, transport(this is the most stressful, it is during transit that most death losses and tissue bruises occur), weighing, driving, water spraying and immobilization.
- The severity of effects of these treatments depend on the climate, equipment used, personnel etc.
- Undesirable effects include carcass bruising, dark cutting meat, and PSE meat.

Immobilization Method

- Immobilization of meat animals, except those slaughtered for kosher meat, is accomplished by carbon dioxide, electric shock and captive bolt (or projectile) immobilization.
- These processes reduce stress responses compared to exsanguination without immobilization.
- But overall effectiveness is dependent on careful design and operation of equipment used.
- Most systems are designed to cause animals to be rendered unconscious without stopping action of the heart, so that it can aid the bleeding process.
- "Deep stunning" systems stops heart action but also minimize reflex struggling, which can produce hemorrhage in muscle tissue.

- ☆ Immobilization should be followed, as quickly as possible, by rapid bleeding to prevent animals from regaining consciousness, and to release blood pressure.
- ☆ Unless bleeding is accomplished within few seconds of immobilization, the meat may exhibit a condition known as *blood splash,* which consists of blood spots (petechial hemorrhages) that can be removed.
- ☆ These problems can be minimized by use of proper voltage and correct placement of electrodes.

Postmortem Effects

Temperature

- ☆ Temperature at which freshly slaughtered animal carcasses are stored may bring about distinct changes in rate of chemical reactions occurring in muscle tissue.
- ☆ Temperature differences of 10°C may cause rates of these reactions to change by a factor of three or more.
- ☆ It is desirable to reduce muscle temperature after death as quickly as possible, to minimize protein denaturation and to inhibit growth of microorganisms, but one needs to avoid extremely rapid reduction as it may cause undesirable consequences.
- ☆ Two conditions, known as *thaw rigor and cold shortening* have been recognized resulting from low temperatures in muscles before onset of rigor mortis.
- ☆ Thaw rigor is a severe type of rigor mortis that develops when muscle that was frozen pre-rigor is thawed.
- ☆ Cold shortening develops when muscle is chilled below 15°C-16°C before onset of rigor mortis, complete disappearance of I band is seen in cold-shortened muscle, beef and lamb are most susceptible.
- ☆ Contraction is caused by sudden release of Ca^2z into the sarcoplasm and may cause a physical shortening of 80 per cent of original length, accompanied by release of large quantities of meat juices and severe toughening.
- ☆ Severe shortening and early onset of rigor mortis may be induced by maintaining muscle at relatively high temperature (upto 50°C). thus *Heat Rigor* is produced,which is a result of of a rapid depletion of ATP stores. Consequently, there appears to be an optimum temperature at which muscle should be held during the onset of rigor mortis to minimize shortening, toughening and other undesirable effects of the rigor process.

Accelerated Processing

- ☆ It is the performance of some processing steps such as cutting, bone removal, or grinding immediately after slaughter.
- ☆ Interval of time between slaughter and meat grinding affects the physical properties of their finished products.

- Meat ground pre-rigor and mixed with curing ingredients,including salt has superior water-binding properties and maximum juiciness. Additionally, exposure of pre-rigor meat to salt during grinding inhibits glycolysis and extent of pH decline even more than grinding alone.
- Less refrigerated storage space is required rapid processing, and products reach consumers with fresh flavour.
- In most kinds of meat, removal of bones and excess fat before chilling reduces energy requirements for chilling and provides more precise control of chilling rate.
- Using accelerated processing enables the industry to minimize time between animal slaughter and meat consumption, these processing systems require less refrigeration than conventional systems, and they provide products to consumers in the freshest form possible

Carcass Electrical Stimulation

- Electrical stimulation (ES) of freshly slaughtered carcasses has been used successfully to improve tenderness and meat quality in turkey, lamb, beef, and veal. Several mechanisms apparently come into play to produce desirable effects.
- Even though knowledge of underlying bases for the practice is incomplete, widespread industry application has taken place.
- ES accelerates the rate of postmortem pH decline and hastens rigor mortis.
- Meat tenderization by ES has been attributed to at least 3 factors:
  - i. Cold shortening prevention through acceleration of glycolysis and rigor onset before temperatures reach the cold shortening range.
  - ii. Accelerated proteolytic activity through enhanced calcium release.
  - iii. Physical disruption of fiber structure through extreme muscle contractions.
- Tenderization by ES is mostly due to prevention of cold shortening.
- ES is most appropriate for carcass of young animals that have not been fed high- energy diets or that lack inherent tenderness.

Factors Affecting Quality of Meat Products

Whether or not a poultry product meets the consumer's expectations depends upon the conditions surrounding various stages in the bird's development from the fertilized egg through production and processing to consumption. Although there are a number of characteristics that determine the overall quality of meat.

The following discussion will focus on appearance(color), texture and flavour.

1. Appearance (Colour)

Poultry meat colour is affected by factors such as:

- Bird's age
- Sex

- ✰ Strain
- ✰ Diet
- ✰ Intramuscular fat
- ✰ Meat moisture content
- ✰ Pre-slaughter conditions
- ✰ Processing variables

Colour of meat depends upon: the presence of the muscle pigments myoglobin and haemoglobin.

Discoloration

- ✰ Discoloration of poultry can be related to the amount of these pigments that are present in the meat, the chemical state of the pigments, or the way in which light is reflected off of the meat.
- ✰ The discoloration can occur in an entire muscle, or it can be limited to a specific area, such as a bruise or a broken blood vessel. When an entire muscle is discolored, it is frequently the breast muscle. This occurs because breast muscle accounts for a large portion of the live weight (about 5 per cent), it is more sensitive to factors that contribute to discoloration, and the already light appearance makes small changes in colour more noticeable.

Extreme Environmental Temperatures

Or stress due to live handling before processing can cause broiler and turkey breast meat to be discolored. The extent of the discoloration is related to each bird's individual response to the conditions.

Table 9.2: Colour Changes in a Bruise Over Time for Broiler Muscle (Gregory, 1992)

Age	*Colour*
2 minutes	Red
12 hours	Dark Red-Purple
24 hours	Light Green-Purple
36 hours	Yellow-Green-Purple
48 hours	Yellow-Green (Orange)
72 hours	Yellow-Orange
96 hours	Slightly Yellow
120 hours	Normal, Flesh Colour

Bruising

- ✰ Another major cause of poultry meat discoloration is bruising.
- ✰ Approximately 29 per cent of all carcasses processed in the United States are downgraded (reduced quality), and the majority of these defects (28 per cent) are from bruises (AMS, 1995).

- ☆ The poultry industry generally tries to identify where (field or plant), how, and when the injuries occur but this is often difficult to determine.
- ☆ The colour of the bruise, the amount of 'blood' present, and the extent of the 'blood clot' formation in the affected area are good indicators of the age of the injury and may give some clues as to its origin.
- ☆ A bruise will vary in appearance from a fresh, 'bloody' red color with no clotting minutes after the injury to a normal flesh color 120 hours later.
- ☆ The amount of 'blood' present and the extent of clot formation are useful in distinguishing if the injury occurred during catching/transportation or during processing.
- ☆ Injuries that occur in the field are usually magnified by processing plant equipment or handling conditions in the plant.

2. Tenderness (Texture)

- ☆ After consumers buy a poultry product, they relate the quality of that product to its texture and flavour when they are eating it.
- ☆ Whether or not poultry meat is tender depends upon the rate and extent of the chemical and physical changes occurring in the muscle as it becomes meat.
- ☆ When an animal dies, blood stops circulating, and there is no new supply of oxygen or nutrients to the muscles.
- ☆ Without oxygen and nutrients, muscles run out of energy, and they contract and become stiff. This stiffening is called rigor mortis. Eventually, muscles become soft again, which means that they are tender when cooked.
- ☆ Anything that interferes with the formation of rigor mortis, or the softening process that follows it, will affect meat tenderness.
- ☆ For example, birds that struggle before or during slaughter cause their muscles to run out of energy quicker, and rigor mortis forms much faster than normal. The texture of these muscles tends to be tough because energy was reduced in the live bird.
- ☆ A similar pattern occurs when birds are exposed to environmental stress (hot or cold temperatures) before slaughter.
- ☆ High pre-slaughter stunning, high scalding temperatures, longer scalding times and machine picking can also cause poultry meat to be tough.

Tenderness of portioned or boneless cuts of poultry is influenced by the time post-mortem of the deboning:

- ☆ Muscles that are deboned during early postmortem still have energy available for contraction. When these muscles are removed from the carcass, they contract and become tough.
- ☆ To avoid this toughening, meat is usually 'aged' for 6 to 24 hours before deboning.

- ☆ However, this is costly for the processor.
- ☆ When poultry is deboned early (0 to 2 hours post-mortem), 50 to 80 per cent of the meat will be tough.
- ☆ On the other hand, if the processor waits 6 hours before deboning, 70 to 80 per cent of the poultry meat will be tender.

Post-Slaughter Electrical Stimulation

- ☆ The poultry industry has recently started using post-slaughter electrical stimulation immediately after death to hasten rigor development of carcasses and reduce 'aging' time before deboning.
- ☆ This is different from energy depletion in the live bird, which causes meat to be tough.
- ☆ When electricity is applied to the dead bird, the treatment acts like a nerve impulse, and causes the muscle to contract, use up energy and enter rigor mortis at a faster rate.
- ☆ In the live bird, the same treatment causes meat to be tough but after death, the treatment causes tender deboned poultry meat within two hours post-mortem instead of the four to six hours required with normal aging.
- ☆ Although electrical stimulation is still in the developmental stages, it seems that processors using it can debone carcasses right out of the chiller and save on their equipment costs, time, space and energy requirements.

3. Flavour

- ☆ Flavour is another quality attribute that consumers use to determine the acceptability of poultry meat.
- ☆ Both taste and odour contribute to the flavour of poultry, and it is generally difficult to distinguish between the two during consumption.
- ☆ When poultry is cooked, flavour develops from sugar and amino acid interactions, lipid and thermal oxidation and thiamin degradation.
- ☆ These chemical changes are not unique to poultry but the lipids and fats in poultry are unique and combine with odour to account for the characteristic 'poultry' flavour.
- ☆ Few factors during production and processing affect poultry meat flavour.
- ☆ This means that it is not only difficult to produce a flavour defect but it is difficult to enhance flavour during production and processing.

Factors Affecting Flavour of Meat

- ☆ Age of the bird at slaughter (young or mature birds) -major
- ☆ Minor effects on meat flavour are related to:
    - Bird strain
    - Diet

- Environmental conditions (litter, ventilation, etc.)
- Scalding temperatures
- Chilling
- Product packaging and
- Storage

However, these effects are too small for consumers to notice.

III. Meat Colour

Meat colour important as it attributes to eye-appeal. A colour has three attributes-hue, chroma, value.

Hue

That normally think of as a colour-yellow, green, red, blue etc. It is the wave length of the light radiation.

Chroma

Refers to purity or saturation-depth or intensity of the fundamental colour with respect to the white light mixed in with it.

Value

(Brightness, luminosity) overall reflectance of the colour-in the other words it reflects the extent to which the hue is diluted with black.

- ☆ Three primaries are –red, blue and green. Any colour may be matched exactly by a suitable mixture of three primaries.
- ☆ Tristimulus value- the relative amounts of the primaries required to match a given colour.
- ☆ Instruments used to measure colour:
    1. Lovibond Tintometer (Colorimeter)
    2. Hunter Colorimeter (tricolorimetric system)
    3. Portable colour comparator-developed by Steinhauf (1964), Lohse and Pfan (1964)

Fresh Meat Colour

Fresh meat colour is due to myoglobin and haemoglobin. Myoglobin is a conjugate protein, consists of a typical amino acid protein chain and a non-protein haeme molecule.

The colour of fresh meat does not influence its palatability and nutritive value, yet it is regarded as a reflection on the quality by the consumers.

- ☆ The conjugate protein myoglobin provides the red colour of the muscle and serves as a storage site for oxygen in muscle.

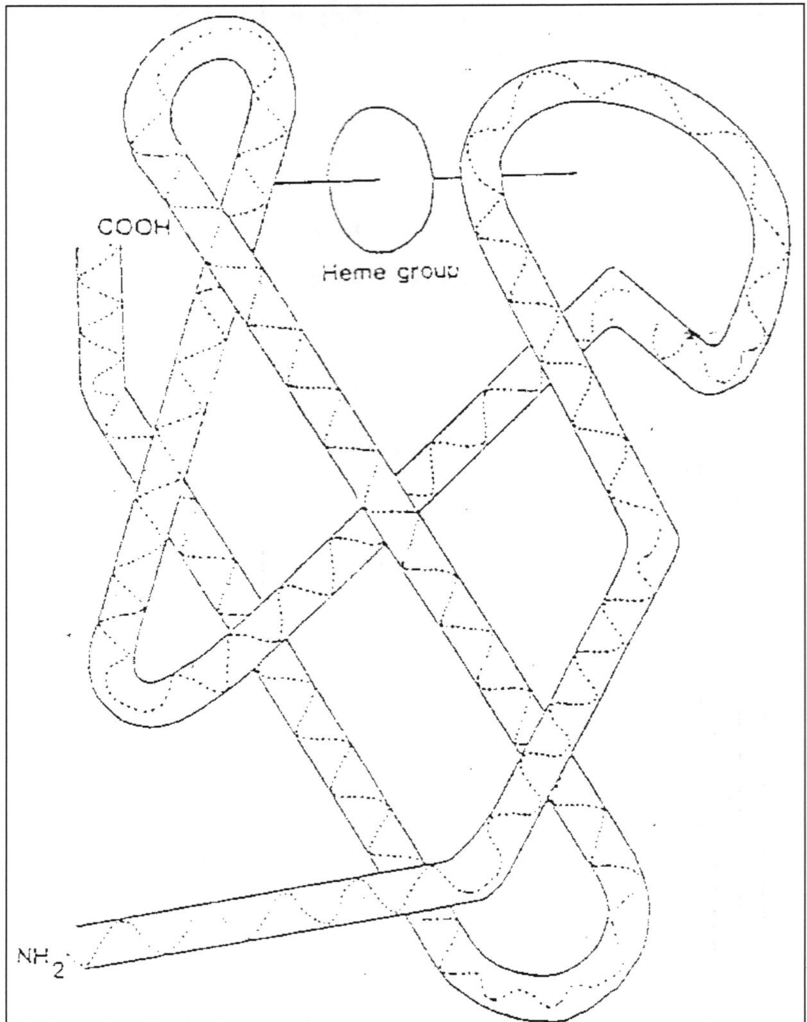

Myoglobin

- Myoglobin (and its various chemical forms) is not the only pigments in muscle but is generally in large enough quantity to colour the tissue. Other pigments of important to living tissues (contribute little to the total colour) are hemoglobin cytochromes, cyanocobalamin (B_{12}), flavins etc. Cytochrome is an enzyme involved in oxidative phosphorylation, contain iron but contribute very little to meat colour.
- Differences in Mb – due to variations in species, breed, age, sex, type of muscle and training exercise etc.

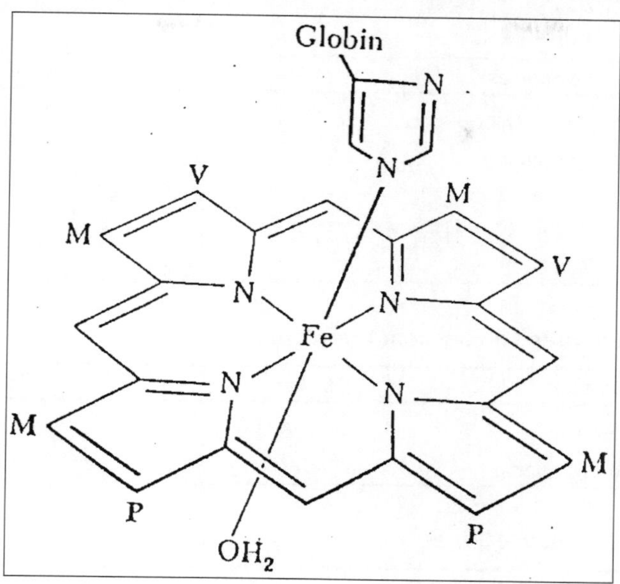

Table 9.3: Effect of Species on per cent Myoglobin and Colour

Sl.No.	Species	Per cent Mb
1.	Rabbit	0.02
2.	Sheep	0.25
3.	Pigs	0.06
4.	Cattle	0.50
5.	Blue Whale	0.91
Sl.No.	*Species*	*Colour*
1.	Beef	Bright, cherry red
2.	Fish	Gray white to dark red
3.	Horse	Dark red
4.	Lamb/mutton	Light red to brick red
5.	Pork	Grayish pink
6.	Poultry	Gray white to dull red
7.	Veal	Brownish pink

Table 9.4: Effect of Age on per cent Myoglobin

Age/Species	Per cent Myoglobin
5 month old pig	0.03
6 month old pig	0.038
7 month old pig	0.044

Contd...

Table 9.4–*Contd...*

Age/Species	*Per cent Myoglobin*
12 days calf	0.07
3 yr steer	0.46
Veal	0.1- 0.3
Beef	0. 4-1.0
Old beef	1.6-2.0

Table 9.5: Effect of Breed on per cent Myoglobin

Breed	*L.dorsi*	*Psoas*
Draught horse	0.46	0.82
Thorough bred horse	0.77	0.88

Table 9.6: Effect of Muscle Types

Muscle Types	*Per cent Mb in Pork Muscles*
L.dorsi	0.044
Ps. Major	0.082
Rectus femoris	0.086
Triceps	0.089
Extensor carpi radialis	0.099

Red and White Fibers

Due to different ratios of red to white muscle fibers – differ in Mb per cent,

Red fiber – higher affinity to Sudan Black B dye because of higher phospholipids.

Table 9.7: Percentage of Red Muscle Fibers and Mb per cent in Dark and Light Pork Muscles

Muscle Fiber Type	*Per cent Red Muscle Fiber of Total Fiber*	*Per cent Mb in Moisture Fat Free Tissue*
Light muscles		
Semimembranosus (light portion)	20	0.33
Biceps femoris (outside part)	25	0.35
L. dorsi	25	0.30
Gluteus medius	27	0.33
Dark muscles		
Rectus femoris	40	0.50
Sirratus ventralis	42	1.20
Inside Biceps femoris	45	0.70
Dark semitendinosus	47	1.20
Trapezius	47	1.10

Table 9.8: Myoglobin and Related Characteristics of Light and Dark Portions of Semitendinosus Muscle

Characteristics	*Light Portion*	*Dark Portion*
Per cent Mb	0.15	0.40
Red fibers per cent of total fibers	14.8	42.7
Succinic dehydrogenase activity (units/g tissue)	1.29	2.89
Glycogen (mg/g)	3.40	3.85
Lactic acid (mg/g)	4.66	3.68

- Succinic dehydrogenase – higher in Red Fiber, this enzyme is associated with oxidative metabolism of the fiber. Red Fiber depends upon O_2 for energy production as compared to White Fiber
- Low conc. of lactic acid in Red Fiber, metabolism aerobically, glycogen – pyruvate.
- White Fiber higher sarcoplasmic proteins *e.g.* enzymes involved in anaerobic glycolysis of glycogen.
- Rigor mortis develops earlier in light muscles that dark muscles.
- Sarcomere length greater in dark muscles. So greater degree of P.M. contraction in W.F.
- Pork more light muscles, so rapid pH fall after slaughter.
- The oxidative enzymes remains potentially active even after extended refrigeration and may interfere with the state of the myoglobin pigments.
- Whale muscle has an exceptionally high conc. Mb. reflecting its aquatic life.
- Muscles carry out sustained work – high Mb. as compared to those in short bursts.
- Muscles of Horse more Mb than rabbit.
- Muscles of racing horse more Mb than draught horse
- Muscles of Bulls more Mb than cows.
- Muscles of steer more Mb than calves
- Muscles of diaphragm more Mb than L. dorsi
- Muscles of free range animals more Mb than stall-fed animals

Chemistry of Myoglobin

Meat pigments mainly have two proteins *i.e.* Hemoglobin(Hb) – pigment of blood and Myoglobin(Mb) – pigment of muscles. In well bled tissues Mb constitutes 80-90 per cent of total pigments. The two pigments are similar in structure, except that Mb molecule is one fourth as large as Hb.

Mb molecule consists of a haematin nucleus attached to a protein component of globulin type called globin. The mol. wt. is about 17000. The haematin portion comprises of a ring of four pyrrole nuclei linked together by methene bridge (-CH=) and coordinated with a central iron atom.

The haem moity of Mb (Porphyrin ring with iron atom in ferrous state)

Heme Pigment found in Myoglobin

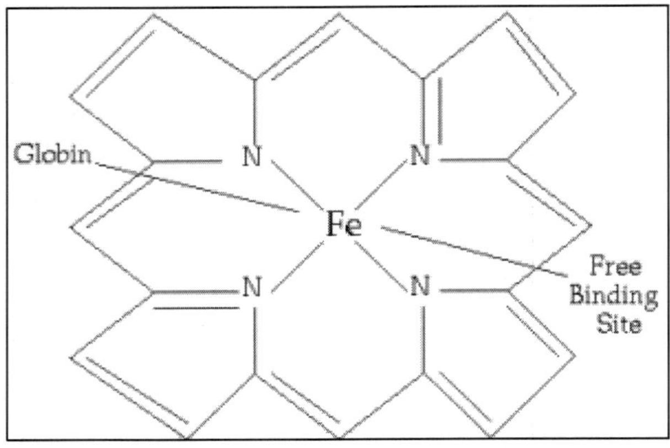

Haemoglobin (Hb) contains four haem groups and has a mol. wt. of 64,500. The similarity between the two substances suggest that Hb consists of four units each resembling Mb.

Hemoglobin has a quaternary structure characteristic of many multi-subunit globular proteins.[23] Most of the amino acids in hemoglobin form alpha helices, connected by short non-helical segments. Hydrogen bonds stabilize the helical sections inside this protein, causing attractions within the molecule, folding each polypeptide chain into a specific shape.[24] Hemoglobin's quaternary structure comes from its four subunits in roughly a tetrahedral arrangement.[23]

In most vertebrates, the hemoglobin molecule is an assembly of four globular protein subunits. Each subunit is composed of a protein chain tightly associated with a non-protein heme group. Each protein chain arranges into a set of alpha-helix structural segments connected together in a globin fold arrangement, so called because this arrangement is the same folding motif used in other heme/globin proteins such as myoglobin.[25][26] This folding pattern contains a pocket that strongly binds the heme group.

A heme group consists of an iron (Fe) ion (charged atom) held in a heterocyclic ring, known as a porphyrin. This porphyrin ring consists of four pyrrole molecules cyclically linked together (by methine bridges) with the iron ion bound in the center.[27] The iron ion, which is the site of oxygen binding, coordinates with the fournitrogens in the center of the ring, which all lie in one plane. The iron is bound strongly (covalently) to the globular protein via the imidazole ring of F8 histidine residue (also known as the proximal histidine) below the porphyrin ring. A sixth position can reversibly bind oxygen by a coordinate covalent bond,[28] completing the octahedral group of six ligands. Oxygen binds in an "end-on bent" geometry where one oxygen atom binds Fe and the other protrudes at an angle. When oxygen is not bound, a very weakly bonded water molecule fills the site, forming a distorted octahedron.

Even though carbon dioxide is carried by hemoglobin, it does not compete with oxygen for the iron-binding positions, but is bound to the protein chains of the structure.

The iron ion may be either in the Fe^{2+} or in the Fe^{3+} state, but ferrihemoglobin (methemoglobin) (Fe^{3+}) cannot bind oxygen.[29] In binding, oxygen temporarily and reversibly oxidizes (Fe^{2+}) to (Fe^{3+}) while oxygen temporarily turns into superoxide, thus iron must exist in the +2 oxidation state to bind oxygen. If superoxide ion associated to Fe^{3+} is protonated the hemoglobin iron will remain oxidized and incapable of binding oxygen. In such cases, the enzyme methemoglobin reductase will be able to eventually reactivate methemoglobin by reducing the iron center.

In adult humans, the most common hemoglobin type is a tetramer (which contains 4 subunit proteins) called *hemoglobin A*, consisting of two α and two β subunits non-covalently bound, each made of 141 and 146 amino acid residues, respectively. This is denoted as $\alpha_2\beta_2$. The subunits are structurally similar and about the same size. Each subunit has a molecular weight of about 16,000 daltons,[30] for a totalmolecular weight of the tetramer of about 64,000 daltons (64,458 g/mol).[31] Thus, 1 g/dL = 0.1551 mmol/L. Hemoglobin A is the most intensively studied of the hemoglobin molecules.

In human infants, the hemoglobin molecule is made up of 2 α chains and 2 γ chains. The gamma chains are gradually replaced by β chains as the infant grows.[32]

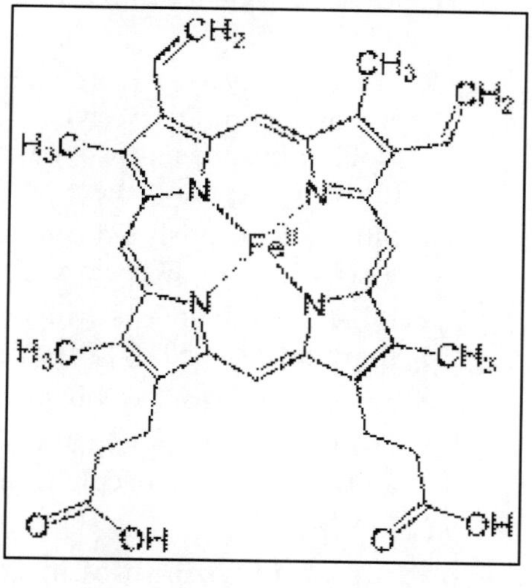

The four polypeptide chains are bound to each other by salt bridges, hydrogen bonds, and the hydrophobic effect.

- ☆ Iron is in the ferrous state in the middle of porphyrin ring.

  The iron atom is endowed with six coordination bonds which represents six bond orbitals in which the atom accepts six electron pairs from other atoms. Four pairs are donated by Nitrogen atoms of porphyrin. Fifth pairs are donated by Nitrogen atoms of histidine molecule in the peptide chain of globin. Sixth position provides the site for complexing of any atom which has an electron pair to donate.
- ☆ Sixth position provides for the function of molecule.
- ☆ The willingness of the atom to donate its electrons determines the types of complex bond formed.

Less willing sharers forming ionic bonds.

More willing sharers forming covalent bonds.

Ionic Bond

The chemical bond formed between two atoms by the transfer of one or more valence electrons from one atom to the other is called the ionic bond. This bond is also called electrovalent or polar bond.

Covalent Bond

The chemical bond between two atoms in which the electrons (in pairs) are shared by both the participating atoms is called covalent bond.

It is this willingness of the atom to share or the bond type formed is the most important factor in determining the final character and colour of the complex.

- ✰ In myoglobin the donator is oxygen in a water molecule but the bond is ionic.
- ✰ With Ferrus ion, complex with molecular oxygen the bond is stronger covalent bond and this becomes still stronger with CO and further still stronger with NO.

Bond Types and Colour

Various known complexes of heme and globin have iron in either ferrous Fe^{++} or ferric Fe^{+++} state. Covalent complexes are of greatest concern for meat colour (Table 9.1).

- ✰ The iron may exist in both reduced and oxidized forms. In Fe^{++} state it can combine with O_2 and NO_2. The ability to combine with O_2 is lost when globin portion is destroyed and the tendency for iron to oxidize to Fe^{+++} form is then greatly increased.
- ✰ Mb has a purplish red color and characterized by a diffused absorption band with max. at 555nm.
- ✰ When molecular O_2 is available oxyMb is formed, it is bright red and gives sharp peaks at 535-545 and 575-585 nm.
- ✰ The formation of oxyMb is called as oxygenation and not oxidation
- ✰ Oxidation of myoglobin involves a change of iron from Fe^{++} to Fe^{+++} state and Met Mb is formed. It has a dull brown colour. Absence of peak is at 505 nm.

Formation of Oxymyoglobin and Metmyoglobin (MMb) in Fresh Meat

- ✰ Molecular O_2 is constantly associating with and dissociating from the haem complex in competition with oxygen consuming systems and at the same time Mb is constantly being oxidized to Met Mb which in turn is reduced to Mb.
- ✰ The relative proportion of three pigments depend on O_2 partial pr, pH, temp. and moisture per cent.
- ✰ Low O_2 pr. (1-20mmHg) favour MMb formation.
- ✰ In fresh meat before cooking the most important chemical form is oxyMb. It occurs on the meat surface only and imparts bright red colour. The cytochrome enzymes are capable of utilizing O_2 for a considerable period PM. Although there is no O_2 in the depths of meat, O_2 can diffuse inwards from meat surfaces exposed to air. A point of balance is established between

Table 9.9: Pigments Found in Fresh (F), Cured (Cu) or Cooked Meat (CM)

Sl.No.	Pigment	Mode of formation	State of Iron	State of Hematin Nucleus	State of Globin	Colour
1.	Myoglobin (F)	Redn. of MMb, deoxygenation of oxy Mb	Fe^{++}	intact	native	Purplish red
2.	Oxy Mb (F)	Oxygenation of Mb	Fe^{++}	intact	native	Bright red
3.	Met Mb (F)	Oxdn. of Mb and oxy Mb	Fe^{+++}	intact	native	Brown
4.	NO Mb or Nitroso Mb (Cu)	Mb + NO (nitric oxide)	Fe^{++}	intact	native	Bright red (pink)
5.	Nitroso MMb (Cu)	MMb + NO	Fe^{+++}	intact	native	Crimson
6.	MMb nitrite (Cu) (NO_2)	MMb + excess nitrite (NO_2)	Fe^{+++}	intact	native	Reddish brown
7.	Globin myohaemo chromogen (CM)	Effect of heat, denaturing agent on Mb, oxy Mb, irradiation of globin haemichromogen	Fe^{++}	Intact, usually bound to denatured protein other than globin.	Denatured, usually detached	Dull red
8.	Globin myohaemi chromogen (CM)	Effect of heat, denaturing agent on Mb, oxy Mb, MMb, haemochromogen	Fe^{+++}	Intact usually bond to denatured protein other than globin.	Denatured usually detached	Brown (sometimes grayish)
9.	NO myohaemo chromogen (CM)	Effect of heat, denaturing agent on NOMb	Fe^{++}	Intact	Denatured	Bright red (pink)
10.	Sulph Mb	Effect of H_2S and O_2 on Mb	Fe^{++}	Intact but one = bond saturated	Native	Green
11.	Met sulph Mb	Oxdn sulph Mb	Fe^{+++}	Intact but one = bond saturated	Native	Red
12.	Chole globin	Effect of H_2O_2 on Mb or oxy Mb, effect of ascorbic acid or other reducing agent on oxy Mb	Fe^{++}or Fe^{+++}	Intact but one = bond saturated	Native	Green
13.	Nitrihaemin	Effect of large excess nitrite and heat on nitroso MMb	Fe^{+++}	Intact but reduced	Absent	Green
14.	Verdohaem	Effect of reagents as is 7-9 in excess	Fe^{+++}	Porphyrin ring opened	absent	green
15.	Bile pigments	Effect of reagents as in 7-9 in excess	Fe absent	Porphyrin ring destroyed chain of porphyrins	absent	Yellow or colourless

the rate of diffusion and uptake by cytochrome enzymes and by Mb to form oxy Mb.

- ✰ The depth of penetration of O_2, d is given by

  $$d = \sqrt{2CO^{D}/AO}$$

  where

  CO = O_2 pr. on the surface

  D = coefficient of diffusion

  AO = consumption of O_2.

- ✰ The bright red colour of oxy Mb will predominate and be apparent to observer when the ratio of oxy Mb: Mb is 1:1 *i.e.* about 84 per cent of the total depth of O_2 penetration.
- ✰ D varies in different muscles (different respiratory activities). Thus after exposure of cut surfaces to the air for 1 hr at 0°c, the depth of oxy Mb was found to be

  0.94 mm in horse psoas, where resp. activity high.

  2.48mm in horse L. dorsi, where resp. activity low.

  d = 4 mm in bacon – because resp. enzymes are inactivated by high salt conc.

- ✰ Decrease in D (coefficient of diffusion) < resp. activity for a given fall in temp., the depth of bright red colour layer of oxy Mb will be greater at 0°C than at 20°C. Therefore colour of meat surfaces become somewhat brighter when stored at low temperature.
- ✰ The formation of MMb – in a layer below the surface where O_2 pr. favourable.
- ✰ Light rays of shorter wave length accelerate oxdn.
- ✰ When oxidisable substrates of cytochrome enzymes become exhausted MMb is formed in deeper layers.
- ✰ When about 60 per cent of Mb in surface layers is convereted to MMb, meat assumes a more or less dark red to dark brown colour. The time taken to reach this pt. varies with animal in respect of the same muscle. It depends upon the activity of the cytochrome enzymes, content of NAD and the amount of substrate *e.g.* succinate.
- ✰ The oxidation of purplish red Mb or of bright red oxyMb to brown MMb is accelerated by
  1. Any factor causing denaturation of globin.
  2. By the absence of reducing mechanism
  3. By low O_2 tension.

However the above circumstances enhance the stability of the red colour of cured meat by converting NOMb in NO haemochromogen.

More Common Heme Pigments of Muscle and their Relationship in Uncured Meats

Mb and oxy Mb are found in fresh meat. MMb due to excessive holding or storage period.

	Mb	Haematin nuclcus intact.
In	oxy Mb	protein in native state
	MMb	but the colour and valency of iron vary.

- ☆ Oxdn. Of Mb in presence of reducing agents results two pigments of green colour.

  Mb + H_2S and O_2 converts to green sulphmyoglobin.

  Mb + H_2O_2 and ascorbic acid converts to green chole globin.
- ☆ Sulph Mb may convert Mb, but not choleglobin.
- ☆ Choleglobin rapidly breaks down to yield globin iron and a tetrapyrrole.
- ☆ Sulp. Mb formation – in meat with ultimate pH >6.0 since at lower < 6.0 pH bacteria capable of produce H_2 unable to liberate H_2S.
- ☆ If these conditions are intensified, the porphyrin ring may be opened although the iron remains, globin is absent, green verdohaem is formed.
- ☆ On further or more intense exposure, iron will be lost from porphyrin, forming the chain of pyrroles characterizing colourless or yellow bile pigments.

Table 9.10: Chemical State of Myoglobin

Bonds	*Compound*	*Color*	*Name*
Fe^{++} Ferrous (covalent)	H_2O	Purple	Reduced myoglobin
	O_2	Red	Oxymyoglobin
	NO	Cured pink	Nitric oxide myoglobin
	CO	Red	Carboxymyoglobin
Fe^{+++} Ferric (ionic)	–CN	Red	Cyanmetmyoglobin
	–OH	Brown	Metmyoglobin
	–SH	Green	Sulfmyoglobin
	$-H_2O_2$	Green	Choleglobin

Metmyoglobin Reducing Activity (MRA)

Reduced myoglobin –> oxymyoglobin –> metmyoglobin –> reduced myoglobin –> etc.

Differs according to muscle: some high in MRA (*Longissimus dorsi*), some low in MRA (*Biceps femoris*).

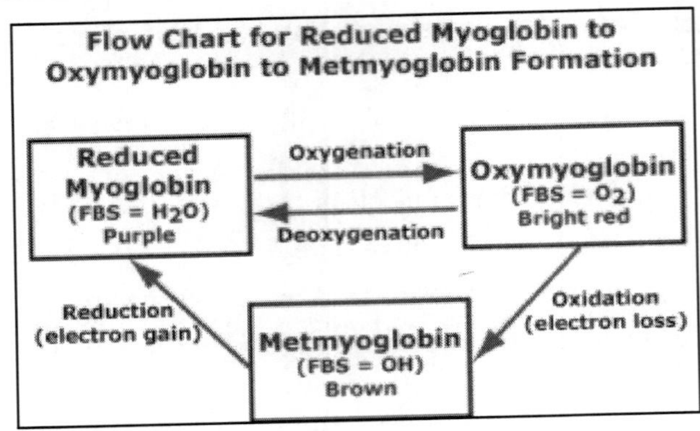

Activity of Bacteria

Pigment	Catalyst	New pigment
Oxymyoglobin	Oxidation + bacteria →	Metmyoglobin (-OH)
Metmyoglobin	Bacteria →	Choleglobin (-H_2O_2)
Metmyoglobin	Bacteria →	Sulfmyoglobin (-SH)

Packaging of Fresh Meat and Meat Colour

Because the bright red colour of oxyMb is desirable, most prepackaged fresh meat is placed in oxygen permeable wrap. But after a few days even at chill temperature some of surface pigments begin to oxidize to MMb or to Myohaemichromogen through incipient denaturation of the globin moiety. This originally discouraged central packaging of fresh meat in O_2 permeable wraps.

If meat is vacuum packed: no O_2 can get in surviving activity of cytochrome enzymes reduces the small amount of MMb formed in these circumtances replacing it by purplish red Mb. Vacuum packed meats in O_2 impermeable shrinkable film can be stored under chill conditions for several weeks. They can be allowed to reoxygenate before sale, thus restoring the bright red colour of oxyMb when the film is removed. Centralized prepackaging of fresh meats has been establish on such a basis.

To avoid browning due to MMb formation, ascorbic acid or niacin can be used. Nicotinamide slows the rate of MMb formation. Ascorbic acid reduces oxidized pigments as soon as it forms. Use of Ascorbic acid and nicotinamide is forbidden in USA. Brown pigments reduced by this way do not have reoxygenation capacity. Meat of pH above 6 is unsuitable for holding in evacuated gas impermeable packs since bacteria production of H_2S leads to formation of green sulph Mb.

Colour of Cooked Meat

Principles

Pigments of cooked meats is brown globin haemichromogen, and in case of bacon, a smoked product, is red NO haemochromogen. Brown pigment of cooked meat is a desirable attribute of meat quality.

- ☆ Colour of cooked uncured lean meat depends largely upon the nature and amount of myoglobin derivatives and decomposition products that are present.
- ☆ Cooked meat from older animals is darker than cooked meat from younger animals.
- ☆ Cooked meat from active animals or from high O_2 demand muscles is darker than that of less active animals or muscle with low O_2 demand.
- ☆ Final colour depends upon pigment changes during cooking. These changes due to cooking method, temp. and time duration. Colour changes gradually from deep red or pink to a lighter thin, finally if a high enough temp. a gray or brown colour.
- ☆ Rarely pink colour due to oxy Mb.
- ☆ Brown colour due to nos. of pigments – denatured haeme compounds, decomposition and polymerization of carbohydrates, fats and proteins.
- ☆ The visual colour changes are related to internal temp.

  Below 60°C (140°F) – little or no change (rare)

  65 – 70°C – decreasing pinkness (medium)

  At 75°C – complete loss of pinkness (well done)
- ☆ Meats cooked slowly in a moist atmosphere near the temp. of boiling water have a uniform gray colour with no browning of outer surface.
- ☆ Browning of cooked meat by slow heat and in canning is due to denaturation and oxdn. of Mb and is different from the surface browning of broiled or roasted meat.
- ☆ The colour of fat portion of meat changes very little during cooking except for surface browning, which contribute greatly to the attractive appearance of meat cooked by dry heat. This surface browning is due to decomposition and polymerization with its carbolydrates and protein decomposition products.
- ☆ When cooked or cured meat is cut, the thin layer of fat spread over the surface sometimes give greenish iridescence to surface as a result of light refraction. This does not indicate spoilage.

Cooked Colour Problems

Premature Browning

- ☆ Usually caused by highly oxidized meat or meat that is exposed to high-oxygen atmospheres

- Meat will turn brown around 130°F internal temperature
- Reason why colour is not a good indicator of cooked meat

Persistent Pinkness

- Usually caused by high pH meat
- Product will stay pink (uncooked colour) even with degrees of doneness that should ensure appropriate cooked endpoint are followed.

Cured Meat Colour

Mb + nitrite - Nitrite oxide Mb. Nitrite used in curing solution is Sodium nitrite.

- Nitric oxide (NO) is the impt. decomposition products from the added nitrite in curing solution, enters directly into curing reaction or color fixation reaction with Mb.
- The nasic chemical reaction involved in meat curing as follows:

  Mb + NO - NO Mb

  The haem pigment can follow many chemical pathways in the curing reactions.
- The ultimate pigment desired in most heat processed cured meats is nitrosyl hemochrome.
- Under some conditions nitrosylhemochrome may oxidized to green, yellow or colourless porphyrin.
- The green pigment formation is undesirable and may be due to bacterial action or chemical oxidation by peroxides, hypochlorites or other agents.
- Light catalyzes these oxidative changes, cured meat surfaces fade rapidly under strong light.

Non-Microbial Discolouration (NMD)

- Benefit of curing is the conversion of oxygen sensitive meant pigments to more stable cured meat pigment.
- Main cause of NMD is oxygen.
- Factors affecting NMD is oxygen.
  1. Amount of pigment actually converted to nitrosomyoglobin.
  2. Quantity of O_2 available for reaction with pigment
  3. Storage temp.
  4. Intensity of lighting.
- At least 70 per cent of meat pigments available for curing should be cured.
- Fading is an oxidative process accelerated by light and influenced by storage temperature.
- Vacuum packaging lengthens shelf life of cured meat. The low levels of O_2 in vacuum packages result in protecting processed meat from rapid onset of microbial spoilage, rancidily and colour fading.

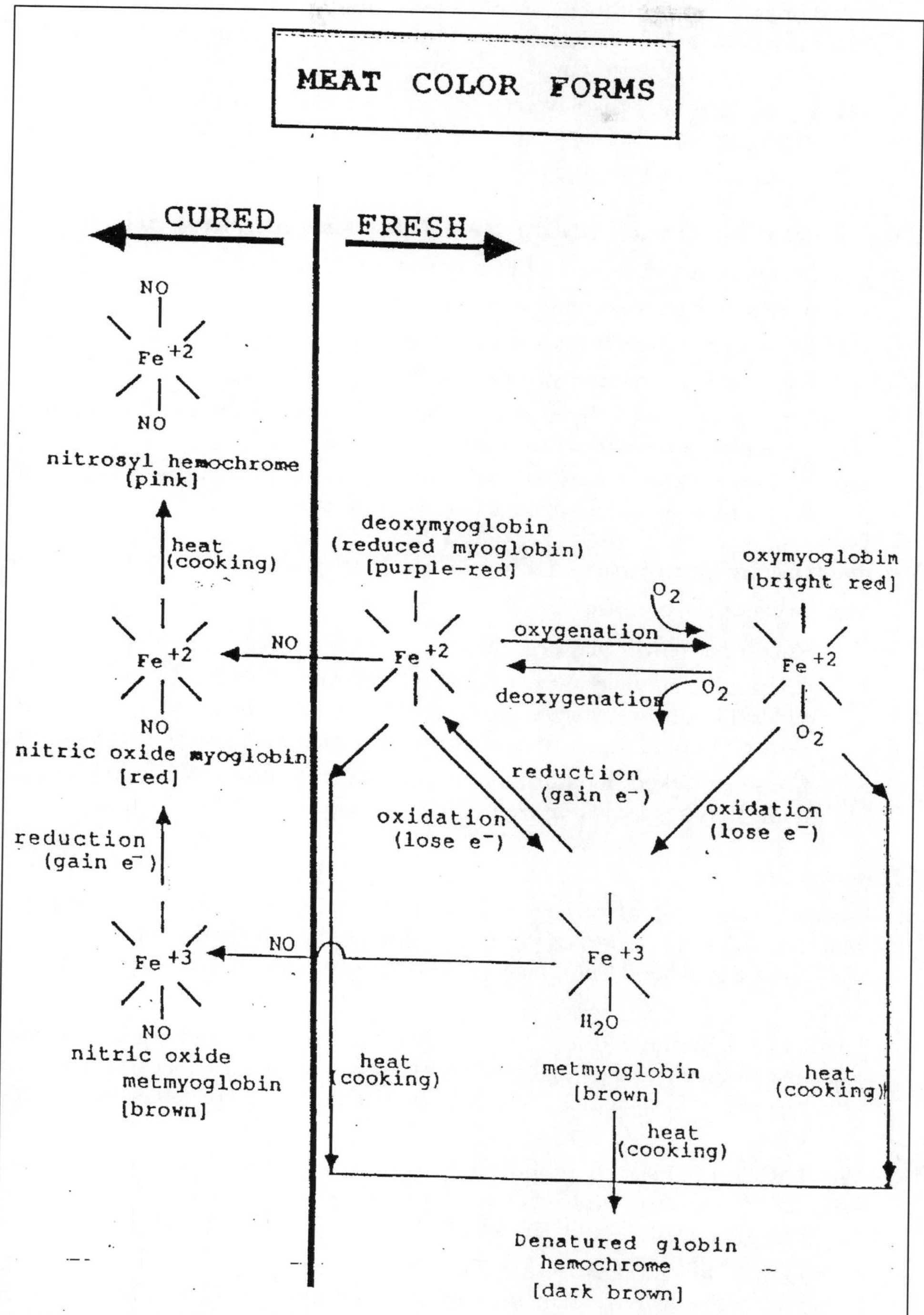
MEAT COLOR FORMS
CURED
FRESH
NO
Fe +2
NO
nitrosyl hemochrome
[pink]
heat
(cooking)
deoxymyoglobin
(reduced myoglobin)
[purple-red]
oxymyoglobin
[bright red]
O2
oxygenation
NO
Fe +2
Fe +2
Fe +2
deoxygenation
O2
NO
O2
nitric oxide myoglobin
[red]
reduction
(gain e⁻)
oxidation
(lose e⁻)
oxidation
(lose e⁻)
reduction
(gain e⁻)
NO
Fe +3
Fe +3
H2O
NO
nitric oxide
metmyoglobin
[brown]
heat
(cooking)
metmyoglobin
[brown]
heat
(cooking)
heat
(cooking)
Denatured globin
hemochrome
[dark brown]

- ☆ For maximum prevention of deterioration, both microbial and non-microbial, meat products shown be stored as close to 28°F as possible. However in practice, cured meats are generally stored between 38° to 45°F.
- ☆ Light, especially display case illumination catalyzes the oxdn. of cured meat pigments and can accelerate the fading rate.
- ☆ Hence cure meat should not be exposed to strong light.

Discolouration: Dark Cutting Beef (Increase ultimate pH)

- ☆ Surviving activity of cytochrome enzyme will be greater.
- ☆ Much of water associated with muscle.
- ☆ Muscle fibers tightly packed presenting a barrier to diffusion of oxygen.
- ☆ Layer of bright red oxyMb very small.
- ☆ Unpleasant, purplish red Mb predominate to such an extent that meat will appear dark *e.g.* dark-cutting beef, "glazy bacon".
- ☆ Appear dark because surface will not scatter light to the same extent as will the more open surface of meat of lower ultimate pH.

White Muscle Condition in Pigs (PSE Pork)

Meat is very pale, because of

1. Relative absent of Mb
2. Chemical change in pigment due to rapid rate of pH fall *i.e.* ultimate low pH while post-mortem temp. is still high. Mb is exposed to conditions causing its oxidation to MetMb (brown) which has a low colour intensity.
3. Cause a marked denaturation of sarcoplasmic and myofibrillar proteins and a very severe loss in water binding properties of the proteins.

References

1. Maton, Anthea; Jean Hopkins, Charles William McLaughlin, Susan Johnson, Maryanna Quon Warner, David LaHart, Jill D. Wright (1993). *Human Biology and Health*. Englewood Cliffs, New Jersey, USA: Prentice Hall. ISBN 0-13-981176-1.
2. Sidell, Bruce; Kristin O'Brien (2006). "When bad things happen to good fish: the loss of hemoglobin and myoglobin expression in Antarctic icefishes". *The Journal of Experimental Biology* **209** (Pt 10): 1791–1802. doi:10.1242/jeb.02091. PMID 16651546.
3. Weed, Robert I.; Reed, Claude F. and Berg, George (1963). "Is hemoglobin an essential structural component of human erythrocyte membranes?". *J Clin Invest.* **42** (4): 581–8.doi:10.1172/JCI104747. PMC 289318. PMID 13999462.
4. Dominguez de Villota ED, Ruiz Carmona MT, Rubio JJ, de Andrés S (1981). "Equality of the in vivo and in vitro oxygen-binding capacity of haemoglobin in patients with severe respiratory disease". *Br J Anaesth* **53** (12): 1325–8. doi:10.1093/bja/53.12.1325. PMID 7317251.

5. Costanzo, Linda S. (2007). *Physiology*. Hagerstwon, MD: Lippincott Williams and Wilkins. ISBN 0-7817-7311-3.
6. Epstein, F. H.; Hsia, C. C. W. (1998). "Respiratory Function of Hemoglobin". *New England Journal of Medicine* **338** (4): 239–247. doi:10.1056/NEJM199801223380407. PMID 9435331. edit
7. Jump up to:[a] [b] [c] [d] [e] Biagioli M, Pinto M, Cesselli D, *et al.* (2009). "Unexpected expression of alpha- and beta-globin in mesencephalic dopaminergic neurons and glial cells". *Proc. Natl. Acad. Sci. U.S.A.* **106**(36): 15454–9. doi:10.1073/pnas.0813216106. PMC 2732704. PMID 19717439.
8. "Max Perutz, Father of Molecular Biology, Dies at 87". *The New York Times.* February 8, 2002
9. Engelhard, Johann Friedrich (1825). *Commentatio de vera materia sanguini purpureum colorem impertientis natura* (in Latin). Göttingen: Dietrich.
10. Adair, Gilbert Smithson (1925). "A critical study of the direct method of measuring the osmotic pressure of hmoglobin". *Proc. R. Soc. Lond.* A 108 (750): 292–300. doi:10.1098/rspa.1925.0126.
11. Hünefeld F.L. (1840). *Die Chemismus in der thierischen Organization*. Leipzig.
12. Funke O (1851). "Über das milzvenenblut". *Z Rat Med* **1**: 172–218.
13. "A NASA Recipe For Protein Crystallography" (PDF). *Educational Brief.* National Aeronautics and Space Administration. Archived from the original on 2008-04-10. Retrieved 2008-10-12.
14. Hoppe-Seyler F (1866). "Über die oxydation in lebendem blute". *Med-chem Untersuch Lab* **1**: 133–140.
15. Perutz, M.F.; Rossmann, M.G.; Cullis, A.F.; Muirhead, H.; Will, G.; North, A.C.T. (1960). "Structure of H".*Nature* **185** (4711): 416–422. doi:10.1038/185416a0. PMID 18990801.
16. Perutz MF (1960). "Structure of haemoglobin". *Brookhaven symposia in biology* **13**: 165–83.PMID 13734651.
17. A Syllabus of Human Hemoglobin Variants (1996). Globin.cse.psu.edu. Retrieved on 2013-09-05.
18. Hemoglobin Variants. Labtestsonline.org. Retrieved on 2013-09-05.
19. Uthman, MD, Ed. "Hemoglobinopathies and Thalassemias". Retrieved 2007-12-26.
20. Reed, Leslie. "Adaptation found in mouse genes." Omaha World-Herald 11 Aug. 2009: EBSCO. Web. 30 Oct. 2009.
21. "Mammoths had 2anti-freeze2 blood". BBC. 2010-05-02. Retrieved 2010-05-02.
22. "Hemoglobin Synthesis". April 14, 2002. Retrieved 2007-12-26.
23. Jump up to:[a] [b] van Kessel *et al.* (2003) "2.4 Proteins – Natural Polyamides." Chemistry 12. Toronto: Nelson, p. 122.

24. "Hemoglobin Tutorial." University of Massachusetts Amherst. Web. 23 Oct. 2009.

25. Steinberg, MH (2001). *Disorders of Hemoglobin: Genetics, Pathophysiology, and Clinical Management*. Cambridge University Press. p. 95. ISBN 0-521-63266-8.

26. Hardison, RC (1996). "A brief history of hemoglobins: plant, animal, protist, and bacteria". *Proc Natl Acad Sci USA* **93** (12): 5675–9. doi:10.1073/pnas.93.12.5675. PMC 39118. PMID 8650150.

27. "Hemoglobin." School of Chemistry – Bristol University – UK. Web. 12 Oct. 2009.

28. WikiPremed > Coordination Chemistry Retrieved on July 2, 2009

29. Linberg R, Conover CD, Shum KL, Shorr RG (1998). "Hemoglobin based oxygen carriers: how much methemoglobin is too much?". *Artif Cells Blood Substit Immobil Biotechnol* **26** (2): 133–48.doi:10.3109/10731199809119772. PMID 9564432.

30. Hemoglobin. Worthington-biochem.com. Retrieved on 2013-09-05.

31. Van Beekvelt MC, Colier WN, Wevers RA, Van Engelen BG (2001). "Performance of near-infrared spectroscopy in measuring local O2 consumption and blood flow in skeletal muscle". *J Appl Physiol* **90** (2): 511–519. PMID 11160049.

32. Jump up to:[a] [b] "Hemoglobin." MedicineNet. Web. 12 Oct. 2009.

33. "Hemoglobin Home." Biology @ Davidson. Web. 12 Oct. 2009.

34. "Hemoglobin saturation graph". *altitude.org*.

35. King, Michael W. "The Medical Biochemistry Page – Hemoglobin".

36. Voet, D. (2008) *Fundamentals of Biochemistry*, 3rd. ed., Fig. 07_06, John Wiley and Sons

37. Ahrens, Thomas; Kimberley, Basham (1993). *Essentials of Oxygenation: Implication for Clinical Practice*. Jones and Bartlett Learning. p. 194. ISBN 0867203323.

38. Pin S, Alpert B, Michalowicz A. (1982). "Oxygen bonding in human hemoglobin and its isolated subunits: A XANES study". *FEBS Lett.* **147** (1): 106–10. doi:10.1016/0014-5793(82)81021-1.PMID 7140986.

39. Pin, S.; Valat, P.; Cortes, R.; Michalowicz, A.; Alpert, B. (1985). "Ligand binding processes in hemoglobin. Chemical reactivity of iron studied by XANES spectroscopy". *Biophysical Journal* **48** (6): 997–1001. doi:10.1016/S0006-3495(85)83862-5. PMC 1329432. PMID 4092074. edit

40. Bianconi A, Congiu-Castellano A, Dell'Ariccia M, Giovannelli A, Burattini E, Durham PJ (1985). "Increase of the Fe effective charge in hemoproteins during oxygenation process". *Biochemical and Biophysical Research Communications* **30** (1): 98–102. doi:10.1016/0006-291X(85)91775-9.PMID 4038310.

41. Childs PE (2001). "Haemoglobin – a molecular lung: 2". *Chemistry in Action* (65). ISSN 0332-2637.

42. Chen H, Ikeda-Saito M, Shaik S (2008). "Nature of the Fe-O2 bonding in oxy-myoglobin: effect of the protein". *Journal of the American Chemical Society* **130** (44): 14778–14790.doi:10.1021/ja805434m. PMID 18847206.

43. Chou KC (1989). "Low-frequency resonance and cooperativity of hemoglobin". *Trends Biochem. Sci.*14 (6): 212–3. doi:10.1016/0968-0004(89)90026-1. PMID 2763333.
44. Jensen, Frank B (2009). "The dual roles of red blood cells in tissue oxygen delivery: oxygen carriers and regulators of local blood flow". *Journal of Experimental Biology* (The Company of Biologists) **212**(Pt 21): 3387–3393. doi:10.1242/jeb.023697. PMID 19837879.
45. Hall, John E. (2010). *Guyton and Hall textbook of medical physiology* (12th ed.). Philadelphia, Pa.: Saunders/Elsevier. p. 502. ISBN 978-1416045748.
46. Nelson, D. L.; Cox, M. M. (2000). *Lehninger Principles of Biochemistry*, 3rd ed. New York, NY: Worth Publishers. p. 217, ISBN 1572599316.
47. Guyton, Arthur C.; John E. Hall (2006). *Textbook of Medical Physiology* (11 ed.). Philadelphia: Elsevier Saunders. p. 511. ISBN 0-7216-0240-1.
48. Lecture – 12 Myoglobin and Hemoglobin on YouTube
49. Rutjes, H. A.; Nieveen, M. C.; Weber, R. E.; Witte, F.; Van den Thillart, G. E. E. J. M. (20 June 2007). "Multiple strategies of Lake Victoria cichlids to cope with lifelong hypoxia include hemoglobin switching". *AJP: Regulatory, Integrative and Comparative Physiology* **293** (3): R1376–R1383.doi:10.1152/ajpregu.00536.2006.
50. Gronenborn, Angela M.; Clore, G.Marius; Brunori, Maurizio; Giardina, Bruno; Falcioni, Giancarlo; Perutz, Max F. (1984). "Stereochemistry of ATP and GTP bound to fish haemoglobins". *Journal of Molecular Biology* **178** (3): 731–742. doi:10.1016/0022-2836(84)90249-3. PMID 6492161.
51. Weber, Roy E.; Frank B. Jensen (1988). "Functional adaptations in hemoglobins from ectothermic invertebrates". *Annual Review of Physiology* **50**: 161–179.doi:10.1146/annurev.ph.50.030188.001113. PMID 3288089.
52. Rang, H.P.; Dale M.M., Ritter J.M., Moore P.K. (2003). *Pharmacology, Fifth Edition*. Elsevier. ISBN 0-443-07202-7.
53. Wiester, M. J.; Winsett, D. W.; Richards, J. H.; Doerfler, D. L.; Costa, D. L. (2002). "Partitioning of benzene in blood: Influence of hemoglobin type in humans and animals". *Environmental health perspectives* **110** (3): 255–261. doi:10.1289/ehp.02110255. PMC 1240765.PMID 11882476. edit
54. "Hemoglobin Variants". *Lab Tests Online*. American Association for Clinical Chemistry. 2007-11-10. Retrieved 2008-10-12.
55. Huisman THJ (1996). "A Syllabus of Human Hemoglobin Variants". *Globin Gene Server*. Pennsylvania State University. Retrieved 2008-10-12.
56. Kikuchi, G.; Yoshida, T.; Noguchi, M. (2005). "Heme oxygenase and heme degradation". *Biochemical and Biophysical Research Communications* **338** (1): 558–567. doi:10.1016/j.bbrc.2005.08.020.PMID 16115609. edit
57. "hemoglobinopathy" at *Dorland's Medical Dictionary*
58. hypoxemia. Encyclopædia Britannica, stating *hypoxemia* (*reduced oxygen tension in the blood*).

59. Biology-Online.org –> Dictionary » H » Hypoxemia last modified 29 December 2008
60. William, C. Wilson; Grande, Christopher M. and Hoyt, David B. (2007). "Pathophysiology of acute respiratory failure". *Trauma, Volume II: Critical Care*. Taylor and Francis. p. 430. ISBN 978-1-4200-1684-0.
61. McGaffigan, P. A. (1996). "Hazards of hypoxemia: How to protect your patient from low oxygen levels".*Nursing* **26** (5): 41–46; quiz 46. PMID 8710285. edit
62. "Definition of Glycosylated Hemoglobin." Medicine Net. Web. 12 Oct. 2009.
63. Madsen, H; Ditzel, J (1984). "Blood-oxygen transport in first trimester of diabetic pregnancy". *Acta Obstetricia et Gynecologica Scandinavica* **63** (4): 317–20. doi:10.3109/00016348409155523.PMID 6741458.
64. Hemoglobin at Medline Plus
65. Padmanaban, P.; Toora, B. (2011). "Hemoglobin: Emerging marker in stable coronary artery disease". *Chronicles of Young Scientists* **2** (2): 109. doi:10.4103/2229-5186.82971. edit
66. Society for Biomedical Diabetes Research. SI Unit Conversion Calculator.
67. Handin, Robert I.; Lux, Samuel E. and StosselBlood, Thomas P. (2003). *Blood: Principles and Practice of Hematology*. Lippincott Williams and Wilkins, ISBN 0781719933
68. Hemoglobin Level Test. Ibdcrohns.about.com (2013-08-16). Retrieved on 2013-09-05.
69. Although other sources can have slightly differing values, such as haemoglobin (reference range). gpnotebook.co.uk
70. Murray S.S. and McKinney E.S. (2006). *Foundations of Maternal-Newborn Nursing*. 4th ed., p. 919. Philadelphia: Saunders Elsevier
71. "Hematocrit (HCT) or Packed Cell Volume (PCV)". *DoctorsLounge.com*. Retrieved 2007-12-26.
72. Frasca, D.; Dahyot-Fizelier, C.; Catherine, K.; Levrat, Q.; Debaene, B.; Mimoz, O. (2011). "Accuracy of a continuous noninvasive hemoglobin monitor in intensive care unit patients*". *Critical Care Medicine***39** (10): 2277–2282. doi:10.1097/CCM.0b013e3182227e2d. PMID 21666449. edit
73. Ferrari, M.; Binzoni, T.; Quaresima, V. (1997). "Oxidative metabolism in muscle". *Philosophical Transactions of the Royal Society B: Biological Sciences* **352** (1354): 677–683.doi:10.1098/rstb.1997.0049. PMC 1691965. PMID 9232855. edit
74. Madsen, P. L.; Secher, N. H. (1999). "Near-infrared oximetry of the brain". *Progress in neurobiology***58** (6): 541–560. doi:10.1016/S0301-0082(98)00093-8. PMID 10408656. edit
75. McCully, K. K.; Hamaoka, T. (2000). "Near-infrared spectroscopy: What can it tell us about oxygen saturation in skeletal muscle?". *Exercise and sport sciences reviews* **28** (3): 123–127.PMID 10916704. edit

76. Perrey, S. P. (2008). "Non-invasive NIR spectroscopy of human brain function during exercise".*Methods* **45** (4): 289–299. doi:10.1016/j.ymeth.2008.04.005. PMID 18539160. edit

77. Rolfe, P. (2000). "Invivonear-Infraredspectroscopy". *Annual Review of Biomedical Engineering* **2**: 715–754. doi:10.1146/annurev.bioeng.2.1.715. PMID 11701529. edit

78. This Hb A_{1c} level is only useful in individuals who have red blood cells (RBCs) with normal survivals (*i.e.*, normal half-life). In individuals with abnormal RBCs, whether due to abnormal hemoglobin molecules (such as Hemoglobin S in Sickle Cell Anemia) or RBC membrane defects – or other problems, the RBC half-life is frequently shortened. In these individuals, an alternative test called "fructosamine level" can be used. It measures the degree of glycation (glucose binding) to albumin, the most common blood protein, and reflects average blood glucose levels over the previous 18–21 days, which is the half-life of albumin molecules in the circulation.

79. Mehagnoul-Schipper DJ, van der Kallen BF, Colier WN, van der Sluijs MC, van Erning LJ, Thijssen HO, Oeseburg B, Hoefnagels WH, Jansen RW (2002). "Simultaneous measurements of cerebral oxygenation changes during brain activation by near-infrared spectroscopy and functional magnetic resonance imaging in healthy young and elderly subjects". *Hum Brain Mapp* **16** (1): 14–23.doi:10.1002/hbm.10026. PMID 11870923.

80. L. Int Panis, B. Goddeeris, R Verheyen (1995). "The hemoglobin concentration of Chironomus cf.Plumosus L. (Diptera: Chironomidae) larvae from two lentic habitats". *Netherlands Journal of Aquatic Ecology* **29** (1): 1–4. doi:10.1007/BF02061785.

81. Weber RE, Vinogradov SN (2001). "Nonvertebrate hemoglobins: functions and molecular adaptations". *Physiol. Rev.* **81** (2): 569–628. PMID 11274340.

82. Zal F, Lallier FH, Green BN, Vinogradov SN, Toulmond A (1996). "The multi-hemoglobin system of the hydrothermal vent tube worm Riftia pachyptila. II. Complete polypeptide chain composition investigated by maximum entropy analysis of mass spectra". *J. Biol. Chem.* **271** (15): 8875–81.doi:10.1074/jbc.271.15.8875. PMID 8621529.

83. Minic Z, Hervé G (2004). "Biochemical and enzymological aspects of the symbiosis between the deep-sea tubeworm Riftia pachyptila and its bacterial endosymbiont". *Eur. J. Biochem.* **271** (15): 3093–102. doi:10.1111/j.1432-1033.2004.04248.x. PMID 15265029.

84. Liu L, Zeng M, Stamler JS (1999). "Hemoglobin induction in mouse macrophages". *Proceedings of the National Academy of Sciences of the United States of America* **96** (12): 6643–7.doi:10.1073/pnas.96.12.6643. PMC 21968. PMID 10359765.

85. Newton DA, Rao KM, Dluhy RA, Baatz JE (2006). "Hemoglobin Is Expressed by Alveolar Epithelial Cells". *Journal of Biological Chemistry* **281** (9): 5668–76. doi:10.1074/jbc.M509314200.PMID 16407281.

86. Nishi, H.; Inagi, R.; Kato, H.; Tanemoto, M.; Kojima, I.; Son, D.; Fujita, T.; Nangaku, M. (2008)."Hemoglobin is Expressed by Mesangial Cells and Reduces Oxidant Stress". *Journal of the American Society of Nephrology* **19** (8): 1500–1508. doi:10.1681/ASN.2007101085.PMC 2488266. PMID 18448584. edit

87. Boh, Larry (2001). *Pharmacy Practice Manual: A Guide to the Clinical Experience*. Lippincott Williams and Wilkins. ISBN 0-7817-2541-0.

88. Holden, Constance (2005). "Blood and Steel". *Science* **309** (5744): 2160.doi:10.1126/science.309.5744.2160d.

89. Moran L, Horton RA, Scrimgeour G, Perry M (2011). *Principles of Biochemistry*. Boston, MA: Pearson. p. 127. ISBN 0-321-70733-8.

IV. Meat Flavour

Flavour is one of the most important quality attributes of meat. Meat flavour is defined as a complex sensation arising as a result of two distinct responses *i.e.* taste and aroma as well as the less defined contribution from the pressure and heat sensitive areas of the mouth. Food can be made to look very appealing, nutritious and of suitable texture but still not consumed if it has an unpleasant flavour. The factors that exerts greatest influence of flavour is Odour. If odour is lacking the flavour is primarily a function of the taste sensation, bitter, sweet, sour and salt. Studies of meat flavour consequently had been concentrated mainly on odorous compounds of meat and their precursors.

Raw Meat Flavour

- ☆ Odour just like serum and blood like taste.
- ☆ In general has a salty, metallic, bloody taste and sweet aroma resembling serum.
- ☆ The raw meat contains volatile components but their flavour notes are much weaker and different.
- ☆ Cooking or processing develops the flavour of meat which is due to compounds formed during the heat treatment from precursor in raw meat.

Flavour Precursors in Meat

- ☆ The components in raw meat which develop Meat flavour are soluble in cold water.
- ☆ Proteins do not contribute to meat flavour
- ☆ Water soluble proteins do not contribute to meat flavour.
- ☆ Addition of glucose to soluble or insoluble proteins did not produce meat like aroma conclusion is that only low molecular wt. compounds are the precursors for the development of cooked meat flavour.

The Extracts of Meat from Freshly Killed Animal Contain

- ☆ Amino acids
- ☆ Peptides

- ☆ Nucleotides and
- ☆ Reducing substances like
- ☆ Glucose, glucose 6-phospahte
- ☆ Focuctose-6-phosphate
- ☆ Diphosphopyrimidine nucleotide

The extract from aged muscle (conditioned)

Glucose, fructose and ribose are present but sugar-phosphate are in traces

- ☆ After browning –all the sugars and diphosphopyridine nucleotides disappear.
- ☆ The increase in flavour is due to the increase in inorganic phosphate; loss of organic phosphate and decrease in reducing substances.

Expt: With model system showed that heating of amino acid and their complete synthetic beef extracts produced neither browning nor meaty odour in the absence of reducing sugars. With glucose- the beef extract did not give browning at room temperature, but on heating flavour of beef extract developed. Ribose-5-phosphate reacts most readily liberating inorganic phosphates and causing rapid browning with mixtures of amino acids.

The primary reactions which occur on heating include:

1. Degradation of sugars
2. Pyrrolysis of proteins and amino acids
3. Lipid degradation

Additionally interaction of two or more precursors may occur as in case of Streekers degradation, Maillard reaction and, Various protein lipid interactions. Much of the experiments showed that the development of brown colour and meaty flavour is result of Maillard reaction. Maillard reaction: Reaction of protein + reducing sugars – resulting in nutritional damage to food proteins during processing and storage. The reaction of proteins with reducing sugars is the major source of nutritional damage to food proteins during processing and storage. This reaction is termed a Maillard reaction. This reaction was named after the French chemist Louis Maillard (1912) who first described the formation of brown pigments or Melanoidins when heating a solution of glucose and glycine (amino acid). It now comprises of reactions of addehydes, ketones and reducing sugars with amines, amino acids, peptides and proteins.

In foods the reactions generally occurs between the reducing sugars and amino acids and proteins. Most amino groups are represented by $-NH_2$ group of lysine and to a very small extent by the α-amino group of the N-terminal amino acids. In addition, most food stuffs contain a certain proportion of free amino acids, whose reactions are often more useful and relevant to flavour formation than to loss in nutritive value.

Maillard reactions are complex and as yet not fully understood although they do appear to follow a common pathways which can be divided conveniently into early and advanced Maillard reactions.

The Primary Steps are

Reducing Sugar + Amino Compound

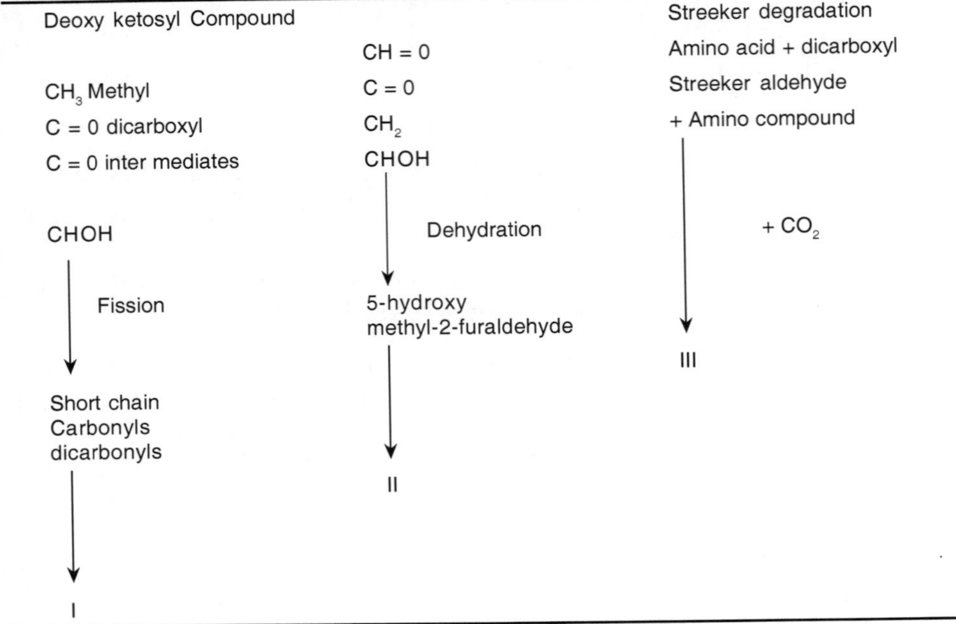

Melanoidin formation by the polymerization of intermediate compounds production of N-heterocyclics.

- ☆ Ist Pathway: Flavour compounds such as Acetalehyde, pyruvaldelyde, diacetyl and acetic acid are formed.
- ☆ IInd pathway: dehydration of 3-deoxy hexosomes leads to hydroxyl methyl furaldehyde (HMF)-dark brown nitrogen containing compounds as pyrazines and pyrolles.
- ☆ IIIrd pathway: Streeker's degradation which involves the degradation of free amino acids by the dicarboxyls formed in the Ist pathways.

$$\text{Amino acids} \xrightarrow{\text{Degraded}} \text{Corresponding aldehydes} \longrightarrow CO_2 \text{ (1 carbon atom lost in form of } CO_2\text{)}$$

This transamination reactions are important to incorporate the Nitrogen into the melanoidins.

Flavour of Cooked Meat

Due to mixture of compounds including

1. Non-volatile or water soluble compounds with taste tactile properties.

2. Potentiators and synergists
3. Volatiles which give rise to odour properties.

Natural flavour constituents: the most important taste compounds in meat are

1. Inorganic salts (salty taste)
2. Hypoxanthin (Bitterness)
3. Sugars (sweetness)
4. Organic acids (sour taste)

Nucleotides, amino acids and peptides (Anserine and carnosine)

Detection of Volatile Compounds in Lean Meat on Heating

Cooked beef, pork, lamb or whale the usual technique is to reflux a mixture of ground meat with water and then the volatiles generated are swept with a stream of nitrogen and then condensed in traps of cold water and identified by GLC

Table 9.11: Volatile Compounds from Cooked Meat (GLC)

Sl.No.	*Carbonyls*	*Acids*	*Other Compounds*
1	Formaldehyde*	Formic acid*	
2	Acetaldehyde*	Acetic acid*	CO_2
3	Propionaldehyde*	Butyric acid	NH_3
4	n-hexanol	Iso-butyric acid*	Methylamine
5	Iso-buteraldehyde*	**Alcohols**	4-hydroxy-5-methyl-3-Furanone
6	Iso-valeraldehyde*	Methanol	
7	Acetone	Ethanol	4-hydroxy-2, 5-
8	Methyl-propyl ketone	**Sulphur compounds**	Dimethyl-3-furanone
9	Methyl-ethyl ketone	H_2S	
10	diacetyl	Methyl mercaptans*	
	Dimethyl sulphide		
	Ethyl mercaptans*		

* Compounds produced by Streeker's degradation of amino acids.

The acids are produced by air oxidation of corresponding aldehydes. All the compounds identified have odour or tastes of various kinds and often very repulsive, but blended together and in minute amounts they contributes to the overall meat aroma. As the volatiles listed above arise on heat treatment of watery meat extract it may be assumed that the precursors are sugar and amino acids present in the raw meat.

The carbohydrates of meat are also important in producing flavour. On heating, they looses elements of water in two stages at 180° and 220°C forming Furfural from pentoses, Hydroxy methyl furfural (HMF) from hexoses. At about 300°C there is caramelization with formation of a number of odorous compounds including– Furans, alcohols and aromatic hydrocarbons.

Flavour Potentiators or Enhancers

Two compounds in meat are of importance for the taste without imparting a particular flavour note by themselves. (1) Monosodium glutamate (2) Disodium insinate. They are called as flavour enhancers. They do not react with falvour components in meat but in some way sensitizes or effect the taste nerve endings. The enhancing effect depends on the structure of the compounds.

COO^-	Glutamic acid has two acid groups – neutralizing
H_3N C.H.	both will give a disodium salt -
CH_2 CH_2 COO^- (glutamic acid)	Disodium glutamate, which has no flavour enhancing effect as compared to Monosodium glutamate(MSG)-which is formed during ageing of meat.

Inosinate is important as a flavour enhancer. This is formed by deamination of AMP (Adenosine monophosphate) in a chain of reactions which converts AMP to Hypoxanthine during ageing of meat.

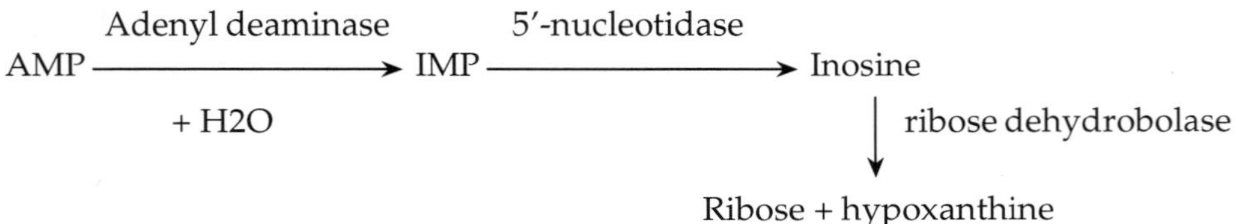

- Only IMP has a taste effect whereas AMP and Inosine have practically none.
- Hypoxanthine gives bitter note

Lipid Contribution to Meat Flavour

Fatty acids on oxidation produces carbonyl compounds that are potential flavour contributors. Carbonyls are partially come from amino acids and partly from lipids.

- Heating of fat from beef and pork in vacuum or in nitrogen gives non-meat aromas but if heated in air gives characteristics odour of meat *viz.* pork and beef. Thus fat oxidation is important in flavour developments.
- Composition is triglycerides phospholipids and FFA are important. FFA are more easily oxidized.
- Carbonyls are more in beef and pork and absent in lamb. Conc. of carbonyls differ considerably between species.
- Chicken fat – higher content USFA than pork hence a wider spectrum of carbonyls in chicken responsible for poultry flavour.

- ☆ The off flavour referred as warmed over flavour in cooked meat and stored meat is probably caused by the oxidation of phosphoslipids of muscle by both haem and non- haem iron.
- ☆ Natural flavour components are Anserine and carnosine.

Compounds responsible for **boar taint** is a steroid 5α- androst-16- ene-3- one or (Androsterone)

Sulphur Compounds

Produces desirable flavour and undesirable flavour

H_2S is the basic component for sulphur containing amino acids like cystein, cystine, methionine. The odour threshold of H_2S in water is 10 PPM. Freshly cooked chicken meat has 20 to 100 times more H_2S than threshold value.

Aroma and Flavour of Meat

Meat from older animals has a stronger odour than meat from younger animals of the same species. "Piggy" or "sex" odour is occasionally found in pork. Meat stored unfrozen develop gamy or aged aroma in aged beef: prolonged storage under unfavorable conditions cause proteolytic or putrid odours due to protein decomposition; sour or tainted odour from microbial growth and rancid odour due to fat oxidation – rancid odour described as tallowy for beef, mottony for mutton, and stale, cheesy, acrylic, fishy or oily for pork.

During cooking – intensified by heating *e.g.* a piggy odour in pork. The additional holding period results in an increase in the "sulfury" flavour component, cooked unaged beef – "metalic" and "astringent" flavour, veal flavour is "Sweet", "Sour" or "flat". Pork flavour is "bland" and "sweet". Broiled lamb – predominant animal flavour and a greasy mouth coating effect and after taste.

Chemistry of Meat Flavour

Raw meats have a mild serum like flavour that in no way resembles the flavour of cooked meat. It is when meat is heated that reactions take place that produce meaty aromas. Probably the same precursor systems are responsible for the meat flavour charcterieteristics of different methods of cooking. Investigations of meat flavour have been characterized by a dual approach:

1. A study of flavour precursor system.
2. An analysis of the meat flavour volatiles.

1. Precursors

Howe and Barbella (1937) considered both lean and fat important and related time and temperature of heating to the quality of the flavour. Crocker (1948) concluded that heating meat fibers produced typical meat aromas and that a non-typical, low intensity flavour was obtained by heating expressed juices. Jones (1952) reported that cooking lean meat produced little flavour and attributed the flavour to the fat. Barylko-Piekielva (1957) stated that meat flavour was not derived solely from muscle fibers. Kranlich and Pearson (1958) reported that heating expressed mfluids from raw beef produced a typical meat aroma. Hornstein *et al.* (1960b) blended ground lean beef with cold water at 0°C (32°F), centrifuged the slurry and heated both the extract and residue to 100°C (212°F) - the extract produced typical aroma while the heated residue was essentially odourless. They concluded that regardless of the site the flavour precursors of lean meat were water soluble and further the insoluble protein fraction contributed little, if anything to meaty aromas.

Horstein and Crowe (1960) Partially freeze-dried a cold water entract of fat free lean beef, then dialyzed this a concentrate against water at 0°C (32°F). the freeze-dried difusate produced typical roast beef aromas on heating. The freeze dried dialysate, constituting sarcoplasmic proteins did not produce meat like aromas when heated. The diffusate further separated by ion-exchange chromatography into an amino acids fraction and a neutral fraction containing reducing sugars. Neither of these fractions on heating produced meat aromas. However when recombined and heated did result in the development of meat like aromas. It was concluded that a nonenzynatic browning reaction between amino acids and reducing sugars present in lean beef was essential for the dev. of meat like aromas.

Wood and Bender (1957) and Bender *et al.* (1958) analysed commercial beef muscle extract and an extract of fresh beef muscle for non-protein constituents. They concluded that the development of meaty aromas in meat extract was a result of Maillard reaction, a reaction between amino acids and reducing sugars Batzer *et al.* (1960, 1962) dialyzed a water extract of raw ground beef, reported that flavour precursors were present in the diffusate. This diffusate was redialyzed – a fraction was obtained that on heating produced an aroma of cooked beef. This fraction contained a glycoprotein and inosinic acid, the latter being considered as meat falvour enhancer. Also reported amino acid sequence in a molecule are apparently responsible for the meat flavour. Wasserman and Gray (1965) repeated the fractionation procedure of Batzer *et al.* (1960). Two fractions were separated which when heated produced meat aromas. Only one of these fractions studied in detail, seventeen amino acids were identified, no reducing sugar were reported.

Mabroak *et al.* (1967): blended the ground beef muscle with water, freeze-dried the resulted slurry, extracted the freeze-dried material with petroleum ether to ensure it complete lipipd-free. The lipid free material blended with water, centrifuged and the extract dialyzed. The diffusate on heating produced meaty aromas. The diffusate was separated by gel permeation chromatography into 12 separate fractions. Meat like aromas were strongest in fractions 3, 4, 5 and 6 and were associated with ninhydrin positive material and carbohydrates. Fraction 5 and 6 exhibited greatest odour intensity in either fraction the only carbohydrate present was 2-deoxy-D-ribuse. Methionine was present in fraction 5 and methionine + cystcic acid in fraction 6. The association of sulfur-containing amino acids was not clear cut. Hornstein *et al.* (1960b, 1963). Same procedure looked for flavour precursor in lean pork and lamb. In each case the flavour precursor was water soluble, non-protein substances with ion exchange chromatography – two sub fractions, one is amino acids and other is reducing sugars. Heating the separate sub fractions did not produce flavour however recombination produced meaty aromas.

Macy *et al.* (1964a, 1964b) analyzed diffusate obtained from pork, beef and lamb. Glutathione was identified in lamb but not in pork and beef. Cystic acid and ornithine were found in pork and beef but not in lamb. The result indicate that ribose may be most active in promoting browning and flavour development.

We can draw the flowing conclusions from these precursor studies:

1. The flavour precursors of meat are water soluble.
2. A non-enzymatic browning type reaction between reducing sugars and amino acids is largely responsible for development of characteristic meat flavour.
3. The similarity in amino acid and carbohydrate composition of beef, pork and lamb may account for the similarity in flavour of the lean meat from these species.
4. Specific glycoprotein may in part contribute to meat flavour.
5. Intact fibrillar and sarcoplasmic protein as such do not contribute to meat flavour.

2. Volatile Compounds

Stahl (1957) and Merrit *et al.* (1959) investigated the volatile compounds recovered from raw beef. These compounds were isolated by vacuum distillation, separated by gas liquid chromatography (GLC) and identified by mass spectrometry. Hornstein *et al.* (1960 b) and Hornstein and Crowe (1960) studied the volatiles that were obtained by heating under high vacuum, a lyophilized extract of lean beef. Bender and Balance (1961) investigated the volatiles isolated from a commercial beef extract heated to 60°C (140°F). Yueh and Strong (1960) and Kramlich and Pearson (1960) examined the volatiles produced by refluxing for several hours, a slurry of ground beef in water. Hirai *et al.* (1968) meat was cooked in water then blended to form slurry, fed at 70°C (158°F) into an all glass, specially designed high vacuum distillation apparatus, isolated by flash vaporization, collected in a series of cold traps, extracted with ether and separated by GLC. 2 of the 18 fractions collected had a characteristics boiled beef odour. The oxazoline and trithiolan exhibited cooked beef odours. α-dicarbonyl compounds resulting from reducing sugars can react with α-amino acids to yield aldehyde containing one less carbon atom than the parent α-amino acids oxidation of aldehyde can produce the corresponding acids *e.g.* 2-methyl propanal lead to 2-methyl propionic acid. Streacker degradation of methionine produced methional which in turn break down to methyl mercaptan and acrolein. Auto-oxidation of unsaturated fatty acids present in intramuscular fat can form hydrocarbons and oxidation of these produce acids.

Jacobson and Koetler (1963) Studied on roasting lamb compounds identified includes acetaldehyde propanal n-hexanal 3-methyl 2-butanone, ammonia and hydrogen sulfide. Same compounds identified in beef volatiles. Hornstein and Crowe (1963) studied the flavour of lean lamb and Hornstein *et al.* (1963) flavour of lean whale meat. Trimethylamine was recovered from whale meat, reinforce the concept that lean meat flavour is similar regardless of species.

Table 9.12: Compounds Identified in Cooked Veef Volatiles

Hydrocarons	*Alcohols*
n-Hexane (5)	Methanol (3,5)
n-Dodecane (5)	Ethanol (3,5)
n-Pen tadecane (5)	n-Propanol (5)
n-Hexadecane (5)	n-Butaiol (5)
n-octadecane (5)	n-Pentanol (5)
I-Undecane (5)	n-Hexanol (5)
I-Pentadecane (5)	n-octanol (5)
	Isobutanol (5)
	Isopentanol (5)
	2-Hexenol (5)
	1-Penten-3-oil (5)
	1octen-3-oil (5)

Sl.No.	*Aldelydes*	*Acids*
1.	Formaldehyde (4)	Formic (1)
2.	Acetaldehyde (2,3,4)	Acetic (1)
3.	Propanal (3)	Propionic (1)
4.	2-methyl propanal (3)	Butyric (5)
5.	n-pentanal (5)	Hexanoic (5)
6.	3-methyl butanal (3)	2-methyl propionic (1)
7.	n-Haxanal (4,5)	Lactic (4)
8.	n-Heptanal (4,5)	**Esters:**
9.	n-Octanal (4,5)	Ethyl acetate (5)
10.	n-Nonanal (4,5)	**Ethers:**
11.	n-Hexadecanal (5)	Hexyl ether (5)
12.	2-Octenal (5)	**Lactones:**
13.	E-Methyl-2-hepten-1-al (5)	α-Valerolactone (5)
14.	Hepta-2-en-1-al (4)	**Aromatics:**
15.	Octa-2-en-1-al (4)	Benzene (5)
16.	Nona-2-en-1-al (4)	Toluene (5)
17.	Deca-2-en-1-al (4)	n-Propyl benzene (5)
18.	Undeca-2-en-1-al (4)	Benzaldehyde (5)
19.	Deca-2, 4-dienal (4)	O-Methyl benzaldelyde (5)

Sl.No.	Ketones
1.	Acetone (1,2,3,4)
2.	2-Butanone (3)
3.	4-Octanone (5)
4.	3-Nonanone (5)
5.	3-Dodecanone (5)
6.	Diacetyl (1,4,5)
7.	Acetoin (5)
8.	**"S" Compounds:**
9.	Methylmercaptan (2,4)
10.	Ethyl mercaptan (3)
11.	Dimethyl sulfide (1,3,5)
12.	Methyl propyl sulfide (5)
13.	Methyl alyl sulfide (5)
14.	Diallyl sulfide (5)
15.	Hydrogen sulfide (1,3,4)
16.	**"N" Compounds:**
17.	Ammonia (1,4)
18.	Methyl amine (4)

The number in parentheses indicate the source of the data:

1. Yueh and Strong (1960)
2. Kramlich and Pearson (1960)
3. Bender and Balance (1961)
4. Hornstein and Crowe (1960, 1963)
5. Hirai *et al.* (1968)

Lipid Studies

Hornstein and Crowe (1960, 1963) concluded that in terms of flavour, lean meats are alike. Pork, beef and lamb have different flavours. So they looked fat as a source of species flavour differences suggested that lipid oxidation is important in the development of beef and pork flavour but not in the lamb flavour. Hornstein *et al.* (1960) - carbonyl compounds were converted to their 2,4 dinitrophenyl hydrazone devivatives and then separated and identified by the method of Gaddis and Ellis (1959). Lamb has virtually no FFA containing more than one double bond. Pork and beef prior to heating have approximately 4 per cent and 23 per cent respectively of FFA containing multiple unsaturation. Heating increases this only slightly unsaturated carbonyl compounds particularly the 2,4-dienals which are potent flavour compounds present in higher concentration in pork fat volatiles than in beef volatiles.

Wasserman and Talley (1968) organoleptically evaluated the hypothesis that the lean meat of various species have essentially the same basic flavour and that the specific species flavour is due to the fat. Hotnstein and Crowe (1964) - Lipid affect meat flavour by virtue of fatty acid composition, also by serving as a reservoir for odouriferous fat soluble substances.

Craig *et al.* (1962) concluded that the compound (s) responsible for this off-odour was present in the unsaponifiables.

Patterson (1968) identified the compounds responsible for "boar" odour as 5-α-androst-16-ene-3-one.

Conclusion

Efforts have been made to identify the precursor systems responsible for the development of meaty flavours. The nature of the volatile compounds developed on heating has been investigated. The distinctive contribution of the lean and lipid portions of meat to flavour have also been studied.

Precursor studies have been shown that proteins per se contribute little to meat flavour but that amino acids and reducing sugars are important meat flavour precursors.

Lipid studies indicate that fat may effect meat flavour in two ways. Fatty acids on oxidation produce carbonyl compounds that are potent flavour contributors. Fat may also act as a storage depot for odoriferous compounds that are released on heating. The volatiles derived from fat may be responsible for the characteristics differences that are associated with the flavour of beef pork and lamb.

Approximately 75 compounds have been identified in the volatiles derived from beef. The organoleptic evaluation of these compounds requires greater attention. Whether the simple carbonyl compounds sulfur compounds acids and alcohols are the major flavour contributors or simply provide distinctive meat flavour nuances.

V. Water Holding Capacity (WHC) of Muscle

Introduction

The properties of fresh meat dictate its usefullness to the merchandiser, its appeal to the purchaser or consumer and its adaptability for further processing. The water holding capacity of muscle tissue has a direct effect on the shrinkage of meat during storage. When the tissues have poor water holding properties, the loss of moisture and consequently the loss of weight during storage **(shrink)** is great. This moisture loss occur from the exposed muscle surfaces of carcasses during storage. The retail meat cuts may loose some of their moisture even after packaging in moisture proof wrapping. The free water may exude from the cut surfaces and accumulate around the meat causing a wet, unattractive retail package. This production of visible meat juice is known as **weep**. Water holding capacity is especially critical in the meat ingredients of the manufactured products that are subjected to heating, grinding and other processes. Achieving proper protein/water ratio is important for palatability and adequate yield of finished product weight.

Chemical Basis of Water Holding Capacity

In the muscle, water exists in the bound, immobilized and free forms. Due to the distribution of their electrons, water molecules are not electrically neutral, but have a positive and negatively charged "ends" (they are polar) thus they can be associated with electrically charged reactive groups on the muscle proteins. Of the total water in the muscle, 4-5 percent is **bound water.** It remains tightly bound even during the application of a severe mechanical or other physical force. Other water molecules are subsequently attracted to the bound molecules in layers that become successively weaker as the distance from the reactive group on the protein become greater. Such water may be termed as **immobilized water**. The quantity so immobilized depends on the amount of force exerted physically on the muscle. Water that is held only by surface forces is known as **free water.**

Bound Water	*Immobilized Water*	*Free Water*
Hydrophilic group on the muscle proteins attract water, form tightly found layer.	Less orderly molecular orientation toward the charged group.	Held only by capillary forces, their orientation is independent of charged groups.

Biochemistry of Meat Hydration or Water Holding Capacity

Muscle binds its 75 per cent water. Water-holding capacity or hydration of meat is closely related to taste, tenderness, colour and other features of meat quality. Water-holding capacity also influence meat quality during processing operations – storage, transport, ageing, grinding, salting, curing, heating, freezing, thawing and drying etc. Weight losses of meat is also associated with the binding of water within muscle tissues. Hence, it has got scientific as well as economic interest.

Definition of Water Holding Capacity of Meat

Hydration:- average amount of water carried by unit weight of protein when the protein molecules migrate through a solution.

Water-holding capacity (WHC):- the ability of meat to hold fast to its own or added water during application of any force (pressing, heating, grinding etc.). Water liberated by some such method may be termed "loose water" and the water retained by the tissue be termed "bound water". WHC can be expressed as amount of loose water related to the total content of moisture in muscle or amount of bound water related to muscle or muscle proteins.

Basic Concepts of Meat Hydration

A. Binding of Water by Muscle Proteins

Muscle proteins are responsible for the binding of water in meat. 34 per cent of muscle proteins are water soluble, remaining proteins are structural substances structural or fibrillar proteins which consist of:

Myosin 34-38 per cent (show specific interaction with water), Actin 13-15 per cent, X-Protein 7 per cent,

Stroma proteins 15-17 per cent. Tropomysin – similar to myosin also present.

WHC mainly concerned with myosin and actin or actomyosin complex.

How is water bound by the muscular protein?

by hydrophilic groups – two types

a) Polar groups of the side chain of proteins *viz.* carboxyl, amino, hydroxyl, and sulfhydryl groups.
b) Undiscounted carbonyl and imido-groups of the peptide bonds. The binding of water is due to the dipolar character of water.

B. Water-Holding Capacity of Meat

4-5 per cent is tightly bound water is muscle protein-influenced by changes in the structure and charges in the protein. Strong influence of changes of protein charges and structure on WHC of meat may affect only the "free" water which is not bound is mono and multi molecular layers. As far as "free" water is concerned, water retained within the protein structure perhaps, immobilized by "capillary condensation" which is forced out with very low pressure. The amount of "free water" immobilized within the tissue is strongly influenced by the spatial structure of the muscle tissue – tightening the network of proteins decreases immobilized water and increases easily expressible water, while loosening the protein structure has opposite effect. This "stereo effect" is influenced by changes of protein charges by attraction or repulsion of charged groups. At certain pH values or in the presence of certain ions, muscle can take up in "immobilized form" 700-800g water per 100g protein.

Factors Affecting Meat Hydration

I. Fundamental Factors

I.A. Protein Charges (influence of pH)

Minimum hydration at pH 5.0. The pH at which the WHC has a minimum (5.0) corresponds approx. to the isoelectric point (1.P.) of actomyosin. The normal pH of meat is more in the basic range of I.P. Small change in meat pH may cause relatively great changes of WHC. According to "zwitterion" theory, the swelling effects of acids or bases on protein gels in due to a cleavage of the electrostatic cross linkages between the peptide chains of the protein molecule.

Proton donator (acid)

$$R\text{-}COO^- + NH_3\text{-}R' + H^+A \longrightarrow R\text{-}COOH + NH_3\text{-}R' + A.$$

Proton acceptor (base)

$$R\text{-}COO\text{-} + NH_3 - R' + B \longrightarrow R\text{-}COO\text{-}\ NH_2\text{-}\ R' + H^+B$$

Here counter charges are eliminated, the protein net charge is increased. There is repulsion between protein groups with same charge (+ve or – ve) and thus the space between the peptide chains is enlarged, so more water can penetrate. An excess of acid decreases the WHC of muscle. Here the marked binding of anion (*e.g.* chloride ions in case of HCl) probably screens the +ve charges of the amino and imidazole groups – the repulsion between these charged groups is lowered, the peptide chains can approach more closely – consequently more water is immobilized.

In basic range of I.P.:- decrease of viscosity of actomyosin with increasing pH in the basic range of I.P. is due to an increasing "screening of the protein charges by binding of the counter ions reducing the electrostatic repulsion.

The pH hydration curve shows – an increase of protein net charge will result in an increased repulsion of the peptide chains and consequently an increase in meat hydration; *vice versa*, an increase of electrostatic and hydrogen bonds between the peptide chains will cause a tightening of the protein network and therefore a decrease in meat hydration.

I.B. Metals

100g of beef muscle contain about 25mg Mg, 5mg calcium and 4.2mg zinc. These bivalent metals have their influence on WHC.

In rigor and post-rigor muscle some of these ions are tightly bound. It is known that polyvalent cations decrease the hydration of proteins, linking together the peptide chains by forming cross linkage and cause tightening of structure.

Potassium and sodium are present in large amount (300-400mg K and 40-70mg Na per 100g fresh beef muscle). Potassium ions are remarkably absorbed by myosin and actomyosin not by actin. These ions are bound weakly compared to bivalent ions. At the same ionic strength Na^+ cause greater hydration than K^+ in the basic range of I.P.

II. Animal Factors Affecting Meat Hydration

II. A. Species, Sex, Age, Grade, Breeding, Muscle Species

WHC is higher in pork than beef. After a one week storage, prepacked beef showed a higher weight loss than pre packed lean pork. It is due to different physiological conditions in the digestive tract of cattle and pigs, also preslaughter treatments and histological structure of muscle influence differences in species.

Age and Sex:- Pork = age and sex, no influence on WHC

Cattle = age and sex, significant different

The poultry meat has a much lower hydration, veal has a better WHC than meat of older animals. WHC decreases with increasing live weight and increasing age. The meat of cows has a higher WHC than that of bull. Schon and Scheper (1960) found the following series in increasing WHC.

Bull> Ox, Heifer > Cow > Calf > Pig.

Muscles

In frog: adductor muscles have a lower swelling ability than the abductor muscles.

Cattle: Vol. of drip from M.longissinus dorsi after freezing and thawing is about twice than that from the Psoas at the same pH. M.longissinus dorsi > M. adductor for WHC.

Pig: M.gluteus medius > M.gluteus accessories and M.gluteus profundus.

M.Longissimus dorsi < Posoas muscle (Grau 1956) 24hrs after slaughter M. adductor > M.longissimus dorsi.

Grade of Animal and WHC

Canner beef has a significantly lower WHC than first grade beef.

Schon (1957) – WHC is lower in lower-grade pork than medium-grade pork.

II. B. Pre Slaughter Treatments and Conditions

B (i) Exercise, Stress

Exercise of both fasted and full-fed hogs lowered the initial content of glycogen and increased both ultimate pH and hydration. The effect was greater in gluteus medius than than gluteus accessories and gluteus profundus muscle.

Temperature of slaughter: Pork slaughtered at 0°C had pH and WHC values 24 hrs after slaughter were significantly higher than those slaughtered at normal temp. Reason was excitation due to extreme temp. and decrease level of muscle glycogen.

B. (ii) Medicaments

Insulin tetany increases WHC, but caused taste to deteriorate. Steers and bulls implanted with diethylstilbosterol gave meat hydration different than normal animals. But treating medicaments were not promising because animals should not be subjected to convulsions and agonizing stress.

B. (iii) Feeding

Cattle: the hydration minimum (I.P.) of muscle (M.longissinus dorsi 3-4 days post-mortem) is in the pH range 5.1-5.5 for heifers fed green fodder and in the pH range 4.8-5.1 after stall feeding.

Hogs: A diminution of proteins in pigs feed decreases the WHC of pork particulars if soy protein is replaced by fish protein. Feeding sugar produces pork with a relatively low pH with WHC higher than control group – the effect is osmotic, for this at least 1kg sugar 3-4 hrs before slaughter is required.

B (iv) Watery Meat Diseases

Mulbery heart diseases – degenerated pork binds 21-30 per cent less water than normal pork

III. Post-Mortem Changes in Meat Hydration

meat immediately after slaughter has a very high WHC. Hydration drops very markedly within a few hours, reaches a minimum in 24 to 48 hrs and increased slowly with increase time of storage.

a. Effect of Adenosine Triphosphate

As long as ATP is not broken down it exerts a hydrating and softening effect on muscle but while it is being decomposed, it causes dehydration and contraction. The function of ATP is due to a complex binding of alkaline earth metals built into the structural muscle protein. The ability of phosphates in muscle to form complexes with calcium increases as follows:

glucoss 6-P < inosine monophosphate << ADP < ATP.

b. Phase of Rigor Mortis

Immediately after slaughter a part of the alkaline earth metals present in muscle are complex-bound by ATP for this reason muscle tissue has a high WHC. During the first hours post mortem activity of calcium ion increases, because of fall in pH. ATPase starts to work with full activity – splitting of phosphate – cause dehydration of muscle.

IV. Influence of Processing on Hydration of Meat and other ingredients

IV.a. Influence of Salts

Salts such as sodium chloride, phosphates or citrate affect the WHC of meat quite strongly.

(i) Neutral Salts

Sodium chloride increases WHC and the swelling of Meat. In the acidic range of muscle I.P. (pH 5.0) the dehydrating effect of anion is stronger and that of cation is weaker in relation to low strongly the ion is bound to the structural muscle proteins. In the basic range of I.P. the situation is inverse. The stronger the ion is bound the stronger is the hydrating effect of the anion and the weaker is the hydrating effect of cation. – binding depend upon interaction between the slat ions and the protein ions.

Acid range (I.P.)

$R\text{-}NH_3^+ \xrightarrow{+A^-} {}^+H_3N\text{-}R'\ R\text{-}NH_3^+\ A^-\ {}^+H_3N\text{-}R'$ tightening of protein structure.

(Repulsion) (no repulsion) decrease of WHC

Basic range of (I.P.)

$R\text{-}NH_3^+ \xrightarrow{+A^-} {}^-OOC\text{-}R'\ R\text{-}NH_3^+A^-\ {}^-OOC - R'$ widening of the muscle structure.

(attraction) (no attraction) increase of WHC and swelling.

(ii) Effect of Cations

With increase pH, binding of cations increases.

Salts of weak acids: Salts of weak acids *e.g.* polyphosphates and citrates are used as additives in meat processing. The more strongly the salts of weak acid increased the pH of the tissues, the more strongly they increase the WHC of meat. Polyvalent anions are the most effective, so poly- phosphates, oxalate and citrate increase muscle hydration very strongly.

Reaction: ion exchange, elimination of alkaline earth metals bound on muscle protein – so increase muscle hydration.

(iii) Presalting Effect

It is possible to prevent the rapid loss of WHC after slaughter by salting the ground or cut meat during the first hours after death. In this way one can preserve high hydration of muscle at least for one week. It depends upon enough ATP remaining in the muscle at the time sodium chloride (2 per cent) is added.

(iv) Curing

The influence of salt (Sodium chloride) on the WHC of large pieces of Meat depends on the rate at which the salt penetrates the meat. That rate, in turn depends on the WHC of muscle when pH of meat increases the penetration of salt is lower because increase hydration of muscle making the structure more closed.

Curing: the influence of salt (sodium chloride) on the WHC of large pieces of meat depends on the rate at which the salt penetrates the meat. That rate, in turn depends on the WHC of muscle. When pH of meat increases the penetration of salt is lower because increase hydration of muscle making the structure more closed.

(v) Combined Effect of Sodium Chloride and Polyphosphates or Ascorbic Acid

NaCl + poly phosphates – considerable increase of meat hydration that is maintained to a certain extent after heat denaturation. This effect decreases with increasing temperature in the range of 0-20°C.

IV.b. Influence of Heating

In the range of 0-25°C the WHC of meat decreases with increasing temperatures. Heating of meat releases juices, the amount depend upon the temperature and that the loss influences the juiciness and texture of meat. Heating between 30 and 40°C, a mild denaturation occur, resulting an unfolding of protein chains.The hydration is somewhat increased in the acidic range. Rigidity of muscle by heating starts at about 35°C, similarly to the coagulation of pure actomysoin.

A stronger denaturation starts at 40°C and countries to 50°C – a decrease of electrostatic repulsion between the peptide chains causing a tighter network of protein structure and a lower WHC (at pH > I.P.). At pH < I.P. loosening of protein structure and consequently an increase of WHC. In the range of temp. 50°C-55°C change of hydration is delayed markedly. Hydration is decreased between 55°C-80°C.

IV.c. Influence of Grinding

The more intensive the grinding, the higher is the WHC of the ground tissue. Meat ground in a meat grinder, thus has a lower WHC than meat ground in a blender. With increasing time of grinding the WHC of meat increase.

V. Influence of Hydration on Meat Quality

A. Taste (Juiciness)

Meat will be the more juicy

a. The less juice is released during cooking

b. The more tightly the juice is bound to the coagulated tissues.

Meat having higher WHC in the raw state will bind its water faster during heating than meat having low WHC.

Factors increasing WHC decrease saltiness of meat. The conc. of both free ion Na^+ and Cl^- responsible for the salty taste. Salty taste is less, when more salt ions are bound by the muscle proteins.

B. Consistency (Tenderness)

The more the aged meat is hydrated the greater is the distance between the peptide chains in the protein structure and the more soft and tender is the meat. The increasing tenderness of meat during ageing is accompanied by an increasing WHC. Tenderization of meat by enzymes also raises the hydration of meat. Splitting of protein chains during ageing and the influence of connective tissue are important factors for tenderness. So correlation between WHC and tenderness is not true in all cases.

C. Colour

Beside myoglobin and hemoglobin, WHC also has considerable influence on the colour. A high WHC, caused by a high ultimate pH value is of primary importance in accounting for the colour of "dark-cutting beef".

– Chapter 10 –

Tenderization of Meat

I. Meat Tenderness

Introduction

Tenderness is one of or the most discussed features in meat. It is a real challenge for the scientific community and for the meat industry to achieve products with standardized and guaranteed tenderness, since these characteristics are exactly what consumers want in a meat product (Koohmaraie, 1995).

The United States meat industry has identified solving the problem of inconsistent meat tenderness as a top priority. This requires a detailed understanding of the processes that affect meat tenderness and, perhaps more importantly, the utilization of such information by the meat industry (Koohmaraie, 1996).

Of the six meat palatability factors (tenderness, juiciness, flavour, aroma, color, texture), tenderness is generally considered the most important palatability factor by the consumer.

In recent years, the meat industry has made great progress in improving tenderness both through genetics improvement and meat science technology.

In addition, the red meat industry could also achieve higher financial gain from producing more tender meat because of the higher selling price associated with tender meat (*e.g.*, fillet or porterhouse steak)compared with tough cuts (*e.g.*, chuck steak) in the market. Therefore, improving customer satisfaction and maintaining the consistency of meat products is a major concern and challenge for the meat industry (Behrends *et al.*, 2005).

A considerable amount of research and resources have been focused on investigations attempting to improve meat tenderness, and have achieved success to various degrees.

Tenderness

Means easily crushed, chewed, fragile or cut part.

Major components of meat that contribute to Tenderness

- ✰ Primarily Connective Tissue
- ✰ Muscle fibers
- ✰ Adipose tissue

Objectives

1. To identify the tender, intermediate and tough major muscles of the carcass.
2. To demonstrate the reasons for differences in tenderness among muscles.
3. To show the relative differences in chemical and histological measurements between tough and tender meat
4. To identify factors responsible for ensuring acceptable tenderness of meat.
5. To show how different biochemical and other postmortem factors affect meat tenderness.

Factors Affecting Tenderness

(1) Genetics

Genetics is one of the main reasons such a wide difference in tenderness often exists among identical grades and cuts of meat.

there are breed differences in tenderness, the differences are not very large, and relate mainly to a reduced 'calpain enzyme system' (responsible for post mortem aging) in *Bos indicus*. Recently (2002) a variant of the calpain 1 gene has been identified that codes for part of the calpain protease enzyme system (micro calpain). The gene variant is relatively widespread in beef herds, but exerts its influence most when the animal carries only the variant form (dominant). This specific gene, even when fully expressed, still only accounts for 20 per cent of tenderness.

Differences between sires within a breed are probably more important, particularly for Bos indicus and this might relate in large part to which sires are dominant for the highly active form of the Calpain 1 gene.

So it was found that different Brahman breeding bulls gave calves with different muscle tenderness.

(2) Breed, Species and Age

Beef usually is the most variable in tenderness followed by lamb, pork, and veal. The tenderness variation from species to species is due primarily to the chronological age of the animal at time of slaughter. Beef normally is processed at approximately 20 months of age, lamb at 8 months, pork at 5 months, and veal at approximately 2 months of age.

Within a given species such as beef, age of the animal at slaughter also influences tenderness. Beef normally is slaughtered between 9 and 30 months of age. Usually the meat from the animals is fairly tender; however, if a female beef animal has been used for breeding purposes, meat from such an animal becomes progressively less tender as the animal gets older.

Cows up to 15 years of age may be processed for beef steaks and roasts, but ideally these should be tenderized because of the increased probability of less tender meat in older animals.

The decrease in tenderness with increasing age is due to the changing nature of collagen (gristle), the connective tissue protein found in meat. Collagen becomes more complex and stronger with advancing age and thus is more resistant to tenderization from moist-heat cooking.

Bos indicus (Brahman, Sahiwal, etc.) breeds tend to be tougher than Bos taurus breeds (Angus, Hereford, etc.). Bos indicus has greater amounts of calpastatin, a protein that interferes with post mortem degradation of muscle.

Pork and lamb from older animals normally are processed into sausage items, so toughness due to age usually is not a problem.

(3) Feeding

Contrary to popular belief, what the animal is fed does not directly influence tenderness. In the case of beef, an indirect effect of feeding on tenderness may be observed. Animals that are finished with grain tend to reach a given slaughter weight sooner than animals that are finished to the same slaughter weight on pasture. Thus, grain-fed animals usually are slightly more tender because they are slaughtered at a slightly younger age.

(4) Influence of Stress

Stress prior to slaughter is one of the most important influences on ultimate meat tenderness., studies of pH have shown that high pH meat is darker but less consistently tender than normal pH meat. The pH of living animals is around pH 7, but after death the sugars in the muscles are converted to lactic acid, lowering the pH. A normal, non - stressed animal has muscle pH of around pH 5.5 after death (24 hours after slaughter all the sugars have been converted).

(5) Muscle to Muscle

Within any species, there is a considerable variation in tenderness among muscles. For example, tenderloin is much more tender than the fore shank or heel of round in beef. This difference is due in part to the amount of connective tissue in the various cuts. The tenderloin usually has a small amount of connective tissue compared with the fore shank or heel of round. The amount of **connective tissue** present is due to the function of the muscles in the live animal. The fore shank and heel of round are used quite heavily in locomotion (movement) and therefore have relatively large amounts of connective tissue. Conversely, the tenderloin provides a support function in the animal and therefore has less connective tissue.

Another source of muscle-to-muscle variation in tenderness is the amount of stretch or tension applied to each muscle while the carcass is being chilled. This stretching is due to the weight of the carcass and prevents shortening (contraction) of the muscle, which in turn results in more tender meat. The major muscle in the rib and the loin is stretched more during the chilling process than are the major muscles in the round; therefore, cuts from the rib and loin are more tender than cuts from the round. This is the major reason the tenderloin is the most tender muscle in the carcass.

Table 10.1: Relative Rank in Tenderness

Tender	*Intermediate*	*Tough*
Psoas major	*Biceps femoris (sirloin)	Deep pectoral
Infraspinatus	Rectus femoris	Latissimusdorsi
Gluteus medius	Adductor	Trapezius
Longissimusdorsi	Semitendinosus	Superficial pectoral
Triceps brachii	Semimembranosus	

* Biceps femoris (round).

Table 10.2: Top Ten "Tender" and "Tough" Cuts in Shear Force (pounds) from the National Beef Tenderness Survey

"Tender" Cuts	*Shear Force*	*"Tough" cuts*	*Shear Force*
Tenderloin steak	5.7	Top round steak	11.7
Top blade steak	6.7	Eye of round steak	10.3
Top loin steak	7.2	Bottom round steak	9.7
Rib roast	7.3	Rump roast	9.5
Rib steak	7.4	Eye of round roast	9.2
Ribeye steak	7.5	Chuck roll steak	9.2
Chuck roll roast	7.6	Chuck tender steak	9.0
Clod roast	7.9	Top round roast	9.0
Round tip roast	7.9	Bottom round roast	8.9

Source: Morgan *et al.* (1991).

Shear force = Pounds of force to shear one-half-inch cores, removed parallel to the muscle fibers, of cooked muscle from steaks and roasts.

Differences among Muscles Because

- ✰ Actomyosin effect
- ✰ Sarcomere length
- ✰ Muscle fiber diameter
- ✰ Sarcomere/fragment
- ✰ Concentration of stromal proteins
- ✰ Size of elastin fibrils
- ✰ Solubility of collagen

- ☆ Bulk density or lubrication effect
- ☆ Amount of marbling
- ☆ Distribution of marbling

Table 10.3: Traits of "Tender" and "Tough" Meat

Trait	*"Tender"*	*"Tough"*
Sarcomere length	3.6 μm	1.8 μm
Muscle fiber diameter	40 μm	80 μm
Sarcomere/fragment	6	15
Amount of stromal protein	3 mg/g	8 mg/g
Size of elastin fibrils	.6 μm	4.0 μm
Collagen solubility	28 per cent	6 per cent
Amount of marbling	7 per cent	2 per cent
Distribution of marbling	Extensive	Collected

(6) Influence of Pre-Slaughter Electrical Stunning

Where animals are routinely rendered unconscious by electrical stunning immediately prior to slaughter, the muscles are positively affected from the tenderness point of view, mainly through mechanically fracturing some of the 'giant', intermediate and shorter muscle fibers of meat. Cattle varieties bred from the tropical *Bos indicus*(breeds such as Brahmin, Santa Gertrudis) do not seem to as affected, with only the 'giant fiber' component fracturing, the intermediate and short fibers remaining unaffected. *Bos Taurus* the European and English cattle breeds (Angus, Hereford, Charolais, Galloway, Salers, Shorthorn etc.) are more markedly affected by electrical stimulation.

(7) Quality Grade

Age of the animal also plays a major role in tenderness as it applies to quality grading in beef. The quality grades of beef are USDA Prime, Choice, Select, Standard, Utility, and Commercial. Carcasses from young animals (up to 40 months of age) are eligible for USDA Prime, Choice, Select, Standard, and Utility grade designations. Carcasses from beef animals older than 40 months are eligible for USDA Commercial

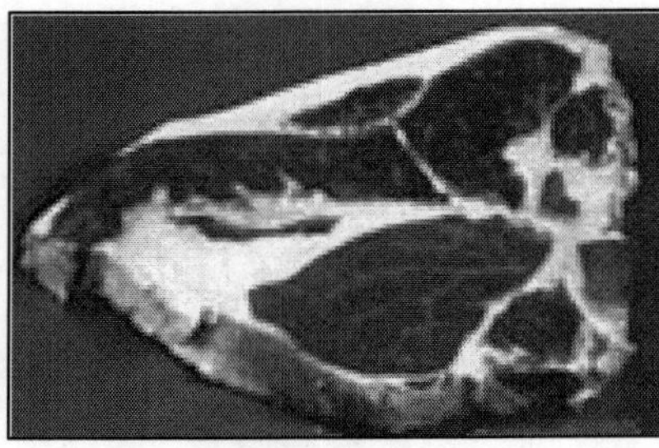

Porterhouse Steak.

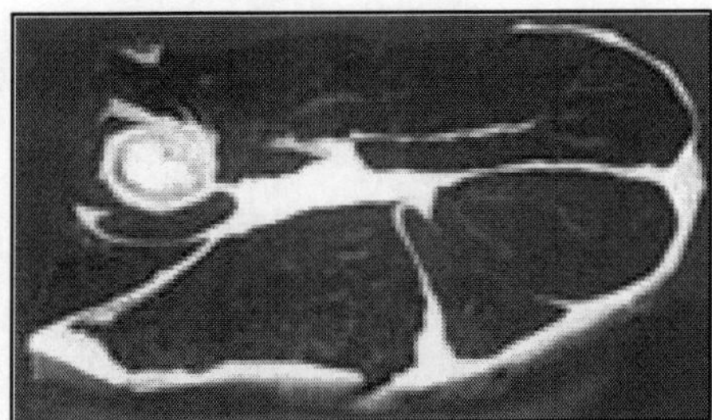

Round Steak.

and Utility grade designations. Normally beef in the young grade designations is more tender than beef from USDA Commercial or Utility grade carcasses and, therefore, is much more common in the market place. Prime has more marbling than Choice and Choice has more than Select.

Marbling, the visible specks of fat in the lean, also is a factor used in determining the USDA quality grade. However, information in the last decade indicates that marbling exerts only a small influence on tenderness of meat, primarily by acting as a lubricant during chewing.

(8) Carving

Muscles, muscle bundles, and muscle fibers are all surrounded by connective tissue. When cuts are made from carcasses and wholesale cuts, **the normal procedure is to cut at right angles to the length of the muscle**. This procedure severs the maximum amount of connective tissue and distributes the bone more evenly among all cuts in that area. Likewise, consumers should carve cooked meat at right angles to the length of the muscle fibers or "against the grain" to achieve maximum tenderness. Cutting with the grain results in "stringiness" and thus less tenderness.

Common Practices For Enhancing Tenderness

(1) Chilling Rate

Immediately after slaughter, many changes take place in muscle that convert muscle to meat. One of the changes is the contraction and stiffening of muscle known as rigor mortis. Muscle is very tender at the time of slaughter. However, as rigor mortis begins, muscle becomes progressively less tender until rigor mortis is complete. In the case of beef, 6 to 12 hours are required for the completion of rigor mortis, whereas in the case of pork, only 1 to 6 hours are required.

The carcass is chilled immediately after slaughter to prevent spoilage. If the carcass is chilled too rapidly, the result is **"cold shortening"** and subsequent toughness. Cold shortening occurs when the muscle is chilled to less than 60°F before the completion of rigor mortis. If the carcass is frozen before completion of rigor mortis, the result is "**thaw rigor"** and subsequently extremely tough meat. Under normal chilling conditions, it appears that unprotected carcasses with less than 0.50 inch of fat over the rib eye probably will have some reduced tenderness because of cold shortening. Aging a carcass affected by cold shortening or thaw rigor will not alleviate the detrimental effects on tenderness caused by these two conditions. To ensure more tender meat, home slaughtered animals and wild game should be protected from very rapid cooling during the first 6-12 hours after death.

(2) Freezing

Freezing rate plays a small role in tenderness. When meat is frozen very quickly, small ice crystals form; when meat is frozen slowly, large ice crystals are formed. While the formation of large crystals may serve to disrupt components of the muscle fibers in meat and thereby increase tenderness very slightly, the large ice crystals result in an increased loss of juices upon thawing. This increase in loss of juices results in meat that is less juicy upon cooking and therefore usually is perceived as being less tender.

(3) Thawing

Thawing meat slowly in the refrigerator generally results in greater tenderness compared with cooking from the frozen state. Slow thawing minimizes the toughening effect from cold shortening (when present) and reduces the amount of moisture loss. Thawing in a microwave is accomplished by using a lower power setting or by manually alternating cooking and standing times. During the standing time, some of the heat from the thawed areas moves toward the frozen area.

(4) Aging

After the completion of rigor mortis, changes take place in muscle that result in the beef becoming progressively more tender. The increase in tenderness is due to natural enzymatic changes taking place in the muscle. The increase in beef tenderness continues only for approximately 7 to 10 days after slaughter when the beef is held at approximately 35°F. Beef held at higher temperatures will tenderize more rapidly, but it also may spoil and develop off-flavours.

Individual muscles respond differently, in extent of tenderization improvement, to post mortem ageing periods because of differences in rate and extent of pH decline and in activity of calpains and thus in the extent of proteolytic degradation. Beef can be **"wet-aged"** (held for periods of time in vacuum packages) or **"dry aged"**(held for periods of time with no protection or package) to allow more complete degradation of myofibrils via loss of integrity of sarcomeres at the Z-lines). Dry aging improved tenderness more than did wet aging, while It was also found that no difference in

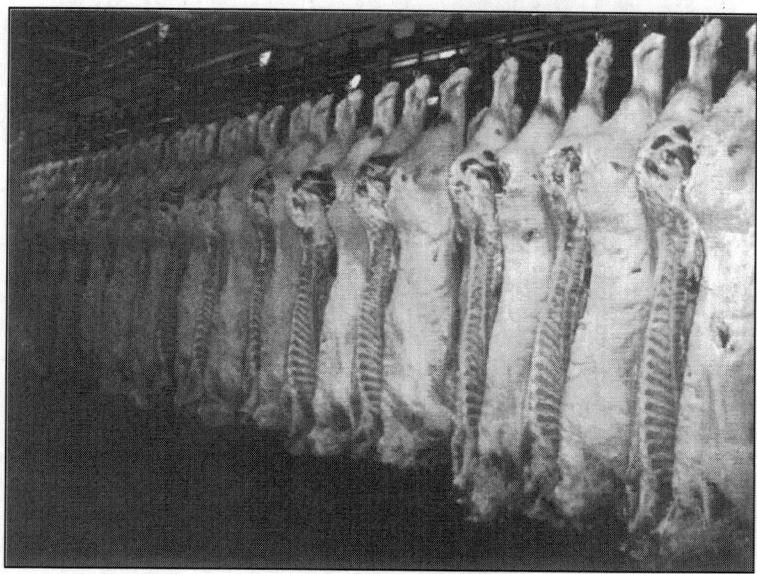

Dry Ageing.

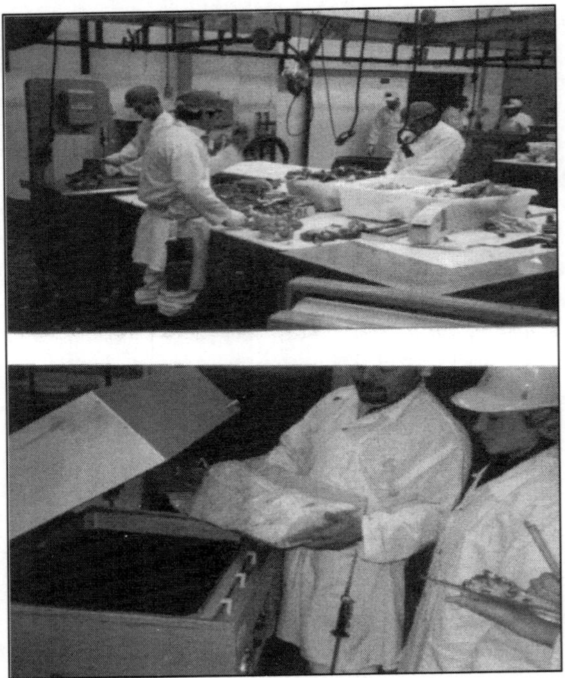

Wet Ageing.

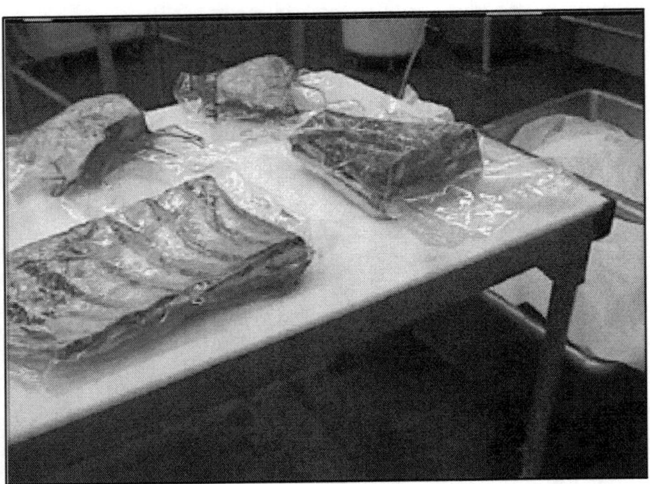

tenderization between the these two method. Lamb and pork are rarely aged. A lack of tenderness usually is not encountered because of lamb and pork's relatively young age when slaughtered.

(5) Electrical Stimulation

Electrical stimulation of the hot carcass immediately after slaughter is an innovation being used in the meat industry to increase tenderness. Beef carcasses are subjected to approximately one minute of high voltage electrical current. The result is an improvement in tenderness of many cuts of the carcass. An improvement in tenderness of cuts from carcasses of older cows also has been observed when electrical stimulation has been applied. Electrical stimulation speeds up the post-mortem conversion of muscle to meat and thus reduces the incidence of "cold shortening". The use of electrical stimulation in the beef industry is widespread.

that beef muscles will be more tender if the carcass during the harvesting process– is subjected to electrically induced contraction/relaxation cycles (12 or so, induced by about 450 volts of AC, at about 2amps). High-voltage ES changes the rate of post mortem pH decline in muscle, creates tears and fissures in muscle fibers, speeds up activities of both cathepsins and calpains, and expends energy, thereby lessening sarcomere shortening occasioned by development of rigor mortis.

Two recent studies of ES have verified the tenderization effect of ES even at low voltage. The studies show that tenderization is due to prevention of excessive muscle shortening during rigor development (minimizing sarcomere shortening),enhanced proteolysis by release of calcium ions at a higher carcass (and muscle) temperature, and physical disruption of the structure of the muscle fiber.

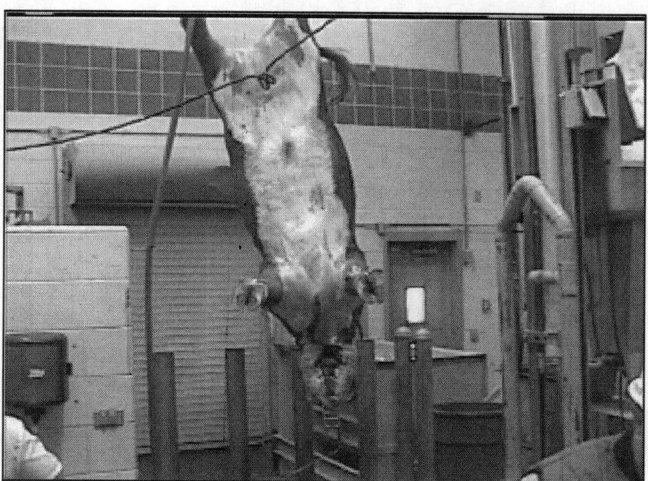

(6) Change in Carcass Suspension

Stretching of the muscle during chilling of the carcass affects tenderness. This has different effects on different muscles according to their anatomical location in the carcass.

The original study of muscles from horizontally placed versus vertically suspended carcass sides demonstrated that when muscles shortened there were corresponding decreases in sarcomere length, increases in muscle fiber diameter and decreases in tenderness. This led to the development of a procedure for carcass suspension from the obturator foramen of the pelvis (*i.e.*, Tender stretch).

Pelvic suspension of beef carcasses is not used widely in industry because it requires changes in plant layout and cutting procedures. It is a procedure, however, than can be used in home slaughtered animals or wild game such as deer.

Tender stretch suspension of carcasses improves the tenderness of muscles of the round because the hind-shanks pull downward, preventing those muscles from shortening (as done in standard Achilles-tendon suspension) and improves the tenderness of the *longissimus* muscle because the forequarter pulls down, straightening and stretching the spine and keeping that muscle from shortening.

Early studies and a more recent study, demonstrate that Tender stretch suspension increases the tenderness of the *longissimus* muscle by 24 to 25 per cent.

Use of Tender stretch suspension changes carcass conformation making commercial handling more difficult, but a novel cutting procedure for preparing

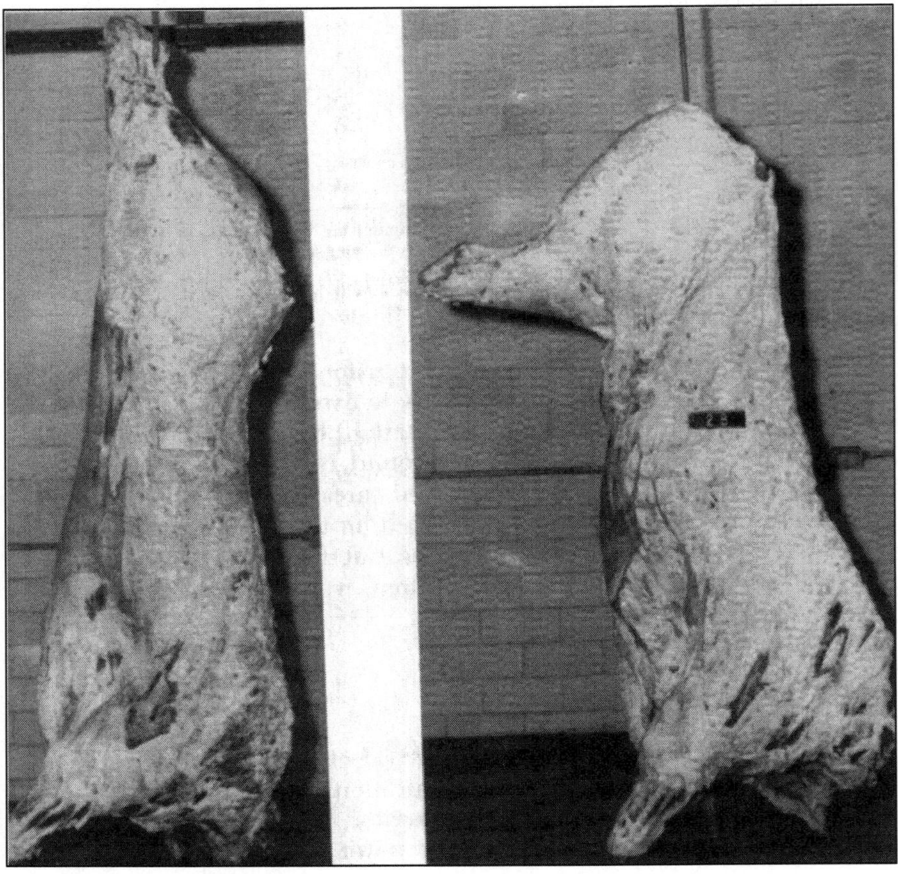

Texas Tender Stretch.

supermarket cuts results in a 2.6 per cent yield advantage for Tender stretch versus conventionally suspended carcasses.

(7) Cooking

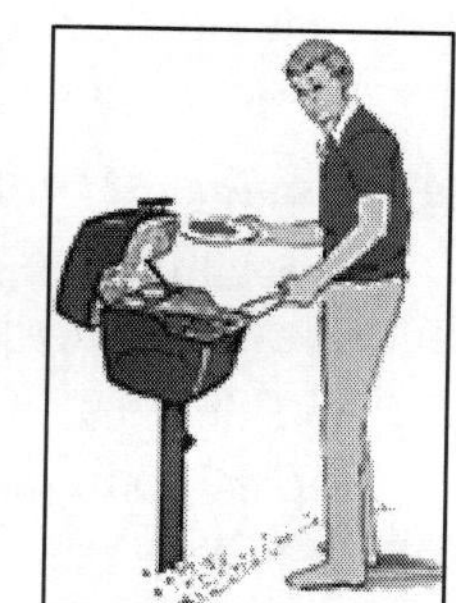

As cooking progresses, the contractile proteins in meat become less tender, and the major connective tissue protein (collagen) becomes more tender. Thus, for cuts that are low in connective tissue–such as steaks and chops from the rib and loin–the recommended method of cooking is dry heat, including pan frying, broiling, roasting, or barbecuing. Dry heat raises the temperature very quickly and the flavour of meat will develop before the contractile proteins have the opportunity to become significantly less tender.

For cuts with a high amount of connective tissue–such as those from the fore shank, heel of round, and chuck–the recommended method of cooking is long and slow at low temperatures using moist heat such as braising. The application of moist heat for a long time at low temperatures (275-325°F) results in conversion of tough collagen into tender gelatin and makes this type of cut more tender compared with dry heat cooking of one of the less tender cuts of meat.

Degree of doneness significantly affects tenderness. As the lean is heated, the contractile proteins toughen and moisture is lost. Both decrease tenderness. Tender cuts of meat cooked to a rare degree of doneness (140°F) are more tender than when cooked to medium (155°F), and medium in turn is more tender than well-done (170°F). Degree of doneness is especially important in the case of beef. Some people, however, do not like the flavour of rare beef and thus choose to cook their beef well-done. They should be aware that by doing so, tenderness is greatly reduced in what normally are tender cuts of meat (tenderness will be improved in less tender cuts when cooked well-done by moist heat).

When consumers switch to a grade of beef with less marbling than what they have been accustomed to, care should be taken not to overcook. In most cases, beef with little marbling requires less cooking time than higher grade beef. However, consumers often fail to make this time adjustment and the result is overcooked beef that lacks tenderness. Some consumers cook low fat beef in the frozen state for the same time as they would higher fat, thawed beef. This procedure helps prevent overcooking.

It is recommended that pork be cooked to approximately 160°F or 170°F internal temperature for desirable flavour. Although this temperature range corresponds to well-done in beef, pork still may be slightly pink. Since *Trichinella spiralis* (trichina) is destroyed at 137°F, an internal temperature of 160-170°F for pork is definitely safe. Therefore, it is not necessary to cook pork beyond this stage of doneness; further cooking will result in dehydration, loss of juiciness, and unnecessary toughening. It usually is recommended to cook lamb to well-done (approximately 160-170°F internal temperature) because the flavour is more desirable compared with lower temperatures.

(8) Marinading

Marinading is a way consumers can improve tenderness and add taste variety to the meat component of meals. The tenderizing action of marinades occurs through the softening of collagen, increased water uptake, and the hydrolysis and breakage of the cross links of the connective tissue. Several processes use for marination--

(a) Infusion of Substances into Carcasses

Three kinds of solutions have been investigated–one containing only calcium chloride (hereafter called "**Calcium Activated Tenderization")** – pre-rigor infusion or post-rigor injection of a solution of calcium chloride into muscle.

Second comprised of dextrose, maltose, glycerine and polyphosphates (hereafter called **"Glycolytic Rate Enhancement")**

Third containing saccharides, sodium chloride, phosphates, vitamins C and/or E.

Early studies of Calcium Activated Tenderization were predicated on the fact that because the high blood calcium levels improve the natural enzymatic aging of meat after death and enzyme m-calpain does not decline during post-mortem storage of carcasses or cuts, it could be activated, post mortem, by calcium chloride, which would tenderize the muscles. So with giving cattle oral 'drenches' of calcium before slaughter, infusing calcium into the carcass through veins and arteries, and injecting calcium (usually as calcium chloride salt0.3 mol) directly into the primal beef cuts. All have increased the tenderness of the meat. With oral calcium a few hours before slaughter improving tenderness by about 1 kg shear force (after aging for 4-7 days) over untreated animals.

So Calcium Activated Tenderization improved tenderness in some trials but could induce bitter and metallic off-flavours. It has not been used in commercial practice.

(b) The Effect of Salt on the Tenderness of Meat

Salt is used on meat as a tenderizer. Salt has several effects on meat to aid in tenderizing. The different methods in which salt is applied will add more or less tenderness when cooked. Overall, salt has a hydrating effect on meat as it retains water. Whether it's kosher salt, sea salt or iodized salt, the purpose is for taste and tenderness.

Salting Hours Before Cooking-Applying salt on meat 24 hours or longer before cooking is recommended to tenderize meat and create a balance of saltiness. Before meat is salted, the muscle fibers are wound-up, coiled proteins. Salting meat ahead of time relaxes and uncoils the proteins, similar to the tenderizing action that occurs with marinades.

Salting Right Before Cooking-Salt creates limited tenderness in meat if applied immediately before cooking. The salt draw outs some of water from the meat seeping into the fibers as it dissolves. Cooking meat immediately after salting does not allow all the meat to seep through and is less tender. Meat salted for **at least an hour** at room temperature is more tenderized.

Brining-Salt used in brining meat works similar to osmosis. The meat is immersed in a large pot of salty water for over a day in the refrigerator. The salt forces through the meat and absorbs into the fibers as it breaks down the protein coils. The meat becomes plumpy with flavour retaining juice during the cooking process.

Curing-Salt is the main ingredient in curing, which is a process of adding flavour and creating an antimicrobial to stop spoilage and contamination. The curing method is very specific in regard to the length of time and cooling temperature. Salt is applied to the meat until it is completely absorbed, locking in all water. This process helps age the meat and makes it last longer than fresh meat.

(c) Organic Acid

Organic acids have been shown to increase tenderness.Commonly used acids are acetic acid,lactic acid and citric acid.Acid cause the tissue break down, allow absorbtion of more moisture, more juicer end products and weaken the sac(*i.e.*, sarcolemma) that surrounds the muscle fiber.

(d) Phosphates

phosphates enhance water-holding capacity of muscle; phosphates and ammonium hydroxide raise the pH of muscle.

(9) Enzymes

Enzymes of fungal or bacterial origin (*e.g.*, fungal amylase, protease) confine their action to muscle fiber protein while those from tropical plants (*e.g.*, Papain from Papaya, Bromelin from Pineapple,Ficin from Fig, Actinidine from kiwifruit) contain both colleagenase and elastase. Any of these enzyme preparations can tenderize meat, provided the right amount of it can penetrate evenly into the meat tissue. Meat can be tenderized by marinating or injecting it with solutions of papain bromelin, ficin or actinidine.

The tropical plant enzymes do not reach their optimum temperature of activity until the range of 70 to 85°C is attained. During cooking unless conditions (time/ temperature) are carefully

Controlled.The limitation of vegetable enzymes is that their action is sometimes restricted to the surface of meat.

Enzeco® Bromelain

Protease from the fruit of pineapple (*Ananas comosus*) characterized by its controlled selective hydrolysis over a wide range of conditions.

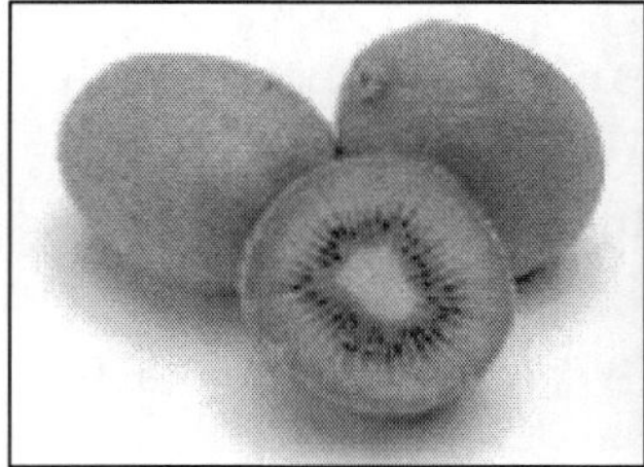

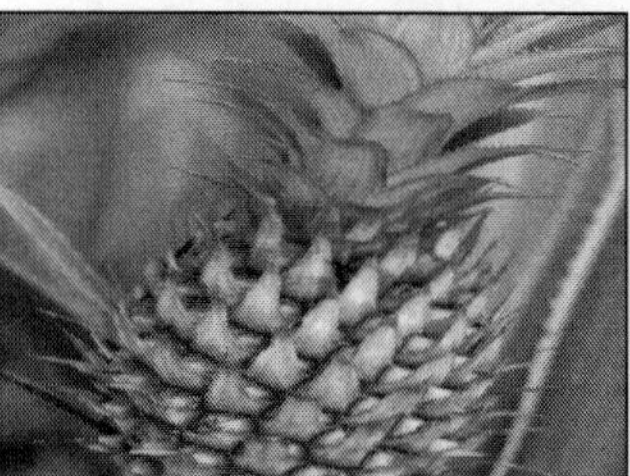

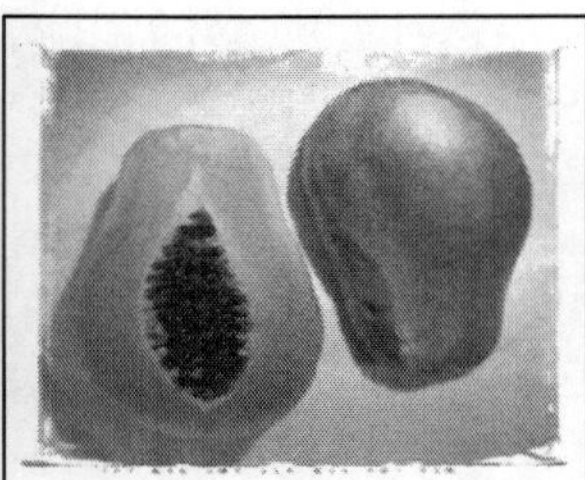

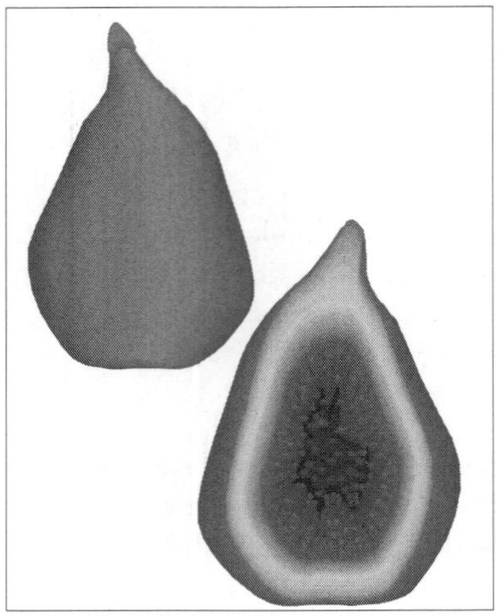

Panol® Purified Papain

Purified, standardized, soluble papain powder obtained from the fruit of papaya (Carica). Will rapidly hydrolyze a variety of proteins over a wide range of conditions.

Liquipanol® T100

Specially formulated liquid papain.

Enzeco® Dual Protease

A special combination of bromelain and papain available as a powder. Particularly useful for tenderizing seafood such as clam and squid.

Enzeco® Ficin 100

Derived from the latex of ficus glabrata fig tree, it has a rapid rate of reaction and a low temperature of inactivation.

Enzeco® Fungal Protease 300

A highly concentrated fungal proteolytic enzyme produced from Aspergillus oryzae. Available as a powder.300,000 HUT/gram.

Enzeco® Neutral Bacterial Protease 160K

Derived from *B. subtilis*, this enzyme preparation was approved for use as a meat tenderizer in 1999. The enzyme has similar temperatures of inactivation as Ficin but is much less expensive and is in more consistent supply.

As a starting point we recommend 1000 to 3000 Milk Clot Units per pound of meat.

Trypsin, Chymotrypsin and pepsin enzymes from animal sources are also widely used.

These enzyme can be applied in two ways:

1. Directly in powder form for surface application or in solution form. The method is most effective on thin steaks or cuts. disadvantages of the technique are lack of uniform action, discoloration and granulation.
2. Injecting the enzyme into jugular vein before 10-15 minutes of slaughter of animal and dose is carefully controlled according to breed, age, sex and weight of an animal. Disadvantage of this method are overtenderness of some organs like heart, liver and tongue.

(10) Mechanical

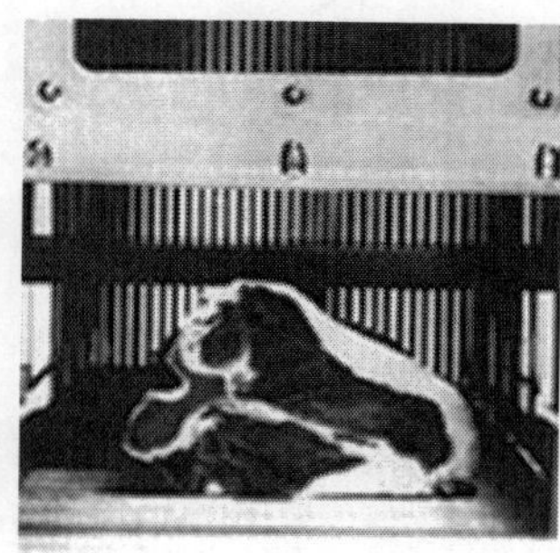

Mechanical severance – scoring, dicing, cubing, grinding or chopping.

Grinding is a very popular means of increasing tenderness of meat, especially beef.

The Cubing is another means of mechanically tenderizing meat. The small blades of a cuber simply sever connective tissue in boneless retail cuts so that the connective tissue is broken into smaller pieces.

Blade or needle tenderization of cuts recently has increased in popularity. This method of tenderization is employed on wholesale cuts that are in turn processed in the normal manner into retail cuts. Very sharp blades or needles is an effective means for disrupting the structural integrity of myofibrils, muscle fibers and muscle bundles, of severing fibrils of collagen, reticulin and elastin and thereby, increasing tenderness of muscles.

It may or may not increase drip loss and/or cooking loss. There have been recent concerns about blade/needle tenderization taking E. coli O157:H7 into the interior of cuts allowing it to survive cooking.

Machines with multiple blades and/or needles that penetrate meat as it passes through on a conveyor. First machine was Jaccard (most people call the process "Jaccarding").

(11) The Hydrodyne Process

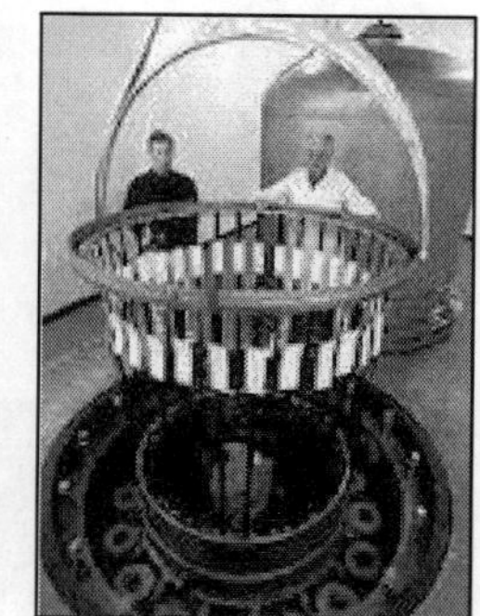

Scientists have discovered that placing a carcass in water and then setting off a controlled explosion in the water instantly tenderizes the carcass. The supersonic shock waves instantly fracture the muscle fibers and destroys most of the Z-lines to greatly improve tenderness. However, this process seems to be still at the experimental stage. In the long run, this process may be able to guarantee tender meat, every time.

(12) Influence of Vitamin D Supplementation

Scientist have demonstrated that animals fed or injected with Vitamin D (7.5 million IU of Vitamin D3) for 7 days before slaughter have more tender meat. It is

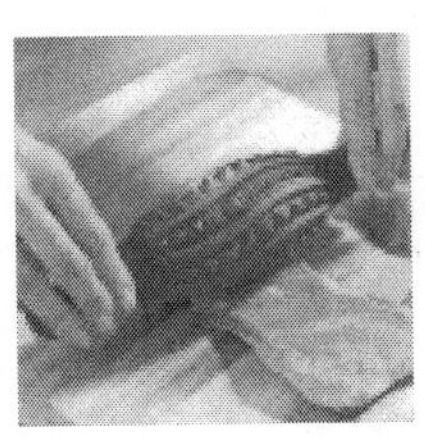
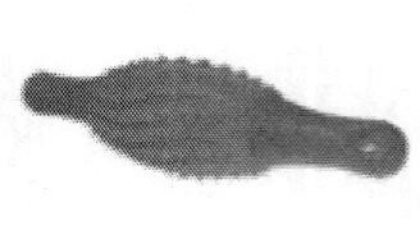
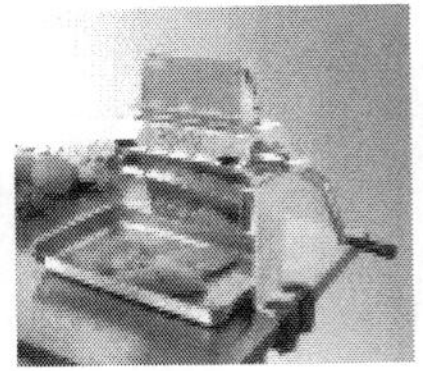
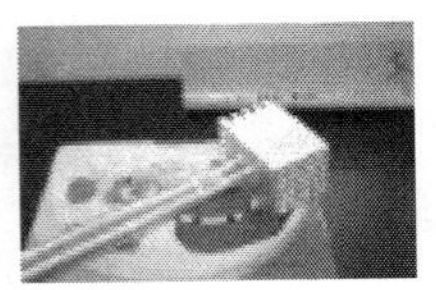
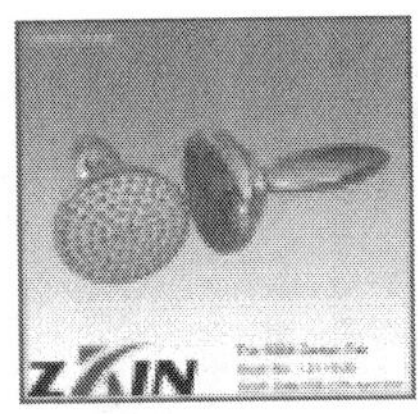
ZHIN
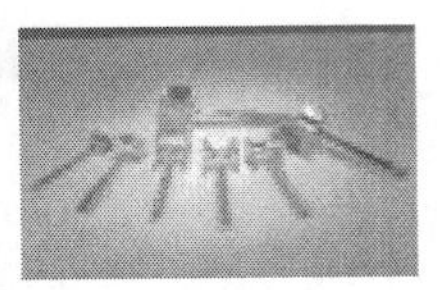
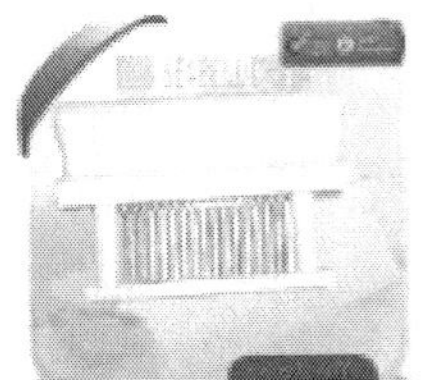
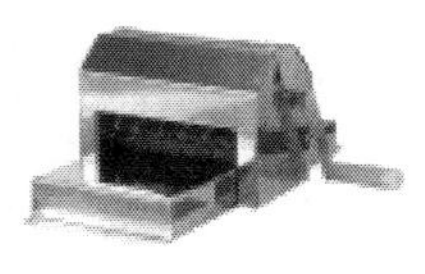
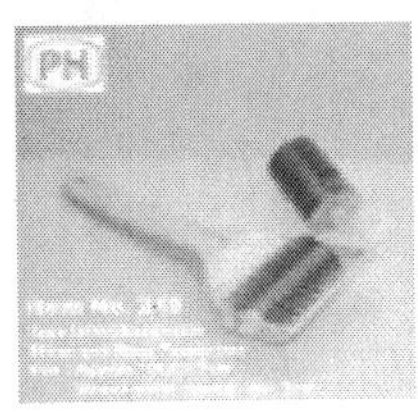
PH
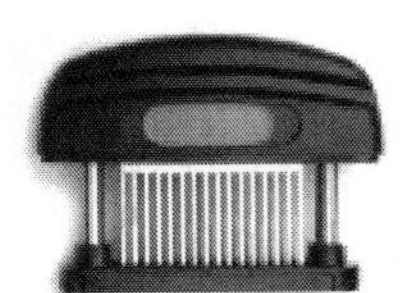
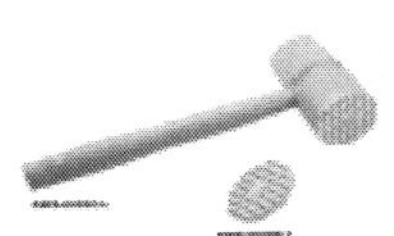
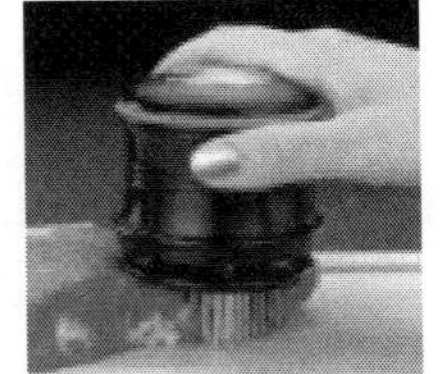
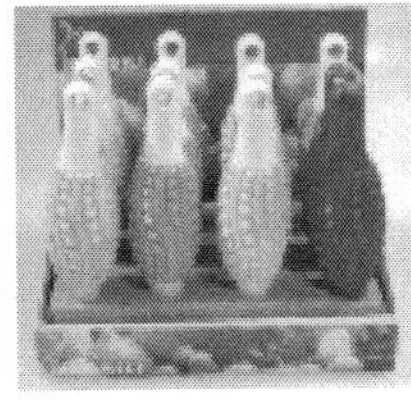
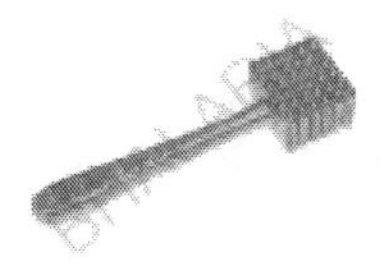
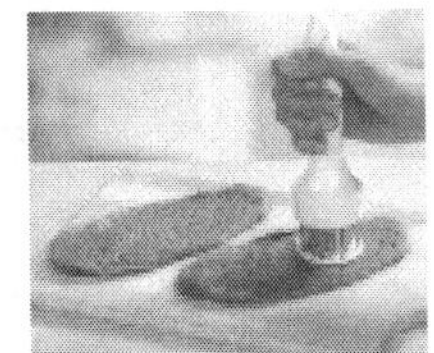
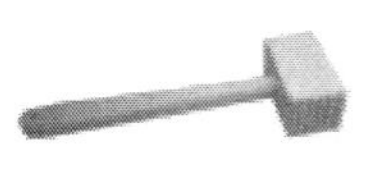
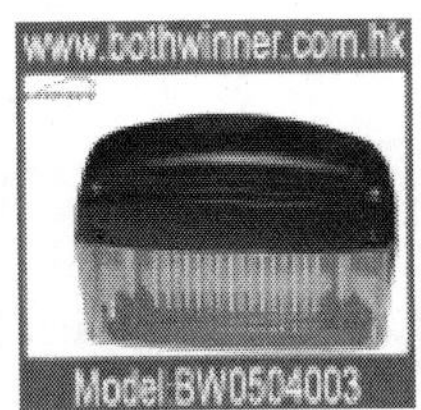
www.bothwinner.com.hk
Model:BW0504003
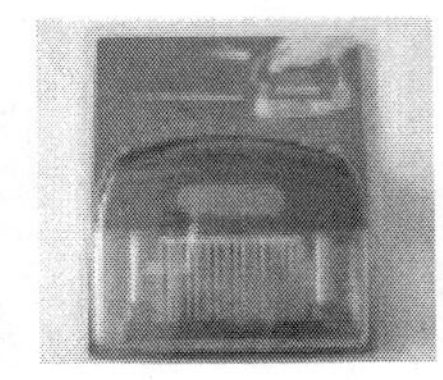
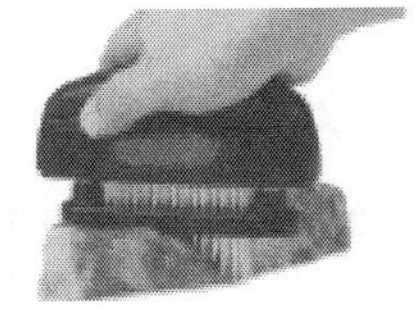
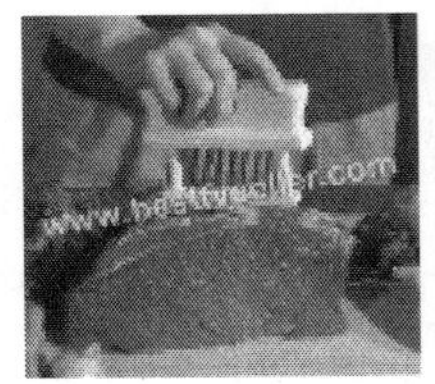
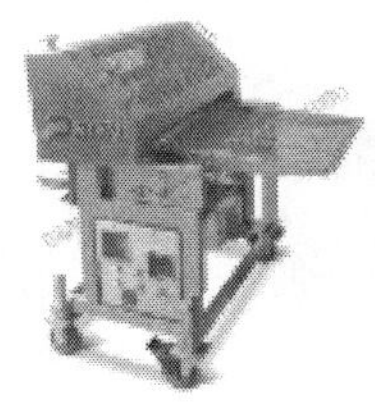
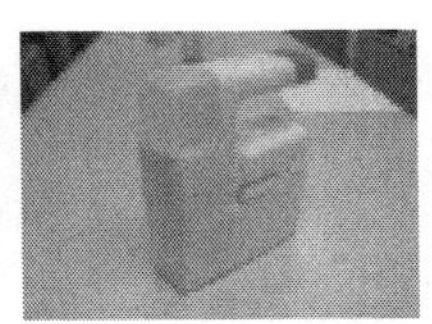
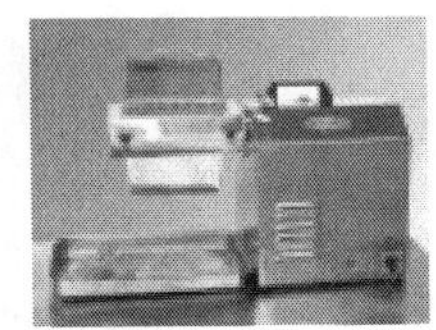
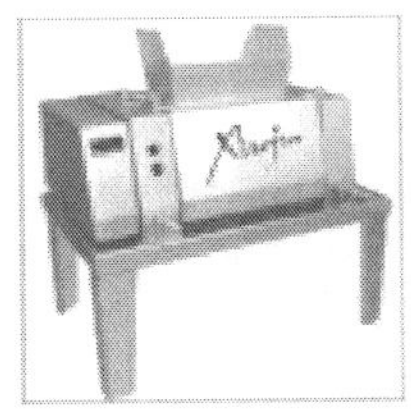

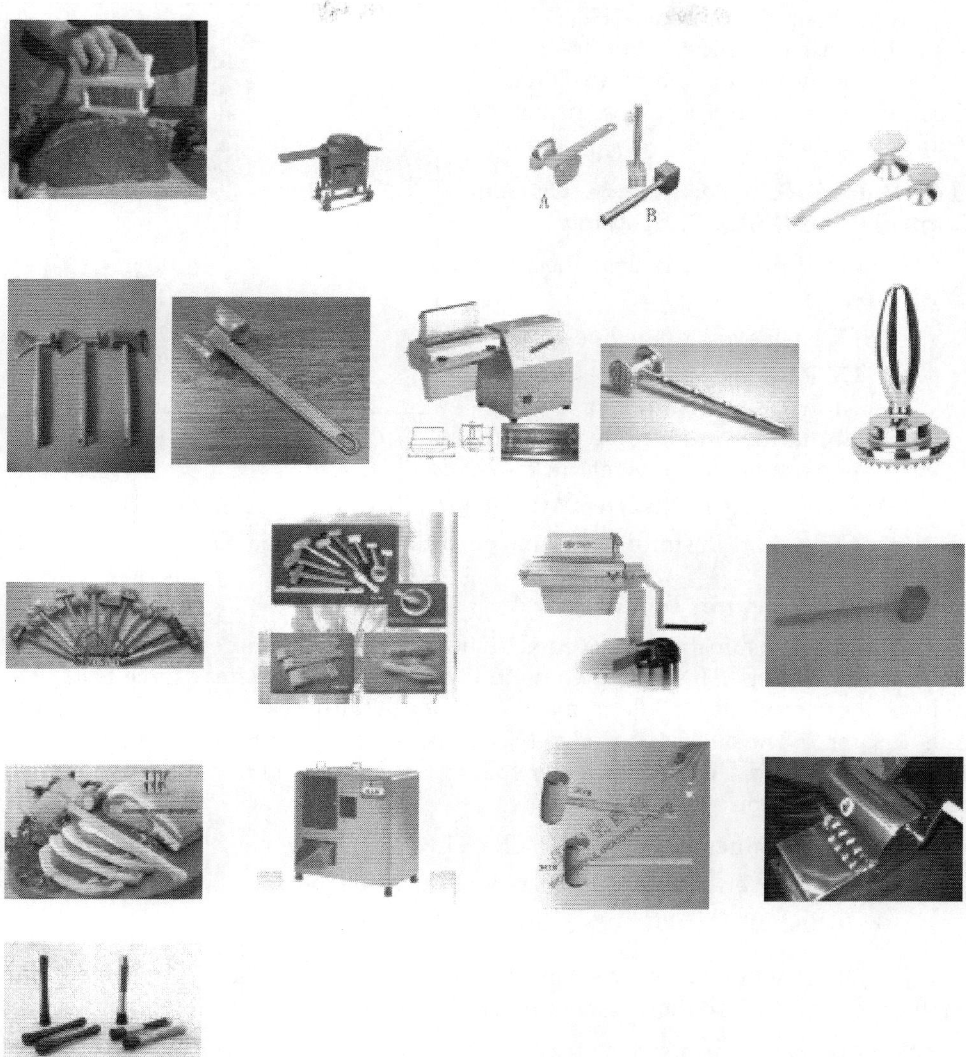

suspected that the Vitamin D greatly increases blood calcium levels (both absorbtion and retention), which in turn assist the naturally occurring enzymes which break down muscle fiber when meat is aged after death (the 'calpain proteolytic enzyme system').

(13) High Pressure Processing

Research conducted in the early 1970s demonstrated that it was possible to subjecting the muscles of freshly harvested animals to very high pressures (100 Mpa) for short periods of time (2 to 4 minutes). Others combined heat and high pressure processing to improve tenderness, and reported that such treatment was efficacious because of effects on myofibrillar proteins or on the sarcolemma.

Hydrodynamic pressure (HDP) wave technology uses an underwater detonation of explosives to generate a hydrodynamic shock wave pressure front as a means for tenderizing meat.

(14) Palatability Assurance Critical Control Point (PACCP) Systems

A PACCP program is described that consists of:

- CCP1–Genetics (sire lines)
- CCP2–Preharvest Cattle Management(age, castration, implants, time-on-feed, health, and a subcutaneous fat thickness target)
- CCP3–Early Postmortem Management(high voltage electrical simulation)
- CCP4–Late Postmortem Management(aging for 21 days).

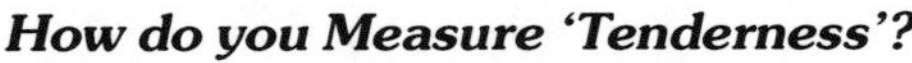

How do you Measure 'Tenderness'?

Scientists measure the force needed to shear muscles. The more force needed, the tougher the meat is. This is known as **the 'Warner-Bratzler shear force test'**. It's units of measurement are kilograms of force needed to shear a 1 cubic centimeter muscle sample. The steak is cooked to 160 o F and at least 8- ½ inch cores are removed from the steak and a Warner-Bratzler shear machine is used to measure the force required to shear the core.

- **Shear values less than 7** – VERY TENDER
- 7 to 10 – tenderness decreases as shear value increases
- 10 and up – tough.

The other method used is a **straight sensory panel test**, where ordinary people eat the meat and record their perception of it's tenderness.

Some people determine tenderness by how easily the teeth sink into the piece of steak upon first bite. Others determine tenderness based upon the number of chews before the piece is swallowed.

Perception of Tenderness

It is described by the following conditions with in meat during mastication.

1. Softness to tongue and cheek
2. Resistnce to tooth pressure
3. Easy of fragmentation
4. Mealiness
5. Adhesion
6. Residue after chewing

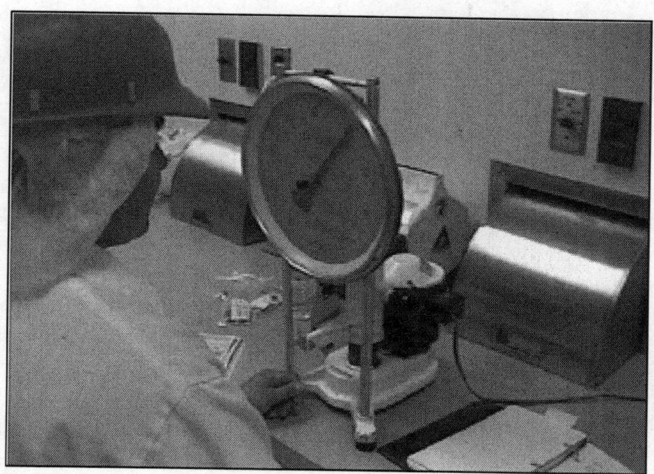

Coring for Shear Force Measurements.

The Future

Consumer say they will pay more for reliably tender meat.Marrying automated shear testing of cooked samples of critical indicator cuts - such as the rib eye steak - with computerized tracing by bar codes on each animals ear tag will help identify 'more tender herds' and 'best handling and management practise'. In this way, both better genetics and best animal feeding and handling practices can be solidly and confidently identified. Those who manage their farming practices, breeds, trucking conditions, and preslaughter yarding conditions to produce identifiable and brandable tender meat

References

A.M. Pearson, and T.R. Dutson chapter no.11- Quality Attributes and Their Measurement in Meat, Poultry and Fish Products (Hardback)Publisher: Aspen Publishers Inc., U.S.ISBN 13: 9780834213050 ISBN 10: 0834213052

www.ars.usda.gov/is/AR/archive/nov99/beef1199.htm; www.aps.uoguelph.ca/~swatland/ch2_3.htm www.ansi.okstate.edu/meats/Article.htm

www.beefresearch.org/./Post-www.extension.umn.edu/distribution/nutrition/DJ0856.html

www.jarvm.com/articles/Vol1Iss2/Polidori.htm journals.cambridge.org/production/action/cjoGetFulltext?fulltextid.

Harvest per cent 20Practices per cent 20for per cent 20Enhancing per cent 20Beef per cent 20Tenderness. meat.tamu.edu/tender.html

meats.marc.usda.gov/MRU_WWW/Protocol/WBS.pdf

www.naiber.com/Publications/RILP/tenderness.pdf - www.naturalhub.com/buy_food_meat_tenderness.htm

savell-j.tamu.edu/pdf/es.pdf

www.uco.es/organiza/servicios/./25_13_47_889BiochemicalLuciano.pdf

II. Artificial Tenderization Methods of Meat

Introduction

Tenderness of meat is one of its most important palatability attributes. Perception of the tenderness of meat to the palate consists of initial ease of penetration of meat by the teeth, the ease with which meat breaks into fragments and the amount of residue remaining after chewing. Even if the meat possesses a good colour or odour and taste if it is tough it is objectionable to the palate. Hence it is undoubtedly the most sought for quality attributes. Tenderness of meat is dependent on two structural components namely (1) **connective tissue** and (2) **myofibrillar components.** The toughness caused by connective tissue is called **'Background Toughness.'** Connective tissue is composed of collagen, elastin, reticulin and ground substance. As the age of the animal advances intramolecular and intermolecular cross links are formed in collagen molecules which contribute towards toughening of meat. The toughness caused by myofibrillar components is termed as **"actomyosin toughness"** or **"myofibrillar toughness."** The changes which occur in myofibrils are due to calcium activated proteases, the ***calpains***,and lysosomal cysteine proteases,the ***cathepsins.*** When meat is stored above freezing point at 0°C and 3°C,all the changes that usually occur at higher temperatures take place but at a reduced rate. The action of bacteria is retarded but not arrested at these temperatures, while the proteolytic enzyme of muscle fiber is active and brings about a desirable change known as ***conditioning*** or ***ripening***, which is manifested by a marked increase in flavour, juiciness,and ***tenderness*** of the meat. Tenderness of the meat is influenced by the breed, age, nutrition and amount of connective tissue present between the muscle fibers.

Different Articifial Tenderisation Methods

1. Mechanical Tenderisation
2. Manual Tenderisation
3. Salts
4. Acids
5. Enzymes
6. Electrical Stimulation
7. Vacuum Tumbling
8. Ultrasonography
9. Cooking
10. Carving
11. Freezing
12. Thawing

1. Mechanical Tenderization

Meat can be tenderised mechanically by a number of methods, including grinding, cubing, needling, and pounding. These actions physically break the muscle cells and connective tissue, making the meat easier to chew. Grinding and cubing meat simply increases the surface-area-to-volume ratio, causing teeth to have less work to do. Needling uses a special piece of equipment to send numerous needle like blades into the meat, separating the tissues. Because of the equipment required to do this, it is not done at consumer level. Another method of mechanical tenderisation, which is more easily done in the home, is simply pounding the meat with special hammer that breaks apart its surface tissue. Meat, which has been mechanically tenderized, retains more of its natural appearance, shape, color, and weight.

2. Manual Tenderization

Manual tenderizers are made in two styles - Hammer and Push. Both are designed to do one thing; Tenderize meat by: Breaking/cutting muscle tissue of tough cuts of meat or punching holes (forking) in the meat to provide easier and quicker access for marinades and meat tenderizing enzymes used in the chemical method. Hammering the meat with a hammer type device breaks the meat's connective tissue and some meat fabric deterioration or granulation will occur. Push style units work like the mechanical units except the cutting knives are pushed into the meat when the user applies force to the handle. The push type that has blades will cut the connective thus tenderizing the meat as well as providing access points into the meat for the chemical tenderizers (marinades). A push style with round prongs will provide access holes for the chemical tenderizers(marinades), which in turn tenderize the meat.

3. Salts

Tenderness can also be increased by the addition of salts in the form of potassium, calcium, or magnesium chlorides. These salts retain moisture and break down the component that surrounds the muscle fibres, resulting in the release of proteins. Polyphosphates are sometimes added to the salts to improve the meat's juiciness by increased water retention ability and if added to processed meats, it also increases firmness, emulsion stability and antimicrobial activity.

4. Acids

Meats can be made more tender by applying marinades containing acids or alcohol, which break down the outside surface of meat. The various acids found in marinades include vinegar, wine and lemon, tomato, or other fruit juices. Not only do marinades tenderize the meat, but they increase flavour and also contribute to colour. The maximum benefit of a marinade can be obtained by increasing the surface area of meat. This may be done by cutting the meat into small pieces. Marinades penetrate only the surface of the meat and are therefore not effective at tenderising large cuts of meat or poultry.

Direct contact is the important point, since it is necessary for the chemical reaction to occur. This means that soaking a piece of meat in a marinade will only penetrate just so far into the surface of the meat. If you marinate a large cut of meat in a tenderizing marinade, you end up with a mushy exterior and an unaffected center. Puncturing the meat for the marinade to penetrate gives an uneven result, with the further undesirable side effect of allowing the meat to lose even more juices while cooking. Thus, flat cuts of meat benefit most from tenderizing marinades. Place meat in a heavy zip-top bag with the air squeezed out and turn it often to be sure all surfaces benefit from the marinade.

5. Enzymes

The two most often used meat tenderising enzymes are ***papain*** and ***bromelin***. Other sources of enzymes have been cited for meat tenderization such as ***Bacillus subtulis, Aspergillus oryzae, ficin(from fig)*** and even ***pancreatin*** derived from pancreatic gland. ***Papain*** is usually produced as a crude, dried material by collecting ***latex*** from ***fruit of papaya*** tree. Further purification is done to obtain purified papain and supplied as dried powder or as a sterilized liquid. ***Bromelain*** is prepared from the ***stump or root*** portion of the ***pineapple*** plant. Bromelain products are all supplied as powders.

An even distribution of enzymes can be achieved by injecting these tenderising enzymes into the blood stream of animals ten minutes before slaughter. This optional treatment sends enzymes travelling to all the muscles through the circulatory system, but they are not activated until meat from the animal is exposed to heat during preparation. This ante mortem use of meat tenderising enzymes is no longer used now.

Post mortem application of these enzymes is generally acceptable. In home use, these enzymes are sprinkled on meat, which is then pierced with a fork to drive the enzymes below the surface, where they hydrolyze muscle cell proteins and connective tissue when activated by the heat of preparation. The enzymes are not active at room temperature. The activity temperature for papain is about 131 to 170°F which is reached only during heating. Exceeding 185°F denatures the enzyme, thus inhibiting its activity. The temperature of inactivation of bromelin is around 160°F.Uniform distribution is hard to achieve with the use of commercial tenderizers and any attempt to get more of the enzymes to penetrate by adding excessive amounts of it can cause the meat to have an unappetizing, mealy, mushy texture.

6. Electrical Stimulation

The meat of beef, cattle and sheep,but not swine,becomes more tender when a current of electricity is passed through the carcass after slaughter and before onset of rigor mortis.Electrical stimulation speeds up rigor mortis by accelerating glycogen breakdown and enzyme activity,which disrupts protein structure,making the meat more tender.In this way,the meat can be immediately cut up without any loss of quality.

The obvious consequence of applying an electrical current to a carcass is to induce vigorous muscular contractions and, in response to the increased energy expenditure, cause a dramatic acceleration of pH decline. Electrical stimulation (ES) of a beef carcass can routinely drop the muscle pH by 0.5 units over a period of 60 seconds of stimulation, a process that could require 3 or more hours in the absence of stimulation (Ducastaing, Valin, Schollmeyer and Cross, 1985). This represents a 180-fold acceleration in the rate of muscle glycolysis and a clear indication of the tight coupling between the rate of glycolysis and ATP turnover in muscle tissue. In addition to the pH drop during stimulation (pH), there can also be an acceleration in the subsequent rate of glycolysis following stimulation (pH/t) above that seen in unstimulated muscles (Chrystall and Devine, 1978). However, this effect tends to be associated with high voltage stimulation (HVS) systems (typically 1000V and above) and is not necessarily triggered by low voltage stimulation (LVS) systems.

7. Vacuum Tumbling

Vacuum-tumbling applies gentle mechanical action in combination with a vacuum that assists in distributing the added ingredients throughout the meat. Vacuum-tumbling is very commonly used in value-added meat products, but it is not used in enhanced fresh pork and beef products. If fresh, enhanced pork and beef products are tumbled, salt-soluble proteins are extracted, water-holding capacity increases, the brine is more readily bound into the meat, and texture becomes softer, more rubberier, and the texture has been described as more processed-meat like.

Vacuum Tumbling removes the air from a rotating drum and "tumbles" the product inside the drum. This "tumbling" under a vacuum allows the meat pores to open up and accept the marinade and water. The tumbling action of a few minutes allows for a greater pickup up of water and spice - 10 per cent - 20 per cent compared to 1 per cent - 2 per cent when soaking for 48 hours Anwar *et al.* (2001) injected beef top loin steaks with up to 10 per cent of a solution containing water, 0.25 per cent sodium phosphates and combinations of either potassium lactate and sodium diacetate. They found that after injection, even up to 30 minutes of vacuum-tumbling increased the processed meat- like texture of top loin steaks. They used vacuum-tumbling less than 30 minutes in combination with blade -tenderization to assist in even distribution of the injection solution into steaks.

8. Ultrasonography

Ultrasound, when used at **low frequencies** and high intensities has the potential of improving tenderness of meat. Application of ultrasound at high intensities to provoke changes in physical and chemical properties of meat and meat products has attracted the interest of research workers for the past few decades because it is a pure physical technique. A study at the University of Queensland is designed to investigate the effects of high power ultrasound treatment on the tenderness, colour, water loss, cook loss, thermal and ultrastructural properties of eye round and strip loin obtained from mature steers. The ultrasound radiation has inherent qualities of heat production and pressurisation.

The **tenderness** was found to be increased due to the ultrasound treatment as measured by the Warner Bratzler shear force device (objective tenderness) and the hardness of the muscles was also significantly reduced after the treatments. Other quality parameters tested were not compromised by the ultrasound treatment(*e.g.* drip loss, cook loss and colour). Conventional applications of ultrasound such as medical imaging, cleaning and measuring fat depth of carcasses are well established.

The sonochemical and sonomechanical effects of sound waves (20 kHz -100 kHz) at a sufficiently high power range (100 W-10 kW) radiated through food (aqueous or semisolids) can alter the intrinsic property of the foods. High power ultrasound has the potential to be used efficiently in food processing in place of chemicals, high temperatures and pressures and longer processing times undernormal processing conditions.

Ultrasound treatment reduces the **denaturation** temperature of **collagen** of both muscles. This effect can be attributed to the fragmentation of collagen macromolecules upon ultrasonication, reducing the denaturation temperature of extracted collagen (Nishihara and Dotty, 1958).

9. Cooking

As cooking progresses, the contractile proteins in meat become less tender, and the major connective tissue protein (collagen) becomes more tender. Thus, for cuts that are low in connective tissue–such as steaks and chops from the rib and loin–the recommended method of cooking is **dry heat**, including pan frying, broiling, roasting, or barbecuing. Dry heat raises the temperature very quickly and the flavour of meat will develop before the contractile proteins have the opportunity to become significantly less tender.

For cuts with a high amount of connective tissue–such as those from the fore shank, heel of round, and chuck–the recommended method of cooking is long and slow at low temperatures using **moist heat** such as braising. The application of moist heat for a long time at low temperatures (275-325°F) results in conversion of tough collagen into tender gelatin and makes this type of cut more tender compared with dry heat cooking of one of the less tender cuts of meat.

Degree of doneness significantly affects tenderness. As the lean is heated, the contractile proteins toughen and moisture is lost. Both decrease tenderness. Tender cuts of meat cooked to a rare degree of doneness (140°F) are more tender than when cooked to medium (155°F), and medium in turn is more tender than well-done (170°F). Degree of doneness is especially important in the case of beef. Some people, however, do not like the flavour of rare beef and thus choose to cook their beef well-done. They should be aware that by doing so, tenderness is greatly reduced in what normally are tender cuts of meat (tenderness will be improved in less tender cuts when cooked well-done by moist heat).

When consumers switch to a grade of **beef** with less marbling than what they have been accustomed to, care should be taken not to overcook. In most cases, beef with little marbling requires less cooking time than higher grade beef. However, consumers often fail to make this time adjustment and the result is overcooked beef that lacks tenderness. Some consumers cook low fat beef in the frozen state for the same time as they would higher fat, thawed beef. This procedure helps prevent overcooking.

It is recommended that **pork** be cooked to approximately 160°F or 170°F internal temperature for desirable flavour. Although this temperature range corresponds to well-done in beef, pork still may be slightly pink. Since ***Trichinella spiralis*** (trichina) is destroyed at 137°F, an internal temperature of 160-170°F for pork is definitely safe. Therefore, it is not necessary to cook pork beyond this stage of doneness; further cooking will result in dehydration, loss of juiciness, and unnecessary toughening. It usually is recommended to cook lamb to well-done (approximately 160-170°F internal temperature) because the flavour is more desirable compared with lower temperatures.

10. Carving

Muscles, muscle bundles, and muscle fibers are all surrounded by connective tissue. When cuts are made from carcasses and wholesale cuts, the normal procedure is to cut at right angles to the length of the muscle. This procedure severs the maximum amount of connective tissue and distributes the bone more evenly among all cuts in that area. Likewise, consumers should carve cooked meat at right angles to the length of the muscle fibers or "against the grain" to achieve maximum tenderness. Cutting with the grain results in "stringiness" and thus less tenderness.

11. Freezing

Freezing rate plays a small role in tenderness. When meat is frozen very quickly, small ice crystals form; when meat is frozen slowly, large ice crystals are formed. While the formation of large crystals may serve to disrupt components of the muscle fibers in meat and thereby increase tenderness very slightly, the large ice crystals result in an increased loss of juices upon thawing. This increase in loss of juices results in meat that is less juicy upon cooking and therefore usually is perceived as being less tender.

12. Thawing

Thawing meat slowly in the refrigerator generally results in greater tenderness compared with cooking from the frozen state. Slow thawing minimizes the toughening effect from cold shortening (when present) and reduces the amount of moisture loss. Thawing in a microwave is accomplished by using a lower power setting or by manually alternating cooking and standing times. During the standing time, some of the heat from the thawed areas moves toward the frozen area.

References

1. http://nr.stpi.org.tw/ejournal/proceedingB/v22n3/97-107.pdf
2. http://www.meatims.org/download/Reassessing per cent 20the per cent 20Principles per cent 20of per cent 20Electrical per cent 20Stimulation.pd
3. http://www.allcookingtips.com/2007/12/29/artificial-tenderizing-meats/
4. http://www.elsevier.com/wps/find/simple_search.cws_home
5. http://homecooking.about.com/od/specificdishe1/a/marinadescience.htm
6. http://pdfcast.org/pdf/effect-of-papain-and-bromelin-on-muscle-and-collagen-proteins-in-beef-meat
7. http://en.wikipedia.org/wiki/Beef
8. http://books.google.coms

– *Chapter 11* –

Chemical Residues in Meat and their Effects on the Health of the Consumer

I. Fate of Chemical Residues in Meat Products and their Effect on the Consumer Health

Introduction

A large number of drugs used to control or prevent infections or to promote growth are considered essential by some authorities in modern animal production systems. Additional chemicals may be added to food to ensure maximum utilization and to delay deterioration.However, there is growing consumer resistance to the presence of unwanted residues in food.

The principal concerns are

1. Drug Resistance
2. Toxicity
3. Potential Allergy

Drugs are intended to be toxic to various forms of parasites and as such may have inherent toxic, **mutagenic, teratogenic or carcinogenic effects**.Penicillin ranks highly among the known allergens and can evoke an allergic reaction in consumers eating sufficient residual drugs. Residues can occur for a variety of reasons. Clearance rates for drugs can vary. Conditions that prolong the process can lead to tissue residues at slaughter. Drugs are also sometimes administered to food –producing animals at a dose rate in excess of the recommended level by unauthorized routes or at more frequent interval than specified. These therapies can alter the withholding time required to ensure that tissues are clear of residues. The pharmokinetics of specific preparation has a major effect on persistence in the animal tissue and is dependent on several factors. Formulations can give slow or rapid release.Current trends favour the use of slow – release formulations, both to prolong therapeutically – active concentrations of therapeutic drugs in tissue and to minimize the stress involved in repeated handling of animals.

The therapeutic product that cause concern fall into number of categories. The major ones are antimicrobials, which are a diffuse group containing several classes of compounds used to treat or prevent bacterial infection. The **pesticides** are also a diffuse group including **anthelmentics used for the activities against roundworms, tapeworms, and flukes, ectoparasiticide, used to kill external parasite such as mange, sheep scab mites or lice and antiprotozoals which are most commonly used for the control and treatment of coccidiosis and babesiosis.Hormones** are used for therapeutic purposes in various fertility treatments or for growth promotion and are administered as injection or implant. One general category include **tranquilizer, β agonists.**

Animals are exposed to many environmental contaminants including **herbicides, heavy metals and fungicides.** In preservation and processing of food,**additives** are employed to prevent the onset of spoilage, to promote binding properties and to enhance flavour and nutritive value.These additives include antioxidants, emulsifiers, humectants,firming agents, sequestrants, colouring agents, stabilizers, sweeteners, tenderizers.etc.

For all chemicals which may produce residues it is essential to establish an acceptable daily intake in the diet. Calculation of this acceptable daily intake depends on the toxicology of the compounds. These toxicological effects are determined by acute and chronic studies involving genotoxicity, teratogenicity, neurotoxicity, carcinogenicity, neurotoxicity and effects on the immune and reproductive systems.

RESIDUE is defined as a substance having a pharmacological action, of their metabolites and of other substances transmitted to animal products and which are likely to be harmful to human health.

Almost all chemicals administered knowingly or unknowingly to animals result in some trace residue remaining in the carcass. Increasingly, laboratory technology is able to detect these minute traces It is therefore important to differentiate between safe and unsafe residual concentrations rather than to insist on zero residues

The Safe Use of Veterinary Medicines

The following advice to farmers has been issued by the veterinary medicine directorate of the UK ministry of agriculture, fisheries and food

1. Source of medicines
2. Administration of medicines
3. Withdrawal times
4. Record keep

Acceptable Daily Intake (ADI)

It is an estimate of the amount of a food additive, expressed on a body weight basis, that can be ingested daily over a lifetime without appreciate health risk

Maximum Residue Levels (MRL)

It is the maximum acceptable human intake of residues over a lifetime.

Detection Limit

It is defined as the concentration corresponding to a measurement level three standard deviations above the mean value.

Sources of chemical contamination of meat

The introduction of chemical in meat occur when animal is alive or during processing or storage of meat. A range of possible source of contamination and likely contaminants are outlined below

1. **Environmental contamination:** It generally involves chemicals which tend to persist in the environment *e.g.* heavy metals and organ chlorine pesticides.
2. **Feed and water additives:** may involve chemicals which use to treat animals, the feed or the water for *e.g.* antibiotic or antibacterial agent, growth promoters, insecticidal or fungicidal feed treatment, ant algal treatment of water.
3. **Feed contaminants:** It may be the result of environmental contamination of the raw material used in feed production or other chemical used in, or associated with the feed production for *e.g.* organochlorines pesticides, heavy metal, aflatoxins, solvents used in some rendering system

   Chemicals used directly on livestock

   ☆ Internal and external parasite treatment

   -*e.g.* dips, pour on insecticides, drenches etc.

   Veterinary drugs

   Chemicals applied indirectly to livestock

   ☆ Crop or pasture aerial spray

   e.g. insecticides or herbicides.
4. **Chemicals** arising from contamination during processing and packaging of meat

   ☆ Contaminants of processing surface *e.g.* Sanitizing agents

   ☆ Contamination of packaging materials prior to use *e.g.* insecticides etc. used in storage areas containing wrapping material which come in contact with meat

   ☆ Chemicals present in packaging material

Table 11.1: Antibiotic Maximum Residue Level (MRL) for Bovines

Compound	*Target Tissues*	*Concentration (μg/g)*
Sulphonamides	Muscle, Liver, Kidney, Fat	100
Benzyl penicillin	Muscle, Liver, Kidney, Fat, milk	504
Ampicillin	Muscle, Liver, Kidney, Fat, Milk	504
Apramycin	Muscle, Fat	1000
	Liver	10000
	Kidney	20000
Cefquinone	Kidney	200
	Liver	100
	Muscle	50
	Fat	50
Cloxacillin	Muscle, Liver, Kidney	300
	Fat, Milk	30
Erythromycin	Liver, Kidney, Muscle,	400
	Fat	40
Florenicol	Muscle	200
	Kidney	300
	Liver	3000
Spiramycin	Liver, Kidney, Fat	300
	Muscle	200
	Milk	200
Streptomycin	Kidney	1000
	Muscle, Fat, Liver	500
	Milk	200
Tetracycline	Kidney	600
	Liver	300
	Muscle	100
	Milk	100
Tilmicosin	Liver, Kidney	1000
	Muscle, Fat	50
Trimethoprim	Muscle, Liver, kidney, Fat, Milk	50
Tylosin	Muscle, Liver, Kidney,	100
	Fat, Milk	50

Source: Meat Hygiene by J.F. Gracy, D.S. Collins, R.J. Huey.

Table 11.2: Maximum Residue Level (MRL) for Comon Anthelmentics

Anthelmentics	*Species*	*Target Tissue*	*Maximum Residue Level (μg/kg)*
Levamisole	Bovine, ovine,	Muscle, kidney, fat, liver	10
	porcine, poultry		100
Ivermectin	Bovine	Liver	100
		Fat	40
	Ovine	Liver	15
	Porcine	Fat	20

Contd...

Table 11.2–*Contd...*

Anthelmentics	*Species*	*Target Tissue*	*Maximum Residue Level (µg/kg)*
Abamectin	Bovine	Liver	20
Doramectin	Bovine	Liverfat	1525
Eprinomectin	Bovine	Muscle, fat Liver Kidney	30 600 100 30
Moxidectin	Bovine, ovine	Fat Liver Muscle, kidney	500 100 50
Closantel	Bovine Ovine	Muscle, liver Kidney, fat Muscle, liver Kidney Fat	1000 3000 1500 5000 2000
Febantel, Fenbendazole	All food- producing species	Liver Muscle, kidney, fat	1000 10
Oxfendazole	Bovine, ovine	milk	10
Triclabendazole	Bovine, ovine	Muscle, kidney, liverfat	15050
Thiabendazole	Bovine, ovine, caprine	muscle	100
Netobimin	Bovine, ovine, caprine	Liver Kidney Muscle, fat Milk	1000 500 100 100

Source: Meat Hygiene by J.F. Gracy, D.S. Collins, R.J. Huey.

Effect of Various Processing Methods on Chemical Residues

Various methods of meat processing used by humans are cooking, boiling, roasting, frying, freezing, irradiation, smoking etc. various studies have been done to see the effect of all these methods of processing on the chemical residues present in the meat product

Effect on Pesticide Residue

With meats, the only potential for residue removal lies in trimming away fat and/or its rendering during cooking. Several studies have shown that organ chlorine insecticide residues in meat (chicken) are generally present in rendered fat at approximately the same concentration as those in tissue fat. Pesticide reduction in chicken during cooking was found to depend upon cooking temperature. Cooking in water at 190 to 200° F. for three hours removed about 45 per cent of the DDT, dieldrin and heptachlor residues; lindane removal was more complete. Autoclaving for three hours at 15 psi (temperature equivalent 250° F.), however, removed over 95 per cent of the DDT, dieldrin and lindane and 90 per cent of the heptachlor residues. Frying and baking of chicken were also evaluated for DDT and lindane removal; 50 to 75 per cent losses were obtained. Some conversion of DDT to DDD occurred with each of the cooking methods, and this increased during the higher temperature methods. With other pesticides, cooking in water at 121° C. removed 63 per cent of chlordane residues and all of the Telodrin, but other residues were not affected. In contrast to these findings with chicken, cooking of beef under various conditions was not very effective in reducing DDT residues. With the exception of frying and pressure cooking (35 and 50 per cent, respectively), relatively little removal occurred. One imagines this might reflect the smaller relative loss of fat during the cooking of beef in comparison to chicken. The higher temperatures associated with frying and pressure cooking, by causing greater fat removal, may have contributed to the more substantial losses of residue associated with such methods. It may be concluded that appreciable reduction of most organochlorine residues contributed to the diet by meats might be achieved through intensive cooking. The effectiveness depends upon whether the fat removal is substantial and whether fat drippings are used later Studies are carried on fermentation of Meat products such as sausages having DDT 5 ppm It is observe that Fermentation process in meat products reduced the pesticide residues by10 per cent and these reductions were due to the activity of meat starter (Abou-Arab, 2002)

Effect on Antibiotic Residues

Antibiotics are normally administered by veterinarians for treatment, prevention of infection disease in farm animals and it is an important measure when raising animal under intensive husbandry methods production In addition, they are routinely used at sub-therapeutic levels as animal feed additives for their growth promoting properties. Study was conducted to see the effect of method of cooking on the residues of antibiotic in meat. For this enrofloxacin was selected.Enrofloxacin is a synthetic fluoroquinolone antimicrobial agent. In veterinary medicine, it is administered orally to turkeys and chickens, for the treatment of infections of the respiratory and alimentary tract. The recommended doses are 10 mg Enrofloxacin/kg bw/day for 3 to 10 days (chickens and turkeys). Currently, levels of drug residues in raw food (meat and animals products) are regulated. Maximum residue limits (MRL) for the fluoroquinolone, Enrofloxacin, and its metabolite, ciprofloxacin, legally permitted in food under European Union regulations (EEC, 1990). European Union (EU) countries established a maximum residue level (MRL) of 30 ng/g of muscle, liver and kidney for sum of Enrofloxacin and ciprofloxacin. They are used as the mainstream screening methods for systematic detection of antibiotic residues in food and they determine the presence of antibiotics in the sample and identify the specific antibiotic group. Screening methods have acceptable false positive result rates and allow detection of a wide spectrum of antibiotics. Their other advantages are the option to analyze a large number of samples simultaneously and the relatively short time needed for preparation of samples as no purification procedures are required. They cannot be used to identify individual antibiotics. A positive result should be confirmed with chemical or physical methods. Microbial methods are relatively inexpensive, easy to use, do not require expensive equipment and can be efficiently adopted by laboratory staff. On the basis of other researches, the plate seeded with *Escherichia coli* is suitable for detection of fluoroquinolones residues Between 1995 and 1999, Rose and his co-workers demonstrated that residues of a range of veterinary drugs have varying degrees of stability during cooking and, therefore, the cooking influences the level of risk posed by such residues Since the most of food producing animals are always cooked before consumption and the variations in Enrofloxacin levels in the tissue are dependent on the type of cooking.

Test Procedure for Raw and Cooked Samples

The test organism that was used in this study is *E. coli* and the used agar Medium was Muller Hinton agar and this medium was adjusted to pH = 6 with sodium hydroxide and acid autoclaved as indicated by the manufacturers. Sterile Petri dishes (diameter 90 mm) were filled with 25 ml of the prepared culture medium then we seeded *E. coli* in plates. Raw sample disks (diameter 2 mm) were put on each plate; also, we put a paper disk for negative control. After all samples were put onto the plates, plates were incubated at 37°C for 24 h. A positive raw sample is indicated by a complete inhibition of growth in an annular zone not less than 2 mm wide around the disc. Less than 2 mm of inhibitory zone indicated negative result. Results of inhibition zones diameter was read by digital caliper after incubation of plates. The positive raw samples were selected for cooking processes (boiling, roasting and microwaving) then the test for cooked samples were performed just like raw samples after complete cooking of them. Also, we placed 0.01 ml of boiling fluid on plates after the boiling process of samples for detection of residues.

Results

Comparison of the effects of different cooking methods on the mean diameter of inhibition zones (mean ± SE) around raw and cooked samples are shown in Table 11.1 We saw that all cooking processes can lead to a reduction in diameter of inhibition zones in cooked samples rather than raw samples. Comparison of the effect of each cooking process on the mean inhibition zones diameter (mean ±SE) around different tissues samplesare shown in Table 11.2. All of the tissues had a reduction in their inhibition zone diameter in each cooking method. Only the difference between the mean inhibition zones of boiled muscle and liver was not significant (Table 11.2).

Discussion

The microbiological detection methods are used to establish whether and where antimicrobial residues accumulate in the tissues of commercial animal farming. They are essentially a qualitative screening test, which detects any tissues substance with the property of bacterial inhibition. The advantages of these tests are quite simple, inexpensive, sensitive, reliable, and they do not have need for high skill of operator. In the microbial test, observation of inhibition zones is possible when antibiotics residue is above MRL because this test cannot detect amounts of residues below or around allowable amounts. According to the results of our study, maximum mean inhibitory zone in all cooked samples regarding to microwaving process and minimum inhibitory zone related to boiled samples in the cooked muscle and gizzard samples and roasting process in the cooked liver samples (Table 11.1). The cooked muscle and liver have the most and lowest detectable remaining residue in boiling fluid, respectively (Table 11.2). These results proved that, most of the residues were excreted from tissue to cooking fluid in the boiling process. The most reduction of Enrofloxacin residue in cooked muscle and gizzard samples related to boiling and roasting processes for cooked liver samples and the highest detectable amount of residues belonged to microwaving process in all cooked samples (Table 11.1). Difference between the residues of raw and cooked muscle samples and difference between the residues in various cooking processes from viewpoint of significance are shown in Table 11.1 ($P<0.01$). Also, the differences between the residues of different tissues in each cooking process was significant except between the boiled muscle and liver samples ($P<0.01$) (Table 11.2). Based on a research about the effect of different cooking processes (microwaving, roasting, boiling, grilling and frying) on Enrofloxacin residues in the breast and whole leg of chicken, the scientists mentioned that the extraction of residues took place when the chicken pieces were boiled at 100°C for 10 min or micro waved at 800 W for 3.5 min and there was a reduction in concentration and the lost amount of residue from the tissue found in water or exudates and the amount of residue increased with roasting at 200°C for 10 min and grilling for 10 min because the lower moisture content of the treated piece caused an apparent concentration of the quinolone residue. The results of boiling and microwaving in this research confirm the findings of our study about the decrease of Enrofloxacin activity, after cooking but there is no consistency with our results about roasting processes and we can relate this variation to the difference in roasting time in our research that it was 40 min for muscle samples for complete cooking and another reason can be related to the detection method that we used; qualitative microbiological method instead of HPLC (High Performance Liquid Chromatography) method as a quantitative method. The results of our study are consistent with other studies about the fate of drug residues. According to a study on the stability of antibiotics in a pork

Table 11.3: Comparison of Mean Inhibition Zones Diameter (mean±SE) between Raw and Cooked Samples in different Cooking Procedures.

	Muscle	*Liver*	*Gizzard*
Raw	24.6±0.99c	19.3±2.24b	20.2±0.55c
Boiled	7.1±0.87a	9.3±1.30a	6.30±0.94a
Boiling fluid	14.7±1.02b	12 ±2.99ab	13.6±0.98b
Microwaved	16.3±1.20b	11.9±3.27ab	16.9±1.13bc
Roasted	7.6±0.31a	5.9±0.81a	6.80±0.25a

a, b and c: Means with different superscripts differ significantly ($P<0.01$).

Table 11.4: Comparison of Mean Inhibition Zones Diameter (mean±SE) in Liver, Muscle and Gizzard Samples in each Cooking Method.

	Boiled	*Boiling Fluid*	*Microwaved*	*Roasted*
Muscle	7.1±0.87a	14.7±1.02a	16.3±1.20a	7.6±0.31a
Liver	9.3±1.30b	12±2.99a	11.9±3.27a	5.9±0.81a
Gizzard	6.30±0.94a	13.6±0.98a	16.9±1.13a	6.8±0.25a

a and b: Means with different superscripts differ significantly ($P<0.01$).

meat-kidney liver mixture after the sterilization step (134°C for 20 min), it was proven that, the mean remaining activity of Enrofloxacin residue reduced to 68 per cent after cooking or in a study on Norfloxacin residue in the liver and muscle samples of poultry

According to the results and findings of another research about effects of different cooking procedures on antibiotic residue in food stuff, we can conclude that cooking processes cannot annihilate the total amounts of this drug but it can only decrease their amounts and most of the residues in boiling process are excreted from tissue to cooking fluid during the boiling process. Thus, exposure to residues may be reduced by discarding any juices which come from the edible tissues as they are cooked. Between the various agents affecting antibiotics residue after the cooking process, it was found that cooking time and temperature can play major roles about antibiotic residue reduction while cooking food. Also, additional separate residue detection experiments on the metabolites of these drugs must be done, that can be produced after cooking and toxicology experiments must be performed for detection of their effects on human bodies.

Residues and Health Risk

Among all residues, pesticides receiving most interest worldwide in recent years. Though violative level of pesticides are relatively uncommon, a low violation rate even remain an important public health consideration because of their wide spread use in meat and poultry production, their persistence in environment and varying toxicity. The United Nations has estimated that about 2 million poisoning and 10, 000 deaths occur each year from pesticides, with about three-fourth of this occurring in **developing countries.** The acute and malicious consumption involving higher dose results in death whereas, chronic insidious intake lead to elevated cancer risk and disruption of body's reproductive, immune, endocrine and nervous system. The carcinogenicity of organochlorine (OC) pesticides has been studied in a number of laboratory animals including non-human primates. Lifetime or limited period of time treatment of mice with DDT induced liver tumors including malignant metastasizing hepatoblastomas. DDT also increased incidences lung tumors and lymphoma in mice, liver tumors in rats and adrenal adenomas in hamster. However, DDT did not induce DNA damage in bacteria or cultured rodent and human cells. It induced chromosomal aberration in mouse but not in rat bone marrow cells. DDT and its metabolites inhibited gap-junctional intracellular communication. Other areas of concerns are childhood brain cancer and cancers of nervous system. Studies suggest an increase in risk in brain cancer, leukemia, Wilm's tumors, Ewing's sarcoma and germ cell tumors associated with paternal occupational exposure to pesticides prior to and during pregnancy. However, maternal occupational exposure during pregnancy was less frequent but was also associated leukemia, Wilm's tumors and germ cell tumors. Pesticides can suppress immune system, as epidemiological evidence shows an association between pesticide exposure and increase incidence of human disease, particularly those disease to which immuno-compromised individuals are especially prone. The endocrine disrupter includes atrazine and alachlor. However, there is strong need of sufficient data for complete health hazard evaluation in this context.

In contrast to pesticides, exposure from veterinary drug residues rather most common as are directly injected or fed to the animals. The overuse of antimicrobials such as tetracyclines, sulfonamides, amino glycosides, β-lactam derivatives etc. in animal production or their residues in food system pose potential allergic reactions in sensitized individuals, but sub therapeutic and therapeutic levels may perturb human gut micro flora. The tetracyclines are incompletely absorbed from the gastrointestinal tract; they reach readily high concentrations in the intestine, producing perturbations of the intestinal microflora within 48 h of daily treatment. Experience with tetracyclines in human medicine indicates that therapeutic levels of tetracyclines can perturb the intestinal microflora by inducing emergence of resistant strains and altering the metabolic activity of the microflora, its resistance to colonization by pathogenic, opportunistic or resistant microorganism barrier effect and its ecological balance, without any identified deleterious effect. Immunodepression and phototoxicity may also occur in animals and human beings besides superinfections related to tetracyclines. Treatment with oxytetracycline during the second month of pregnancy presents a teratogenic risk to the foetus. As an undesirable side effect, OTC not only discolours the primary and permanent teeth but also causes hypoplasia in developing teeth when administered to the infants, mothers during last two trimesters of pregnancy and children under 12 years of age. However, unwanted risk is highest when OTC is given to neonates and babies prior to the first dentition. Sulphonamides' (sulfadimidine and sulfamethoxazole) can induce thyroid, adenoma and hyperplasia in laboratory animals. It has also potential carcinogenic character. To reduce bacteria resistance to sulfonamides to get synergistic effect, pyrimethamines such as trimethoprim and oriprim are used in combination. The National Research Council and Institute of Medicine have noted a link between the use of antibiotics in food animals and the development of bacterial resistance to these drugs causing human diseases. Similarly, scientist at Centre for Disease Control and Prevention (CDC) began tracking a new type of *Salmonella* called Newport 9+ which is resistant to nine antibiotics including ceftriaxone, one of the few drugs that kill most bacteria and the drug of choice for children when *Salmonella* enter the blood stream. Nonetheless, toxicity of these antimicrobial chemicals includes aplasia of bone marrow, the emergence of resistant bacteria within animals and the transfer of **antibiotic resistance** gene to human pathogens. The appearance of resistance among pathogenic organisms such as *Salmonella* DT-104 and *Campylobacter* is of more concern. *E. coli* is an opportunist pathogen capable of infecting people via the food chain and causing enteric infections in young children and travelers as well as range of other infections. Enteric infections with *Salmonella*, *E. coli* or *Campylobacter* rarely warrant antibiotic treatment and so one might argue that the problem is not nearly as important as Methicillin Resistant ***Staphylococcus aureus*** (MRSA) or other major human resistance problems. However, treatment failure has been reported and the livestock industries cannot ignore the problem. Enterococci have only been thought of as food borne organisms since discovery of Vancomycin Resistant Enterococci (VRE) in pigs and poultry and there is some dispute that their spread occurs from animals to people.

Similarly, uses of hormonal compound like DES in meat production known to have strong carcinogenic effects and are banned from use for food producing animal. On the other hand, beta-adrenergic agonist (clenbuterol, salbuterol, cimeterol) act through binding to receptor on target cells and act by repartitioning energy from fat to lean meat production. This compound in excessive amount leaves residues in meat and thereby adverse reaction in consumers requiring hospital treatment. Thus, health risks of veterinary medicinal products and their metabolites are very difficult to define and their presence of above the violative level is illegal and subject to financial penalties in many countries.

The health implications from heavy metals lead to kidney damage, **cardiovascular disease**s, induction of hypertension, **growth inhibition**, interference in haeme synthesis, irreversible changes in brain and nerve cells and also some of these residues are known to be carcinogenic in nature. The pulmonary and nervous systems and skins are the main target organs of arsenic contamination. Cadmium associated with kidney damage and lead considered to has been associated with learning deficits in children. Copper and zinc are essential micronutrients but in higher amount may impact metallic taste to the product resulting unacceptability of the product Like other residues mycotoxin also mutagenic, carcinogenic, teratogenic or hepatotoxic to most experimental and domestic animals and man. Aflatoxin B_1 the most important mycotoxin in view of occurrence and toxicity, is a potential hepatocarcinogen in various species of laboratory animals tested, among which are fish, birds, rodents and monkey.

References

Biswas.A.K, Kondaiah.N, Anjaneyulu.A.S.R, Mandal.P.K;(2010) Food Safety Concerns of Pesticides, Veterinary Drug Residues and Mycotoxins in Meat and Meat Products. Asian Journal of Animal Sciences, 4: 46-55.

Blackman.N.L. Meat Quality Control, 186,187

Gracy J.F., Collins D.S and Huey R.J :(2009) Meat Hygeine, Ed Tenth, 299 to 303,306,315

Javadi.A, Mirzaie.H, Khatibi.S.A. (2011) Effect of roasting, boiling and microwaving cooking methods on Enrofloxacin residues in edible tissues of broiler, 214-217

Kaushik.G., Satya, S., Naik, S.N. (2008) Food processing a tool to pesticide residue dissipation – A review, 29

Street. J.C. (1969) Vol 100, Current Views on Pesticides, 156,157

II. Effect of Processing on Veterinary Drug, Hormone and Pesticide Residues

Veterinary Residues are the very small amounts of veterinary medicines that can remain in animal products and therefore make their way into the food chain.

Hormones residues are agents which are found in meat because these are injected before slaughter for increasing market value.

Hormones specially steroidal hormones are used to increase body weight of animal

Pesticide residues are obtained in meat from feed of animal.

Pesticides having high affinity to accumulate in body fat of animals and amount of this storage in body fat varies in different species and it is proportional to concentration in diet.

Table 11.5: Pesticide Residue in Meat

Residue	*Meat*	*MRL mg/kg*
Chlorpyrifos	Meat of goats and sheep	1
	Cattle meat	1
	Poultry meat	0.01
Carbaryl	Meat (from mammals otherthan marine mammals)	0.05
	Poultry meat	0.05
Carbendazim	Cattle meat	0.05
	Poultry meat	0.05
Carbosulfan	**Meat (from mammals other**than marine mammals)	0.05
	Poultry meat	0.05
Carbofuran	Meat (from mammals otherthan marine mammals)	0.05
	Poultry meat	0.08

DDT and BHC are main organochlorides found in Indian market meat.

Table 11.6: DDT and BHC Residue in different Meats

Meat Source	*DDT*	*BHC*
PIG (Ludhiana)	0.6	0.12
CHICKEN (Ludhiana)	0.084	0.031
Sheep (Ludhiana)	0.015	0.013
GOAT (Ludhiana)	0.056	0.002
GOAT(Izatnagar)	0.390	–
BUFFALO(Izatnagar)	1.833	–
GOAT(Hyderabad)	0.150	–

Whatever may be residues in meat the amount of pesticide residues ingested by human is quite different as method of cooking or processing and use of cooking juice reduces pesticides in appreciable amount.

Change in Pesticide on Processing

- It was observed that cooking influences the level of pesticide residues in food.
- Breakdown of DDT and DDE takes place during normal processing of chicken and it was up to 90 per cent.
- Breakdown down of DDT and DDE to lindane level reduced during both methods of cooking but tissue losses DDT greater when steaming or frying is done

- ☆ Baking, frying, steaming, heating in closed container reduced the level of residues in tissues containing lindane, endrin, hepatochlor, and dieldrin.
- ☆ Lindane and hepatochlor epoxide reduced considerably during heating but amount of endrin, diendrin were not affected
- ☆ Steaming and pressure cooking reduces lindane and dieldrin
- ☆ Thermal processing at 104° decreases DDT amount
- ☆ Ham processing reduce HCB level by 42 per cent
- ☆ Food safety is an area of growing worldwide concern on account of its direct bearing on human health.
- ☆ The presence of harmful pesticide residues in food has caused a great concern among the consumers. Hence, world over to tackle food safety issues, organic farming is being propagated. However, due to several reasons, diffusion and acceptance of this approach in developing countries has been very slow.
- ☆ Therefore, it is important in the transient phase that some pragmatic solution should be developed to tackle this situation of food safety. Food processing treatments such as washing, peeling, canning or cooking lead to a significant reduction of pesticide residues.
- ☆ In this background this paper reviews the common food processing operations along with the degree of residue removal in each process.
- ☆ The processes reviewed include: baking, bread making, dairy product manufacture, drying, thermal processing, fermentation, freezing, infusion, juicing, malting, milling, parboiling, peeling, peeling and cooking, storage, storage and milling, washing, washing and cooking, washing and drying, washing and peeling, washing peeling and juicing and wine making.
- ☆ Extensive literature review demonstrates that in most cases processing leads to large reductions in residue levels in the prepared food, particularly through washing, peeling and cooking operations
- ☆ Meat processing technology comprises the steps and procedures in the **manufacture of processed meat products**.
- ☆ Processed meat products, which include various different types and local/regional variations, are food of animal origin, which contribute valuable animal proteins to human diets.
- ☆ Animal tissues, in the first place *muscle meat* and *fat*, are the main ingredients, besides occasionally used other tissues such as *internal organs, skins* and *blood* or *ingredients of plant origin*.
- ☆ Meat processing involves a wide range of physical and chemical treatment methods, normally combining a variety of methods.
- ☆ Meat processing technologies include:
- ☆ Cutting/chopping/comminuting (size reduction)
- ☆ Mixing/tumbling

- ✰ Salting/curing
- ✰ Utilization of spices/non-meat additives
- ✰ Stuffing/filling into casings or other containers
- ✰ Fermentation and drying
- ✰ Heat treatment
- ✰ Smoking
- ✰ **Effect of deep frying on furazolidone residues**
- ✰ This study investigated the effect of deep frying (210oC/15 min) on furazolidone residues in liver and muscle tissues of chicken.
- ✰ Furazolidone was administered (2 mg/kg body weight) orally to chicken daily for five days.
- ✰ The hens were then sacrificed at 1, 5, 24 168 and 264 h after treatment stopped and liver and muscle tissue samples obtained.
- ✰ The samples were deep fried, blended with distilled water and then centrifuged at 6000 rpm for five minutes
- ✰ The supernatant was analyzed for the concentration of the drug using a using the Delvotest SP microbiological assay.
- ✰ A detection limit of 11.0 g/ml was obtained with spiked liver tissues contaminated with Furazolidone.
- ✰ Furazolidone residues were detected in fried liver and muscle tissues 264 h post treatment.
- ✰ It was concluded that furazolidone drug residues in chicken liver and muscle tissues were not destroyed by deep frying.
- ✰ Effect of cooking on biologically active antibiotic residues in meat
- ✰ Five antibiotics, ampicillin, chloramphenicol, oxytetracycline, streptomycin (Streptomycin and sulphadimidine were used in the injectable forms and administered at therapeutic levels once daily on three consecutive days.
- ✰ The levels used per kilogram body weight were 7 mg/kg(ampicillin),5mg/kg(chloramphenicol),5mg/kg(oxytetracycline),2 mg/kg (streptomycin) and 14 mg/kg (sulphadimidine).
- ✰ Two bovine animals, aged 7-12 months(weight range 190-300 kg) were used perantibiotic, except in the cases of streptomycin, where only one test animal was used
- ✰ Each animal was injected intramuscularly in the neck area and within two hours after the third injection, was slaughtered.
- ✰ Each carcass was skinned, eviscerated, split into two sides and left to hang at 4 °C for 5-7 days
- ✰ After the hanging period, one sirloin roast (average weight 15-2 kg) and three steaks (average 400-500 grams each) were cut from each carcass side.
- ✰ Roasting commenced with the recommended cooker setting of 176 °C

- ☆ The results of the microbiological assays of each antibiotic were recorded in millimeters as zones of inhibition.

Table 11.7: Cooking Effect on Ampicillin Residues in Meat

Carcase Side	*Sample*	*Temperature*	*Total Cooking Time*	*Anuular Zone Reduction in Diameter*
	Streak Rare	56 and 45	10	7.8 and 4.6
Right and left	Streak medium	71 and 90	20	30 and 33
Right and left	Streak well done	90 and 92	30	81.8 and 77.2

Cooking effects on sulfonamide residues in chicken thigh muscle net change by cooking on residues of sulfadiazine (SDZ), sulfamethoxazole (SMX), sulfamonomethoxine (SMM) and sulfaquinoxaline (SQ) in chicken muscles.

- ☆ These sulfonamides (SAs) were fed to chickens at a dietary concentration of 100 mg/kg (each drug) for 7 successive days. On the 7th day of feeding, they were killed and thigh muscles were collected.
- ☆ Muscle was ground, mixed and formed into 10-g "meatballs".
- ☆ SA residues were determined by high-performance liquid chromatography. By using the usual cooking methods, boiling, roasting and microwaving, the muscles containing SAs were treated for the specified times.
- ☆ Net residues in the muscles cooked by boiling were reduced 45–61 per cent in 12 min.
- ☆ In roast cooking, the SMX, SMM and SQ residues, except for SDZ, were reduced 38–40 per cent in 12 min. No significant reduction of SDZ was found.
- ☆ By the microwave cooking, the four SAs residues were reduced 35–41 per cent in 1 min.
- ☆ Reducing half-lives of SAs in chicken muscles cooked were estimated as follows: 9.3 min for SDZ and 13.2 min for SMX, SMM and SQ in boiling; 18.3 min for SMX, SMM and SQ in roasting; 1.6 min for all the SAs in microwaving
- ☆ The aim of this study was to investigate the depletion of residues of cyadox in chicken muscle over time.
- ☆ The heat stabilities of cyadox (CYX) and its two metabolites, 1,4-bisdesoxycyadox (BDCYX) and quinoxaline-2-carboxylic acid (QCA), in water, cooking oil, and as incurred residues in chicken muscle were investigated.
- ☆ CYX was shown to be unstable with a half-life of about 37.7 min in 100 °C water.
- ☆ In hot cooking oil at 180 °C, all three compounds were unstable. CYX decreased quickly and was not able to be detected after heating for 2 min.

- Diode-array analysis of CYX standard solution in cooking oil indicated that a portion of BDCYX was formed.
- The residues of CYX and BDCYX deteriorated rapidly in frozen storage, while that of QCA changed slowly. Muscles containing CYX residues were boiled, microwaved, or fried for the specified times.
- During boiling, CYX and BDCYX were reduced 94 per cent and 81 per cent in 10 min, respectively.
- During microwave cooking, CYX and BDCYX were reduced 54 per cent and 47 per cent in 2.5 min, respectively.
- During frying, CYX and BDCYX were reduced 86 per cent and 76 per cent, respectively.
- No significant reduction of QCA was found for the three cooking methods.
- The half-lives of CYX residues in cooked chicken muscles were estimated as follows: 2.22 min for CYX and 4.44 min for BDCYX by boiling; 6.66 min for CYX and 9.36 min for BDCYX by microwaving.
- The effects of various cooking methods (boiling, baking and microwaving) on residues of malachite green (MG) and its major metabolite, leucomalachite green (LMG), in incurred carp muscles were investigated. Moreover, the stability of MG and LMG standard solutions under boiling in water and in oil was examined.
- The MG and LMG residues in cooked meat were determined by liquid chromatography with visible and fluorescence detectors.
- The results showed that in muscles cooked by boiling or baking MG concentration was reduced by 54 per cent in 15 min while LMG was stable in these conditions.
- By microwave cooking MG residues were reduced by 61 per cent after 1 min. Microwaving was the only method of cooking when a loss of LMG was observed (40 per cent in 1 min).
- Both MG and LMG standard solutions were stable in boiling water at 100 °C. In cooking oil, MG was reduced by 49 per cent after 10 min and less than 3 per cent of the original MG remains after 90 min at 150 °C.
- No losses of LMG were observed over a time period of 120 min in cooking oil at 150 °C. Upon increasing the temperature to 210 °C and holding for 120 min, MG was rapidly reduced by 97 per cent after 10 min.
- LMG under the same conditions was reduced by 18 per cent after 10 min. No further loses of MG and LMG were observed after 120 min.

Pesticide, Antibiotic and Hormone Residues in Food are Harmful

Pesticides

- There are adverse health effects of chronic exposure.

- There is substantial toxicologic evidence that repeated low-level exposure to organophosphate (OP) pesticides may affect neurodevelopment and growth in developing animals.
- For example, animal studies have reported neurobehavorial effects such as impairment on maze performance, locomotion, and balance in neonates exposed (italic)in utero(/italic) and during early postnatal life.
- Possible mechanisms for these effects include inhibition of brain acetylcholinesterase, down regulation of muscarinic receptors, decreased brain DNA synthesis, and reduced brain weight in offspring.

Hormones

- In some countries, abuses in the use of these substances have occurred and hormonal treatment has left high residues in poultry, veal and eggs which have resulted in breast enlargement, premature cessation of pubertal development and ovarian cysts in children.
- Growing scientific evidence highlights the dangers of exposing people to hormones.
- Hormone residues in meat and meat products can disrupt the natural "endocrine equilibrium" (hormone balance) which exists within everyone's body.
- Any disruption of this equilibrium can result in multiple biological effects with potentially harmful consequences for human health.
- Risks include neurobiological (endocrine) effects, developmental effects, immunotoxicity, reproductive and immunological effects, genotoxicity and carcinogenicity.

Adverse Effects of Veterinary Drug Residues

- A number of possible adverse health effects of veterinary drug residues have been suggested.
- These include the following:
  - Allergic/toxic reactions to residues.
  - Chronic toxic effects occurring with prolonged exposure to low levels of antibiotics.
  - Development of antibiotic-resistant bacteria in treated animals. These bacteria might then cause difficult-to-treat human infections.
  - Disruption of normal human flora in the intestine. The bacteria that usually live in the intestine act as a barrier to prevent incoming pathogenic bacteria from getting established and causing disease. Antibiotics might reduce total numbers of these bacteria or selectively kill some important species.

References

Camilibary K and Smith JS 1994.Effect of pH and cooking temperature as stability of organophosphate pesticide in beef muscle.J.Agric.and Food chemistry 7:826

McCracken, A. and O'Brien, J.J. (1976b). Comparison of two methods for detecting residues in slaughter animals. Research in Veterinary Science 21, 361-363.

McCracken, A., O'Brien, J.J. and Campbell, N. (1976a). Antibiotic residues and their recovery from animal tissues. Journal of Applied Bacteriology 41, 129-135.

Peric, M. and Dakic, M. (1973). Resistance of penicillin and streptomycin to exposure to heat Tehnologija Mesa 6, 162-164.

www.fao.org/docrep/meeting/005/x7616e/x7616e0n.htm

III. Pesticides, Veterinary Drugs and Mycotoxins Residues in Livestock Products

Residues in the widest sense may be defined as undesirable substances present in meat. These substances are chemical or biological in nature and have always been present in a small amount or can be introduced into the environment by various technological practices, can arise as a result of incorrect storage of food stuff, can get in to the food chain due to modern agricultural practices and thus introduced into the foods or they may be results of medicines given to the animals or of processing methods.

Surveillance/monitoring on the occurrence of residues in meat and their products were relatively a neglected area until last decade. But with the advancement of technological intervention regarding livestock rearing, disease control and intensive crop production system, the chances of residues in foods of animal origin increased tremendously. This results a potential risk of various life threatening diseases such as cancer, leukemia, reproductive disorder besides disruption of body's immune, endocrine and nervous system. The growing awareness of public perception about this reduces the confidence among the consumers and resultant adverse impact on global economy. Ideally, meat food should be completely free from such types of contaminants. This is a utopian goal considering current agricultural and technological practices. Many develop countries in the world have already been tracking this problem by fixing statutory limitations of pesticides, veterinary drug residues and microbial toxins in meat and meat products, and their enforcement through monitoring setup to ensure safe food supply to consumers. Monitoring of such types residues in food of animal origin can reveal current status of contamination, thus enabling preventive and control measures to be initiated before contamination becomes so serious or wide spread that threatens human health or causes serious economic losses.

Source of Exposure

Pesticides have unique status of all food residues because these compounds are regularly used in agricultural fields to meet worldwide food demands. It is estimated that, without pesticides, world production of food would be reduced by 30 per cent.

Despite the obvious benefits, however, occasional misuse of such chemicals has resulted in intoxication of animals and/or accumulation of residues in livestock products. Among all pesticides, organochlorine (OC) compounds such as DDT, lindane or hexachlorobenzene, heptachlor, heptachlor epoxide, aldrin/dieldrin are mostly persistent in the environment and cause major health hazard effects. Some of these compounds such as mercury, arsenic etc. also contain toxic elements which, when break down in the soil, produce the actual residues. The industrial chemicals (chlorinated hydrocarbons) such as PCB, the dioxin, or perchlorethylene (PER) play the main parts, but organometal compounds such as tetraethyl lead in fuel, benzopyrene and other substances are also important.

In contrast to pesticides, residues of veterinary medicinal products are most common in food of animal origin as are directly exposed to the animals. But this could be avoided, if use properly with sufficient withdrawal period of times. Drug residues in meat occur, when these are used via parental or oral route or as feed additives in food animals. The range of veterinary medicinal products used in regular animal husbandry practices is extremely wide, ranging from teat dips to hormones. Approximately 42 per cent of all veterinary pharmaceuticals used world-wide are used as feed additives, 19 per cent are used as anti-infectives, 13 per cent as parasiticides, 11 per cent are used as biologicals and 15 per cent represent other pharmaceuticals. All they are administered to animals either by injections (intramuscularly, intravenous, subcutaneous) or orally in the feed and water, topically on the skin, and by intra-mammary and intra-uterine infusions. Injectables were responsible for 46 per cent of the violative residues in meat followed by oral administration at 20 per cent (feed, water and bolus) and intra-mammary infusions at 7 per cent. Several other factors have contributed to the residues problem such as poor treatment records or failure to identity the animals and result from the use of a drug in same manner that is inconsistent with the labeling. This occurs primarily through not observing label of withdrawal times as well as "extra-label" use of drug.

The microbial residues mostly mycotoxins, metabolites of toxigenic molds (fungi) are present in feedstuffs. During the course of evolution organisms have accustomed themselves to certain toxic contents in foods. However the direct consumption of mycotoxin-contaminated cereal grains is much more probable than exposure to residues in food of animal origin because livestock and poultry have the ability to dilute or detoxify these chemicals.

Detection of Residues

Pesticides

Conventional Methods

A number of analytical techniques such as colorimetric method, thin layer chromatography (TLC), high performance- thin layer chromatography (HP-TLC), gas liquid chromatography (GLC), gas chromatography- mass spectrometry (GC-MS), high performance liquid chromatography (HPLC), liquid chromatography-mass spectrometry-mass photometry (LC-MS-MS) etc are established for detection and quantification of pesticide residues in animal tissues. However, colorimetric and

TLC method are limited only for qualitative determination due to its low sensitivity. GLC or GC-MS though normally used for determination of non-volatile compounds (organochlorine and organophophorus pesticides), but can also effectively utilizing for determination of thermo-labile compounds such as synthetic pyrethroid and *N*-methyl carbamate pesticides.

Modern Methods

Although conventional techniques such HPLC/MS and GC/MS gives satisfactory analytical results for pesticide determination, new assays and sensors for cheaper and faster on-site analysis are being developed. Enzymatic sensors, based on the inhibition of a selected enzyme, are the most extended biosensors used for the determination of these compounds. Biosensors based on enzyme inhibition although sensitive, are not selective and cannot, therefore, be used for quantification of either an individual or a class of pesticides.

Veterinary Drugs

Conventional Methods

For determination of veterinary drug residues in foods, currently six types of detection methods are commonly used. These include microbial growth inhibition assays, microbial receptor assays, enzymatic colorimetric assays, receptor binding assays, chromatographic methods and immunoassays. But microbial growth inhibition assays and later two methods are popular for monitoring of antimicrobial residues in meat and meat products as are capable of detecting a broad range of these drugs. Researchers also evaluated a number of common bacterial inhibition test for screening antimicrobial drug residues in tissues. They found that screening for tetracycline was excellent with German three-plate test, the European Union four-plate test and new Dutch kidney test in stead of swab test on premises (STOP), calf antibiotic and sulfa test (CAST) and the fast antibiotic screen test (FAST).

Modern Methods

Most of the biosensors developed are aimed at determining them in biological or food samples. The Surface Plasmon Resonance (SPR) technique has been developed and demonstrated for on-line/at-line detection of veterinary drug residues in milk, porcine bile and bovine urine, including a commercial handling robot. This sensor operates in real time and it may detect up to 8 different veterinary drugs simultaneously with a throughput of up to 600 samples per day.

Mycotoxins

Conventional and Modern Methods

TLC and HP-TLC is regularly using for determination of micotoxins in foods. However, a great number of specific sensors for bacterial toxins and mycotoxins have been developed for food and environmental control. Thus, an integrated optical sensor has been reported for the analysis of aflatoxin B in corn. A light-addressable potentiometric immunosensor based on the commercial device for the analysis of saxitoxin and ricin has also been described. An impedance- based immunosensor has been prepared by using an ultrathin platinum film with an immobilized layer of antibodies against the staphylococcal enterotoxin B. A rapid and sensitive immunosensor for the detection of the Clostridium botulinum toxin A has also been developed. This fiber optic-based biosensor utilizes the evanescent wave of a tapered optical fiber where antibodies antitoxin A has been covalently immobilized at the distal end. The toxin could be detected by means of a rhodamine label, within a minute at concentrations as low as 5 ng/ml.

Residues and Health Risk

Among all residues, pesticides receiving most interest worldwide in recent year. Though violative level of pesticides are relatively uncommon, a low violation rate even remain an important public health consideration because of their wide spread use in meat and poultry production, their persistence in environment, and varying toxicity. The United Nations has estimated that about 2 million poisoning and 10,000 deaths occur each year from pesticides, with about three-fourth of this occurring in developing countries. The acute and malicious consumption involving higher dose results in death whereas, chronic insidious intake lead to elevated cancer risk and disruption of body's reproductive, immune, endocrine, and nervous system.

The carcinogenicity of organochlorine (OC) pesticides has been studied in a number of laboratory animals including non-human primates. Lifetime or limited period of time treatment of mice with DDT induced liver tumors including malignant metastasizing hepatoblastomas. DDT also increased incidences lung tumors, and lymphoma in mice, liver tumors in rats and adrenal adenomas in hamster. However DDT did not induce DNA damage in bacteria or cultured rodent and human cells. It induced chromosomal aberration in mouse but not in rat bone marrow cells. DDT and its metabolites inhibited gap-junctional intracellular communication.

Other areas of concerns are childhood brain cancer and cancers of nervous system. Studies suggest an increase in risk in brain cancer, leukemia, Wilm's tumors, Ewing's sarcoma and germ cell tumors associated with paternal occupational exposure to pesticides prior to and during pregnancy. However, maternal occupational exposure during pregnancy was less frequent but was also associated leukemia, Wilm's tumors and germ cell tumors.

In contrast to pesticides, exposure from veterinary drug residues rather most common as are directly injected or fed to the animals. The over use of antimicrobials such as tetracyclines, sulfonamides, amino glycosides, β-lactam derivatives etc. in animal production or their residues in food system pose potential allergic reactions in sensitized individuals, but sub therapeutic and therapeutic levels may perturb human gut micro flora. The tetracyclines are incompletely absorbed from the gastrointestinal tract; they reach readily high concentrations in the intestine, producing perturbations of the intestinal microflora within 48 hours of daily treatment. Experience with tetracyclines in human medicine indicates that therapeutic levels of tetracyclines can perturb the intestinal microflora by inducing emergence of resistant strains and altering the metabolic activity of the microflora, its resistance to colonization by pathogenic, opportunistic or resistant microorganism barrier effect and its ecological balance, without any identified deleterious effect.

Immunodepression and phototoxicity may also occur in animals and human beings besides superinfections related to tetracyclines. However, sulfonamides can induce thyroid, adenoma and hyperplasia in laboratory animals. It has also potential carcinogenic character. To reduce bacteria resistance to sulfonamides to get synergistic effect, pyrimethamines such as trimethoprim and oriprim are used in combination.

The National Research Council and Institute of Medicine have noted a link between the use of antibiotics in food animals and the development of bacterial resistance to these drugs causing human diseases. Similarly, scientist at Center for Disease Control and Prevention (CDC) began tracking a new type of *Salmonella* called Newport 9+ which is resistant nine antibiotics including ceftriaxone, one of the few drugs that killed most bacteria and the drug of choice for children whose *Salmonella* enter the blood steam. Nonetheless, toxicity of these antimicrobial chemicals includes aplasia of bone marrow, the emergence of resistant bacteria within animals and the transfer of antibiotic resistance gene to human pathogens. The appearance of resistance among pathogenic organisms such as *Salmonella* DT-104 and *Campylobacter* is more concern. *E. coli* is an opportunist pathogen capable of infecting people via the food chain and causing enteric infections in young children and travellers as well as range of other infections. Enteric infections with *Salmonella, E. coli* or *Campylobacter* rarely warrant antibiotic treatment and so one might argue that the problem is not nearly as important as methicillin resistant *Staphylococcus aureus* (MRSA) or other major human resistance problems. However, treatment failure has been reported and the livestock industries can not ignore the problem. Enterococci have only been thought of as food borne organisms since discovery of vancomycin resistant enterococci (VRE) in pigs and poultry and there is some dispute that their spread occurs from animals to people.

Similarly, uses of hormonal compound like DES in meat production known to have strong carcinogenic effects and are banned from use for food producing animals. One the other hand, beta-adrenergic agonist (clenbuterol, salbuterol, cimeterol) act through binding to receptor on target cells and act by repartitioning energy from fat to lean meat production. This compound in excessive amount leaves residues in meat and thereby adverse reaction in consumers requiring hospital treatment. Thus, health risks of veterinary medicinal products and their metabolites are very difficult to define and their presence of above the violative level is illegal and subject to financial penalties in many countries.

The health implications from heavy metals lead to kidney damage, cardiovascular diseases, induction of hypertension, growth inhibition, interference in heamsynthesis, irreversible changes in brain and nerve cells and also some of these residues are known to be carcinogenic in nature. The pulmonary and nervous systems and skins are the main target organs of arsenic contamination. Cadmium associated with kidney damage and lead considered to has been associated with learning deficits in children. Copper and zinc are essential micronutrients but in higher amount may impact metallic taste to the product resulting unacceptability of the product.

Like other residues mycotoxin also mutagenic, carcinogenic, teratogenic or hepatotoxic to most experimental and domestic animals and man. Aflatoxin B_1 the most important mycotoxin in view of occurrence and toxicity, is a potential hepatocarcinogen in various species of laboratory animals tested, among which are fish, birds, rodents and monkey.

Regulation

In 1979, a US General Accounting Office (GAO) report identified 143 drugs and pesticides as likely to leave residues in raw meat and poultry. Of these, 42 are known to cause or are suspected to causing cancer, 20 are suspected teratogens, and 6 are suspected mutagens. In the ensuing 24 years these numbers have probably risen.

The regulation of residues handled by each country throughout the world has a tendency towards uniform approach. But much greater enforcement has been seen with the passage of WTO and Sanitary and Phytosanitary measures. In the United States, pesticide use is regulated under FIFRA (US, Federal Insecticide, Fungicide and Rodenticide Act) on the basis of risk-benefit standard. This balancing takes into account "the economic, social and environmental cost as well as potential benefits of the use of any pesticide in relation to its efficacy, inherent toxicity to mammals, wild-life and plants". A given pesticide may have many different uses, but required individual approval by the U.S. Environmental Protection Agency (EPA) under FIFRA. In fact, in the United States, pesticide regulation is under auspices of three government agencies, the Environmental Protection Agency (EPA), the Food and Drug Administration and the United States Department of Agriculture-Food Safety Inspection Services (USDA-FSIS). The FDA and USDA-FSIS are responsible for monitoring pesticide residues in foods based on level set by the EPA. The FSIS is responsible for meat and poultry products and FDA covers all other types of raw commodities and processed food products. However, regulation of pesticides in European Union is done on the basis of their toxicological properties. The council directive of the European Economic Community 91/414/EEC specified criteria for plant protection products in relation to acceptable daily intake (ADI) for man, acceptable operator exposure level (AOEL), acute reference dose, and maximum admissible concentration in water (Anadon *et al.,* 2001). The international organizations such as Codex Alimentarius Commission (CAC) have also set their standards using the term maximum residue limits (MRLs) and acceptable daily intake (ADI) levels of various pesticide residues in meat and meat products.

In contrast to pesticides, the USDA-FSIS and the FDA are responsible for monitoring meat and poultry products for animal drug residues. The USDA-FSIS conducts the National Residue Programme (NRP) to prevent animals containing violative amounts of drug residues from market samples through extensive on-site sampling technique (FSIS-USDA, 1998). The samples are also sent to FSIS field laboratories for further testing. The FDA Center for Veterinary Medicine (CVM) is responsible for approving new animal drugs, setting tolerances, and enforcement action depends on results of FSIS findings. Other international organizations include the European Agency for the evaluation of medicinal products (EMEA), Office International des Epizootics (OIE) and Consultation Mondiale de I' Industrie de la

Sante Animale (COMISA). Many countries have specialist groups involved such as FDA in USA, the Bureau of Veterinary Drugs in Canada and the Veterinary Products Committee of Ministry of Agriculture, Fisheries and Foods in the United Kingdom.

In India, regulations of residues are governed under different Acts/Rules, that is, Insecticides Acts, 1968; Environmental (Protection) Act, 1986; Hazardous (Management and Handling) Rules, 1989; Water (Prevention and Control of Pollution) Act, 1974; Air (Prevention and Control of Pollution) Act, 1981; Prevention of Food Adulteration Acts, 1954; The Factories acts, 1948; Bureau of Indian Standards Act, 1986; Drug and Cosmetic Act, 1940. The Ministry of Agriculture (GOI) regulates the manufacture, sale, import, export and use of pesticides through the Insecticides Act. Central Insecticides Boards (CIB) constituted under the section IV of the Act advises central and state governments on technical matters. The registration committee (RC) constituted under section V of the Act approves the use of pesticides and new formulations to control the pest problem associated with various crops or ectoparasiticides measure onto the animals. The monitoring of residue level in food comes under the purview of Ministry of Health and Family Welfare (GOI). The Central Committee on Food Standards (CCFS), a statutory committee under the PFA Act, 1954, Ministry of Health and Family Welfare, is responsible for laying down standards for various food items. The essential parameters required for dietary exposure assessment at the national/international level are (a) food consumption data (b) food chemical data (c) methods for estimating dietary exposure, (d) priority setting function of dietary exposure methods and (e) extent of over estimation, uncertainty and variability.

Statutory Limits/Risk Assessment of Residues

International Organization such as Codex Alimentarius Commission have taken initiation of harmonization of chemical residues in food through establishment of statutory limitations *viz.* maximum residue limits (MRLs), acceptable daily intake (ADI) levels, acute reference dose (ARfD), No Observed Adverse Effect Levels (NOAEL) etc. However all these statutory limitations are important principals for risk assessment of residues in foods. For statutory limits of residues, the terms tolerances or maximum residue limits (MRLs) are frequently used by regulatory agencies. But both the term tolerances and MRLs are synonymous, former is used in United States other countries, while later is used in Canada and the European Union. The term MRL may be defined as the maximum concentration of marker residue (*e.g.* parent compound, metabolites etc.), expressed in parts per million (ppm) or parts per billion (ppb) on fresh weight basis, that is legally permitted or recognized as acceptable in or on food. The MRLs are established on the basis of package of toxicology and residue data and these are referred to as safety file and the residue file. The toxicology data are used not only to characterize the biological properties of the molecules, but also to identify a suitable 'no observed effect levels' (NOELs), which in turn is used to calculate an acceptable daily intake (ADI), the quantity, which if consumed over a human lifetime will have no adverse effect on consumer health. This in turns expressed on a body weight basis and can be considered the safety standard for that compound. The MRL is then elaborated from this ADI along with knowledge of the depletion kinetics of the residues in the animal or its meat and with reference to standard intake values for particular types of food. The identification of NOELs, the calculation of ADI values and the establishment of MRLs is a complex scientific process involving toxicology, pharmacology, microbiology, residue kinetics and analytical chemistry but the MRL is established at a magnitude which ensures that the ADI will not be exceeded by the consumer when eating food of animal origin. Another term total residue levels (TRL) refers to the safe concentration of total residues that corresponds to the MRL.

The term acceptable operator exposure level (AOEL) and acute reference dose (ARfD) also practiced most commonly by European Union. The AOEL is defined as the maximum amount of active substance to which the operator may be exposed without any adverse health effect and is based on the highest level at which no adverse effect is observed in tests in the most sensitive relevance animal species. The AOEL is expressed as mg of chemical/kg body weight of the operator. On the other hand, the ARFD of a chemical is an estimate of the amount of substance in food or drinking water, expressed on the body weight basis, that can be ingested over a short period of time, usually during 1 meal or 1 day, without appreciable health risk to the consumer, based on all the known fact at the time of evaluation. This calculated reference dose is compared to an estimate or measurement of exposure in the risk assessment process.

IV. Pesticides and Veterinary Drug Residues in Food of Animal Origin and their Impact on Human Health

The indiscriminate use of toxic chemicals poses a considerable risk to human health due to the presence of the residues in foods and resultantly wide spread contamination of the environment. The degradation of the life-saving components *viz.* air, water and land is making a constant threat to the very existence of life on the earth. Pesticides, drug residues, Heavy and toxic metals are pivotal amongst these contaminants, because of their toxicity, long half life, accumulation in nature and circular course in biosphere. These compounds are not biodegradable and tend to persist for years in the environment and move to other parts of the environment. Most of pesticides, can accumulate in the environment and cause damage to ecosystems and human health. A consistent and effective strategy needs to be derived to reduce these impacts and long-term effects on the environmental components.

Residues are defined as substance that remain in food along with degradation products, derivatives, metabolites, other toxicological contaminants arising from the use of pesticides, drug and hormonal preparations, antibiotics and industrial chemicals. The increase in productivity in animal husbandry often involves the use of chemicals that are physiologically, pharmacologically and toxicologically very potent. When animals are exposed to these chemicals these may leave residues in the animal food products.

Pesticide Residues

Pesticide word means a substance which is used to kill pests and it may be defined as any substance employed for preventing, attracting, repelling or controlling any pest during the production, storage, transport, distribution and processing of food, agricultural commodities or animal feeds or which may be administered to animals for control of ectoparasites. The presence of pesticides in the environment *viz.*, soil, air, water, plant, animal and human tissues etc. has been demonstrated world over. The pesticide spreads into the environment and has detrimental effect on human health through the contamination of soil, air and water resources. This has resulted in situations posing health risks to humans and the other forms of life and can easily be used as trade barrier in WTO regime.

Pesticide residues mean any specified substances in food, agricultural commodities, or animal feed resulting from use of pesticides. The term includes any derivatives of pesticides such as conversion products, metabolites, reaction products and impurities considered being of toxicological significance (Codex Alimentarius Commission 1993).

The organochlorine pesticides like DDT, HCH, chlordane, heptachlor, endosulfan, aldrin, dieldrin and endrin etc are very lipophilic in nature, are not readily excreted by animals except milk, which makes OCl highly persistent and bio accumulative. The organophosphates and carbamates are comparatively less soluble, degradable and excreted in urine, faeces, and breathe of animals, so they are less persistent but exhibit higher acute toxicity. Due to lipophillic nature of OCI these tends to accumulate in the fatty tissues. When these are consumed by the organisms of higher tropic level of food chain, the pesticides show a trend of bio accumulation and biomagnification *i.e.* animals that are at the top of food chain in an ecosystem tend to accumulate higher residues of pesticides than animals/plants, which are at the lower tropic levels. Through their persistence and lipophilicity, the pesticides and their residues may concentrate in the adipose tissues and in the blood serum of animals leading to environmental persistence, bioconcentration and biomagnification through the food chain.

Animal feed containing pesticides is the main source for accumulation of these residues in tissues of animals, although inhalation of polluted air and absorption through intact skin also may take place. Organochlorine pesticides are lipophillic in nature, so after ingestion through contaminated feed and fodder, they accumulate in fat and usually do not get converted to the water-soluble metabolites inside the animal body. As their concentration exceeds a certain threshold level, pesticides are translocated to mammary glands and are secreted in milk as residues.

The levels of residues vary in different species of food animals and are proportional to the concentration of pesticides in their diet. The occurrence of pesticides or residues in edible food is a risk that has been main focus of public concern. On comparison of pesticide residues detected in food in India and world it was surprising to see that only 2.5 per cent of food commodities in India are free of pesticide residues as compared to 80 per cent at world level. The indiscriminate use of pesticides poses considerable risk due to presence of the residues in agricultural and animal husbandry practices. Therefore, the awareness and need for regular screening of various animal products such as milk and meat is imperative in the interest of trade and consumers society.

Human Health Hazards of Pesticides Residues

The persistent misuse and abuse of pesticides reflects poorly on their occupational and safety standards, regulation and enforcement and knowledge of the hazards. This has resulted in situations posing health risks to humans and the other forms of life and can easily be used as trade barrier in WTO regime. The World Health Organization estimates that 20,000 women, men and children die of accidental pesticide poisonings each year; three million are non-fatally poisoned and nearly three-fourths of a million new people each year experience chronic effects from exposure.

In chronic poisoning the person is repeatedly exposed to toxic agents over a long period, but only a low dose enters the body each time. Normally, no symptoms develop in relation to each exposure. Instead, victims gradually become ill over a period of months or years. This occurs when the toxic substance either accumulates in body tissues or causes minor irreversible damage at each exposure. After a long time, enough poison has been accumulated in the body to cause clinical symptoms. Chronic effects of long-term pesticide exposure include: impaired memory and concentration, disorientation, severe depressions, irritability, confusion, headache, speech difficulties, delayed reaction times, nightmares, sleepwalking, drowsiness and insomnia. Animal experiments indicate that exposure to cholinesterase-inhibiting chemicals can induce damage to the liver, kidneys and brain. Whether affecting adults or children, consequences of chronic pesticide exposure may only appear later in life, or even in the next generation, and include learning difficulties, behavioral and reproductive defects *e.g.* accelerated puberty, infertility, and increased susceptibility to cancer. Other long-term effects are teratogenic and mutagenic

Pesticide residues have been reported to cause cancer, epilepsy, liver and kidney dysfunctions, somatic growth, depression, neuritis and testicular cancer. OCI like DDT and PCB have been responsible for breast cancer and decreased fertility in human beings. DDT and HCH are widely recognized as neurotoxic substances affecting the peripheral and central nervous system, respectively and causing hyper excitability of nerves and muscles. The inductive and stimulating effects of OCP such as DDT and dieldrin on mixed function oxidase and cytochrome P 450 has been connected with the formation of free radicals which cause damage to DNA. ppDDE a metabolite of DDT was found in brain samples from persons affected by neurological disorders. In leukemia or lymphoma patient's concentration of OCP in bone marrow were found to be high as compared to normal cases. The extensive and annual birth defects in children in the USA exposed in utero to chlorpyriphos, included defects of brain, eyes, ears, palate, teeth, heart, feet nipples and genitalia have been reported. Organophosphorus pesticides cause a significant increase in sister chromatid exchanges in mammalian cell lines. The chemicals such as DDT, PCBs, HCH and HCB as well as some other inducers of drug metabolizing enzymes are also known as promoters in experimental hepatocarcinogenesis.

The indiscriminate use of pesticides poses a considerable risk due to presence of the residues in agricultural and animal husbandry practices, therefore the awareness and need for regular screening of various animal products such as milk and meat is imperative in the interest of trade and consumers society. Though Govt. has imposed ban or restricted the use of various pesticides, a rigorous monitoring system on animal food products has to be introduced in India, so that dairy industry could be effectively involved to produce residue free food for consumers and export

Veterinary Drug Residues

The concern over the presence of veterinary drug residues in food has been increasing world wide. The presence of these Veterinary Drug Residues in food has become an issue of intense international concern and debate in recent years. Consumer's awareness through media has expressed desire of a consumer for a residue free animal product supply.

It is not possible to give an unequivocal assurance that the use of antibiotics, hormones and other veterinary drugs as NSAID, antiparasitic drugs etc. in food production will not result in residues that may be hazardous for some individuals. If the directions for the 'safe' use these substances are not followed (for example, if too much is used or it is applied at the wrong time) then there is the potential for hazardous residues to enter the food chain. Just as some people may be sensitive to particular foods, food ingredients or food additives, some may be sensitive to residues of these drugs in food.

Antibiotic Residues

The widespread use of antibiotics has contributed to the control of diseases and nutritional well being of livestock. Antibiotics have been used by dairyman and veterinarians in dairy cattle management for over more than five decades. Antimicrobials administrated through various routes especially intra mammary infusions; deliver high concentrations of antibiotics directly into the mammary gland. The contamination of otherwise usable milk by left over antibiotic is a frequent sequel to disease treatment in milk producing animals. Antimicrobials are also commonly used to improve performance and growth promoters as feed additives especially in the poultry industry. Residues in foods of animal origin are a priority for the milk and meat industry because higher standards of food safety assurance are being required by our society. Antibiotics are neither inactivated during pasteurization, boiling, sterilization, nor destroyed during cooling, chilling and freezing which further increases the importance of this problem. Momentary heating of the milk to 80°C likewise does not affect the biological activity of tetracyclines, chloramphenicol, or streptomycin. So the indiscriminate use of antibiotics (Extra label usage, Failure to observe withholding times, overuse in agricultural production) poses a serious threat to human health. The presence of antibiotics in milk in even minute quantities has created problems in dairy industry.

Impact of Antibiotic Residues on Dairy Industry

1. Inadequate curdling of milk, improper ripening of cheeses during their manufacture.
2. Decreased acid and flavour production during the manufacture of butter milk and similar products.

3. Diminished starter culture growth when propagated in reconstituted skim milk.
4. Affecting validity of certain quality control tests.
5. These can result in inferior products that must be discarded.

The persistence of residues in milk, poultry meat and eggs should be avoided because of many distinct concerns.

1. Residues are illegal.
2. The milk/meat are from treated animals and may contain large numbers of potential pathogens.
3. There may be biologically active metabolites of drugs.
4. Antibiotic residues may cause allergic reactions *e.g.* penicillin, streptomycin, tetracycline, novobiocin.
5. Emergence of bacterial resistance to daily intake of antibiotic residues through milk is another observed risk to human health causing treatment failure, protracted therapeutic regime, and treatment cost escalation, etc.
6. Certain antibiotics like chloramphenicol are known to cause aplastic anaemia over long term use which can lead to death.
7. Tetracycline group of antibiotics reportedly cause staining of denture (especially in children of 7 – 8 years) as they combine with calcium and are deposited in the bones and teeth.
8. Photosensitization and decreased immune response are other major impacts of antibiotic residues on human health.

The Food and Drug Administration (FDA) considers antibiotic contaminated milk as adulterated. In order to safeguard human health, the World Health Organization (WHO) and the Food Agriculture Organization have set standards for acceptable daily intake and maximum residue limits in foods.

Discarding contaminated milk represents a considerable economic loss in itself. Failure to discard such milk may lead to severe penalties if antibiotic is detected in the supply submitted for sale. In addition, legislative requirements are becoming more exacting both in terms of the range of substances covered and the lower residue levels to which test systems must measure.

Hormones

Hormones can be used to accelerate the growth rate of animals so that they can reach market earlier. The most effective growth promoters are natural sex hormones or substances which imitate the action of the natural hormones. If hormones are used appropriately, the residues in food should be very low or undetectable and not result in a significant hormonal effect. In some countries, abuses in the use of these substances have occurred and hormonal treatment has left high residues in poultry, veal and eggs which have resulted in breast enlargement, premature cessation of pubertal development and ovarian cysts in children. In view of these potential health hazards it is important that foods are monitored for hormone use and residue levels.

Hormone implants containing estradiol benzoate/progesterone were first approved in and 1956 by the U.S. Food and Drug Administration (FDA) for increasing growth, feed efficiency, carcass leanness of cattle. Later, other implants containing testosterone, zeranol, trenbolone acetate, and combinations of these hormones were developed and approved for use in cattle by the FDA. Currently, five hormones (progesterone, testosterone, estradiol-17, zeranol, and trenbolone acetate) are approved for implants in cattle in the U.S.A. But these implants have been officially prohibited in Europe since 1989. Hormone implants are widely used in the U.S.A., Australia, and Canada.

While a variety of hormones are produced by our bodies and are essential for normal development of healthy tissues, synthetic steroid hormones used as pharmaceutical drugs, have been found to affect cancer risk. For example, diethylstilbestrol (DES), a synthetic estrogen drug used in the 1960s was withdrawn from use after it was found to increase the risk of vaginal cancer in daughters of treated women. Lifetime exposure to natural steroid hormone estrogen is also associated with an increased risk for breast cancer. Hence, consumers are concerned about whether they are being exposed to hormones used to treat animals, and whether these hormones affect human health.

The levels of naturally produced hormones vary from animal to animal, and a range in these levels is known to be normal. Because it is not possible to differentiate between the hormones produced naturally by the animal and those used to treat the animal, it is difficult to determine exactly how much of the hormone used for treatment remains in the meat or the milk. Studies indicate that if correct treatment and slaughter procedures are followed, the levels of these hormones may be slightly higher in the treated animal's meat or milk, but are still within the normal range of natural variation known to occur in untreated animals. Scientists are currently trying to develop better methods to measure steroid hormone residues left in edible meat from a treated animal.

There is a concern about milk-related allergies. Digested or broken down fragments of proteins absorbed through the stomach can cause the immune system to produce antibodies, which sometimes can lead to milk-related allergies.

There is also a concern that because of increased milking, hormone-treated cows may become more prone to infection of the udders, called mastitis. This could lead to more antibiotics being used to treat the cows, in turn leading to more residues of antibiotics to remain in the milk. Frequent exposure to antibiotic residues through milk or dairy products is a health concern for people over the long term. Some increase in incidence of antibiotic residues was observed in cow's milk following the use of rbGH. An Expert Committee at FDA's Center for Veterinary Medicine has obseved that rbGH use may cause a slight increase in mastitis, dairy management practices that are currently in use should prevent any increase in antibiotic residues in milk.

NSAID Residues

Despite widely used differing chemical structures, most NSAID (Non-steroidal anti-inflammatory drugs) share three basic properties: they are anti inflammatory, antipyretic and analgesic. Studies indicate that NSAID do not accumulate in high concentrations in tissues in food producing animals. Milk concentrations are specially low, being limited to both plasma protein binding and pH of milk, which is more acidic than plasma. Tissue concentration of most NSAID is lower than plasma level except phenylbutazone and its metabolite oxyphenbutazone. FDA has prohibited extra label use of phenylbutazone animal and human drugs in female dairy cattle, 20 months of age or older from May 29, 2005. With this action the use of any phenylbutazone in adult dairy cow becomes violation of Food Drug and Cosmetic Act and one of FDA'S highest regulatory priorities.

— Part II —

Poultry and Fish Technology

– Chapter 12 –

History and Development of Poultry Meat and Egg Processing Industry

Introduction

The value output in livestock sector (1999-2000) in India is Rs 130234 crores which is 32.11 per cent of the value output of total agriculture *i.e.* Rs 405576 crores. The gross domestic product (GDP) from livestock is 5.5 per cent and GDP (Agriculture) is 24.85 per cent of the total GDP of the country. The share of livestock products in terms of percentage of agriculture sector has increased form 22.9 per cent to 35.95 per cent and percentage of GDP increased from 8.66 per cent to 9.33 per cent during the previous years (1980-81 to 1994-95).On the other hand the plan investment in Animal Husbandry sector is only 5 per cent of agriculture though the livestock products share of GDP is increasing year by year. Poultry Industry is an agro-based farming activity and contributes Rs 11,000 crores to the national GDP. The lower investment in the animal husbandry sector by the government in spite of the significant contribution speaks of the political negligence to the livestock sector.

Poultry production has increased rapidly all over the world including India in recent years. The main reasons include economical price, health conscious diets, and availability of variety products and successful scientific adoption of poultry enterprise. In India poultry has made better progress than any other livestock species mainly due to the entrepreneurship of poultry farmers. Beside, poultry is the most efficient converter of grain and by-products into meat with added advantages of high reproductive rate, short generation interval and quick turn over of the input costs leading to a lower cost of meat per unit weight to other species.

Poultry meat is considered as white meat and has many unique properties. It is preferred to red meat, it has more nutrients per unit number of calories, excellent flavour, easy to digest, lower fat content, high ratio of unsaturated fatty acids to saturated fatty acids excellent source of protein, fair source of vitamins and minerals, more tender so require less cooking and retain more nutrients, better functional properties (WHC, SSP, Fat retention in product), preferred in convalescent diets and assumed to have curative power (*e.g.* chicken soup). So there is need to know the present status, challenges and strategies for promotion of poultry processing industry in India for sustainable poultry farming.

Present Status of Poultry Processing Industry

The domestic poultry market size is estimated at more than Rs. 47,000 crore and the growth trend is likely to continue for the present decade as demand has been growing steadily on back of favourable socio economic factors like healthy GDP growth, rising purchasing power, changing food habits, and increasing urbanization.

The poultry sector in India has undergone major shift in structure and operation during last two decades transforming from a mere backyard activity into a major commercial activity with presence of large integrated players with successful implementation of contract poultry farming on a large scale. This transformation involved sizeable investments in breeding, hatching, rearing and processing activities.

Farmers in India have moved from rearing country birds in the past to rearing hybrids such as is Hyaline, Shaver, Babcock, Ross, etc which ensure faster growth of chicks, low mortality rates, excellent feed conversion and sustainable profits to the poultry farmers. The industry has been supported by indigenous advancements in genetic capabilities, veterinary health, poultry feed, poultry equipment, and poultry processing sectors. India also leads in producing specialized products like Specific Pathogen Free (SPF) eggs in Asia, which act as key inputs for manufacturing poultry vaccines and health products.

Indian poultry sector has been growing at around 8-10 per cent annually over the last decade and at more than 15 per cent in last three years. The production capacity has responded with increased integration and increased penetration of contract poultry farming.

ICRA's assessment based on industry feedback indicates that the domestic broiler meat demand is expected to grow at around 15-18 per cent while table egg demand is expected to grow at 5-7 per cent over medium to long term.

There have been concerted efforts in recent years from large integrators as well as Government bodies to promote increased processing of poultry products (in form of frozen/chilled chicken) and at the same time increasing acceptability of dressed chicken in domestic market. The processed chicken market is expected to grow at a much stronger pace of more than 25 per cent albeit on a low base. Transition from a predominantly live bird/wet market to a chilled/frozen market is crucial for the future expansion of domestic poultry industry as well as to increase presence in international trade.

India ranks 5th in the egg and 15th in the broiler production in the world and has 2.5 per cent of world poultry population. India produces about 41 billion eggs and 1000 million commercial broilers with growth rate of 10 per cent and 20 per cent respectively. The share of fowls in total egg production of India is 95.12 per cent (28.18 per cent desi fowls +66.93 per cent improved fowls) while the share of ducks is only 4.88 per cent (4.43 per cent desi ducks + 0.45 per cent improved ducks). There are more than 1 lakh layer farms and more than 75,000 broiler farms with flock size of 5000 to 30,000. According to 2001 figures, poultry meat production was 0.6 million tonnes per annum It constitutes 12 per cent of total meat (4.92 million tones) production in India. Human population is expected to double in Asia and Africa by 2020. So there is a vast scope of production of poultry meat and eggs in our country. The poultry industry yields approximately 3 MMT of manure, the organic fertilizer. The market share of poultry meat has gone up from 4 per cent to 13 per cent in the last two decades.80 per cent of chicken is sold as live birds,15 per cent dressed in small processing units and only 5 per cent in modern mechanized processing plants. At present there are 38 semi-automatic/fully automatic chicken processing plants and 7 egg powder plants which are of export oriented with capacity of 5 millions eggs per day. Most of the processing plants are operated under the installed capacity.The birds are sold alive mostly on the roadside, unregistered/unlicensed meat shops and dressed in front of the consumers by unskilled and untrained persons, unhygienically without caring for the meat quality. It is difficult to see the inhuman seen of handling these birds during slaughtering. Such activities inhibit many persons to consume meat. Out of the dressed chicken product 75 per cent is sold as hot dressed, chilled or frozen carcasses and remaining 25 per cent as cut up deboned and value added products. The per capita per annum availability of poultry meat is little more than 800gm and for egg is 40 numbers against the recommended (NIN) level of 1kg meat and 180 eggs per annum per person, respectively.

Indian Poultry Meat Sector: Existing Situation

In the year 2011, India has produced 2.2 million tons of poultry meat which is 2.44 per cent of the total poultry meat (Table 12.1) produced around the World (90 MT). About 0.57 MT of poultry meat worth 494 crore has been exported from India in the year 2012 13 (APEDA, 2013). As much as 8085 per cent of eggs and chicken produced in the country are estimated to be from the organized sector. The organized sector includes contract farming and independent farming. In India 70 per cent of production is from contract farming. In India, typically broilers are marketed at the weight of 1.8 to 2.2 kg in different parts of the country. This weight is generally achieved in 3540 days. With rise in feed prices, the feed efficiency has become the most important trait for the customers. The broiler diets typically used in India would have energy levels of about 3000 Kcal with about 2022 per cent protein, depending on the prices of the ingredients.

When it comes to breeding, feeding and management, the poultry Industry in India is very well organized with strong backward integration. However, processing and further processing of poultry is still struggling to catch up with modern production practices. With vast majority of chickens marketed live, the shift from wet market to centralized processing plants inline with developed countries is not happening. Birds are sold on live weight basis and freshly dressed at the shop. Consumers in India chose birds on birds appearance and meat yield is just a perception. However, in processing sector where chicken is sold to Institutions and quick service restaurants, meat yield is important. But almost 96 per cent of broilers produced in India are sold live and fresh dressed as whole. About 2 per cent is sold as frozen either as whole chicken or as cutup parts. Another 2 per cent is further processed as deboned meat for quick service restaurants.

Table 12.1: Meat Production (million tonnes) in India and World in 2011

Species	*India*	*World*	*Proportion (per cent)*	*Ranking in the World*
Buffalo meat	1.50	3.50	42.85	I
Goat meat	0.60	5.22	11.49	III
Chicken	2.20	90.00	2.44	IX
Beef	1.08	63.03	1.71	
Mutton	0.29	8.17	3.54	
Pork	0.33	108.64	0.30	

Evolution of Poultry Industry in India

In 1980's chicken was known as country chicken with limited availability and consumption only among the rich population. Gradually, organized poultry came in, prices became affordable, and the availability went up. This increased the availability of chicken at retail shops in Metro cities, District and Taluk places. But still for major chunk of population living in villages, the availability of chicken is nil. These villagers have to depend on backyard or desi birds grown locally and have to pay higher prices and thus limit the consumption. Almost onethird of the Indian population either does not have access to, or cannot afford to buy chicken. Another onethird of the population is vegetarian and the rest of onethird population consumes chicken during festivals or as a weekly dish. The number of hotels serving the nonvegetarian food has gone up which shows the increased consumer interest and preference for meat and meat products. Food habits are changing especially among younger generation and in the coming days the consumer base will increase. It is expected that, chicken consumption may become biweekly or daily in the coming years.

Organized retail sector in India is expected to reach USD 184 billion by 2020 and play an instrumental in development of food/meat industry. Organized retailing ensures the availability of food throughout the year and reduces the wastage. Further, with foreign direct investment it is expected that retailers should invest 50 per cent in new warehouse, cold chain and modern transport facility.

Due to liberalization, urbanization, fast growing economy and government policies, the meat consumption habits are changing among Indian consumers especially in metros, cities and smaller towns. Large meat processing companies like

Venky's Xprs, Fresco Pollo, Suguna Daily Fresh, Australian Country Chicken, Kentucky Fried Chicken (KFC), McDonald, MaryBrown, Subway, GodrejTyson, Sumeru, Falcon Foods, Vista Food Processors, Alchemist, Meat Products of India Ltd., etc. have entered into meat processing and catering to the demands of certain percentage of population. By late 2010, KFC has around 100 stores in the country and by 2015 it is aiming to open 500 stores mainly in smaller towns and cities. Suguna Daily Fresh is planning to open 100 retail outlets for chilled chicken and readytoeat grilled chicken in next 3 years. Venky's Xprs has opened its outlets in Pune, Mumbai and Hyderabad and planning to expand. The Venkateshwara Hatcheries (VH) Group, Sagri Foods, Shalimar Poultry Group are coming up with stateof theart large scale poultry processing plants with a slaughter capacity of 30006000 birds/hour. GodrejTyson has created the infrastructure to market poultry products in most of the western and southern cities in India. The evolution of modern retail outlets with better packaging, labeling, chilling and cold chain facilities will hopefully address the drawbacks of the existing situation. Realizing the Indian quick service restaurant market which is worth $ 13 billion, several food majors viz, Denny's Corp, Pollo Tropical Carrols Restaurant, Applebee's and Johnny Rockets, Wendy's, etc. are entering India. Few large players like METRO, SPAR Hypermarket, Wal Mart, etc. have already entered into retail sector.

Poultry Processing Trend In India

- ☆ Over a dozen modern mechanized poultry processing plants
- ☆ 5 per cent slaughtering by these mechanized plants
- ☆ 15 per cent slaughtering by small poultry processing units
- ☆ Rest sold as live bird/deskinned carcass at retail meat shops
- ☆ 2/3rd of dressed chicken sold as hot dressed/chilled/frozen whole carcass
- ☆ 1/3rd of dressed chicken further-processed as cut-ups/deboned/ground meat/marinated/ready-to-eat products

Vertically integrated poultry producers/EOUs/Multinational food chains/ Domestic Food processors/Fast-food outlets – Driving force in value-added products business

Scope for Processed Poultry Meat Products

While the poultry sector is growing at about 10 per cent annually, the processed meat sector is growing at nearly 30 per cent. The market for processed meat is just 45 per cent of the total chicken consumption segment in India. Processed meats have 3 major buyers: quick service restaurant chains who purchase processed meats from certified plants; 510 per cent of restaurants have moved towards processed chicken and retail consumers (45 per cent). For retail consumers, the limitation is availability of processed chicken according to their need. Consumer preferences differ according to cooking style and dish. Very few modern retail outlets sell processed meat. Therefore, customization of meat and meat products to meet the specific demands of consumers is required. Sale of unpacked, but customized products in branded shops will succeed, rather than branding the product for few more years.

Dairy has moved to packed concept mainly because availability of fresh products has reduced and customer trust of the product in the packed form has increased. In poultry, even in metros, consumers do not store meat in the refrigerator and use it over a period of time. They prefer to buy the product fresh from a meat shop and cook it immediately. In such a market, branding of the shop helps. Godrej Tyson Foods has recently launched new frozen south Indian styled unleavened bread stuffed with minced chicken "Chicken Kheema Paratha". Reliance retail has picked 45 per cent stake in "2 Sisters Food Group" (UK based company) and planning to market chilled and frozen chicken with a brand "CHICKEN CAME FIRST". In the year 2012 I has 300 KFC and 180 Pizza hut with brand "YUM" and by 2015 India is expected to have 1000 KFC's, Pizza Huts and Taco Bell restaurants in more than 100 cities.

Table 12.2: Egg Processing Trend In India

Sl.No.	*Processing Units*	*Location*	*Capacity/Day*	*Products*
1.	Food and inns	Pune	1 lakh	Whole egg powder
2.	Balaji food and feed ltd	Hyderabad	10 lakhs	Whole egg, albumin, yolk powder and lysozyme
3.	SKM egg products export (India) Ltd.	Erode	12 lakhs	–Do–
4.	Ovobel foods ltd.	Bangalore.	6 lakhs	–Do–

Only 5-6 per cent of eggs produced converted into dehydrated/frozen egg products

Clean/graded/branded/designer table eggs – recent introduction

Export Scenario

India has marginal presence in poultry exports market, though Middle East and Africa provides strong potential.The poultry products exported from the country include poultry meat, live poultry, hatching eggs, table eggs, egg powder, frozen eggs and value added products. As regards the value of export, maximum foreign exchange was earned from hatching eggs followed by egg powder and frozen eggs. The export was initiated in 1990.The value of export of poultry products was only Rs 15 crores in 1998 which was increase to Rs 130 crores in 2001-2002.In the international trade the share of the country is 8 per cent and 2 per cent of total output of 70.4 million tonnes poultry meat and 52.5 million tones table eggs in the world. The percent contribution of different poultry products include frozen broiler 0.02 per cent, shell eggs 0.21 per cent, frozen liquid egg 4.015 per cent and egg powder 2.80 per cent of the global trade.

India's poultry export is marginal with current exports estimated at less than Rs. 500 crore annually. India's poultry exports are dominated by table eggs, mainly to the Middle East and Africa, with minimal sales of processed items. Intermittent outbreaks of bird flu in pockets of India since 2006 have hampered exports. Further with domestic demand outstripping supplies, manufacturers were not required to look for export segment. Outbreak of 'bird flu' in one corner of the country affects export of poultry from whole of India, as India is considered as one zone for disease out breaks. Bird flu cases occur frequently after a gap of six to eight months and the industry has been urging the government to mark out bird flu-prone areas to avoid any bans on poultry products in case of an isolated outbreak.

With India becoming one of the largest poultry producers and increasing investments in processed chicken manufacturing along with focus on improving cold chain infrastructure, Middle East, Africa and SAARC nations provide strong export potential. Further value added items like egg powder and SPF eggs are already well accepted in European markets though production for these items remains limited. The poultry sector is expected to remain focussed on domestic market. There is a bright chance of poultry products export provided bio-security and food safety measures are strictly implemented.

Food Safety Criterion for Poultry Meat

Diseases caused by foodborne microbial hazards constitute a worldwide public health concern. During the past decade, the incidence of foodborne diseases has increased in many parts of the world and campylobacteriosis and salmonellosis remain the most frequent foodborne zoonosis. Epidemiological reports, however, incriminate poultry meat as a source for outbreaks of human food poisoning. The organisms involved are *Salmonella* spp., *Campylobacter* spp. and, to a lesser extent, *Listeria monocytogenes, Escherichia coli, Staphylococcus aureus, Yersinia enterocolitica, Clostridium perfringens* and *Aeromonas* spp. Contamination of the endproduct with pathogenic microorganisms is a reflection of the contamination of the live birds and, therefore, measures to be taken by industry to avoid contamination of the consumerready product should start at that level. In terms of the critical control point approach of the HACCP concept, the quantitative contribution of critical phases in the production chain towards endproduct contamination should be estimated in order to take the necessary intervention or corrective steps.

Foodborne threats occur for a number of reasons. These include microbial adaptation, changes in the food production systems, including new feeding practices, changes in animal husbandry, agronomic process and food technology, increase in international trade, susceptible populations and travel, change in lifestyle and consumers demands, changes in human demographics and behaviour. The globalisation of food markets has increased the challenge to manage these risks. As consequence over the last decade, the approach to food safety control by governments has been changing. For public health protection and the facilitation of fair trade, international meat community have chosen to follow the framework of risk analysis described by Codex Alimentarius, providing a structured approach to the management of the safety of foods. In the Codex document on Microbiological Risk Management and in ICMSF's Microbiological Testing in Food Safety Management (ICMSF, 2002), the establishment of a food safety objective (FSO) is described as a tool to meet a public health goal, such as an appropriate level of protection (ALOP).

Poultry processors must be ready to meet the requirements of the Food Safety and standards authority of India (FSSAI) guideline and must adopt good manufacturing practices (GMP), Hazard analysis and critical control point (HACCP) and IS022000 standards to meet the challenges and to sustain the competition from global players. Exposure to various quality systems of management, technological innovations and their application in meat and poultry sector is also of utmost importance in this era. Governments should take overview decisions during policy making that help the meat and poultry industry in setting up/modernization of abattoirs by providing technical consultancy for production of hygienic meat and meat products and for utilization of slaughterhouse wastes to prepare animal byproducts with value addition, reducing environmental impacts.

All plants shall have sanitation standard operating procedures (SSOPs). Good manufacturing practices (GMPs), and standard operating procedures (SOPs) may be in place as the foundation of the HACCP program. GMPs are minimum sanitary and processing requirements applicable to all companies processing food. SOPs are stepbystep directions for completing important plant procedures, and should specifically describe the method for conducting and controlling the procedure. SOPs should be evaluated regularly to confirm proper and consistent application and should be modified as necessary to ensure control.

Major Constraints

- ☆ Regional imbalance in poultry production
- ☆ Mix of small/medium/large poultry farms
- ☆ Escalating feed cost
- ☆ Rising chick cost
- ☆ Shrinking profit margin
- ☆ Neglect of rural poultry
- ☆ Demand – supply mismatch : (5 per cent increase in supply leads to 25 per cent decrease in prices and vice-versa)
- ☆ Inadequate infrastructure *viz.* small/medium scale processing equipments, cold-chain and quality assurance measure in domestic market/sales promotion/disease diagnostic labs
- ☆ Threat of dumping
- ☆ Environmental concern

Challenges in Poultry Processing Industry

Key challenges faced by industry include high feed costs combined with supply shortage of corn, inadequate cold chain and transportation infrastructure, high vulnerability to disease outbreaks and highly volatile realizations affecting cash flows. The realisation pressures stem from the low entry barriers, which leads to oversupply situation. Further the marginal penetration of processed chicken (less than 5 per cent) in overall poultry market limits the value-add potential and adds to the volatility of cash flows for the key players in the industry.

i) Poor Processing and Marketing Conditions

Poultry producers are quite often subjected to distress conditions due to vagaries in market prices of broilers and spent hens brought out by the natural market forces of supply and demand and moreover influenced by the vested interests of middlemen.

As a consequence the farmers at last are affected with a reduction in prices to an unreasonably low level. It had been reliably learnt that due to this many small farmers were bound to stop poultry farming. Not only that eggs are not priced as graded eggs. Dirty eggs in open trays pulled by smart carts and exposed to direct sun, hot and humid weather are sold to the consumers without any quality assurance. Similarly poultry meat is processed unhygienically by uneducated and untrained persons without any scientific logic and sold to the consumers without proper packaging and refrigeration even in very hot weather. There is lack of cold chains in the marketing channels and the traders face a great risk to handle such highly perishable food items. Sometimes such undesirable practices cause food borne infection and intoxication to the consumers. Even the educated persons and field veterinary officials, marketing officials and health officials remain almost as silent observers without couraging to implement the government regulations prescribed for post harvest handling and marketing of poultry products.

ii) Profitable Disposal of Adult Birds

Disposal of culled adult layers and adult parent stock breeders is the greatest challenge. Because meat produced from such birds is tough, not suitable for traditional chicken curry in domestic kitchens. So there is a least consumer demand for these birds.

iii) Microbiological Problems

Contamination of poultry meat by food poisoning bacteria such as *Salmonella enteritidis, Salmonella typhimurium, Campylobacter jejuni, Listeria monocytogenes, Escherechia coli, o157:H7, Staphylococcus aureus, Yersinia enterocolitica, Clostridium perfringens, Clostrdium botulinum etc.* is also a big challenge to the growth and development of the poultry industry in our country. The microbial contamination happens at different steps of processing. The most important steps are scald water (Salmonella are destroyed but *Clostridium perfringens* survive), chilling medium (*Campylobacter jejuni* survives better in air chilling than water chilling method) and packaging and storage (in CO_2 flushed bags lactobacilli, clostridia and enterobacteriaceae may grow) and in refrigerated low scald birds there is higher total plate counts and enterobacteriaceae count than frozen high- scalded products.

iv) Quality Deterioration due to Biochemical Changes

Due to the inherent composition of poultry meat (rich in polyunsaturated fatty acids),it is more prone to oxidative changes due to the conditions prevailing during post harvest handling and marketing practices followed in the country. Health conscious people do not like to consume the meat with oxidized radicals like peroxyl radicals, hydro peroxides hydroxyl, oxygen radicals, superoxide anions and their secondary degraded biochemical compounds which cause serious health problems even cancer.

v) Bio-insecurity of Poultry Products

Due to intensive poultry farming and random use of antibiotics, hormones, detergents and sanitizers etc., there is every chance of presence of residual levels beyond permissible limits of the above classes of chemicals in the poultry meat and egg products which are of greater concerns to human health.

Future Thrust and Prospects

Future Thrust

- ☆ Genetic improvement and evolving package of feeding, management and healthcare practices for alternate (diversified) poultry species
- ☆ Development of elite poultry stocks resistance to specific poultry diseases/ tropical adaptability through biotechnological approach
- ☆ Conservation, improvement and utilization of native poultry for promoting small scale rural poultry farming through cluster approach
- ☆ Exploring alternate feed resources/precision feeding/quality assurance of compounded feed/additives
- ☆ Physiological intervention to mitigate heat stress/improve growth, production and reproduction efficiency
- ☆ Evolving efficient marketing network including quality assurance of poultry products along the entire value-chain
- ☆ Appropriate bio-security measures during production, processing and trade
- ☆ Nation-wide assessment of bio- and phyto-contaminants to address food safety concern to promote export trade under WTO regime
- ☆ Effective utilization of poultry by-products as feed, fuel and fertilizer to address environmental concern
- ☆ Effective dynamic linkage between R and D institutions and private sector

The annual per capita poultry meat consumption in India though increasing from 0.7 kg in 2001 to 2.5 kg in 2010 remains one of the lowest globally with vast gap even between NIN (National Institute of Nutrition) recommended levels of 180 eggs and 11 kg of poultry meat per person. This offers a tremendous opportunity for further integration and growth in industry. The domestic broiler meat demand is expected to grow at around 15-18 per cent, while table egg demand is expected to grow at 5-7 per cent in medium to long term.

In the past, chicken was considered to be a delicacy but with the strong gains in poultry production over the years, poultry prices are now lower than other meat prices and consumption among middle-class consumers is expanding rapidly. With increasing urbanization and higher levels of disposable income, poultry meat is increasingly seen as less of a luxury product and more as a daily staple.

Further with changing food habits and increasing exposure to global cuisines, population is increasingly converting to a non-vegetarian diet. Poultry meat is preferred over other meat products as it is considered more hygienic and is available year around throughout the country at relatively lesser prices than fish/mutton. All these factors have led to strong growth in broiler meat and table egg consumption in past few years and the growth trend is expected to continue going forward. Even stronger growth, albeit on a small base, is expected from processed chicken segment and other value added items like fortified eggs, egg powder, etc.

Modern poultry production has remained largely limited to Southern India and Western Maharashtra though States like Haryana, Punjab and some parts of West Bengal have seen increased adoption of poultry farming as alternative source of income for largely agrarian economy.

Further with industry moving from fragmented structure to large scale integrators, contract poultry farming is expected to grow strongly across India. This is expected to provide further production efficiency and scale to the industry though bigger impediment to the growth and profitability in poultry sector is marketing efficiency. The profitability for the key players in the industry has been healthy during last two fiscals and is expected to remain comfortable over short to medium term though increasing feed prices are putting some pressure on margins. Developing efficient distribution system with large investments required in cold chain infrastructure and increasing market acceptability of frozen chicken are going to be the key industry drivers in long term. Integrated players having presence in value added segments like processed chicken, fortified eggs, etc are expected to grow strongly in long term.

Strategies for Promoting Poultry Industry in India

To meet out the prevailing challenges in poultry processing, following strategies must be followed.

i) Hygienic Processing

In order to implement it there should be **immediate ban** of selling of liver birds, roadside slaughter and strongest possible punishment should me given to the culprits disobeying the government rules and regulations regarding slaughtering of birds to prepare for marketing of dressed chickens. Flying squads should be appointed to identify the corrupt officials those who intentionally leave the unlicensed meat shop owners and to take disciplinary action against them.

There should be ante mortem and postmortem inspection in letter and spirit of each bird during slaughter. The typical flow diagram of poultry processing mentioned below must be followed.

ii) Utilization of Adult and Spent Birds

Spent hens, culled cocks and broiler parent stock birds can be profitably utilized by converting them into various value added products. The usual way of utilizing spent hens is to debone the cooked carcasses. The cooked meat is diced and mostly used for canned meat stews, pot-pies and dry soup mixes. Spent hens are therefore known as "**soupers**". The bones, backs, wings and skins are rendered and recycled as animal feed ingredients. Alternatively, efficient utilization of these birds can be done by developing ground or emulsion based convenience food products such as sausages, patties, rolls, steaks, nuggets, blocks, kebabs etc.

iii) Good Manufacturing Practices (GMP)

Practice of GMP is vital in poultry industry before aiming at application of HACCP system. This has to be carried out as per Codex Principles of Food hygiene. Training of production managers is the key issue to avoid contamination to the poultry products.

iv) Hazard Analysis and Critical Control Points (HACCP)

Consumers world over are becoming quality conscious. Growing consumer awareness regarding the safety and quality of food products, changing pattern of lifestyle, markets etc mandates producers to achieve food safety standards to international level.

Consequent to the establishment of WTO regime liberalizing the trade, its member countries have been called upon to confirm their production systems to the food safety standards as given in Codex Alimentarius Commission (CAC) and the International Office of Epizootics (OIE), so as to prevent spread of diseases on account of international movement of plants, animals and their products (SPS agreement).

To achieve an acceptable level of confidence, we need programme that undertake risk assessment and preventive measures. Hazard Analysis and Critical Control Points is one such program proposed by USDA as final rule for pathogen reduction. HACCP 9 CFR part 304 in 1996 often referred as "Mega Reg" HACCP System a well established concept in food safety identifies specific hazards.

To avoid the production of defective items and ensure that the quality of the product is within the limits specified, all aspects of production from raw materials and ingredients to processing stages, storage, sale, distribution, retailing and consumer abuse have to be considered.

HACCP system basically aims at:

1. Identification of hazards (Physical, chemical biological), and assessment of their risks
2. Determination of critical control points (CCPs) at which hazard can be minimized/controlled; CCP_1 indicates the inhibition of growth of microorganisms while CCP_2 denotes reduction in the level of microorganisms,
3. Establishing critical limits and tolerances
4. Monitoring procedures
5. Identification of any corrective action needed when a CCP is not under control
6. Procedures for verification to confirm that the HACCP system is working effectively
7. Documentation of all procedures and records.

v) Irradiation of Poultry Meat

WHO clarified in 1980 the medical acceptability of irradiated foods and reported that no health hazard could result from the consumption of any foods irradiated up to a dose of one mega rad (1M rad = 10Kgy).A dose of 2-3 KGy is adequate to

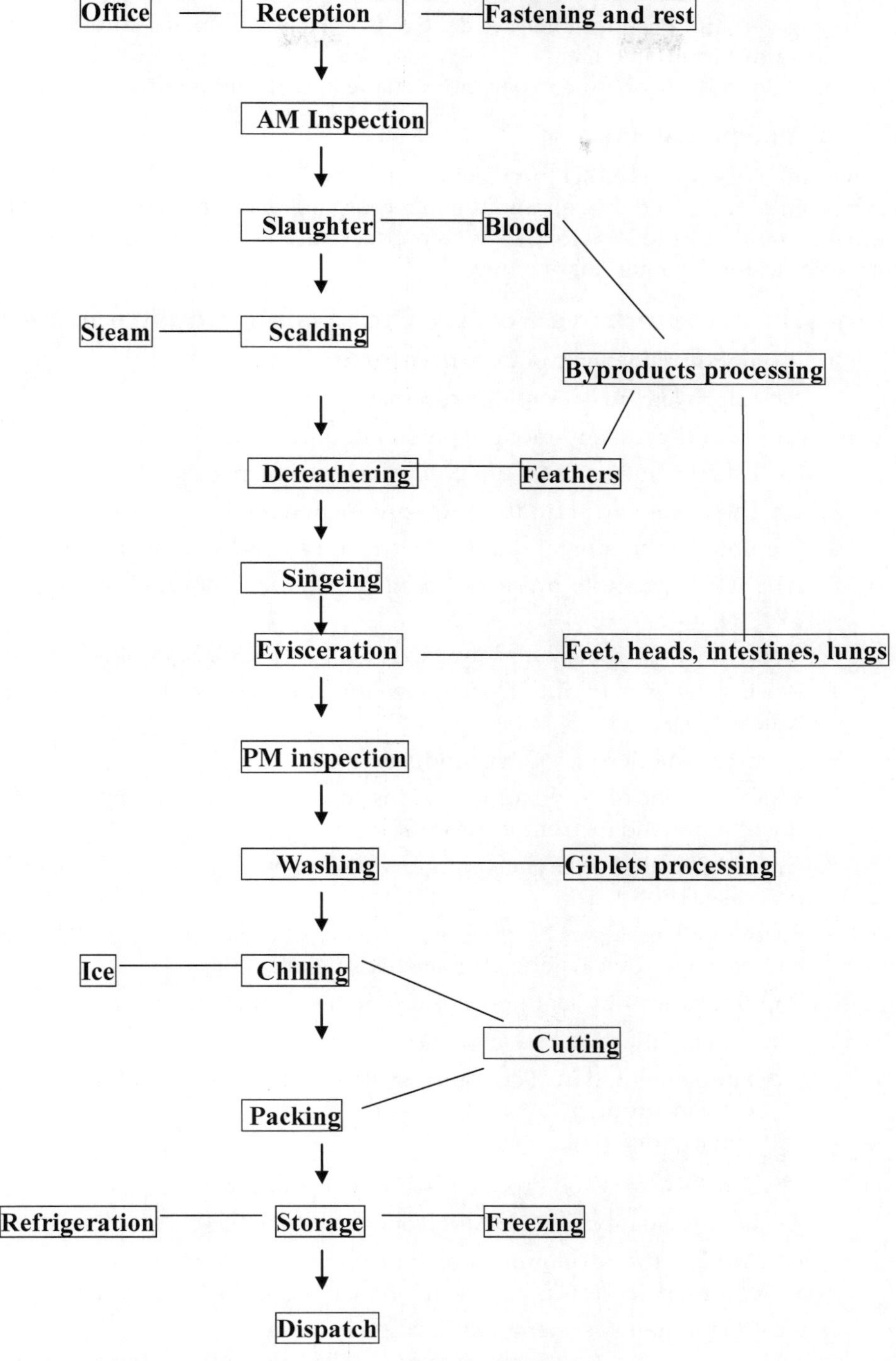

Figure 12.1: Typical Flow Diagram of Poultry Processing.

decontaminate the meat and poultry from Salmonella, Campylobacter, E.coli, Listeria monocytogenes and Pseudomonas. A dose of 0.3-1KGy eliminates parasites from meat. The sale of irradiated meat has been permitted in many countries. Irradiation with a dose op to 10KGy has been permitted in meat, fish, and poultry in India.

vi) Combination Systems

A combination of HACCP, Irradiation and modified atmosphere packaging (MAP) would prove better in eliminating microorganisms from meat and poultry. There is a good scope to look for newer techniques such as electromagnetic waves, ultrasonic etc. for decontaminating meat.

Suggestions to Improve Poultry Processing Industry in India

1. Promotion of hygienic poultry meat production
   - ☆ Improvement of existing processing plants
   - ☆ Adoption of semi-modern poultry dressing plants
   - ☆ Establishment of modern poultry processing plants
   - ☆ Establishment of rural poultry production centers
2. Promotion of small-scale poultry products centers by entrepreneurs
3. APEDA to promote processed poultry products thorough appropriate assistance
4. Government needs to withdraw excise duty on packaged poultry products.
5. Raising the level of duty to minimize the import of poultry products(*e.g.* Chicken legs)
6. Export promotion of poultry products
7. Establishment of cold storage chains to correct adverse effect of price fluctuations and to promote processed poultry products.
8. Growing broilers to larger weights to produce premium quality meats for processed products.
9. Further processing techniques to profitably utilize meat from culled birds and bony cuts (neck, wings, deboned frames etc)
10. Popularization of scientific approach of poultry processing.
11. Consumer education and awareness
12. Strict implementation of operating systems for production of safe poultry meat and its products.
    - ☆ MFPO (1973,1994)
    - ☆ Role Of Meat Food Products Advisory Committee
    - ☆ Export Quality Control And Inspection Act (1963)
    - ☆ APEDA for development of export trade and strengthening quality control systems (Trainings on HACCP. TQM, ISO 9000 series etc)
    - ☆ BIS for quality systems certification in India

- ☆ Ministry Of Food Processing Industry (MFPI) – financial support for upgrading infrastructural facilities in poultry processing plants and supporting R and D programmes in improving the quality of poultry meat products.

13. Long-term policy for a holistic approach for quality control in poultry Food chains from Farm –to-Fork.
14. Involvement of Indian Meat Science Association (IMSA) in organization of quality control systems and food safety aspects.

Conclusion

Immediate needs of the poultry processing sector are to take advantage of liberalized world trade to benefit the Indian poultry industry by harmonization of standards, giving incentives to farmer for quality poultry production and to adopt stringent quality control measures, to develop long term strategies for export, popularize and develop traditional products technology, and regularly monitoring for chemical residues and microbial quality and produce international standard meat products. Training workers to observe sanitation and hygienic requirements while handling meat in slaughterhouses, processing plants and consumer/retail outlets should be taken care of. To guarantee the production of safe poultry meat, knowledge of the capability of microorganisms to colonise the gastrointestinal tract is needed and the use of vaccines, antimicrobials and competitive exclusion microflora as well as the implementation of new processing technology should be encouraged.

References

Codex Alimentarius. http://www.codexalimentarius.org/

Cox JM, Pavic A (2010). Advances in enteropathogen control in poultry production. J Appl Microbiol 108: 745755

FAOSTAT, (2012). FAO statistical yearbook. *http://faostat.fao.org/site/291/default.aspx*.

Keener KM, Bashor MP, Curtis PA, Sheldon BW, Kathariou S 2004: Comprehensive review of Campylobacter and poultry processing. Compr Rev Food Sci Food Safety 3: 105116

Naveena, B.M., Muthukumar, M., Anjaneyulu, A.S.R., Sen, A.R. and Kondaiah, N. (2011). Value Added Chicken Products: An Entrepreneur Guide, Hind Publishers, Hyderabad.

Sahoo, J. 2004. Lead paper entitled "Present status, challenges and strategies for promotion of poultry processing industry in India" presented in XXII Conference of Indian Poultry Science Association and National Symposium on Strategies for promoting commercial poultry farming in Hills, April 7-9, 2004 held at CSKHPKV, Palmpur, Souvenir and Abstract, pp. 229-234.

– Chapter 13 –

Commonly Occurring Anti-Nutrients, and Antibiotics in Poultry Feed Ingredients and its Effect on Egg and Meat Nutrition

Introduction

The anti-nutritional factors (ANFs) may be defined as those substances generated in natural feed stuffs by the normal metabolism of species and by different mechanisms (*e.g.*, inactivation of some nutrients, diminution of the digestive process or metabolic utilization of feed) which exert effects contrary to optimum nutrition.

Substances which either by themselves or through their metabolic products, interfere with food utilization or affect the health and production of animals.

Being an ANF is not an intrinsic characteristic of a compound but depends upon the digestive process of the ingesting animal (Cheeke and Shull, 1985). The utility of the leaves, pods and edible twigs of shrubs and trees as animal feed is limited by the presence of ANFS. In fact, plants contain thousands of compounds which, depending upon the situations, can have beneficial or deleterious effects on organisms consuming them. These compounds, with the exception of nutrients, are referred to as 'allelo chemicals' (Rosenthai and Janzen, 1979). ANFs may be regarded as a class of these compounds, which are generally not lethal. They diminish animal productivity but may also cause toxicity during periods of scarcity or connement when the feed rich in these substances is consumed by animals in large quantities. The ANFS which have been implicated in limiting the utilization of shrub and tree forages include non-protein amino acids, glycosides, phytohemagglutinins, polyphenolics, alkaloids, triterpenes and oxalic acid.

General Characteristics

- ☆ Products of secondary metabolism
- ☆ Found in virtually all plants to some degree
- ☆ Common in tropical forages
- ☆ Defensive role: Bitter, colors, poisonous, odor, antinutritive/ immunosuppressive

Classification

a) Proteins

- ☆ Protease inhibitor
- ☆ Haemagglutinin

b) Glycosides

- ☆ Saponin
- ☆ Cyanogens
- ☆ Glucosinolates

c) Phenols

- ☆ Gossypol
- ☆ Tannins

d) Others

- ☆ Mycotoxins
- ☆ Anti metals
- ☆ Anti vitamins

Proteins

(a) Protease Inhibitor

- ☆ Proteolytic activity
- ☆ Source : soya bean, mung, kidney bean
- ☆ Concentrated in the outer part of cotyledon
- ☆ Types : i) kunitz inhibitor: inhibits trypsin
  ii) Bowman: inhibits both trypsin and chymotrypsin
- ☆ Effect: young chicks fed raw soyabean shows hypertrophy of pancreas.
- ☆ Control : temperature, duration of heating, particle size, moisture level,

(b) Haemagglutinin

- ☆ Also called as lectines.
- ☆ Source : soya bean, castor bean (ricin)
- ☆ Concentrated in both plant and animal tissue.

- Effect: inflammation in intestine, kidney, thyroid gland
- Control : pancreatic juice, dry heat

Glycosides

(c) Saponin

- Generally bitter
- Structure: Contain CHO and non-CHO moiety (aglycone)
- Mode of action: Toxicity results from aglycone release during enzymic degradation
- Sources :Linseed, cassava, sorghum, soya, clover etc
- Sub-Groups
  - Cyanogenic
  - Goitrogenic
  - Coumarin
  - Nitropropanol
  - Carcinogenic
  - Isoflavons (phytoestrogens)
  - Steroidal (Saponins)

Glycosides–Effects

- Phytoestrogens, *e.g.* Formononetinin Red and Subterranean clover
- Female sterility, *e.g.* Genistein in soya
- Estrogenic activity and male sterility
- Have distinctive foaming characteristics *e.g.* in White clover, alfalfa, Brachiaria decumbens and Panicum spp.
- Cause bloat, hemolysis, GIT erosion, inhibit enzyme action

(d) Cyanogens

- Mainly present in the form of cyano genetic glycosides.
- Hydrolysed by prussic acid and HCN
- Not very common in poultry.
- Detoxified by liver.
- Excess cyanide ion cause anoxia, muscle perosis

(e) Glucosinolates

- Source : cabbage, turnips, rutabaga, mustars green
- Produced pungent oddour.
- Effect : depress the synthesis of thyroid hormone(T_4 and T_3),
- Thio glucose group bound to an amino acid.

(f) Gossypol

- Genus : gossipium
- Present in pigment glands of leave
- Complex formation with iron.
- Effect : ascitis, decrease in growth, anorexia, decrease egg size and wt., olive green colour yolk, yellow and brown pigment in liver and spleen

(g) Tannins

Selected Forage Plants with Tannins

Lotus Species

- *Sainfoin*
- *Faba beans*
- *Peas*
- *Sorghum*
- *Calliandra calothyrsus*
- *Leucaena leucocephala*
- *Sesbania sesban*
- *Gliricidia sepium*
- *Acacia* species

Tannins are water soluble phenolic compounds with a molecular weight greater than 500 and with the ability to precipitate proteins from aqueous solution. They occur almost in all vascular plants. Hydrolysable tannins and condensed tannins (proanthocyanidins) are two different groups of these compounds. Generally tree and shrub leaves contain both types of tannins. The two types differ in their nutritional and toxic effects. The condensed tannins have a more profound digestibility–reducing effect than hydrolysable tannins, whereas the latter may cause varied toxic manifestations due to hydrolysis in rumen. Sheep ingesting 0.9g hydrolysable tannins kg/body weight showed signs of toxicity in 15 days. Nevertheless, deleterious effects and episodes of toxicity suggest the inadequacy of defense against high quantities of dietary tannins (Kumar and Vaithiyanathan, 1990).

The mechanism of dietary effects of tannins maybe understood by their ability to form complex with proteins. Tannins may form a less digestible complex with dietary proteins and may bind and inhibit the endogenous protein, such as digestive enzymes (Kumar and Singh, 1984). Tannin-protein complexes involve both hydrogen-bonding and hydrophobic interactions; the precipitation of the protein-tannin complex depends upon pH, ionic strength and molecular size of tannins. Both the protein precipitation and incorporation of tannin phenolics into the precipitate increase with the increase in molecular size of tannins (Kumar and Horigome, 1986). However, when the molecular weight is very large (>5000), the tannins become insoluble and loose their protein precipitating capacity. Hence the measurement of the phenolic prole in terms of total phenols, condensed tannins, their protein precipitating capacity and degree of polymerization become simper active to asses the role of tannins in ruminant nutrition (Kumar, 1983; Lowry, 1990).

Detannification Methods

1. Physical treatments: soaking and cooking
2. Chemical treatments: addition of polyetelene glycol (PEG), Polyvinyl pyrrolidone (PVP), use of formaldehyde, alkaline H_2O_2, $KMnO_4$
3. Solid state fermentation

Mycotoxins

- ☆ MYCO from a Greek Word Mykes means Mould or Fungi
- ☆ TOXIN from a Latin word toxicum means Poison

1. Classification as per source (organism)

- ☆ Aflatoxin(A)- Asperagillus flavus
- ☆ Ochratoxin(O)- A. ochraceous
- ☆ Trichohecenes(T) – Fusarium gr.
- ☆ Zearalenone (Z) –F. moniliformi
- ☆ Citrinin (C) - Pencillium gr.
- ☆ Strigmatocystine – A. vesicular
- ☆ Oosporin (Os) – Chaelornium sp.

2. Classification as per the Effect of the Fungi (Mycotoxicosis)

- ☆ Hepatotoxin – All groups excepts Z.
- ☆ Nephrotoxin – O,C,A
- ☆ Genitoxin – Z
- ☆ Neurotoxin – T
- ☆ Dermatotoxin – T
- ☆ Immunotoxin- A, T,

Mycotoxicosis

- ☆ All organ system affected.
- ☆ All age group affected but youngs are more susceptible.
- ☆ Both the sexs are affected but males are more sensitive.
- ☆ Decrease feed intake.
- ☆ Decrease production and body wt.
- ☆ Abnormal behavior.
- ☆ Reproductive problem like anestrous, RB, Retention of placenta, Metritis.
- ☆ Immune suppression.
- ☆ Hematological changes like decrease Hb, PCV, TLC

- ✫ Oral lesions
- ✫ Death
- ✫ Heamorrage in the vital organs and intestine.

(h) Anti Metals

- ✫ Mainly two types: Phytic acid and oxalic acid
- ✫ Source : Phytic acid -wheat, rice, soyabean, linseed, cotton seed

Oxalic Acid-Plan Foodstuffs

- ✫ Effect digestive disorder, decrease blood calcium level, retarded growth, egg abnormality

(i) Anti Vitamins

- ✫ Antivitamin A
- ✫ Antivitamin E
- ✫ Antivitamin K
- ✫ Antivitamin D
- ✫ Antipyrodoxine
- ✫ Antiniacin
- ✫ Antithiamin

Other Anti-Nutritional Factors

Apart from the ANFs discussed in preceding sections, shrub and tree forage may contain alkaloids, terpenoids, oxalate, indospecine, lignins and certain other ANFs. Alkaloids such as N-methyl-aphenethylamine cause locomotor ataxia of the hindquarters in sheep. Sesbaine causes haemorrhagic diarrhoea. The terpenoids azadirachtin and limonin impart a bitter taste and the leaves of Azadirachta indica are therefore not relished by cattle. Oxalate in the leaves of Acacia aneuramay limit the Ca availability and a negative correlation between digestibility and lignin content in tropical browse has been observed (Bamualin *et al.*, 1980).

Anti-nutritional factors, the potential risks of toxicity and methods to alleviate them in a single plant. Furthermore, lesser known fodder trees and shrubs may contain unknown ANFs and their presence would only be revealed through feeding trials, not by chemical analysis directed at known compounds. 2. Quantification: There is wide variation in the reported concentration of ANFs in the same plant species. This may be either real, because of the changes occurring due to environmental conditions, or may arise because of lack of standardization of methods between laboratories, as well as their destruction in assays. 3. Assessment of biological effects: It is often observed that sensitivity t0ANFs varies between species of animals, different ages and physio- logical stages. Furthermore, the leaves of a particular tree or shrub may contain different group of ANF s and it becomes difficult to separate their biological effects.

Alkaloids

- ☆ Usually basic, bitter and toxic (v. potent) *e.g.* Cocaine, nicotine and caffeine
- ☆ Animal feed sources: Lupins, potatoes contain solanine-based alkaloids
- ☆ Effects: Kidney, pulmonary and liver damage, diarrhea

Ergot Alkaloids and Fescue Toxicosis

- ☆ Most pre 80s tall fescue in US infected with endophyte fungi (Neotyphodium coenophialum) that produced ergot alkaloids *e.g.* clavine alkaloids, lysergic acid amides, and ergopeptines
- ☆ Symptoms
  - Vasoconstriction
  - Foot problems
  - Retained winter coat
  - High body temp and respiration
  - Fat Necrosis
  - Reproductive and birthing problems

Non-Protein Amino Acids

1. Mimosine

- ☆ Found in *Leucaenaleucocephala (20-30 per cent CP)*
- ☆ Metabolic derivative 3,4-DHP (3-hydroxy-4(1H)-pyridone) causes goiter, alopecia, anorexia, gastroenteritis, hepatotoxicity
- ☆ R. Jones discovered that Leucaena toxins are inactivated by a rumen microbe (*Synergistis jonesii*) in Hawaii sheep and has introduced cultures
- ☆ Florida Senopol (origininated from St Croix) cattle are also resistant to DHP

Mimosine, a non-protein amino acid structurally similar to tyrosine, occurs in a few species of Mimosa and all species of closely allied genus Leucaena. Concern has arisen because of the importance of L. leucocephala, in which the level of mimosine in the leaf is about 2-6 per cent and varies with seasons and maturity. In poultry, mimosine causes poor growth, alopecia, eye cataracts and reproductive problems. Levels of Leucaena meal above5–10 per cent of the diet for swine, poultry and rabbits generally result in pooranimal performance.

The mechanism of action of mimosine in producingits effect is not clear but it may act as an amino acid antagonist or maycomplex with pyridoxal phosphate, leading to disruption of catalyticalaction of B6-containing enzymes such as trans-aminases, or may complex with metals such as zinc (Hegarty, 1978). Some of these symptoms may be due to mimosine and others to3, 4 dihydroxypyridine, a metabolite of mimosine in the rumen (Jonesand Hegarty, 1984). Toxic signs like skin lesions also resemble Zn deciency. A solution to the mimosine problem could be the development of low mimosine cultivars. However, low mimosine types are found to be unproductive and of low vigour. The other approach is to feed Leucaena mixed with other feeds.

Phytohemagglutinins

Phytohemagglutinins, otherwise referred to as lectins, are proteins which agglutinate red blood cells. They have been shown to occur in some important fodder trees . The highest concentrations of lectins are found in seeds but, in the leaves, their concentration is low due to translocation. The biological effects of lectins probably result from their affinity for sugars. They may bind to the carbohydrate moieties of cells of the intestinal wall and cause a non-specific interference with nutrient absorption (Liener, 1985). In fodder trees, the lectins of interest arerobin and ricin. Robin, a lectin from Robinia pseudoacacia, has been reported to cause symptoms of anorexia, lassitude, weakness and posterior paralysis in cattle (Cheeke and Shull, 1985). Ricin occurs in castor beans (*Ricinus communis*) which have beenreported to cause poisoning in all class of livestock. Due to ricin, de-oiled castor seed cake (CP 35 per cent) is seldom used as a livestock feed. However, the mature leaves of R. communis have been found suitable for feeding to sheep (Behl *et al.*, 1986); hence precautions against bean contamination are necessary. Castor bean meal can be detoxied by autoclaving at 20 psi for 60 minutes for incorporation in sheep diets Glao *et al.*, 1988).

Anti-Nutritional Factors in Soybean

Among the anti-nutritional factors present in soybean seed, the main ones are protease inhibitors – Kunitz trypsin inhibitor (KTI) and Bowman-Birk inhibitor, and lectins. Protease inhibitors represent 6 per cent of the protein present in soybean seed. Approximately, 80 per cent of the trypsin inhibition is caused by KTI, which strongly inhibits trypsin and therefore reduces food intake by diminishing their digestion and absorption. Another effect of KTI is the induction of pancreatic enzyme, hyper secretion and the fast stimulation of pancreas growth, hypertrophy and hyperplasia. Due to this, raw soybean can not be used for feeding monogastric animals. Heat treatment doesn't completely eliminate these factors and may decrease protein solubility. Despite the efficiency of thermal treatment to reduce protease inhibitors, residual inhibition (10-20 per cent) is maintained (*Carvalho et al.,1998*). By this reason, a part of the breeding program of the Maize Research Institute Zemun Polje is aimed at developing soybean cultivars with reduced trypsin inhibitors content. As a result, two cultivars lacking KTI, Lana and Laura, were released *Srebriæ et al.* (*2008*). The trypsin inhibitor content in these cultivars ranges from 15.01 mg g-1 in Laura to 15.35 mg g-1 in Lana, which is about 50 per cent reduced as compared to the genotypes with standard grain type (*Periæ et al., 2009*). The utilization of these cultivars is a great opportunity for saving energy and preserving valuable nutritional composition of soybean grain, which is of interest in industrial processing. This trait makes them also suitable for direct feeding in adult non-ruminant animals without previous thermal processing. Lectins are proteins that are widely distributed in plant kingdom and have unique property of binding carbohydrate-containing molecules with a high specificity, causing agglutination of red blood cells. Soybean agglutinin (SBA) causes the atrophy of the microvilli, reduces the viability of the epithelial cells and increases the weight of small intestine because of hyperplasia of crypt cells (*Grant*A. Mikiæ et al.1184*et al.*,

1987; Pusztai et al., 1990). The inactivation of soybean lectin by a moist heat treatment is parallel with the destruction of trypsin inhibitors. Soybean lectin is quite resistant to inactivation by dry heat treatment. The soybean genotypes lacking SBA were found *Pull et al.* (*1978*).

References

D'Mello,JPF2000.Farm animal metabolism and nutrition. (Ed.). CAB, Wallingford. P319. Chapter 18

Caygill, J C and Mueller-Harvey 1999. Secondary plant products. Nottingham University press.

Cheeke, P R and Shull L R 1998. Natural toxicants in feeds and poisonous plants. AVI Publ. Co.

Garland T and Barr, C. 1998. Toxic plants and natural toxicants. CAB International

Journal of the Science of Food and Agriculture 37: 37-42 Roscnthal, G.A. and Janeen, D.H.I979. Herbivores. Their Interaction with secondary plant metabolites. Academic Press. New York. Russel, J.B. and Wilson, D.B. 1988.

Potential opportunities and problems for genetically altered rumen microorganisms. Journal of Nutrition 118: 271-279. Russell, R.W. and Lolley, J.R. 1989.

Deactivation of tannin in high tannin milo by treatment with urea. Journal of Dairy Science 72: 2427-2430. Shanna, D.D., Chandra, S. and Negi, SS. 1969. The nutritive value and toxicity of 0111 (Albizziastipulata Bovin) tree leaves. Journal of Research Ludhiana 6: 388-393. Shqueir, A.A., Brown, l).L.,Taylor, S.J Rivkin, 1., Klasing,K.C. 1989.

Effects of solvent extraction, heat added cholesterol on Sesbania ses- treatments and ban toxicity in growing chicks. Animal Feed Science and Tech- nology 27: 127-135. Singh, R.V. 1982. Fodder trees of India. Oxford and IBH Publishing Co., New Delhi pp. 303. Source

Book :Principle of animal nutrition and feed technology by D.V. READY

Book :Feeds and Principle of animal nutrition by G.C. Banerjee

– Chapter 14 –

Quality Identification and Quality Maintenance of Poultry Meat

Quality Identification

A number of state, country, and municipal laws influence quality identification. In many cases the only purpose is to eliminate the sale and use for food for all poultry which is unfit for human consumption; in other cases the laws are an attempt to standardize the different types of poultry offered for sale; and in a few cases laws act as trade barriers. Food and drug laws are similar to the federal Food, Drug and Cosmetic Act. Their prime objective is to prevent the sale or consumption of poultry which is unfit for human consumption

Licensing laws require dealers and poultry processors to obtain a license before buying and selling poultry. Generally the licensee must file a report of his activities or undergo inspection of his place or business or his records. Standardization laws are an attempt to standardize the different types of poultry offered for sale in a given trading area or in a given political subdivision. Laws pertaining to proof of ownership of poultry in transit are an attempt to guard against thievery and to provide a means of identifying the owner for law in enforcement officers. Laws limiting the hours of business make it unlawful to sell or offer poultry for sale at specified times.

Inspection laws require inspection of the poultry at some phase during processing or just prior to delivery or sale. Laws governing the sale of imported poultry attempt to regulate the quality of poultry processed outside the jurisdiction of the state, country, or city where it is offered for sale or consumed.

United States Department of Agriculture Grades and Standards

The U.S. Department of Agriculture Grades and Standards applied by qualified personnel provide as accurate and objective a method of identifying quality as can be devised for practical application. Within the limits of subjective evaluation, they are the same in all areas of country and for all conditions and types of poultry marketed. The grades and standards are a matter of public record and are acceptable evidence in legal cases. They also serve as a basis for establishing state, trade and research specification.

Poultry are classified by the U.S. Department of Agriculture into kinds, classes, grades, weight range, condition, live, dressed, and ready-to-cook. Gading service is provided for the purpose of determining the class, quality, quantity, condition or any combination of the above. Inspection service is provided for determining the condition and wholesomeness of poultry.

Market Class

Before grading, poultry are divided into market classes according to their species, age and sex (Table 14.1). In some cases there age is limited to span of several weeks; in other cases they may be classified simply as young or old. Sex may not be specified where it has no effect on the market quality.

Table 14.1: Market Classes of Poultry

Species	*Class*	*Sex*	*Age*
Chicken	Cornish game hen	Either	5-7 weeks
Chicken	Broiler or fryer	Either	9-12 weeks
Chicken	Roaster	Either	3-5 months
Chicken	Capon	Unsexed male	Under 18 months
Chicken	Stag	Male	Under 10 months
Chicken	Hen or stewing	Female	Over 10 months
Chicken	Cock	Male	Over 10 months
Turkey	Fryer-roaster	Either	Under 16 weeks
Turkey	young hen	Female	5-7 months
Turkey	Young tom	Male	5-7 months
Turkey	Yearling hen	Female	Under 15 months
Turkey	Yearling tom	Male	Under 15 months
Turkey	Mature or old	Either	Over 15 months
Duck	Broiler duckling	Either	Under 8 weeks
Duck	Roaster duckling	Either	Under 16 weeks
Duck	Mature or old	Either	Over 16 weeks
Goose	Young	Either	
Goose	Mature or old	Either	
Guinea	Young	Either	
Guinea	Mature or old	Either	
Pigeon	Squab	Either	
Pigeon	Pigeon	Either	

U.S. Dept. Agr., Agriculture Handbook 31 (1956).

Species

For purpose of grading, poultry are classified into chickens, turkeys, ducks, geese, guineas and pigeons. Each species has definite characteristics which influence cooking methods and organoleptic properties.

Sex

In many cases the various species of poultry are classified according to sex because sex has a definite influence on the quality of the resultant carcass. The flavours, tenderness, juiciness, conformation and finish of an old rooster are quite different from those of a stewing chicken or hen. In other cases where sex has little influence on the carcass, it may not be used as a basis for classifying birds. Two examples are broilers or fryers and geese. Some characteristics of poultry which can be used to determine sex are the larger head, comb and wattles and coarser appearance of males compared to females. Male feathers are long and pointed at the ends with long curved tail feathers in chickens and a curl in the tail feathers of male ducks. In females, the feathers are shorter with a blunt end and a short straight tail. Females have a finer bone structure and a more rounded body, a shorter keel and drumsticks and thighs, comparatively shorter than males. The skin of males is coarser and the feather follicles are larger than females of the same lot. The feather tracts of females carry more fat than males.

Age

The degree of maturity also influences cooking method and organoleptic qualities. There are number of indications of the age of poultry. Young chickens have a pliable, smooth, glossy comb with sharp points; young ducks have a pliable bill. Older birds have faded, worn, broken plumage except those which recently molted. Old birds generally are darker in color and have a coarser texture and hardened muscle fibers, the end of the keel is hardened with no cartilage and the pinbones are not pliable. Young birds have smooth small scales on the shanks, a small, soft oil sac and spurs on the males are small and undeveloped. Young ducks and geese have a soft windpipe which is easily dented.

Grading Live Poultry

United States Standards of quality for individual birds, nevertheless, can be used as criteria for inspecting and determining the quality of live poultry even though each bird in a flock is not individually inspected. Live poultry are examined for health and vigour, feathering, conformation, fleshing, fat, and freedom from defects (Table 14.2). Grading of live birds is not as accurate as grading dressed carcasses, because feathers cover many defects on live birds.

Grading Ready-to-Cook Poultry

Dressed and ready-to-cook poultry are graded for class, condition and quality in that order. Summaries of specifications for standards of quality for the several classes of poultry are shown in Tables 14.3 and 14.4. Official United States grades for individually graded ready–to-cook poultry carcasses are U.S. Development of

Table 14.2: Summary of Standards of Quality for Live Poultry on an Individual Bird Basis (Minimum requirements and maximum defects permitted)

Factor	*A or No. 1 Quality*	*B or No. 2 Quality*	*C or No. 3 Quality*
Health and vigour	Alert, bright eyes, healthy, vigorous	Good health and vigour	Lacking in vigour
Feathering	Well covered with feathers showing luster or sheen Slight scattering of pin feathers	Fairly well covered with feathers Moderate number of pin feathers	Complete lack of plumage feathers on back Large number of pin feathers
Conformation	Normal	Practically normal	Abnormal
Breast bone	Slight curve, 1/8-inch dent (chickens), ¼-inch dent (turkeys)	Slightly crooked	Crooked
Back	Normal (except slight curve)	Moderately crooked	Crooked or hunched back
Legs and wings	Normal	Slightly misshapen	Misshapen
Fleshing	Well fleshed, moderately broad and long breast	Fairly well fleshed	Poorly developed, narrow breast, thin covering of flesh
Fat covering	Well covered, some fat under skin over entire carcass Chicken fryers and turkeys fryers and young toms only moderate, no excess abdominal fat	Enough fat on breast and legs to prevent a distinct appearance of flesh through skin Hens or fowl may have excessive abdominal fat	Lacking in fat covering on back and thighs, small amount in feather tracts
Defects	Slight	Moderate	Serious
Tears and broken bones	Free	Free	Free
Bruises, scratches, and calluses	Slight skin bruises, scratches, and calluses	Moderate (except only slight flesh bruises)	Unlimited to extent no part unfit for food
Shanks	Slightly scaly	Moderately scaly	Seriously scaly

U.S. Dept. Agr., Agriculture Handbook 31 (1972).

Agriculture Grades A, B, C. Wholesale grades are U.S. Extras, U.S. Standards, and U.S. Trades. Individual quality factors consist of conformation, fleshing, fat, freedom from pinfeathers and freedom from defects. The final quality of the bird will be determined by the individual factor applied to it which has the lowest rating. It should be emphasized that standards of quality apply to evaluation of individual birds or carcasses and that grades generally apply to wholesale lots of poultry. Tolerances have been to set up to compensate for human error and variations in interpreting degrees of quality.

For the purpose of encouraging uniformity, specifications for weight have been set up for the various classes even though they are not included in the U.S. Grades.

Condition

Condition refers to any characteristics which makes the carcasses unfit for human consumption.

Craftsmanship

Dressed or ready- to- took carcasses under certain conditions are returned for additional processing, or if this is not possible, they are classified as "No Grade". As such they cannot receive an official U.S. Grade. Some of these conditions are protruding pinfeathers, bruises which require trimming, lung, sex organs or part of the trachea incompletely removed, vestigial or other feathers, extraneous material such as faeces, blood, grease, feed, etc.

Conformation

The same defects which are present on live birds are also found on dressed and ready -to-took carcasses. A bird of A quality must have normal physical conformation with the exception of a slightly curved breastbone or other slightly abnormality. Chickens, ducks, guineas, and pigeons may have as much as a 1/8 inch dent in the breastbone and still qualify as A quality.

Fleshing

Carcasses qualifying as A quality have "well-developed, moderately broad and long breasts, well-fleshed throughout the entire length, with the flesh carrying sufficiently well up to the crest of the breast bone is not prominent. The legs are well covered with flesh."

Fat

An A quality poultry carcasses is well covered with fat over the breast, back, hips, and pinbones, except that chicken broilers or fryers and young tom turkeys may have only a moderate amount of fat covering. A hen, stewing chicken or fowl, although well covered with fat, is free from excessive abdominal fat.

Pinfeathers

Pinfeathers are classified as protruding and non-protruding. Non-protruding pinfeathers are those which although visible have not as yet as broken through the outer skin. Read-to-cook poultry must be free of protruding pinfeathers "visible to an inspector or grader during an examination of the carcasses at normal operating speed" before any quality designation can be assigned. Vestigal feathers (hair like appendages) must also be considered when examining a carcasses for pinfeathers.

Table 14.3: Summary of Specification for Standards of Quality for Individual Carcasses of Ready-to-Cook Poultry and Parts Therefrom (Minimum Requirements and Maximum Defects Permitted)

Factor	*A Quality*	*B Quality*	*C Quality*
Conformation	Normal	Moderate deformities	Abnormal
Breastbone	Slight curve or dent	Moderately dented, curved or cooked	Seriously curved or crooked
Back	Normal (except slight curve)	Moderately crooked	Seriously crooked
Legs and Wings	Normal	Moderately misshapen	Misshapen
Fleshing	Well fleshed, moderately long deep and rounded breast	Moderately fleshed, considering kind, class and part	Poorly fleshed
Fat covering	Well covered–especially between heavy feather tracts on breast and considering kind, class and part	Sufficient fat on breast and legs to prevent distinct appearance of flesh through the skin	Lacking in fat covering over all parts of carcass
Pinfeathers			
No protruding pins and hair	Free	Few scattered	Scattering
Protruding pins	Free	Free	Free

Exposed Flesh[1]

Carcass Weight Minimum	*Maximum*	*Breast and Legs*	*Elsewhere*	*Part*	*Breast and Legs*	*Elsewhere*	*Part*	
None	1 ½ lbs.	None	¾"	(Slight	¾"	1 ½	(Moderate	
Over 1 ½ lbs	6 lbs.	None	1 ½"	trim on	1 ½"	3"	amount of	No
Over 6 lbs.	16 lbs.	None	2"	edge)	2"	4"	the flesh	Limit
Over 16 lbs	None	None	3"		3"	5"	normally covered)	

Discolouration[3]

None	1 ½ lbs.	½	1"	¼"	1"	2"	½"	No limit[4]
Over 1 ½ lbs.	6 lbs.	1"	2"	¼"	2"	3"	1"	
Over 6 lbs.	16 lbs.	1 ½"	2 ½"	½"	2 ½"	4"	1 ½"	
Over 16 lbs.	None	2"	3"	½"	3"	5"	1 ½"	

Contd...

Table 14.3–*Contd...*

Disjoined bones No limit	1	2 disjointed and no broken or	
Broken bones No limit	None	1 disjointed and 1 nonprotruding	
		Broken	
Missing parts Wing tips,	Wing tips	Wing tips, 2nd wing joint and tail	
Wings and tail	Tail[5]		
Freezing defects (when consumer packaged)	Slight darkening over the back and drumsticks. Few small 1/8" Pockmarks for poultry Weighing 6 lbs. or less and ¼" pokmarks for poultry weighing more than 6 lbs. Occasional small areas showing layer of clear or pinkish ice.	Moderate dried areas not in excess of ½ inch diameter. May lack brightness. Moderate areas showing layer of clear pinkish or reddish colored ice.	Numerous pock-marks and large dried areas

From U.S. Deptt. Agri Handbook 31 (1972)

1. Total aggregate area of flesh exposed by all cuts, tears and missing skin.
2. A carcass meeting the requirements of a quality for fleshing may be trimmed to removed skin and flesh defects, provider that no more than one-third of the flesh is exposed on any part and the meat yield is not appreciably effected.
3. Flesh bruises and discolorations such as "blue back" not permitted on breast and legs of A Quality birds. Not more than one-half of total aggregate area of discoloration may be due to flesh bruises or "blue back" (when permitted) and skin bruises in any combination.
4. No limit in size and number of areas of discoloration and flesh bruises if such areas do not render any part of the carcasses unfit for food
5. In geese, the parts of the wing beyond the second joint may be removed at the joint and both wings are so treated.

Table 14.4: Summary of Specification for Standard of Quality for Individual Carcasses of Ready-to-Cook Turkeys and Geese (Minimum Requirements and Maximum Defects Permitted)

Factor	*A Quality*	*B Quality*	*C Quality*
Conformation	Normal	Practically normal	Abnormal
Breastbone	Slight curve or dent	Dented, curved slightly cooked	Seriously crooked
Back	Normal (except slight curve)	Moderately crooked	Seriously crooked
Legs and Wings	Normal	Moderately misshapen	Misshapen
Fleshing	Well fleshed, moderately long and rounded breast	Fairly well fleshed on breast and legs	Poorly fleshed

Contd...

Table 14.4–*Contd...*

Factor	*A Quality*		*B Quality*		*C Quality*
Fat covering	Well covered considering class		Sufficient fat on breast and legs to prevent distinct appearance of fleshthrough the skin		Lacking and fat covering over all parts of carcasses
Pinfeathers	*Breast and Legs*	*Elsewhere*	*Breast and Legs*	*Elsewhere*	
No protruding pins and hair	Pract. free	Pract. free	Few scattered	Few scattered	Scattering
Protruding pins	Free	Free	Free	Free	Free No limit
Cuts, tears, and missing skin[1]	Free	3 in.	3 in.	6 in.	No limit
Discolorations[2]	2 in.	3 in.	3 in.	6 in.	No limit
Disjoined bones	1		1 or 2 if no broken bones		No limit
Broken bones	None		1 None-protruding		No limit
Missing parts	Wing tips and tail		Wing tips, 2nd wing joint and tail		Wing, tips, wings and tail
Freezer burn	Few small (1/4 in. diam.) pockmarks		Moderate-dried areas not in excess of ½ in. in diameter		Numerous pock-markers and large dried areas

From U.S. Department Agr. Handbook 31 (1972)

1 Total aggregate area of flesh exposed by all cuts, tears and missing skin.

2 Flesh bruises and discolorations such as "blue back" not permitted on breast and legs of A Quality birds. Not more than one-half of total aggregate area of discoloration may be due to flesh bruises or "blue back" (when permitted) and skin bruises in any combination.

3 No limit in size and number of areas of discoloration and flesh bruises if such areas do not render any part of the carcasses unfit for food.

Defects

The presence or absence of such defects as cuts, tears, broken bones, skin discoloration, flesh blemishes, bruises, abrasions, and freezer burn all influence the grade placed on a carcass, generally depending upon the severity of the defect and its location on the carcass.

Freezer burn is a discoloration and pock marking of the skin caused by dehydration of the skin during frozen storage.

Quality Maintenance

Introduction

Although the area of poultry technology is limited to the processing and handling of poultry after it leaves the farm, many factors influencing quality have already occurred before the birds are loaded for market. For this reason factors which influence quality during production are discussed as well as those occurring during marketing.

Production Factors

With the initiation of compulsory inspection, many producers and processors found to their dismay that a new cost for handling and processing poultry had been added, that of condemnations. The majority of condemnations are largely results of pathological conditions, which in turn are influenced to a great extent by management practice. Management practices are related to high condemnation rates and that a combination of poor management and adverse weather conditions leads to even higher condemnations.

Housing

Because temperature, humidity and air movement are interrelated it is difficult to determine the effects of a specific variable on the quality of carcasses produced. The field of environmental physiology is one where considerably more information is needed. Abnormally high or low temperatures and humidity or rapid changes in temperature or humidity cause stresses on live broilers which make them less resistant to disease. Such extremes of temperature and humidity also set up other conditions within a poultry house which cause further stress situations.

Broilers and turkeys are housed to prevent abnormally high or low temperatures and to reduce wide fluctuations in temperature. A room temperatures between 60 and 70°F is generally considered the most desirable for poultry.

Ventilation

Air movement helps to control the temperature and humidity inside poultry houses by removing heat and moisture from the house. Ventilation also helps to remove dust and fumes such as carbon dioxide, carbon monoxide and ammonia. More information is needed on the effects of temperature, humidity and the rate and amount of ventilation on the comfort of turkeys and broilers and on the role of air in the transmission of disease.

The following housing conditions were found to be correlated with high condemnations: inadequate ridge ventilators, houses longer that 150ft., over 35 ft. wide, and houses located in low areas. Condemnations were lower in an arrow houses than wide ones and in houses having solid partitions between pens. These same conditions are also correlated with air movement and ventilation.

Insulation

Insulation prevents the loss of warm air in winter and cool air in summer and helps to prevent wide fluctuations in temperature. Because the amount of moisture retained but air under a given set of conditions is influenced considerably by temperature, insulation helps to keep the inside of a poultry house dry. As a result of the insulation the air is warmer and retains more moisture than cold air which causes moisture to condense inside the house.

Litter

Littler absorbs moisture when conditions in a poultry house are damp and releases it during dry periods. It also absorbs some gasses and releases them when damp conditions occur and provides a good medium for the protection and growth of pathogenic organisms, especially when damp. Litter is source of dust and irritation for growing birds when it becomes too dry; when too wet it is cold, damp and uncomfortable and adds an additional stress. Coarse damp litter is also one cause of breast blisters in growing birds.

Disease Control

Condemnations because of disease cause the greatest loss of carcasses during inspection. In several surveys it was observed that those flocks with high condemnations rates did not have a satisfactory disease control program. Particular problems were lack of mortality records, houses not disinfected high mortality during the first week, a disease outbreak during the fifth week, or a flock sick two weeks or longer. Other conditions found in flocks with high condemnation rates were the type of coccidiostat used and early discontinuance of coccidiostat, the combination of vaccines used, severe vaccine reactions, moderate to severe infestations of round worms and a persistence of disease symptoms up to the time of slaughter.

Respiratory diseases are the most important factor related to broiler condemnations.

Other Management Factors

The following factors were also correlated with high condemnation rates: new, inexperienced growers; houses not prepared for chicks; houses not disinfected or not left vacant more than a week; chicks overcrowded under brooders; chicks started at 90°F instead of 95°F and lack of heat during illness. Only three management practices related to feeding were observed. These were dirty feed bins, feeding chicken only once or twice daily, and poor conversion which is probably the combined result of disease outbreaks and other poor management conditions.

With turkeys, clipping poults' wings at hatching time frequently caused infection of the point where the second joint of the wing also had to be removed at processing time and caused the grade of the carcasses to be lowered to B.

Breast blisters are frequently a cause of low grade carcasses. Selection, care and depth of litter, weight of birds at market time, control of disease, ventilation and other management factors all influence keel blisters formation. A considerable number of breast blisters may occur during transportation.

Insects such as lice, mites, ticks and other insects can be certain conditions cause considerable damage to poultry by forming sores and lesions.

Blue back is a condition found on dark feathered varieties of turkeys. It is caused by broken pinfeathers and exposure to sunlight. These two conditions cause patches or blotches of blue pigment under the skin. Although it occurs mainly on the breast, it can occur on any part of the skin. A genetic conditions different from "blue back can also cause formation of melanin pigment in turkeys to the extent that the carcasses are downgraded.

Marketing Factors

Loss in quality in market channels can be caused by handling live birds during the procurement operation, damage to the carcass during processing and loss of quality because of poor or prolonged storage conditions. Although losses in quality during marketing generally do not result in condemnation of a whole carcass, the monetary loss caused by a reduction in yield and grade are considerable.

Handling

Birds although small in size are awkward to handle because they are of an odd shape and they struggle and spread their wings when held by the feet. To prevent the escape of birds previously placed in creates, the crate opening is just slightly larger than the minimum size which is needed to allow entrance of the birds. Injury to a bird can result from careless handling of either individual birds or crates of birds.

Shrinkage

Shrinkage is the loss in weight of live poultry between the time it is picked up at the farm and delivered to the processing plant. The following factors influence shrinkage: The time in transit from loading to market, the ration fed, the sex (males lose more Weight than females) and changes in temperature and humidity. As the length of time from loading increase, the shrinkage also increases but at a decreasing rate. The decreasing rate can probably be explained by the fact that birds generally struggle and excrete when picked up but relax as soon as they are placed in a crate. Birds fed on high fiber rations show the greatest shrinkage. High temperatures also increase the amount of weight lost; high humidity reduces it.

Increase in temperature cause an increase in shrink: Crowding in coops also appears to influence weight loss. In the same study, as the weight per coop increased from 45-49 lb. to 58-68 lb shrinkage increased from 3.5 to 5.0 per cent. The effects of time and distance on the weight losses of broiler are shown in Table 14.5.

Table 14.5: The Effects of Time and Distance on Weight Losses of Broilers

Hours	*Weight Loss*[1]	*Miles*	*Weight Loss*[2]
2	1.1	1-25	1.1
6	2.9	26-50	1.1
10	3.7	51 and over	1.5
14	4.2	Average	1.3
18	4.6		

1 Estimates by King and Zwick (1950)

2 Data from Jeweet (1960)

Bruises

Bruises were second only to fleshing as a defect and were responsible for over 11 per cent of all broilers downgraded from A. Roughly 19 per cent of all broiler had bruises and of this group 30-40 per cent had bruises of sufficient size to cause a lowering of the grade of the carcass. Of the total bruised birds 11.6 per cent were on the breasts and 7.5 per cent on the legs. Fresh bruises were responsible for 56 per cent of all undergrads, with bruises on the breast the most common type of injury.

To reduce bruising, it is recommended to removal feeders and waterers before catching, more care in catching birds, and more supervision in assembling broilers. Bruising was reduced 36 per cent by slaughtering birds direct from the crates rather than transferring them to batteries. Flocks with a large proportion of poorly fleshed birds tended to have fewer bruises than flocks with a higher proportion of well fleshed birds. Some breeds of chickens were found to bruise easier than others.

A sudden lowering of the environmental temperature reduced the susceptibility of birds to bruising and decreased the rate at which bruises healed. On the other hand, birds raised at high environmental temperatures bruised easily but the bruises healed quickly. Bruises on young birds healed faster than those on old birds.

Bruises cause the greatest loss of quality during the marketing operation and that about eight per cent more hens that toms were downgraded because of bruises were responsible for almost 23 per cent of all undergrades.

As bruised tissue ages the blood oxidizes and the bruised area darkens in colour from red to dark red or purple then to green or yellow. In carcasses the bruises change to dark red or purple. Bruised tissue has a greater permeability to penetration of dye and microorganisms than normal tissue. 61 per cent -74 per cent of the bruises examined contained both aerobic and anaerobic bacteria. The age of the bruise, environmental conditions, particularly sanitation, the serverity of the bruise, and the hemogolobin and its degration products all had some influence on the microbial content.

Broken Bones

Broken bones are caused by rough handling during assembly or processing. If bones are broken while the bird is still alive a bruised area results. Broken bones are the third most important factor in causing down grading of eviscerated carcasses.

Processing

Several conditions which result in grade losses or condemnations also occur as result of processing.

Tears

Tears are often caused by birds crowding on top of each other or during processing. Poorly feathered birds are subject to more tears and scratches than well-feathered ones. Old injuries on turkeys from fighting or mating are an important cause of tears. The carcasses are either torn by pickers during dressing or trimmed by the inspector upon processing with resultant B or C grade carcasses.

Poor Bleeding

Improper slaughtering can cause incomplete bleeding and prolonged breathing so that the bird inhales water from the scalding tank. Such birds are considered contaminated and are subject to condemnation. Poorly bled carcasses have poor keeping quality, undesirable flavours and an unappetizing appearance. Such carcasses have red areas over the neck, shoulders, wings and feather follicles which discolour on storage and visceral blood vessels which are greatly engorged.

Rough handling causes an increase in excitement, temperature, and nervous tension. Birds in this condition do not bleed as rapidly or thoroughly as they should, scalding is not as effective and feather removal is difficult. The final results of rough handling are an increase in processing costs and undergrades.

Over Scalding

This condition generally results from stopping the conveyor line when carcasses are moving through the scalder. Such carcasses as a result of being immersed in hot water for a prolonged period, are partially cooked and may be contaminated. The tissues of such carcasses can not be properly cleaned and are susceptible to bacterial growth, decomposition and deterioration. Overscalded carcasses are condemned.

Disfigurement

Occasionally a carcass had a bad tear opened by rubber picker fingers to the extent that the skin is torn off and the flesh is macerated. A similar condition sometimes occurs when the line stops and birds are left hanging in a picker with the fingers revolving.

Contamination

Sources for contamination are numerous. A common occurrence is the contamination of a carcass by oil or grease rubbed in the carcass and spread by picker fingers. Disposition of such carcasses depends upon the type and extent of contamination. Common contaminants are piant, grease, manure, and solvents. Carcasses contaminated with volatile oils and poisons are condemned.

Storage

The results of improper or prolonged storage can range from slight off-flavour to decomposed carcasses.

Freezer Burn

Freezer burn is defined as the development of lighter colored circular spots around feather follicles and discoloured areas of irregular shape on the surface of the skin. Light colored spots are caused by uneven surface drying which depends upon temperature, relative humidity, air circulation and the rate of movement of moisture from the frozen products is in a solid state, little if any moisture moves to the surface to replace that lost by surface evaporation. It is believed that uneven desiccation of the skin occurs because of the layer of fat immediately under the skin.

Feather removal causes uneven desiccation to take place around the feather follicles. Loss of flavour, tenderness and juiciness are the results of extreme freezer burn. Dried out meat becomes tought and hard to cook. Severely freezer burned muscle tissue contains only 50-55 per cent moisture, whereas normal tissues contain about 72 per cent. They stated that the best way to reduce freezer burn was to store poultry wrapped in moisture vapour-proof paper at a low temperature and high humidity. Variations in below freezing temperatures are also reposted to cause freezer burn.

Rancidity

Fresh, pure poultry fat is almost odourless, and tasteless. " The free fatty acid content of poultry fat after storage varies somewhat between birds, but is usually low, and shows no relation to the storage condition at freezing temperatures. The storage temperature is the most important factor determining the extent of peroxide-oxygen formation in poultry fat, the amount increasing with increase in storage temperature." Turkey fat is considerably more unstable than chicken fat.

Off-Flavours

Off-Flavours can be caused by decomposition, rancidity, contamination, feed, and absorption of odors during storage.

Pink Meat in Cooked Poultry

It is a condition in which the meat, especially white meat, turned pink after thorough cooking. Generally the colour extends to a depth of about one-fourth inch and is most often in young birds. The colour is caused by a chemical reaction between carbon monoxide and nitric oxide, which are generated by the cooking flame, and the haemoglobin of the blood in the muscle tissue. Carboxy-hemoglobin and nitric oxide haemoglobin are formed. The pink color does not influence the edibility or palatability of the meat.

– Chapter 15 –

Structure, Chemical, Nutritional and Microbiological Quality of Poultry Meat

Structure of Poultry Meat

Epimysium surrounds whole muscle and Perimysium muscle bundles penetrating septa from epimysium, contain blood vessels and nerves. Endomysium surrounds each muscle fiber. Increase in the quantity of these connective tissue increases toughness of muscle.

Tendon – congregation of connective tissue attached to the bone.

Connective tissues- ground substances + elements.

Three types.

1. Collagen tissue – straight, inextensible, non-branching
2. Reticular tissue – resemble collagen tissue, contain myristic acid
3. Elastic tissue – yellow colour, branching

Tendon: tough band of connective tissue connects the muscle with bone

Ligaments: Support organs or connect two bones or other parts

Aponeuroses: type of muscle attachment to bone in the form of a sheet.

Connective tissue also help formation of adipose tissue and cartilage.

Collagen: arranged in bundles with wavy line filaments, little stretching capacity.

Turns into gelatin when cooked.

Collagen fibers made of fibrils.

A number of protofibrils from collagen fibril.

Aggregation of filaments, primitive fibers and fibrils finally form the collagen fiber.

Collagen molecule is a polypeptide chain with high per cent of glycine residue and hydroxyproline.

The protofibrils are interwoven into a helical structure.

Composed of three polypeptide chains bound together in a helical fashion by intermolecular bonds.

After the polypeptide chains are formed in the ribosome of the fibroblastic cells, certain proline and lysine residues should be hydroxylated to form the collagen fiber.

What stops the synthesis of collagen hydoxylation of proline and lysine?

Ferrous ions and ascorbic acids are required for the activity of oxygenase enzyme which plays important role in hydroxylating the proline residues.

Elastin

Yellow elastic fibers are common in ligaments. The fibers are distributed in a random pattern forming a network with elasticity.

The structure and arrangement of elastic fibers very according to their origin.

Do not undergo hydrolysis on boiling.

The ground substance varies from a soft jelly like structure to that of a tough matrix due to the presence of mucopolysaccharide, chondrocyte cells, hyaluronic acid.

In cartilage chondroitin sulphate is abundant. In soft C.T. and skin-hyaluronic acid.

Adipose tissue: a specialized C.T.

Fat tissues are found scattered or grouped in loose C.T.

Usually seen in subcutaneous C.T., around kidneys, in the omentum around and in between certain muscles and organs.

Muscle Tissue

Essential structural unit is muscle fiber

Diameter of muscle fiber – varies with sex, age, species, plane of nutrition etc.

Consists of a sarcolemmal membrane, Sarcoplasmic reticulum, nuclei, mitochondria, golgi bodies, 'T' system, contractile proteins myofibrils.

Muscle fibers are narrow, cylindrical, tapered and multinucleated

Each muscle fiber is surrounded by sarcolemma, a double layered structure, 50-60 angstrom apart, transmit the contraction force. There may be spiral collagenous structure connecting endomysium and sarcolemma.

Inside sarcolemma occur, the myofibrils which are surrounded by sarcoplasm.

Sarcoplasm contains mitochondria or sarcosomes, sarcoplasmic reticulum, lipid bodies, sarcotubular system (T-system), certain dissolved suspended substance.

Nuclei found just below the sarcolemma, ovoid shape, flattened or elongated, more numerous towards tendinous attachment.

Contain genetic material DNA responsible for behaviour and activity

Principal component are nucleolus, chromatin and nuclear matrix, nucleolus are rich in RNA, chromatin – DNA chromosomal substance.

Chromatin and nucleolus are dispersed in the nuclear matrix.

Nucleolus plays key role in nucleic acid metabolism and protein synthesis.

Mitochondria

Fibrous matrix and crystal components

Functional role – citric acid cycle and oxidative phosphorylation

No. of mitochondria varies from cell to cell depending upon its activity.

Myofibril

Surrounded by membrane bounded tubules and vesicles.

Longitudinal tubules *i.e.* sarcolpasmic reticulum run parallel to the myofibrils and are linked at intervals along the sarcomeres.

The transverse tubules run transversely across the fibrils as invaginations of the sarcolemma (T system)

The two series of tubules do not join but their walls are in contact with each other.

Function of sarcoplasmic reticulum is to conduct impulses from the sarcolemma to the contracile system.

The muscle fiber contains myofibrils, are unbranched, run along its long axis.

Myofibrils are striated – alternate light (I-band) and dark (A-band)

A-band has a central clear zone known as 'H-zones'.

I-band has a central dark zone called Z-line

Distance between two Z-line form the sarcomere – the functional unit of myofibrils

A-band is thicker than I-band

Thick filament contain contractile protein myosin

Thin filament contain contractile protein actin

Cross section of a myofibril reveal that each myosin filament is surrounded by six actin filaments in a hexagonal array.

There is a fine zone in the centre of the myosin filament known as 'M' zone

M-zone contain M-bridges – are linked by thin filaments running between those of myosin and are responsible for central alignment of the myosin in the sarcomere.

Chemical Composition of Poultry Meat

Body tissues – a number of chemical elements, water, protein, fat, carbohydrates

Elements – C, H, O, N form 96 per cent of total body chemical composition

Water forms 67 to 68 per cent of the soft tissues

Fat molecules – C, H, O

Protein – C, H, O + nitrogen sulfur, phosphorus

Inorganic elements – range between 1.5 to 3.4 per cent of body's elemental composition.

Skeletal muscle – principal component of meat – contain water, protein, fat, carbohydrate, inorganic matter.

Water

Largest component, 56-74 per cent, associated with cellular structure, colloidal protein molecules, a medium for transporting nutrients, metabolites from vascular bed to muscle tissues, a medium through which various chemical and metabolic activities occur.

Protein

forms around 20 to 35 per cent of edible meat tissues – it is necessary for the structure and various other vital functions of the muscle tissues.

1. Sorcoplasmic proteins
2. Myofibrillar proteins
3. Stromal protein

Myofibrillar proteins: Consists of myosin, actin, tropomyosin, troponin, M-protein, C-protein, α-actinin and β-actinin; require intermediate to high ionic strength buffers for their extraction.

Sarcoplasmic Proteins

Soluble sarcoplasmic and mitochondrial proteins, myoglobin, haemoglobin, cytochromes, flavoproteins-readily extractable in water or buffers of low ionic strength.

Stroma Proteins

Connective tissues and (collagen, reticulin, elastin) associated fibrous proteins, comparatively insoluble.

Fat

Widely variable ranging between 6.9 to 12.1 per cent depending on the breed, sex, age, feed, environment and other managemental conditions. Primarily made up of neutral lipids (triglycerides) and phospholipids.

Carbohydrates

Usually small quantity. 100g of chicken meat hardly contribute 150 to 300 calories of energy and carbohydrate in it is around 2 per cent of edible tissue. Present as glycogen content of muscle tissue, mucopolysaccharides of connective tissue or intermediate of glycolytic metabolism.

Inorganic Matter

Ranges from 1.0 to 1.3 per cent of the meat tissue. Among many inorganic substances those which are of physiological significance are Ca, Mg, K, Na, Fe, P, S and Cl.

Factors Influencing Composition of Poultry Meat

1. Type of Bird

Chicken hen – the edible portion of meat contain 56 per cent moisture. Turkey – 58 per cent moisture. Same trend for calories and proteins. Broiler meat – 151 calories/ 100g Turkey meat – 268 calories. Turkey white meat (roasted) – 34.3 per cent protein, chicken (roasted) – 31.5 per cent protein. Duck muscle tissue – higher amount of linoleic acid and linolenic acid when compared to turkey and chicken. Goose and Pigeon muscle tissue – higher amount of oleic acid when compared to turkey, chicken and duck.

2. Sex of Bird

Male broiler carcasses – more moisture and protein but less of fat as compared to females *e.g.* Broilers of 59 days contain:

Sex	*Moisture per cent*	*Protein per cent*	*Fat per cent*
Male	63.2	19.3	14.3
Female	60.4	19.0	17.4

Besides, riboflavin content is higher in muscle tissue of male birds than females.

3. Age of the Bird

1. Broilers – 71 per cent Moisture
2. Roaster – 66 per cent Moisture
3. Hens – 56 per cent moisture
4. Broiler (4wk) – thiamine and riboflavin content superior to broiler (8wk). Birds of 28 days – significantly lesser amount of protein and fat as compared to bird aged 59 days.

4. Diets

In almost all birds *i.e.* chicken, turkey, duck carcass; fat increase with rise in dietary fat. A wide calorie: Protein ratio in diet resulted in an increase in fat deposition. Chicks store more vitamin A from alfalfa than from carotene or vitamin A feeding. Increase store of niacin in breast and liver at higher level of niacin intake.

Carcass protein was increased and fat was decreased in a linear manner with the increasing level of dietary protein.

Increasing level of dietary energy resulted in decreased carcass protein and increased carcass fat.

Type of dietary fat influences carcass fat score, carcass composition and cooking loss.

High protein diet resulted in slow growth rate, less body fat than those fed with medium protein diet.

5. Environmental Temperature

Birds subjected to higher environ temperature had reduced growth and feed consumption; but there was no change in moisture or fat of carcass.

However fatty acid composition of the carcass altered.

With increasing ambient temperature and energy level of the diet the carcass fat of the birds went up and the protein content came down.

6. Hormone

12 mg diethylstilbosterol implanted to 7 wk broiler – carcass fat increased to 16.9 per cent against 11.9 per cent in control bird.

Chickens given 0.5 mg DES per day for 28 days contained 8 per cent carcass fat while their control counterparts had only 3.9 per cent fat.

Nutritive Value of Poultry Meat

Poultry meat occupies an important position in our diet from the nutritional point of view.

Low in calories.

A good source of saturated fatty acids(SFA),unsaturated fatty acids(UFA) and essential fatty acids(FA)

Protein content is higher than other types of red meats and the proteins are a good source of essential amino acids.

The muscle fibers of meat are tender, easy to chew or grind, easy to digest.

Flavour of meat is mild that blends well with different seasonings

Carbohydrate content is low so not a good source of energy

Good for the people want to reduce their body weight without sparing protein requirement.

Moisture content: According to USDA, edible portion of chicken broilers contains about 71 per cent moisture, roasters 66 per cent, hens 56 per cent and medium fat turkeys about 58 per cent. Carcasses from young birds have a higher proportions of moisture to tissue than old ones.

Calories

Poultry meat is low in calories in relation to other nutrients present. For this reason poultry is a good foodstuff for weight control diets, convalescents and old people who are not physically active. By eating poultry meat as the source of proteins in a diet, it is possible to reduce caloric intake but at the same time help keep other nutrient requirements in proper balance. Broilers contain 160 calories per 100 gm of meat, roasters 198, hens 300, duck meat 185, and turkey meat 170 calories.

Protein in Diet

Very important because of physiological role of protein – constituent of muscles and vital body fluid; replace wear and tear of tissue, so proteins are body building foods; vital life processes, enzymes, hormones, antibodies – body defense. So sufficient quantity of protein in diet is necessary. Starchy foods (cassava, potato, sweet potato) – very little protein. Fruit – low proteins. Green leaf of vegetables – good source of vitamins and minerals but not protein. Pulses and nuts – rich source of protein. Animal foods – meat, fish, egg are the richest source of protein.

Not only quantity of protein but also its quality matters

Proteins in different foods differ in their nutritive value because of their amino acid composition

Based on the amino acid composition proteins are classified as first, second and third class proteins

Poultry meat provides the first class protein as it contains all the essential amino acids in balanced proportion necessary for promoting growth and maintaining life.

Cereals are deficient in lysine and threonine, pulses are deficient in sulfur containing amino acids *i.e.* methionine, cystein etc.; while poultry meat contain all these essential amino acids. Hence vegetarian diet should be blended with poultry meat. In India availability of total protein/capita/day is 55g. In developed countries availability of total protein/capita is 82-120g. Availability from animal sources in India 4-8.9g/cap/day. Availability in developed countries is 30-75g/cap/day.

Poultry meat is superior in biological value as compared to vegetable proteins. It is not only a good source of protein but it contains more proteins than red meats. Poultry white meat contains 31.5 per cent protein and dark meat contains 25.4 per cent protein. Cooked poultry meat, excluding edible viscera, contains from 25-35 per cent protein depending upon the part of the carcass and the method of preparation. Beef contains 21-27 per cent, pork 23-24 per cent and lamb 21-24 per cent. Poultry meat contains high quality protein. It is easy to digest and contains all the essential amino acids presently known to be required in human diets. The amino acid composition of turkey is similar to chicken, beef and pork. Since poultry contains a higher proportion of proteins than other meats it also contains more amino acids.

Fat in Diet

Important, conc. source of energy. Supplies per unit weight double the energy than protein or carbohydrate. In normal Indian diet– pure fat or oil consumed as such and meat makes very little contribution. Most fat in poultry is sub-cutaneous. The fat content of poultry carcasses varies according to the age, sex and species of poultry as well as the part of the carcass from which the fat is taken. For example, cooked turkey skin contains 33.8 per cent fat whereas the breast meat contains only

6.7 to 8.3 per cent. Unlike red meats, most fat in poultry meat is found under the skin rather than distributed throughout the tissues. Cooked chicken breast meat contains only 1.3 per cent fat, veal cutlets 11 per cent, beef cuts from 13-30 per cent. Not only the amount of fat in a diet is important but also the type of fat *i.e.* saturated/unsaturated. One measure of degree of saturation or unsaturation is the iodine number. Low iodine values indicates saturated fats, high ones unsaturated. Poultry meats contain a higher proportion of unsaturated fatty acids than the fats from red meats but less than fats or oils of vegetable origin. Poultry meat also contain less cholesterol than other foods of animal origin.

Daily intake of fat should be such that it contribute 15 to 20 per cent of calories in the diet.

A total of 40 to 60g of fat can be easily and safely consumed daily.

Essential fatty acids in poultry meat are linoleic, linolenic and arachidonic required for maintaining health, necessary constituent of cell wall, mitochondria and other active metabolic sites.

Table 15.1: Essential Fatty Acids in Poultry Meat

Saturated Fatty Acids (FA) in Chicken Meat – 28.32 per cent, duck meat – 28.33 per cent, turkey meat – 27.0 per cent

	Chicken	*Duck*	*Turkey*
Oleic acid per cent	47.5	39.5	45.0
Linoleic per cent	18.0	24.0	18.0
Linolenic per cent	1.0	1.4	1.0
Arachidonic per cent	0.5	0.2	0.5

Type of fat in diet is important rather than quantity of fat. High per cent of SFA – high blood cholesterol level. In this respect poultry meat scores over red meat as it contains higher proportion of unsaturated F.A. Diet deficient in essential fatty acids – cause perianal i of rritation in children, changes in skin, dryness, thickness, desquamation, oozing, development folds. Common disorder – "phyrnoderma" – charcacterized by presence of horny papular eruptive on posterior and lateral aspects of limbs, back.

Vitamins

Important life processor, essential for health. Poultry good source of B-vitamins, B_{12} niacin – pellagra (Sourness of tounge, pigmnted scaly skin, diarrhoea) requirement of this vit. is 10mg/day. Poultry meat also moderately good source of riboflavin, thiamin. Poultry meat is a good source of niacin and a moderately good source of riboflavin, thiamin and ascorbic acid. Uncooked chicken livers contain 32,500 i.u. of viatmin A, 0.20 mg of thiamine, 2.46mg of riboflavin, 11.8mg of niacin and 20mg of ascorbic acid. Other edible parts of the carcass contain thiamin, riboflavin and niacin but in smaller quantities than found in liver.

Minerals

Poultry meat contains sodium, potassium magnesium, calcium, iron, phosphorus, sulfur, chlorine and iodine - necessary for bones, teeth, soft tissues, essential for body fluids – Na, K, Cl, Muscle – phosphors, Blood – hemoglobin, thyroxine – iodine.

Table 15.2: Nutritive Value of Poultry and Poultry Products

Food No.	Food Description	Measure of edible portion	Weight (g)	Water (%)	Calories (kcal)	Protein (g)	Total fat (g)	Fatty acids: Saturated (g)	Fatty acids: Monounsaturated (g)	Fatty acids: Polyunsaturated (g)
	Poultry and Poultry Products									
	Chicken									
	Fried in vegetable shortening, meat with skin									
	Batter dipped									
868	Breast, ½ breast (5.6 oz with bones)	½ breast	140	52	364	35	18	4.9	7.6	4.3
869	Drumstick (3.4 oz with bones)	1 drumstick	72	53	193	16	11	3.0	4.6	2.7
870	Thigh	1 thigh	86	52	238	19	14	3.8	5.8	3.4
871	Wing	1 wing	49	46	159	10	11	2.9	4.4	2.5
	Flour coated									
872	Breast, ½ breast (4.2 oz with bones)	½ breast	98	57	218	31	9	2.4	3.4	1.9
873	Drumstick (2.6 oz with bones)	1 drumstick	49	57	120	13	7	1.8	2.7	1.6
	Fried, meat only									
874	Dark meat	3 oz	85	56	203	25	10	2.7	3.7	2.4
875	Light meat	3 oz	85	60	163	28	5	1.3	1.7	1.1
	Roasted, meat only									
876	Breast, ½ breast (4.2 oz with bone and skin)	½ breast	86	65	142	27	3	0.9	1.1	0.7
877	Drumstick (2.9 oz with bone and skin)	1 drumstick	44	67	76	12	2	0.7	0.8	0.6
878	Thigh	1 thigh	52	63	109	13	6	1.6	2.2	1.3
879	Stewed, meat only, light and dark meat, chopped or diced	1 cup	140	56	332	43	17	4.3	5.7	4.0
880	Chicken giblets, simmered, chopped	1 cup	145	68	228	37	7	2.2	1.7	1.6
881	Chicken liver, simmered	1 liver	20	68	31	5	1	0.4	0.3	0.2
882	Chicken neck, meat only, simmered	1 neck	18	67	32	4	1	0.4	0.5	0.4
883	Duck, roasted, flesh only	½ duck	221	64	444	52	25	9.2	8.2	3.2
	Turkey									
	Roasted, meat only									
884	Dark meat	3 oz	85	63	159	24	6	2.1	1.4	1.8
885	Light meat	3 oz	85	66	133	25	3	0.9	0.5	0.7
886	Light and dark meat, chopped or diced	1 cup	140	65	238	41	7	2.3	1.4	2.0
	Ground, cooked									
887	Patty, from 4 oz raw	1 patty	82	59	193	22	11	2.8	4.0	2.6
888	Crumbled	1 cup	127	59	298	35	17	4.3	6.2	4.1
889	Turkey giblets, simmered, chopped	1 cup	145	65	242	39	7	2.2	1.7	1.7
890	Turkey neck, meat only, simmered	1 neck	152	65	274	41	11	3.7	2.5	3.3
	Poultry food products									
	Chicken									
891	Canned, boneless	5 oz	142	69	234	31	11	3.1	4.5	2.5
892	Frankfurter (10 per 1 lb pkg)	1 frank	45	58	116	6	9	2.5	3.8	1.8
893	Roll, light meat (6 slices per 6-oz pkg)	2 slices	57	69	90	11	4	1.1	1.7	0.9

Contd...

Table 15.2–*Contd...*

Choles-terol (mg)	Carbo-hydrate (g)	Total dietary fiber (g)	Calcium (mg)	Iron (mg)	Potas-sium (mg)	Sodium (mg)	Vitamin A (IU)	Vitamin A (RE)	Thiamin (mg)	Ribo-flavin (mg)	Niacin (mg)	Ascor-bic acid (mg)	Food No.
119	13	0.4	28	1.8	281	385	94	28	0.16	0.20	14.7	0	868
62	6	0.2	12	1.0	134	194	62	19	0.08	0.15	3.7	0	869
80	8	0.3	15	1.2	165	248	82	25	0.10	0.20	4.9	0	870
39	5	0.1	10	0.6	68	157	55	17	0.05	0.07	2.6	0	871
87	2	0.1	16	1.2	254	74	49	15	0.08	0.13	13.5	0	872
44	1	Tr	6	0.7	112	44	41	12	0.04	0.11	3.0	0	873
82	2	0.0	15	1.3	215	82	67	20	0.08	0.21	6.0	0	874
77	Tr	0.0	14	1.0	224	69	26	8	0.06	0.11	11.4	0	875
73	0	0.0	13	0.9	220	64	18	5	0.06	0.10	11.8	0	876
41	0	0.0	5	0.6	108	42	26	8	0.03	0.10	2.7	0	877
49	0	0.0	6	0.7	124	46	34	10	0.04	0.12	3.4	0	878
116	0	0.0	18	2.0	283	109	157	46	0.16	0.39	9.0	0	879
570	1	0.0	17	9.3	229	84	10,775	3,232	0.13	1.38	5.9	12	880
126	Tr	0.0	3	1.7	28	10	3,275	983	0.03	0.35	0.9	3	881
14	0	0.0	8	0.5	25	12	22	6	0.01	0.05	0.7	0	882
197	0	0.0	27	6.0	557	144	170	51	0.57	1.04	11.3	0	883
72	0	0.0	27	2.0	247	67	0	0	0.05	0.21	3.1	0	884
59	0	0.0	16	1.1	259	54	0	0	0.05	0.11	5.8	0	885
106	0	0.0	35	2.5	417	98	0	0	0.09	0.25	7.6	0	886
84	0	0.0	21	1.6	221	88	0	0	0.04	0.14	4.0	0	887
130	0	0.0	32	2.5	343	136	0	0	0.07	0.21	6.1	0	888
606	3	0.0	19	9.7	290	86	8,752	2,603	0.07	1.31	6.5	2	889
185	0	0.0	56	3.5	226	85	0	0	0.05	0.29	2.6	0	890
88	0	0.0	20	2.2	196	714	166	48	0.02	0.18	9.0	3	891
45	3	0.0	43	0.9	38	617	59	17	0.03	0.05	1.4	0	892
28	1	0.0	24	0.5	129	331	46	14	0.04	0.07	3.0	0	893

Poultry Meat in Special Diets

Poultry meat is an ideal food for infants, young children, adolescents, adults, old people, convalescents and those attempting to control their weight. Because of its high meat yield and low shrinkage during cooking, serving poultry meat fits well on the menu of restaurants, hotels, airlines, hospitals, schools and institutions.

Why chicken is important in hospital diet?

- ☆ Patients and staff like it and readily accept well prepared chicken
- ☆ Adapted to many special diets eg. Broiled and boiled chicken for all age groups and easy to digest.

- Chicken drumsticks are easy to eat for patients who are too young or incapable of handling knives or forks.
- The endless ways in which chicken can be cooked
- The cost per pound of edible meat and the nutrient return for the money spent, chicken is the best buy.
- Chicken also lends itself well to a portion of low-sodium diets.

References

Poultry Meat Processing. Alan R. Sams, Department of poultry Science, Texas A and M university, 2001

Meat and Meat Products Technology (Including Poultry Products Technology). B. D. Sharma, 1999

Meat Products Handbook (Practical Science and Technology) Gerhard Fischer, 2006.

Indian Food Industry, Vol. 20, No. 3, May–Jun '01, Modern Trends in Packaging of Meat and Poultry

Poultry Products Processing: An Industry Guide, Shai Barbut, 2001.

Nutritive Value of Foods. Susan E. Gebhardt and Robin G. Thomas, USDA, Agricultural Research Service Home and Garden Bulletin Number 72, 2002.

Internet source (Indian chicken recipe.com, surf India.com, Patna daily.com)

Nutritive Superiority of Turkey Meat

Where does the Name "Turkey" come from?

Now, a lot of people may think they know what - or who- a turkey is. But to really be in the know, take a look at this. The name turkey was originally applied to an African bird (now known as the guinea fowl) which was believed to have come from Turkey. When the Europeans stumbled on the American turkey, they thought it was the same bird - so they named it "turkey".

How much Turkey do we Eat a Year?

This will amaze you. In 1996, it was estimated that we each ate almost 15 pounds of turkey. Clearly, turkey is heading for our dinner plates more often than just the holidays.

Which is Better: A "Hen" Turkey or a "Tom"?

This is an equal opportunity world. And the answer to this question is - they're equally good! Actually, the designation of "hen" (female) or "tom" (male) is optional on the label and is an indication of size. Toms are larger.

What's the Nutrient Content of Turkey?

There's a lot of good news here. Turkey provides a significant amount of protein as well as other nutrients. Fat, saturated fat and cholesterol are also present, with most of the fat being in the skin. A three ounce serving of baked turkey breast with skin has 160 calories, 6 grams of fat, 65 milligrams of cholesterol and 24 grams of prtein. Without skin: 120 calories, 1 gram of fat, 55 milligrams of cholesterol and 26 grams of protein.

How Long can you Keep Turkey in the Fridge or Freezer?

Fresh whole turkey and fresh turkey parts should be cooked (or frozen) within one to two days of purchase. A whole turkey (uncooked) can be frozen for up to 12 months before quality gradually declines.

When is it "Done"?

For tenderness and doneness, the internal temperature, as registered on a meat thermometer, must reach a minimum of 180°F in the innermost part of the thigh before removing the turkey from the oven. For optimum safety and uniform doneness, we recommend cooking stuffing outside the bird. If you do stuff it, the center of the stuffing must reach 165°F before you remove it from the bird.

How about Safe Grilling and Smoking?

More and more people are heading outdoors to cook the turkey, so it is important to know how to do it safely.

When you grill remember that cooking times vary, depending on many factors, including the size of the turkey and the distance from the coals. We recommend that you don't stuff the turkey. It will cook more evenly and safely without it. Replenish the grill with approximately 15 briquettes every hour. The turkey is done when a meat thermometer in the inner thigh reaches 180° F.

When you smoke you are using both heat and moisture to cook your food. So, be sure to add liquid to the drip pan. Be aware that some smokers has a built-in temperature indicator. If yours doesn't, place an appliance thermometer on the food rack to monitor the air temperature.

When the thermometer reaches 225 to 300° F, place the turkey on the rack, and quickly replace the cover. As with grilling, we recommend that you don't stuff the turkey. Because your take too long for heat to reach the stuffing.

Smoking takes longer than grilling, so follow the manufacturer's estimated cooking times. Add fresh charcoal every hour to maintain temperture of 225 to 300° F and ensure smoke. Also add liquid to the water pan as needed. As with grilling, the turkey is done when a meat thermometer inserted into the inner thigh reaches 180° F.

How Long can you Keep Cooked Yurkey?

Cooked turkey and cooked turkey dishes can be kept in the refrigator for three to four days. After than, freeze them or pitch them. Cooked turkey will maintain quality in the freezer for four months, turkey dishes for four to six months.

Did you know Turkey is a Superfood? It's the only meat included in the bestselling book Superfoods: 14 Foods that will Change your Life by Dr Steven Pratt. He says everyone should try to eat a 100g portion of turkey three or four times a week because it is "the leanest meat source of protein available on the planet".

His other 13 "superfoods" are: tomatoes, broccoli, beans, blueberries, tea, oats, pumpkin, yoghurt, walnuts, spinach, salmon, soy, and oranges. Dr Pratt says: "These foods prevent disease and extend our health span, and perhaps our life span as well." His research shows the foods could prevent or even reverse heart disease, diabetes, dementia and cancer.

See below the nutrients in turkey, which Dr Pratt says are beneficial for healthy hearts and in helping to lower the risk of cancer.

More information can be found at http://www.britishturkey.co.uk

Turkey is one of the lowest fat mainstream meats available and is also lower in fat than many commonly eaten foods.

100g grilled turkey breast meat without skin contains just 155 calories and 1.7g fat.

Turkey contains B vitamins, including Niacin (B3), which helps convert carbohydrate into energy, nerve function and digestion.

100g of raw turkey meat contains 7.9mg of Niacin - that's 61 per cent of the Recommended Nutrient Intake for females and 46 per cent for males.

Turkey is a source of Zinc which is essential for a healthy immune system, healing cuts and grazes, and needed for the body to metabolise fat, protein and carbohydrate.

100g of raw turkey meat contains 1.7mg of Zinc - that's 24 per cent of the Recommended Nutrient Intake for females and 18 per cent for males

Turkey is high in protein, and contains all the essential amino acids closely matched to our body's needs. Nearly all protein found in turkey meat can therefore be used to maintain cellular integrity and function.

100g of Bernard Matthews Honey Roast Turkey contains 23.5g of protein - that's 51 per cent of the Recommended Nutrient Intake for females and 42 per cent for males

Table 15.3: Nutritional Comparison per 100g of different Meats (McCance and Widdowson's The Composition of Food, 1998)

Meat Types	*Energy Value (Kcal)*	*Fat (g)*	*Protein (g)*
Turkey Meat, light meat raw	103	1.1	23.2
Turkey Meat, light meat cooked	132	1.4	29.8
Chicken, light meat raw	116	3.2	21.8
Chicken, light meat cooked	142	4.0	26.5
Pork, trimmed lean average	123	4.0	21.8
Pork, loin chop 30 per cent fat	270	18.6	21.7
Beef, trimmed lean average	123	4.6	20.3
Beef, minced cooked	229	15.2	23.1
Lamb, trimmed lean average	162	8.8	20.8
Lamb, chump steaks, lean and fat grilled	355	29.0	23.5

Turkey is a SuperFood!

Dr. Steven G. Pratt, author of the New York Times Best Seller SuperFoods Rx: Fourteen Foods That Will Change Your Life, has taken fourteen everyday foods that are full of nutrients and vitamins and shows readers how to use these products as part of their everyday meals to help them live healthier lives.

Turkey was named as one of these SuperFoods! After studying the most disease-preventing, anti-aging diets, scientists found that the same nutrients repeatedly came up. Superfoods Rx shows people how to eat well using these fourteen foods so they can feel better, prevent disease, get energized and live healthier lives.

Not only is turkey a delicious source of lean protein, but studies now show that it is linked to providing nutrients that prevent disease and promote a healthy lifestyle. The SuperFoods are rich in nutrients and relatively low in calories and more importantly help prevent diabetes, heart disease and some cancers. Turkey is among the nutrient packed foods promoted by this study because it is the perfect example of a healthy protein source that is very low in fat and provides many nutrients that help build a strong immune system.

Microbiological Quality of Poultry Meat

Introduction

The microbiological safety and quality of poultry meat are equally important to producers, retailers and consumers, and both involve microbial contaminants on the processed product.

Two quite different groups of microorganisms are relevant: on the one hand certain foodborne pathogens and on the other, spoilage organisms that are generally harmless to human health, but, being psychrotrophic, are able to muliply on the product during chill storage. Spoilage results mainly from 'off-odour development, and product shelf-life is determined both by the number of spoilage organisms present initially and the temperature history of the product at all stages of production and subsequent storage and handling (Pooni and Mead, 1984). For chill-stored poultry, Viehweg *et al.* (1989) demonstrated that virtually all the odorous substances found at spoilage could be attributed to microbial growth and metabolism.

Foodborne Pathogens in Poultry Meat

Contamination of poultry meat with foodborne pathogens remains an important public health issue, because it can lead to illness if there are malpractices in handling, cooking or post-cooking storage of the product. In developed countries, foodborne illness causes human suffering and loss of productivity, and adds significantly to the costs of food production and healthcare. It is also a possible cause of mortality, which is even more of a problem in developing regions, where the health status of many individuals is already compromised.

Salmonella and *Campylobacter* spp.

Numerically, the most important agents are Salmonella and Campylobacter spp. Data for the European Union (EU) show that in 2001, there were157 822 reported cases of human salmonellosis and 156 232 cases of Campylobacter enteritis (Cavitte, 2003), although both diseases are known to be under-reported, and the true figures are likely to be considerably higher. While poultry is by no means the only source of the causative organisms, it is widely recognised as a major reservoir in each case, due to symptomless carriage in the live bird (Table 15.3). The problem is exacerbated by modern conditions of intensive rearing, where large numbers of birds are kept together, and high-rate processing, in which carcasses remain in close proximity throughout the operation. Such conditions favour the spread of any pathogens that may gain access to the flock. Moreover, the use of antimicrobials in poultry production, whether for prophylactic, therapeutic or performance-enhancing purposes, contributes to the development of resistance in pathogens, which is increasing, and can have serious consequences for the treatment of human illness from these organisms. With salmonellosis, for example, the testing of 27 000 isolates from human cases in ten European countries in 2000, showed that almost 40 per cent were resistant to at least one antimicrobial, while 18 per cent were multiresistant (Threlfall *et al.*, 2003).

Multiple resistance was most often observed in serotype Typhimurium, including DTs 104 and 204b, and 51 per cent of Typhimurium strains were in this category. Serotypes from humans with multiple resistance include those that are also found in poultry, of which S Paratyphi B variant Java is the most recent example. In the Netherlands, variant Java had increased in poultry from less than 2 per cent of isolates before 1996 to 60 per cent in 2003 (van Pelt *et al.*, 2003). The resistance of Campylobacter to antimicrobials is also rising, especially to fluoroquinolones, which have been widely used in both human and veterinary medicine. Although Salmonella and Campylobacter spp. are the predominant foodborne pathogens associated with poultry and are frequently implicated in human illness from this source, other pathogens also occur, including Clostridium perfringens, Escherichia coli 0157 and Listeria monocytogenes, together with those recognised more recently, such as Arcobacter and Helicobacter spp. (Corry and Atabay, 2001). This review will consider the more important contaminants of poultry meat in relation to product safety and shelf-life. Also discussed is the present status of control measures, including application of the Hazard Analysis Critical Control Point (HACCP) system and the benefits likely to arise from the use of Quantitative Risk Assessment as a management tool in the control of foodborne pathogens and contamination of poultry carcasses and parts with these organisms is well documented and data are available for many parts of the world (*e.g.* Waldroup 1996; Simmons *et al.*, 2003). Most salmonellas found on poultry meat are non-host-specific and are considered capable of causing human food poisoning. The thermophilic campylobacters are mainly *C. jejuni*, which is the principal cause of human campylobacteriosis, but other, so-called 'campylobacteria' also occur frequently, and include species of Acrobacter and *Helicobacter pullorum*. Their potential for causing human illness has been discussed by Corry and Atabay (2001). For processed poultry, both the proportion of positive samples and the number of organisms present per unit sample is greater for Campylobacter than it is for Salmonella, reflecting the greater colonising ability and higher level of intestinal carriage at slaughter (Table 15.3), which can be up to 10^9cfu/g. With Salmonella, there is wide variation in the incidence of positive carcasses, but counts rarely exceed 100 cfu/carcass, well below the level normally associated with food poisoning. However, both types of bacteria include strains that are invasive in poultry and can penetrate internal organs or deep tissues of the bird, where the organisms may be less readily destroyed by cooking. On the surface, campylobacter contamination tends to be relatively high, up to 10^9cfu/carcass. Since the infective dose is only a few hundred viable cells, illness can easily result from handling raw poultry without suitable hygiene precautions, and is a potential hazard for new staff in poultry processing plants.

Table 15.4: Characteristics of *Campylobacter* and *Salmonella*

Feature	*Campylobacter*	*Salmonella*
Host susceptibility	Not age-related	Age-related
Preferred site	Caeca	Caeca
Preferred niche	Mucus in crypts	None
Colonisation type	Persistent	Transient/intermittent
Carriage level	Relatively high	Variable
Invasiveness	Some strains	Some strains
Colonisation genes	Some identified	Some identified

Salmonellas survive well in the environment, but campylobacters appear less well-adapted to survival outside the alimentary tract of warm-blooded animals. Also, growth only occurs under conditions of high moisture, reduced oxygen and an environmental temperature above 30 °C. The organisms are particularly sensitive to drying and the effects of freezing and thawing, which can cause a 1 – 2 log reduction in the level of contamination on poultry meat. However, campylobacters have many different hosts, they colonise at high levels and therefore are shed into the environment in large numbers. There is still much debate about possible survival mechanisms outside the host, including the ability to exist in a supposedly dormant form, in which the organisms appear to be viable, but non-culturable by conventional methods. From the practical viewpoint, campylobacters can persist as contaminants of poultry products throughout the entire supply chain and remain detectable by cultural methods. A key factor in their survival may be their attachment to, or entrapment in, poultry tissues during carcass processing. In this situation, their resistance to adverse conditions, like that of other bacteria, is significantly increased. Thus, the organisms can survive on carcasses during processes such as scalding, washing and water chilling, that might otherwise remove or destroy them As a cause of human food poisoning, this is not among the more dangerous pathogens. It is, however, a spore-forming organism and some strains produces spores that are unusually heat-resistant. Therefore, unlike vegetative bacterial cells, the spores are not necessarily destroyed by normal cooking and may subsequently germinate and outgrow to hazardous levels, if post-cooking storage is inadequate. In fact, most outbreaks involve strains that produce the more heat-resistant spores. In a survey of food-poisoning outbreaks associated with poultry in England and Wales during 1992 - 1999, Cl. perfringens was found to be responsible for 21 per cent of the outbreaks, second only to Salmonella as a causative agent (Kessel *et al.*, 2001). In some instances, the problem arose from consumption of contaminated turkey at Christmas time, when storage of the larger, whole carcasses used for festive meals appears to have been at fault. The organism is an obligate anaerobe that is relatively tolerant to oxygen and can be found in low numbers in the alimentary tract of poultry. When present in meat crevices etc, growth is favoured by conditions in which oxygen has been dispelled by cooking. However, since growth of the organism cannot occur if the meat is held below 15°C, the problem is easily avoided by refrigerated storage.

E. coli 0157

Verocytotoxin-producing strains of *E. coli* (VTEC), cause diarrhoea and haemorrhagic colitis in humans and can lead to potentially life-threatening sequelae, such as haemolytic uraemic syndrome and thrombotic thrombocytopaenic purpura. Although VTEC strains occur in a wide range of O serogroups, the most important in human disease is 0157, which accounts for almost all major foodborne outbreaks in Europe and the USA. In England and Wales, the first case involving this organism occurred in 1982 and reported cases have increased steadily since then, reaching a peak of 1087 in 1997 (PHLS data). While VTEC 0157 is mostly found in ruminant animals, it is occasionally associated with other livestock and various foods of animal origin. To what extent is the organism a matter of concern in relation to poultry? An outbreak in the UK that was associated with eating turkey roll was reported by Salmon *et al.* (1989) and two further outbreaks linked Salmonellas survive well in the environment, but campylobacters appear less well-adapted to survival outside the alimentary tract of warm-blooded animals. Also, growth only occurs under conditions of high moisture, reduced oxygen and an environmental temperature above 30 ° C. The organisms are particularly sensitive to drying and the effects of freezing and thawing, which can cause a 1 - 2 log reduction in the level of contamination on poultry meat. However, campylobacters have many different hosts, they colonise at high levels and therefore are shed into the environment in large numbers. There is still much debate about possible survival mechanisms outside the host, including the ability to exist in a supposedly dormant form, in which the organisms appear to be viable, but non-culturable by conventional methods. From the practical viewpoint, campylobacters can persist as contaminants of poultry products throughout the entire supply chain and remain detectable by cultural methods. A key factor in their survival may be their attachment to, or entrapment in, poultry tissues during carcass processing. In this situation, their resistance to adverse conditions, like that of other bacteria, is significantly increased. Thus, the organisms to chicken dishes were mentioned by Kessel *et al.* (2001). With all three, however, cross-contamination in the kitchen was suspected. Experience suggests that VTEC 0157 is rare in poultry, whether in live birds or on processed products, and, when it has been found, tests for the necessary virulence factors have not always been carried out. On the other hand, strains lacking Shiga toxin genes have been isolated from patients with typical disease symptoms (Schmidt *et al.*, 1999).

In an early survey of retail meats in the USA, Doyle and Schoeni (1987) found VTEC 0157 in 1.5 per cent of 263 samples of chicken and turkey leg meat. Although

Heuvelink *et al.* (1999) could find no VTEC 0157 in chicken faeces, 1.3 per cent of 459 pooled samples from turkeys were positive and one isolate contained genes for type 2 verotoxin, attaching-and-effacing capability and the relevant haemolysin. Because of these virulence factors, the strain appeared capable of causing illness in man. Only turkeys had been kept on the farm in question, so transfer of the strain from other livestock was unlikely. VTEC other than 0157 were found in 12 per cent of retail chicken samples and 7 per cent of turkey samples in the USA by Samadpour *et al.* (1994).

Despite the rarity of VTEC 0157 in poultry, experimental studies have shown that chicks can be readily colonised with a challenge dose as low as 10 cfu/bird (Schoeni and Doyle, 1994) and colonisation may persist for at least three months. Another study (Stavric *et al.*, 1993) showed that the organism was present, following challenge, on caecal mucosa and in the contents of the lumen. The extent of colonisation depended on dose, age, breed and time after exposure. However, colonisation could be reduced by competitive exclusion (CE) treatment, using a culture of faecal material from a pathogen-free donor bird. Hakkinen and Schneitz (1996) obtained a four-log reduction in colonisation, when a commercial CE product was used to treat chicks before challenge.

Since VTEC 0157 is capable of colonising poultry without causing illness in the birds, is present in some wild-bird vectors, survives well in soil and is able to grow in chicken manure held at ambient temperatures, it is surprising that the organism is not found more often in commercial broiler flocks. The significance of non-0157 VTEC, which also appear to occur in poultry, needs to be further investigated.

Listeria monocytogenes

The organism is a leading cause of food-related mortality and morbidity in man, and the majority of cases are believed to be foodborne. The symptoms vary widely and those affected are frequently among the most vulnerable groups in society. Nevertheless, despite the common occurrence of L. monocytogenes in a variety of foods, human listeriosis is relatively rare, which may be due in part to the high infective dose of ca 10^9 viable cells that appears to be necessary in most cases (Smerdon *et al.*, 2001). The organism is common on raw poultry meat and has been found on chicken,turkey, duck and pheasant. Numerous surveys have shown that more than 50 per cent of processed chicken carcasses are likely to be positive, although numbers are usually low, even $< 1/cm^2$ of skin.

The health hazard from contaminated, raw poultry is mainly one of cross-contamination in the kitchen, where the organism may spread to cooked foods or other ready-to-eat items, such as salad vegetables. There is also a potential problem with cooked poultry produced commercially. Although normal cooking destroys listerias, recontamination can occur during post-cooking handling at the factory, even with the most rigorous hygiene control. Since pre-cooked items are not necessarily reheated by consumers before being eaten, and the organism is capable of growth under chill conditions, strict microbiological limit values are considered necessary. At one extreme, in the USA, there is zero tolerance for L. monocytogenes in ready- to-eat poultry products, and periodical recalls of contaminated product batches have cost many millions of US dollars. A different approach is taken in the UK, and counts of Listeria spp. below 20 cfu/g are considered 'satisfactory'. In a recent survey of barbecued chicken sampled at retail (Williams et al.,2002), all 221 samples examined were in this category. Such a low level of product contamination does not suggest that any significant growth of the organism had occurred in positive samples.

Spoilage Organisms

When poultry meat is stored aerobically under chill conditions, the organisms that predominate at spoilage are invariably Pseudomonas spp., accompanied by lower numbers of other Gram-negative bacteria (Table 15.4). Using numerical taxonomy, Arnaut-Rollier *et al.* (1999) found four major clusters of pseudomonads: Ps fragi, Ps lundensis, Ps fluorescens biovars and an unidentified group resembling Ps fluorescens. Other bacteria that are sometimes present include Shewanella putrefaciens and psychrotrophic strains of Enterobacteriaceae. The above organisms are common in soil and water, and are thought to originate from the live-bird environment. Yeasts, too, can be involved in spoilage and may be more important in this respect than was previously thought.

The more recent development of relatively low-cost gas-packaging for poultry has resulted in widespread use of this technology for retail presentation of chilled poultry-meat products. The approach is based on the known inhibitory effects of carbon dioxide atmospheres, in the range 10 - 30 per cent, on the growth of aerobic spoilage bacteria (Mead, 2004). Under these conditions, a different, slower-growing microflora develops (Table 15.5), while pseudomonads, in particular, are suppressed. At spoilage, the predominant organisms are usually lactic acid bacteria, but other Gram-positive and Gram-negative bacteria can occur in relatively large numbers.

Table 15.5: Poultry Meat Spoilage Bacteria under Chill Conditions

Aerobic Storage	*Modified-Atmosphere Storage*
Pseudomonas	Lactobacillus
Acinetobacter	Carnobacterium
Moraxella	Brochothrix
Psychrobacter	Shewanella
	Enterobacteriaceae
* Candida	[psychrotrophic strains]
* Yarrowia	–
* Yeasts	–

Control of Product Contamination

For food to be entirely safe from the microbiological viewpoint, it would need to be free from all pathogenic organisms. It is widely recognised, however, that this is not a realistic goal for raw poultry meat. There is still no economically viable means of eliminating foodborne pathogens in poultry-meat production, without the use of ionising radiation, which is presently unacceptable to many consumers. Therefore, some level of product contamination must be tolerated, although this varies widely from one country to another, especially in relation to Salmonella. In Sweden, which has a small poultry industry, the prevalence of Salmonella-contaminated poultry meat has been less than 1 per cent for many years and the organisms are rarely found in retail samples due to rigorous surveillance and control programmes that are relatively costly to operate (Persson and Jendteg, 1992). Food from which salmonellas are isolated in Sweden is, by law, considered unfit for human consumption. By contrast, countries with larger, more complex poultry industries

find control of Salmonella more difficult and subject to cost constraints. In the UK, improved practices in production and processing have led to a steady decline in the contamination rate, the latest survey of retail chicken showing only 5.7 per cent of samples positive, in comparison with almost 80 per cent some 20 years ago (Report, 1996). This can be attributed largely to controls at farm level, especially in relation to S. Enteritidis, which, however, has increased in incidence recently. Recent data for the USA (Simmons et al.,2003) showed 33.9 per cent of whole carcasses positive for Salmonella over a 20-week sampling period, which contrasts with the national average of less than 9 per cent (Shane, 2004). In the USA and many other countries, detection of Salmonella in a particular lot of poultry does not imply that the lot should be condemned for that reason, bearing in mind that the small number of cells usually present on a contaminated item is unlikely to be a direct cause of human illness. Also, regular rejection of contaminated lots would be economically unacceptable on the scale required. Instead, there is a growing emphasis on the application of preventative measures within the Industry and there is now much reliance on the HACCP system for controlling foodborne pathogens in poultry processing.

The microbiological hazards in the processing operation are well known and are often difficult to control effectively, because of the technological limitations in the process that can lead to cross-contamination of the carcasses being processed. Implementation of the HACCP system does not overcome this drawback, but has a number of clear benefits, including the following:

1. The system ensures regular monitoring of the process as a whole.
2. Hygiene control is optimised, within the above- mentioned constraints, thereby providing evidence of 'due diligence' on the part of the processor, as required by UK food law.
3. Checking of control parameters and recording of results are an integral part of the system.
4. Compliance with hygiene legislation is ensured.
5. Staff awareness of food-safety requirements is increased.
6. As a result of national HACCP implementation, operational standards across the Industry become more uniform.

Although use of the HACCP system in poultry processing is aimed primarily at the control of foodborne pathogens, there is also the potential to reduce contamination of carcasses with spoilage organisms. Pseudomonads, in particular, are largely destroyed during scalding and carcasses are re-contaminated during subsequent stages of processing (Mead, 2004). It is these stages that need to be targeted for control purposes.

Cross-contamination of carcasses with pathogens can occur at virtually every stage of the process and currently there is little evidence that this problem is significantly reduced by the application of HACCP principles. Also unclear is the effect of the HACCP system on levels of carcass contamination, although this will vary according to the type of process used and permitted intervention measures in different countries. The most effective type of process for reducing contamination is likely to be one in which carcasses are immersion-chilled in chlorinated water and then frozen. In the USA, where water-immersion chilling is the norm and super-chlorination of process water is permitted, there is also the option to use a chemical decontamination treatment for carcasses, which may involve substances such as trisodium phosphate, acidified sodium chlorite or peroxyacetic acid (Russell, 2003). In this respect, there is currently a very different situation in the EU, because super-chlorination is not allowed, immersion chilling has been largely replaced by air chilling or evaporative cooling, and any form of chemical decontamination is unacceptable. Therefore, in the case of fresh carcasses that are air chilled, there is no marked reduction in carcass contamination (Allen *et al.*, 2000; Fluckey *et al.*, 2003). Moreover, there is no Critical Control Point at which a significant reduction in pathogen contamination can be guaranteed. However, this unsatisfactory situation may change in 2006 (Report,2003). Without the use of processing aids to improve hygiene, the greatest reductions in carcass contamination are likely to come from technological developments in the process that are designed to improve hygiene, as long as these are acceptable to the Industry. For example, a process for simultaneous scalding and plucking of broilers, although not adopted commercially, reduced levels of Enterobacteriaceae on carcasses by one hundred-fold in experimental trials (Mulder, 1985). On the other hand, a study aimed at reducing Campylobacter contamination by merely optimising existing processing procedures, achieved much smaller improvements (Mead *et al.*, 1995). Possible benefits from physical carcass decontamination treatments that are being developed to reduce levels of Campylobacter are reported.

Mandatory use of the HACCP system in US processing plants, which began in 1997, is coupled with performance standards that include a Salmonella prevalence of 20 per cent for post-chill broiler carcasses (Federal Register, 1996). How cost-effective has this approach been in reducing human salmonellosis? In posing the question, it must be acknowledged that the Salmonella status of processed carcasses depends ultimately on control measures taken on the farm, which are not addressed directly in the legislation. Attempts to meet the requirements of the so-called

'Mega-Reg' have involved a 30 – 40 per cent increase in the use of clean water during processing, and overall costs are said to be several times higher than official forecasts (Ollinger and Mueller, 2003). So far, there is no real evidence that human salmonellosis has fallen in the USA as a result of HACCP implementation.

Furthermore, in the year 1999, there were 32 782 reported isolations of Salmonella from human cases, increasing to 33 310 in 2000 and then decreasing to 31 675 in 2001 (CDC data). Thus, the recent situation has been relatively static.

Microbiological Risk Assessment (MRA)

MRA is a developing concept, which is complementary to the application of HACCP principles. As defined by the Codex Alimentarius Commission (CAC, 1999), it includes hazard identification, exposure assessment, hazard characterisation and risk characterisation. The concept is discussed in relation to poultry by Kelly *et al.* (2003). It is important not only in quantifying the risk of human illness from a pathogen or microbial toxin associated with poultry, but in determining the extent to which the risk can be reduced by specific intervention measures. Thus, the effect of controlling the hazard at a particular Critical Control Point can be quantified with this approach.

Quantitative risk assessments vary in mathematical complexity, depending on the question being asked. Often, they require a diversity of data that is sufficient to account for any variation that occurs. In practice, data sets are usually far from complete and may be subject to considerable uncertainty. This problem is compounded by the dynamic nature of microbial populations, which undergo continuous change. Dealing with uncertainty has been a feature of the development of MRA and is clearly evident in the case of Campylobacter infections associated with chicken consumption. Here, the true extent to which human cases are derived from eating chicken is unknown, it has to be assumed that all strains of the organism have the same potential to cause human illness and that their pathogenic and survival properties are similar. Also, there is a general lack of data on levels of product contamination at different stages of the supply chain and during subsequent handling prior to consumption. Nevertheless, the MRA described by Kelly *et al.* (2003) makes some important predictions and highlights the effects of freezing poultry meat, which, more than other mitigation strategies examined, will reduce both the chance and level of subsequent human exposure.

In another recent MRA (Rosenquist *et al.,* 2003), it is predicted that human campylobacteriosis associated with chicken consumption would decrease 30-fold if levels of Campylobacter contamination on carcasse could be reduced by two log units. Alternatively, flock prevalence would need to be reduced by the same factor. Such reductions would require better on-farm control than is possible at present or a highly effective decontamination treatment for processed carcasses. However, a comparable reduction in human illness was also predicted from possible improvements in kitchen hygiene or, again, by freezing the product. As knowledge of Campylobacter in poultry meat production continues to expand, it is likely that further mitigation strategies will become apparent.

Increasingly, risk assessment is being used as a scientific tool to evaluate human health risks from hazardous agents present in foods. In this respect Munday *et al.* (2003) have identified 36 risk assessments on Salmonella, 18 on Campylobacter and 16 on Listeria, including completed and on-going studies in both developed and developing countries, as well as those undertaken by FAO/WHO on Salmonella and Campylobacter in broilers. However, it is necessary to recognise that MRA is still in its infancy and the degree of uncertainty is high, indicating that much remains to be done to fill the data gaps and refine the mathematical methods involved. Ultimately, MRA will ensure that public health policies have a sound scientific basis and will be directed towards the most effective control strategies.

References

Allen VM, Corry JEL, Burton CH, Whyte RT, Mead GC. Hygiene aspects of modern poultry chilling. International Journal of Food Microbiology 2000; 58:39–48.

Arnaut-Rollier I, Vauterin L, De Vos P, Massart DL, Devriese LA, DeZuler L, Van Hoof J. A numerical taxonomic study of the Pseudomonas flora isolated from poultry meat. Journal of Applied Microbiology 1999; 87:15–28.

CAC Principles and Guidelines for the Conduct of Microbiological Risk Assessment. Codex Alimentarius Commission, FAO, Rome, Italy, CAC/GL-30; 1999.

Cavitte JC. Present and future control of food-borne pathogens in poultry; revision of the European Community legislation on zoonoses. In: Proceedings of the XVI European Symposium on the Quality of Poultry Meat 2003; Saint-Brieuc, France v.1 p 46–58.

Corry JEL, Atabay HI. Poultry as a source of Campylobacter and related organisms. Journal of Applied Microbiology 2001; 90:96S–114S.

Corry JEL, James C, O'Neill D, Yaman H, Kendall A, Howell M. Physical methods, readily adapted to existing commercial processing plants, for reducing numbers of campylobacters on raw poultry. International Journal of Medical Microbiology 2003; 293 Suppl., 35:32.

Doyle MP, Schoeni JL. Isolation of Escherichia coli 0157: H7 from retail fresh meats and poultry. Applied and Environmental Microbiology 1987; 53:2394–6.

Federal Register. Pathogen Reduction; Hazard Analysis and Critical Control Point (HACCP) Systems; Final rule. Department of Agriculture: Food Safety and Inspection Service. Federal Register 1996; 61 (144):38806–38989.

Fluckey WM, Sanchez MX, McKee SR, Smith D, Pendleton E, Brashears MM. Establishment of a microbiological profile for an air-chilling poultry operation in the United States. Journal of Food Protection 2003; 66:272–9.

Hakkinen M, Schneitz C. Efficacy of a commercial competitive exclusion product against a chicken pathogenic Escherichia coli and E. coli 0157:H7. Veterinary Record 1996; 139:139–141.

Heuvelink AE, Zwartkruis-Nahuis JTM, Van Den Biggelaar FLAM, Van Leeuwen WJ, De Boer E. Isolation and characterization of verocytotoxin-producing Escherichia coli 0157 from slaughter pigs and poultry. International Journal of Food Microbiology 1999; 52: 67–75.

Kelly LA, Hartnett E, Gettinby G, Fazil A, Snary E, Wooldridge M.Microbial safety of poultry meat: Risk assessment as a way forward. World's Poultry Science Journal 2003; 59:495–508.

Kessel AS, Gillespie IA, O'Brien SJ, Adak GK, Humphrey TJ, Ward LR. General outbreaks of infectious intestinal disease linked with poultry, England and Wales, 1992 – 1999. Communicable Disease and Public Health 2001; 4:171–7.

Mead GC. Shelf-life and spoilage of poultry meat, In: Mead GC, editor. Poultry meat processing and quality. Cambridge, UK, Woodhead, 2004. p. 283–303.

Mead GC, Hudson WR, Hinton MH. Effect of changes in processing to improve hygiene control on contamination of poultry carcasses with campylobacter. Epidemiology and Infection 1995; 115:495–500.

Mulder RWAW. Decrease microbial contamination during poultry processing. Poultry Misset 1985 march; 52–5.

Munday D, Coburn H, Snary E. Risk Assessments in the Area of Food Safety, Weybridge, UK: Veterinary Laboratories Agency; 2003.

Ollinger Mueller V. The economics of sanitation and process controls in meat and poultry plants. Washington, DC: Unites States Department of Agriculture; 2003. (Agricultural Economics Report no. 817).

Persson U, Jendteg S. The economic impact of poultry-borne salmonellosis: how much should be spent on prophylaxis? International Journal of Food Microbiology 1992; 15:207– 213.

Pooni GS, Mead GC. Prospective use of temperature function integration for predicting the shelf-life of non-frozen poultry-meat products. Food Microbiology 1984; 1:67–78.

Report. Report on Poultry Meat. Advisory Committee on the Microbiological Safety of Food, HMSO, London, UK; 1996.

Report. Proposal for a Regulation of the European Parliament and of the Council laying down specific rules for the organisation of official controls on products of animal origin intended for human consumption. Working Party of Veterinary Experts (Public Health). Council of the European Union, 7368/2/03; 2003.

Rosenquist H, Nielsen NL, Sommer HM, Nørrung B, Christensen BB. Quantitative risk assessment of human campylobacteriosis associated with thermophilic Campylobacter species in chicken. International Journal of Food Microbiology 2003; 83:87–103.

Russell SM. Disinfection of poultry carcasses during scalding and immersion chilling. Turkeys 2003; 51:5–8.

Salmon RL, Farrell ID, Hutchison JGP, Coleman DJ, Gross RJ, Fry NK, Rowe B, Palmer SR. A christening party outbreak of haemorrhagic colitis and haemolytic uraemic syndrome associated with Escherichia coli 0157:H7. Epidemiology and Infection 1989; 103:249–254.

Samadpour M, Ongerth JE, Liston J, Tran N, Nguyen D, Whittam TS, Wilson RA, Tarr PI. Occurrence of Shiga-like toxin producing Escherichia coli in retail fresh seafood, beef, lamb, pork and poultry from grocery stores in Seattle, Washington. Applied and Environmental Microbiology 1994; 60:1038–1040.

Schoeni JL, Doyle MP. Variable colonization of chickens perorally inoculated with Escherichia coli 0157: H7 and subsequent contamination of eggs. Applied and Environmental Microbiology

1994; 60:2958–2962.

Schmidt H, Scheef J, Huppertz HI, Frosch M, Karch H. Escherichia coli 0157:H7 and 0157:H(-) strains that do not produce Shiga toxin: phenotypic and genetic characterization of isolates associated with diarrhea and hemolytic-uremic syndrome. Journal of Clinical Microbiology 1999; 37:3491–6.

Shane SM. The changing face of poultry disease: a twenty-year retrospective. World Poultry 2004; 20(7):26–8.

Simmons M, Fletcher DL, Cason, J.A. Berrang, M.E. Recovery of Salmonella from retail broilers by a whole-carcass enrichment procedure. Journal of Food Protection 2003; 66:446–450.

Smerdon WJ, Jones R, McLauchlin J, Reacher M. Surveillance of listeriosis in England and Wales, 1995 – 1999. Communicable Disease and Public Health 2001; 4:188–193.

Stavric S, Buchanan B, Gleeson TM. Intestinal colonization of young chicks with Escherichia coli 0157:H7 and other verotoxin-producing serotypes. Journal of Applied Bacteriology 1993; 74:557–563.

Threlfall EJ, Fisher IST, Berghold C, Germer-Smidt P, Tschäpe H, Cormican M. Luzzi I, Schneider F, Wannet W, Machado, J Edwards G. Antimicrobial drug resistance in isolates of Salmonella enterica from cases of salmonellosis in humans in Europe in 2000: results of international multi-centre surveillance. Eurosurveillance 2003; 8:41-5.

Van Pelt W, Van Der See H, Wannet WJB, Van De Giessen AW, Mevius DJ, Bolder NM, Komijn RE, Van Duynhoven YTHP. Explosive increase of Salmonella Java in poultry in the Netherlands: consequences for public health. Eurosurveillance 2003; 8:31–5.

Waldroup AL. Contamination of raw poultry with pathogens. World's Poultry Science Journal 1996; 52:7–25.

Williams K, Allen G, Bolton FJ. Survey on the microbiological examination of barbecued chicken. Food Safety Express 2002; 3(3):26–7.

Viehweg SH, Schmitt RE, Schmidt-Lorenz W. Microbial spoilage of refrigerated fresh broilers. VII. Production of off odours from poultry skin by bacterial isolates. Lebensmittel-Wissenschaft und-Technologie 1989; 22:356–367.

– Chapter 16 –

Nutritive Value, Preservation and Packaging Techniques of Shelled and Liquid Eggs

I. Nutritive Value of Egg

Eggs contain about 75 per cent water and are rich source of protein that is of high biological value. The protein quality of the egg is often the standard for the measuring the quality of all other food proteins. Eggs are also an important source of essential unsaturated fatty acids (linoleic 18: 2 n6), oleic acid a monounsaturated fatty acid, iron phosphorus, trace minerals, the fat-soluble vitamins A, D, E and K and many of the water-soluble B vitamins. The egg is potent source of vitamin D but it is low in calcium and devoid of vitamin C.

Egg provides a unique, well-balanced source of nutrients for persons of all ages. Before the advent of the present day baby foods hard cooked egg yolk served as a major supplementary source of iron for young babies. Now in iron enriched, precooked baby cereals, strained meats, and canned egg yolks offer alternative and more convenient sources of iron. However home prepared, hard cooked egg yolks are still a practical and desirable supplement for infants. Egg contributes significantly to the body's nutrient needs during rapid growth, and therefore an excellent food for young children and teenagers.

The high digestibility and concentrated nutrient content of eggs makes them a valuable food source for those recovering from illness. Most bland diet and the first light or soft diet during convalescence from surgery or other illness usually include in eggs. Eggs are valuable and readily acceptable in diets for elderly who may have lower caloric needs but have greater difficulty digesting and absorbing nutrients. Adequate nutrient intake in the elderly is critical to health science age related changes occur in G.I tract, and diet can profound influence the immune system. Eggs are easily digested and absorbed to provide several essential nutrients.

Table 16.1: Values of Nutrient Composition per Egg Edible Portion (50 g)

Nutrients Unit	*Whole egg*	*White*	*Yolk*
Proximate			
Solids, g	13.47	4.6	8.8
Water (per cent)	73.7	87.6	48
Calories	84.0	19.0	64
Proteins, g	6.60	3.88	2.74
Total lipids, g	6.00	–	5.80
Ash, g	0.55	0.26	0.29
Lipid			
Fatty acids, g			
SFA	2.01	–	1.95
USFA	3.26	–	3.22
Cholesterol (mg)	226	–	226
Lecithin, g	1.27	–	1.22
Cephalin, g	0.253	–	0.241
Carbohydrate, g	0.36	0.264	0.10
Fiber, g	–	–	–
Minerals, mg			
Calcium	29.2	3.8	25.2
Magnesium	6.33	4.15	2.15
Iron	1.08	0.053	1.02
Phosphorus	111	8	17
Potassium	74	57	9
Sodium	71	63	28
Vitamins			
Vit. A, IU	264	–	260
Vit. D, IU	27	–	27
Vit. E, mg	0.88	–	0.87
Choline, mg	237	0.46	238
Inositol, mg	5.94	1.52	4.35
Niacin, mg	0.045	0.035	0.010
Riboflavin, mg	0.18	0.11	0.07
Thiamine, mg	0.05	0.004	0.048
Ascorbic acid, mg	0	0	0

The chemical analysis for nutrients in the egg is presented in the Table 16.1. The composition of a large, whole raw egg and of boiled egg is almost same, of course, but that of scramble egg varies slightly due to added milk and fat that may occur during preparation. Though yolk comprises slightly over one-third of he edible portion, but it yields 78 per cent of calories and provides all or most of fat, calcium, phosphorus, iron, zinc, vitamin B_6, B_{12} and A, folic acid, pantothenic acid, and thiamin, and almost half the protein and riboflavin of the whole egg. Protein and riboflavin are less concentrated in the white, but because almost twice as much white as yolk, more than half the total protein and riboflavin are in the white.

Fatty acid composition of the egg yolk is easily modified by adding fat to diet of the hen. Vitamin and trace mineral values can also vary greatly when rations are heavily modified with a particular vitamin or mineral.

II. Preservation of Eggs

As egg is fragile and perishable commodity, it should be handled carefully and marketed as soon as possible. However, in situation of surplus egg production and/ low demand, particularly in summer months, preservation of egg necessary until released to the market. The methods of preservation of shelled eggs are based on the principle of retarding the microbial growth by sealing the pores of the shell to minimize the evaporation of moisture and gases, thus reducing physico-chemical changes in the egg contents for a reasonable length of time. Many methods have been used to counteract the harmful effect of this surface microorganisms and to extend the shelf life. There are number of methods for the preservation of shell eggs and liquid eggs.

Shell Egg Preservation

Dry Packaging

Eggs are kept in earthen pots with clean dry packing material and the pot is buried in wet land. This method is practiced in remote areas particularly rural villages where the access to modern method of preservation is very poor.

Thermal Treatment

This method involves the application of heat and includes flash heat treatment and thermostabilization. Sometimes the latter is followed by simultaneous oil coating for more effective preservation.

Flash Heat Treatment

The eggs are immersed for five seconds in boiling water. The advantage of this method is that it destroys some of the bacteria present on shell surface and does not require any thermostatic control to maintain specific temperature. In this method a thin film of albumen coagulates beneath the shell membrane which seals the shell pores internally.

Thermostabilization

This method is good for fertile eggs since it kills the embryos and therefore is also known as defertilization method. It essentially consists of immersing shell eggs in hot water at 130°F/45C for 30 minutes, at 54°C for 15 min. or 56°C for 10 min or 60°C for 5 min. which tend to coagulate the albumin and then the eggs are cooled under tap water. A pasteurizing effect is also obtained in this process.Treated eggs remain edible for 3-4 weeks even during summer months. Though this method has many advantages such as stabilizing the albumin and sterilization of the egg shell, the egg looses the property of foaming to a remarkable extent.

Immersion in Preservative Solutions

Lime water and water glass can be used for the preservation of eggs in rural area.

1. Lime Water

Lime water is prepared by mixing about 0.5 kg of quick lime (calcium oxide) in about 1litre of boiling water. The mixture is left to settle overnight and the clean supernatant, liquid is poured out into a jar. Sodium chloride 112gms per litre may also be added to increase the specific gravity of water and will minimize the chances of breaking of eggs. To this solution 2.5 litres of cold water is added and filtered through muslin cloth. Eggs meant for preservation should be kept in a jar or earthen pot and pour the lime solution over the eggs till all the eggs are completely immersed. A little mineral oil may be added over this layer to prevent evaporation. Eggs have to be kept for 24 hours in this solution. After 24 hours they are taken out, dried and arranged in filler flats. Eggs can be stored in this method for 2-3 months in a good edible condition at normal ambient temperature. Only disadvantage however is taste of lime can be detected in the eggs.

The preservative effect of lime water is mainly due to the deposition of a thin film of calcium carbonate on the shell surface which partially seals the pores. In addition, the alkalinity of lime water also exerts some preservative effect. The chemical reaction involved in the process is as follows-

$$CaO + H_2O \rightarrow Ca(OH)_2$$

$$Ca(OH)_2 + CO_2 \rightarrow CaCO_3 + H_2O$$

2. Water Glass Method

A 10 per cent solution of sodium silicate is prepared in hot water and allowed to cool. The cooled solution is then poured into a jar containing the eggs till they are immersed completely. The jar is covered and kept in a cool place where the temperature should not be above 70°F. The eggs are dipped for 12 hours in this solution, then taken out and dried at room temperature prior to storage in the filler flats. In this process a thin precipitate of silica deposited on the surface of the shell seals the pores. Besides water glass has some antiseptic properties and does not impart any undesirable taste or odour to the eggs.

3. Oil Coating

Preservation of egg by oil coating is of commercial importance. It preserves the eggs by forming a thin film of oil in the surface of the shell to seal the pores. This treatment is superior to the ones described above in preserving egg quality. The eggs should be oil treated within few hours of laying so as to retain better interior quality. Dirty eggs should be washed before oil coating.

The oil used for coating must be colourless, odourless, free from fluorescent materials and having a specific gravity of about 0.855 to 0.870 at 15°C, viscosity should be between 70-90 and it should remain liquid at low temperature. Vegetable oil, such as Cotton seed, linseed and groundnut oils mixed with an antioxidant, butylated hydroxyl toluene (BHT) at 125ppm level is a good sealing agent. However, refined food grade mineral oil (liquid paraffin) is preferred because of its less susceptibility to oxidative changes during storage. The commercial egg treatment oils are : Heavy paraffin oil (CFTRI), Liquid paraffin, Myvacet 9-40 (CFTRI), Coconut oil, Technical white oil. The rate of CO_2 escape is considerably reduced in oil immersed eggs and eggs are not likely to absorb foreign odours. Egg can be coated by dipping in oil or spraying with it.

In oil dipping, the eggs held in wire baskets and dipped in a bath of oil pre-heated to 45°C for 5 to 7 seconds. The baskets are then taken out and excess oil is drained-off before storage of eggs in filler flat. Oil spray method can be used to replace the oil dipping method as it is more economical and convenient than the latter. The egg coating oil preheated to 55°C, is sprayed on the broader end of the egg shell where pores are in abundance. The oil treatment can also be done by spraying using hand or electrical sprayer. Although it seals about three fourths of the shell surface but is equally effective as oil dipping in maintaining egg shell quality. Eggs can be successfully used in vacuum impregnated method. The egg is first immersed in oil and then subject to reduced atmospheric pressure, when normal pressure is restored the tendency of air to enter the pores of the shell causes the solution also to be drawn in. The oil does not penetrate through the shell membranes.

The oil coated eggs can be safely stored at 5°C, 13°C, 26°C, and 38°C for 120, 60, 28 and 10 days, respectively. The storage time limits for unoiled eggs at these temperatures are 60, 30, 7 and 5 days, respectively.

Over-Wrapping

For over wrapping of eggs, polythene cellophane, polyvinylidene and other transparent, thin but sufficiently strong, films are used. These films should be impervious to gases and moisture. Over wrapping of eggs in different atmosphere like carbon dioxide and vacuum etc. have been tried and found successful in preservation of eggs.

Cold Storage

An egg storage centre with cold storage facilities should be properly designed and always keep clean. It has three main sections such as receiving area for egg brought from the farms, processing area for grading and packaging, and cold stores for storing graded and packaged eggs. These sections should be physically separated for the sake of hygiene and quality control. In some cases, the first two operations are carried out at the packing station from where the eggs are sent to cold storage.

Pre-Storage Treatment

Prior to cold storage, clean eggs are separated from the dirty egg. The latter are washed, graded and packed separately. All the eggs are candled and those having cracked or unsound shell and interior quality defects should not be stored. Eggs of different grades are packed separately, as described earlier, first in filler flats and then in corrugated cardboard egg boxes which are stacked on the shelves provided in cold store. Eggs meant for long period of storage are oil coated by spraying method before packaging corrugated cardboard boxes.

Cold Storage and Duration of Storage

The quality of eggs prior to storage as well as temperature and relative humidity (R.H.) of cold room determine the period of storage. Eggs intended for short storage *i.e.* about a month of storage should be stored at 10-12°C with 75-80 per cent R.H., whereas for long term (3 months), they should be stored at 4-6°C with the same relative humidity. Again for very long term (5-8 months) storage, the temperature of egg storage room should be between -1.7 to 0.5°C with 80-85 per cent R.H. Oil coated eggs will obviously, keep well for a longer period at these storage temperature.

However, in no case, the cold storage temperature should be below -2°C in order to prevent freezing of albumen and associated cracking of shell. Similarly, the R.H. of cold store room should not exceed 85 per cent to prevent mold growth. Samples of egg should be examined periodically to detect spoilage, if any, and ensure efficient functioning of the cold store.

Post Storage Care of Eggs

The egg held in the cold store particularly at low temperature (<8°C) show condensation of water on shell surface which is known as sweating. Hence, they should be placed in an ante-room maintained at a temperature of 15 to 20°C for about 8-12 hours before release to market. Cold stored eggs should preferably, be marketed within 5 days while oil coated eggs within 10 days after removal from cold store.

Liquid Egg Preservation

Freezing and dehydration are the common methods of preserving the quality of liquid egg in term of frozen and dried egg products, respectively for domestic food markets and also for export. They are often sale in the outlets for disposal of surplus eggs.

Freezing

Low temperature inhibits the microbial growth and some physico-chemical reactions and thereby retains the quality of liquid egg. Separated albumen or yolk or whole egg liquid are frozen and marketed for uses in other food products. For the manufacture of frozen egg products, the egg liquid is homogenized, filtered, pasteurized, filled in metal cans or plastic cartons/bags of 2 to 5 kg capacity and quick frozen at -30 to -40°C in a blast freezer before storage at -18°C for 6-8 months. Freezing does not cause any significant change in the functional properties of albumen.

The quality of eggs made from frozen egg albumen is as good as those made from fresh albumen. On the other hand, on freezing of yolk or whole egg liquid appear as a thick, lumpy and tenacious mass. It becomes difficult to mix them with other food ingredients. The amount of gelation is more drastic in frozen yolk than in frozen whole egg liquid. So, egg yolk gelation is affected by rate and temperature of freezing and thawing as well as by storage time and temperature. The freezing point of egg yolk is about -1°C, yet gelation does not occur until a temperature of -6°C is attained. Gelation of plain yolk takes place most rapidly at -18°C. Fast freezing and thawing result in less gelation than slow freezing and thawing because of smaller ice crystals are formed and less dehydration of proteins occurs.

Preservation by Drying (Dehydration)

The removal of water from food inhibits the growth of microorganisms and slows down the chemical reactions in the constituents of food and thus, preserved its quality. This principal is applied in the production of dried egg products from albumen, yolk and whole egg separately depending on their usages in food and non-food industries. If properly dried, they have quality comparable to that of shell eggs. The main advantages of egg dehydration are- easy handling, saving of space, reduce transportation cost and eliminate refrigeration for storage of such products.

Preparation Egg Mélange

The process for conversion of shell eggs into dried egg products consists of washing of eggs and breaking them individually in cups by hand or machine, inspection for odour and blood spot etc, collection of contents as whole liquid, albumen or yolk, albumen or yolk, homogenization, filtration, desugarization, pasteurization and dehydration of egg mélange. Filtration is done to remove chalazae, vitelline membrane and shell particles, if any, from the liquid. Desugaring is the removal of reducing sugar *i.e.* glucose from egg liquid by the use of either glucose-oxidase enzyme or baker's yeast in order to control browning (Maillard) reaction responsible for discolouration, off-flavour development and reduction in the solubility of dried egg products during storage.

It is mandatory to pasteurize egg liquids to destroy all the pathogenic microbes including *Salmonella* spp. and to reduce spoilage organisms as much as possible before dehydration; if the product is intended for use in human foods. The United States Department of Agriculture now requires that liquid whole egg be heated to at least 60°C and held for no less than 3.5 min for the average particles while United Kingdom recommended a pasteurization temperature of 64.5°C for2.5 min. An important advantage of this combination of time temperature conditions is the fact that an enzymatic test for determining the adequacy of pasteurization is available. In India liquid eggs are pasteurized at a temperature of 62.5°C for 3.5 min while in China that are pasteurized at a temperature of 62°C for 2.5 min. Different pasteurization methods are given as under-

Time Temperature Requirements for Pasteurization of different Liquid Egg Products

The purpose of liquid egg product pasteurization is to kill all pathogenic bacteria as well as a numbers of food spoilage bacteria so that it may be safe for human consumption with extended storage life. The most pathogenic bacteria causing human illness through egg products are *Salmonella enteritides, Salmonella typhymurium, Listeria monocytogenes, Yearsinia enterocolitica, Campylobacter jejune* and *Streptococcus feacalis*.

Egg Products	*Temperature (°C)*	*Time (min)*
Albumen	57	3.5
Whole eggs (plain)	60	3.5
Salted whole egg (2-10 per cent)	63	3.5
Sugared whole egg (2-12 per cent)	61	3.5
Plain yolk	61	3.5
Sugared yolk	63	3.5

Test for Adequacy of Pasteurization

Few simple tests have been identified for determination adequacy of pasteurization. These tests include enzyme phosphatase and α-amylase as well as catalase activity test.

Phosphatase Enzyme Activity

So useful for milk not for egg since phosphatase activity remains in whole egg heated to 60°C for 20 min or 70°C for 5 min. Hence the test is not useful for egg products.

Alpha-Amylase Test

Alpha-amylase enzyme is destroyed in whole egg heated to 64°C for 2.5 min. This test is useful for British standard which used 64°C but not suitable for U.S.A. (60°C for 3.5 min).

Catalase Activity Test

It is very useful and ideal for egg products. Since catalase activity of white and whole egg is substantially reduced at 54°C or below. Hence, it is a good indicator of pasteurization efficiency.

Drying Methods

Of the various methods of egg dehydration, such as spray drying, pan drying, belt drying and freeze drying. The first one is most commonly used for the manufacture of whole egg power, albumen or yolk power. Here small droplets of liquid eggs are produced by atomizing them and pass through the hot air chamber of spray drier. Because of very rapid evapouration, egg liquid spray is converted into fine powdered instantly. Flow diagram for preparation of whole egg powder-

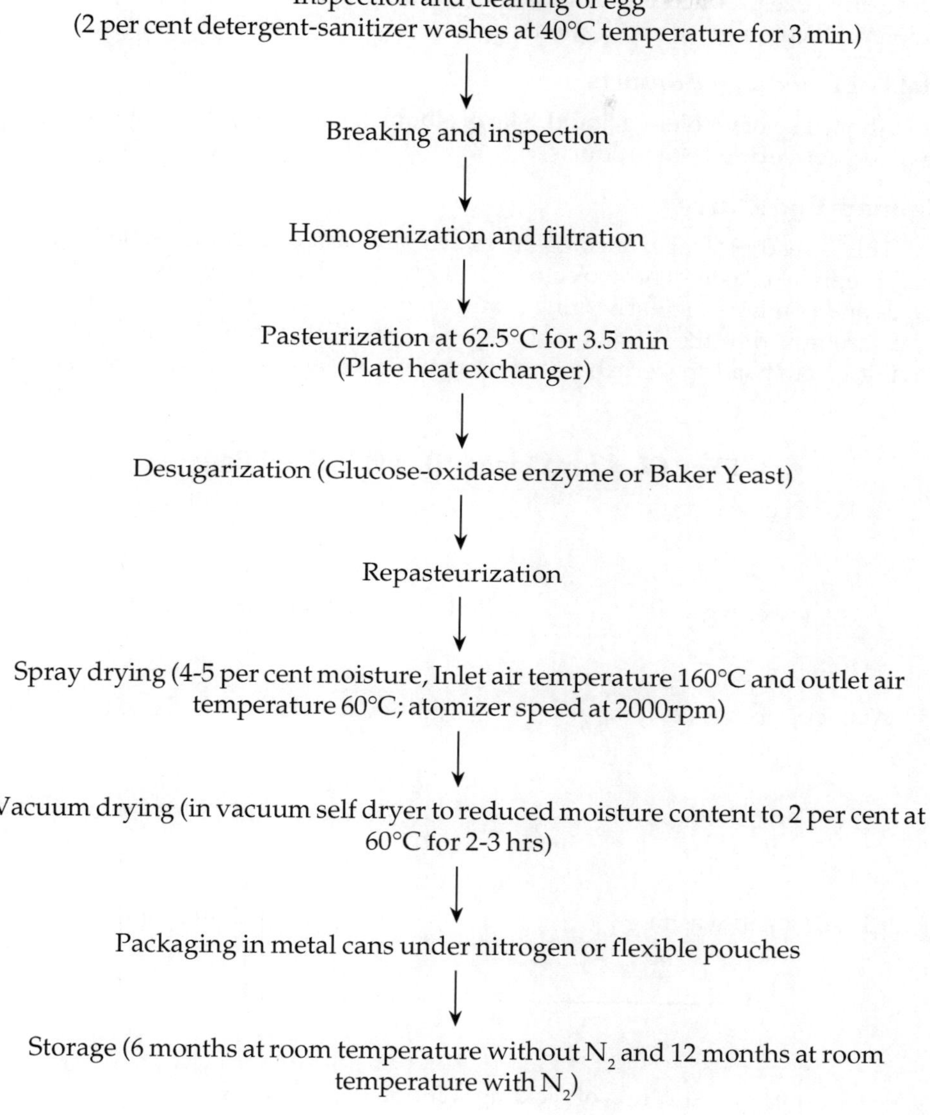

Pan drying is used for producing albumen flakes. A thin layer of liquid albumen is poured shallow metal trays and dried at moderate temperature (54-56°C) in hot air oven or water gasket pan for uniform drying. Belt drying involves spreading of thin layer of liquid egg material on a continuous aluminium belt moving through a hot air steam. A modification of this method is foam drying in which the liquid egg is beaten into foam which is subsequently dried in a thin layer on a perforated belt or mat. This yields a granular egg product. In freeze drying liquid egg is first blast frozen and dried under vacuum at low temperature in a freeze dryer. Although the quality of freeze dried egg products is much superior but the cost of freeze drying is prohibitive factor for its commercial application.

Yield of Dried Egg Products

About 4 kg of whole egg liquid, 8 kg of albumen and 2.2 kg of yolk will yield one kg of respective dried egg products.

Canned Egg Curry

This is ready-to-eat canned egg product. The hard boiled and peeled eggs are fried in edible oil to light brown colour. The gravy is prepared by mixing and frying spices and condiments (garlic, ginger and onion) to suit salt. The peeled eggs and gravy are mixed in the ratio of 55:45 (±5 per cent), filled in lacquered metal cans leaving 1.5 cm head space, exhausted (to remove air) and hermetically sealed. The

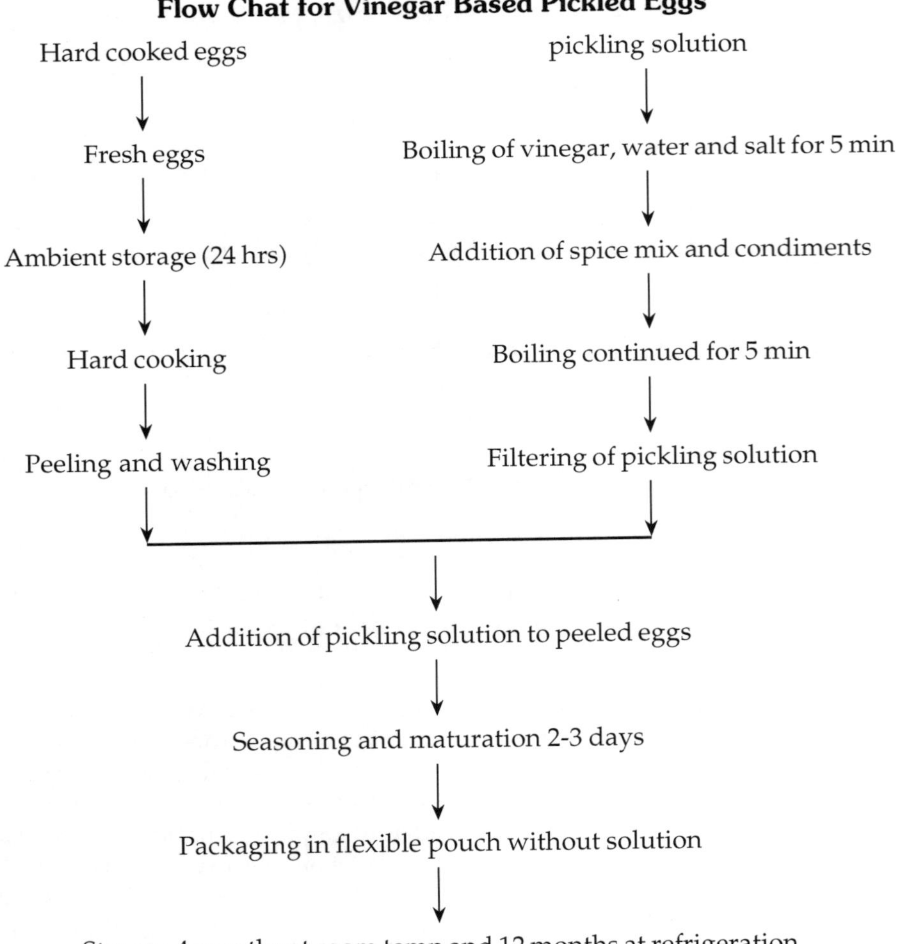

sealed cans are then subjected to retorting (1kg/cm^2 pressure for about 20 min) to ensure sterilization of the product without burning or over cooking. The canned egg curry should have characteristic taste and flavour without any disintegration of eggs during one year of its storage life under ambient storage.

Pickled Eggs

Pickling is an effective means of preserving and marketing quail eggs which weigh about 10 g or small size (40-45 g) chicken eggs as nutritious, ready-to-eat product. Simple, economical and efficient methods have been developed for the preparation of both vinegar and oil based pickled eggs to suit the taste of the consumers. The product does not require refrigeration for storage, transport and marketing, unless intended for very long period of storage. Apart from fast food outlets, pickled eggs can be find an important place in the mid day meal programme of school going children to improve their nutritional status.

Other Egg Products

there are some other convenient eggs and egg based products produced commercially. These include delivered egg, egg roll, egg nog, albumen ring and mayonnaise etc. Delivered eggs are prepared by cutting hard cooked and peeled eggs longitudinally, removing the yolk which is seasoned with salad mixture and then stuffed back into the cavity of each half of albumen. *Egg roll* is cylindrical in shape. It is prepared by cooking a uniform layer of albumen around the centre of yolk in a

Flow Chart for Oil Based Pickled Eggs

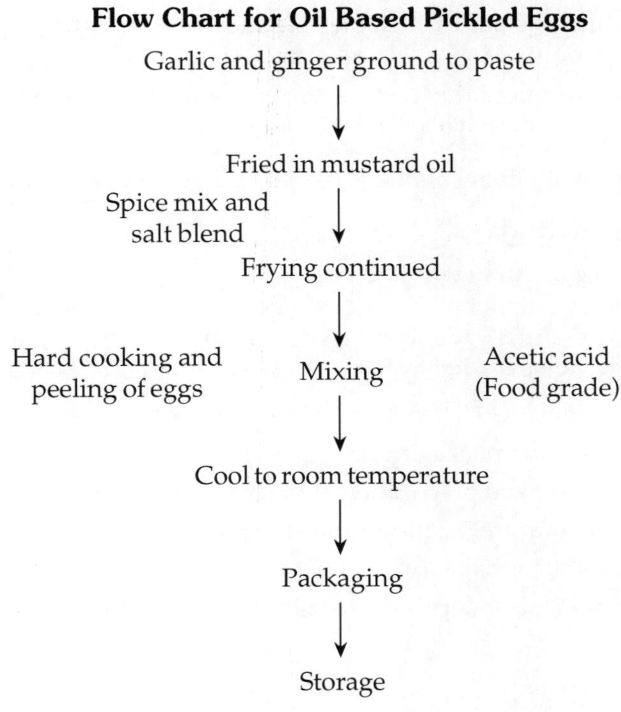

tubular mould. The product is sliced and used in salad dressing. It looks like the central out of a normal hard-boiled egg hard. *Egg nog* is, on the other hand, a nutritious egg based drink. It contains egg, milk, sugar and flavourings and can be served cold or hot. *Albumen ring* is a high protein, crisp snack foods which looks like onion ring. This product is manufactured by cooking egg albumen in ring shaped moulds and then battering, breading and deep fat frying. *Mayonnaise* is a semi-solid egg yolk based product. It is an emulsion of edible vegetable oil (80 per cent), yolk (10 per cent), vinegar and various seasonings in which yolk acts as an emulsifier for the uniform dispersions of oil in non-oily substances so as to stabilize the emulsion.

III. Storage of Eggs

The storage of shell eggs during the main laying season, in order to conserve them for consumption when they are scarce, has been practised for many centuries.

For the successful storage of eggs, the following conditions must be met.

- ☆ The eggs placed in storage must be clean; they must not be washed or wet.
- ☆ Packaging material used should be new, clean and odourless.
- ☆ Loss of water due to evaporation should be reduced to a minimum.
- ☆ The storage room must be free from tainting products and materials and should be cleaned regularly with odourless detergent sanitizers.
- ☆ The storage room must be kept at a constant temperature and humidity must be checked.
- ☆ There should be air circulation in the storage room.
- ☆ Eggs should be stored so that they are allowed to breathe.
- ☆ As far as possible, interior quality should be monitored; there should be a good proportion of thick white, the yolk should stand up well, and the flavour of white and yolk should be good.

If all of the above requirements are to be met, refrigerated storage is necessary.

Cold Storage of Eggs

In the tropics, eggs can deteriorate very quickly unless they are stored at low temperatures. The ideal temperature for storage in such climates is 13°C or lower (usually between 10° and 13° C). Here refrigeration is a necessity for successful commercial storage; however, it may be unavailable or the costs too high.

The most important factors in successful cold storage are as follows.

- ☆ The selection and packaging of eggs.
- ☆ The equipment and preparation of the cold store.
- ☆ Proper temperature, humidity and air circulation.
- ☆ Periodic testing for quality.
- ☆ The gradual adjustment of eggs to higher temperatures when removed from storage.

The Selection and Packaging of Eggs for Storage

Eggs for storage must be clean, of good interior quality and have a sound shell. If they are to be stored for more thana month, they should be equivalent to the U.S. grade A. Therefore, it is best to candle all eggs before storage. It may also be advisable to take a sample and to break out these eggs as a further quality check. The period of time between laying and storage should not be more than a few days. The eggs should be kept cool during that time.

Packaging materials used for storage should be new, clean, odourless and free from damage. When packaging material is reused, it is extremely important that it is clean, odourless and free from damage. It is important that the material used allow the eggs to "breathe" and to be free from tainting odours. It should also be sturdy in the event that the cases have to be stockpiled on top of one another.

The Equipment and Preparation of the Cold Store

The storage room should have a concrete floor that is washable. Walls and ceilings must also be washable. Wooden buildings have been found to be satisfactory, provided they do not impart foreign odours or flavours to the eggs. The room should be scrubbed thoroughly with hot water and soap or an odourless detergent sanitizer before being used. A final rinse with a hypochlorite solution will help greatly in deodorizing the storeroom. A liberal application of freshly slaked lime to unpainted plaster surfaces will also help. The storage room should be aired and dried out thoroughly after cleaning, then closed up and the refrigeration turned on. It is best to allow several days for the temperature and humidity to stabilize before introducing the eggs.

Proper Temperature, Humidity and Air Circulation

Careful and accurate control of the air condition is essential. A temperature between - 1.5° and - 0° C is recommended. At a temperature of - 2.5° C eggs freeze. The room should be well constructed and insulated and the refrigeration should be capable of maintaining an adequate uniform temperature in all areas. The cases of eggs should be separated by wood-strips and kept well away from the walls so as not to obstruct air circulation. Aisles left for the convenience of handling specific egg cases also help air circulation. Periodic ventilation of the storage room is advisable to promote air exchange.

The relative humidity should be between 80 and 85 percept at a cold storage temperature of - 1° C. At cold storage temperatures of about 10° C the relative humidity should be between 75 and 80 percent. In such instances, on average, egg weight loss should not exceed 0.5 percent per month. During the early stages of storage when the packaging material is absorbing moisture at a high rate, the floors should be sprinkled with clean water several times a day. If forced-air circulation is feasible, a controlled temperature water-spray air washer may be used. If the humidity becomes excessive, part of the air can be cycled through a unit containing calcium chloride. Where eggs have been oiled less attention can be paid to the humidity level.

Periodic Testing for Quality

Periodic quality checks are essential if the risk of heavy egg losses is to be avoided. Every month or so a sample of eggs should be selected from the various lots and tested. Usually a sample of about 1 percent of all eggs in storage may be sufficient. For example, if 3000 eggs are kept in storage, 30 eggs sampled from various egg cases will enable a good estimation of the general quality level of the eggs. If there is evidence of excessive deterioration, it is best to dispose of the eggs quickly, after eliminating those that are unfit for consumption.

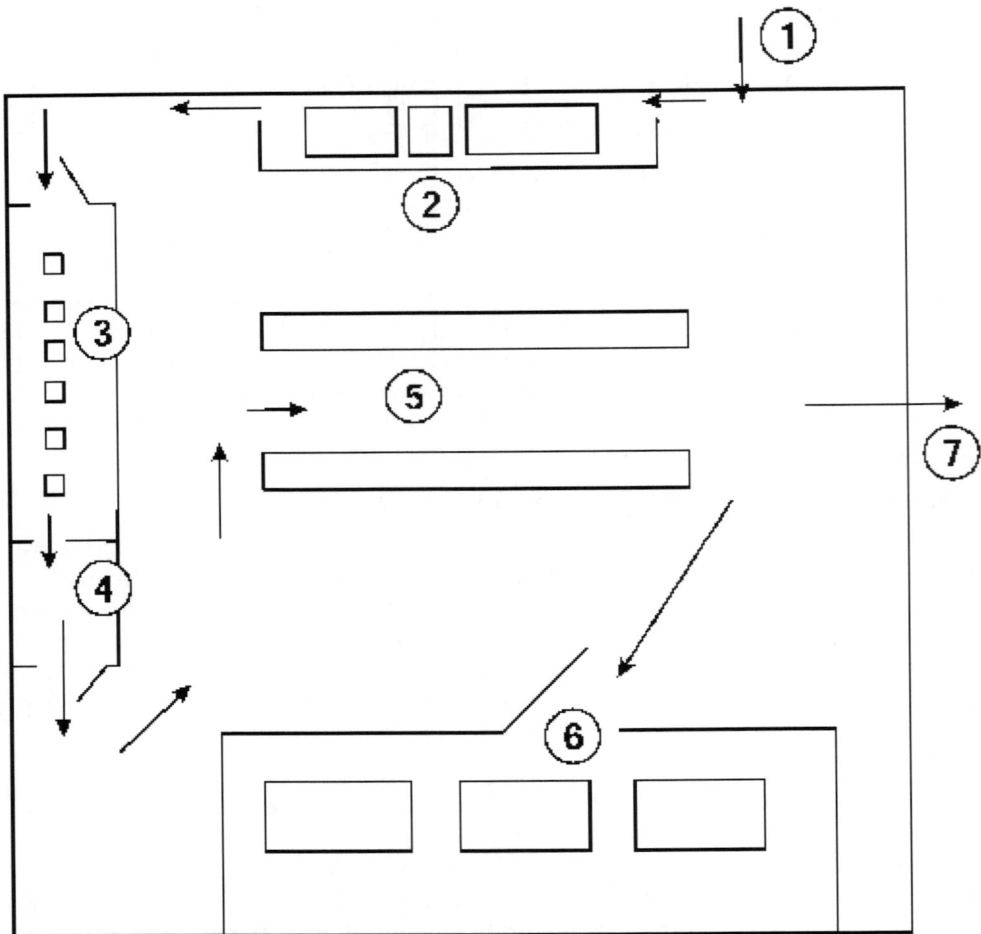

Figure 16.1: Layout of Packaging and Storing Facilities for Shell Eggs.

1. Eggs enter the packing/storage facility; 2. Temporary store room; 3. Candling room; 4. Weighing/cleaning room; 5. Packaging area; 6. Long-term storage; 7. Eggs ready for transport.

The Gradual Adjustment of Eggs to Higher Temperatures

Care must be taken in removing eggs from storage to avoid the condensation of moisture on shells. This is minimized by raising the temperature slowly or by moving the eggs through rooms with intermediate temperatures. If condensation occurs, the eggs should be held under conditions that allow the moisture to evaporate within a day or so.

As indicated earlier, eggs should not be stored with products that may taint them. For the long term, eggs are best stored alone, while for the short term they may be kept with dairy products such as milk and mild-flavoured cheese. The average storage life for eggs is between six and seven months.

The layout for the packaging and storing facility is of great importance for efficient and effective management. The various rooms should be kept clean, well ventilated and, where necessary, refrigeration provided. All personnel working in the facility should wear clean outer garments, use caps or head bands and wash their hands when handling eggs and equipment. All equipment used should be clean.

1. Eggs Enter the Packing/Storage Room

Eggs from production are brought into the packing/storage facility. Eggs can be brought in by hand or by conveyor belt. In intensive egg production, the birds lay eggs that roll out of the cage onto conveyor belts, which transport the eggs directly to the packing/storage facilities. This can be seen in shows how eggs could be stacked for manual movement if brought in by hand from production to the packing/storage facilities.

2. Temporary Storage Room

Here eggs are stored temporarily before they are moved to the candling room.

3. Candling Room

Eggs are brought into the candling room, where candlers verify the interior and external quality of eggs. The small squares represent candling benches. The candling machine in is used in fully mechanized or semi-mechanized systems, where the eggs are brought onto the candling machine by a conveyor belt.

4. Cleaning/Weighing Room

After candling, eggs are transported by conveyor belts to the cleaning/weighing room. Here eggs are cleaned with abrasives, where possible, and sorted by weight. Usually the size indicates which category eggs should fall into - small, medium or large. This can be done by hand; however, automated weighing machinery is available.

5. Packaging Area

After weighing, the eggs are taken to the packaging area. Packaging can be done either by hand or automatically by machinery.

Economics of Cold Storage

There is a tendency to underestimate the difficulties involved in providing good cold storage facilities and to recommend their installation without adequate investigation of their cost and potential economic return. The following factors should be considered when contemplating cold storage.

- ☆ Refrigeration is a complex and highly technical business.
- ☆ Capital investment and operating costs must be estimated.
- ☆ Potential available business must be appraised.

The potential available business must be appraised as well as its distribution over the different seasons of the year and the costs involved. Egg storage to even out the availability of supplies is likely to provide business for only a part of the year. The average - not maximum - price difference between the plentiful and scarce seasons must be calculated. If projected returns do not significantly exceed the costs envisaged for storage, there is little incentive for egg traders to make use of storage.

It must be considered that some egg producers, according to their circumstances and possibilities, maintain yearly production through special breeding and feeding programmes and by providing illumination in the hen laying houses. This may even out the rate of egg production throughout the year and hence long-term storage should not be considered.

IV. Packaging of Eggs and Egg Products

Eggs are provided with natural package-like shell and shell membrane however, the egg is fragile and perishable food stuffs.

Deterioration Factors

1. Weight loss due to escape of moisture and to a very lesser extent to the escape of gases.
2. Loss of CO_2 resulting in thinning of white.
3. Flattening of yolk due to absorption of water from egg white, weakening of vitelline membrane.
4. Spoilage due to microbial contamination (bacteria and fungi)
5. Absorption of foreign odour.

Packaging of Shell Eggs

Nature has given the egg a natural package - the shell. Despite its relative strength, the egg is an extremely fragile product and even with the best handling methods, serious losses can result from shell damage. Economical marketing generally requires that eggs be protected by the adoption of specialized packaging and handling procedures.

Functions of Packaging

Packaging is an important component in delivering quality eggs to buyers. It embraces both the art and science of preparing products for storage, transport and eventually sale. Packaging protects the eggs from:

- ☆ Micro-organisms, such as bacteria;
- ☆ Natural predators;
- ☆ Loss of moisture;
- ☆ Tainting;
- ☆ Temperatures that cause deterioration; and
- ☆ Possible crushing while being handled, stored or transported.

Proper handling and storage, as seen in the previous chapter, help control moisture loss, but appropriate packaging may also help prevent it. Eggs also need to breathe, hence the packaging material used must allow for the entrance of oxygen. The material used must be clean and odourless so as to prevent possible contamination and tainting. Authentic egg packaging materials can be reused, but careful attention must be paid to possible damage, odours and cleanliness. The packaging must be made to withstand handling, storage and transport methods of the most diverse kind and to protect the eggs against temperatures that cause deterioration and humidity. Finally, consumers like to see what they are buying, especially if it concerns fresh produce. An egg package should be designed so that the customers not only recognize the product as such, but can also see the eggs they are buying.

Many factors must be taken into consideration for packaging eggs. It is important to obtain information regarding the necessary requirements for a particular market, such as:

- ☆ Quality maintenance;
- ☆ Storage facilities;
- ☆ Type of transport;
- ☆ Distance to be travelled;
- ☆ Climatic conditions;
- ☆ Time involved; and
- ☆ Costs.

Egg Packages

There are many different types of egg packages, which vary both in design and packaging material used.

Type 1

Packing eggs with clean and odourless rice husks, wheat chaff or chopped straw in a firm walled basket or crate greatly decreases the risk of shell damage.

It is also possible to pack eggs in a simple basket. The basket has no cushioning material such as straw and therefore damage to the eggs may occur more easily. This kind of packaging may be fit for short distance transport.

Type 2

A very common form of packaging is the filler tray. The fillers are then placed in boxes or cases.

Filler trays are made of wood pulp moulded to accommodate the eggs. They are constructed so that they can be stacked one on top of the other and can also be placed in boxes ready for transport. Filler trays also offer a convenient method for counting the eggs in each box, without having to count every single egg. Usually the standard egg tray carries 36 eggs. Therefore, if a box holds five trays, for example, the box has a total of 180 eggs (36 x 5 = 180).

The cases used may be made of sawn wood; however, they are more commonly made of cardboard. When using cardboard cases, special care must be taken in stacking so that excessive weight is not placed on a case at the bottom of a stack.

Fillers can also be made of plastic. The advantages of using plastic egg fillers are that they can be reused and are washable. The fillers can be covered with plastic coverings and be used as packages for final sale to the buyer. More importantly, however, plastic transparent fillers allow for the inspection of eggs without handling or touching the eggs.

Type 3

Eggs can also be packed in packages that are smaller and specific for retail sale. Each package can hold from two to twelve eggs. These cases can be made of paperboard or moulded wood pulp, or can be made of plastic. It is also possible to pack eggs in small paperboard cases and cover them with plastic film. Egg cases have also been developed from polystyrene. The advantages of using polystyrene are superior cushioning and protection against odours and moisture. The package is also resistant to fungus and mould growth.

The use of small cases is restricted by availability and cost considerations. However, small cases are good for retailers and customers. They are easy for the retailers to handle and customers are able to inspect the eggs.

Egg should be properly cleaned and graded prior to packaging. Eggs of different grades should be packed separately with broader end uppermost in trays or cartoons.

1. **Moulded pulp filler flats or moulded plastic filler flats** are most commonly used for packaging of eggs. Moulded filler flats consist of 6 rows of five eggs each.egg trays capacity 20, 24, 30 and 48 eggs. Most common 30 egg tray. The filler flat should be clean. Eggs with broader end up are filled in the filler flats. The flats are then stacked in wooden or plastic crates or baskets or in corrugated shipping containers made up of rigid or corrugated cardboard boxes (collapsible cardboard boxes of two sizes to contain 360 or 210 eggs in filler flats have been devised for transport by rail.
2. **Folded paper board egg cartoons, moulded pulp egg cartoons and moulded polystyrene egg cartoons** may be made of different shape and sizes from these materials. However, the usual practice is to market eggs in one or half a dozen egg size cartoons. Two rows of 6 eggs or one row of 6 eggs per cartoon are the usual retail packs of eggs.

Folded paper board cartoons with interlock dividers could be shaped to hold 3 rows of 4 eggs and the open top may be overwrapped with shrink film, such as PVC, PVDC, or shrinkable PE to enable the buyer to see the product.

Moulded pulp egg cartoons are cheap but it suffers from the drawbacks, like lack of physical strength and unattractiveness. Therefore, to increase the strength, denser pulp or binders are used in wooden pulp prior to moulding. The surface of moulded pulp egg cartoons is also rough and fancy printing is not possible on the rough surface.

On the other hand, moulded plastic (polystyrene foam) egg cartoons offer excellent cushioning, light wheight and good insulation and mechanical strength. The snowy white surface gives good aesthetic appeal.

The egg cartoons are provided with male and female locking grooves or tabs to hold the lid (flat top) with the body of the cartoon.

(1) Bulk Container

Made up of fiber board boxes, plastic or metal or collapsible cardboard boxes. Collapsible cardboard boxes of two sizes to contain 360 egg or 210 eggs in filler flats have been devised for transport by rail. Box containing 360 eggs (30×12) is generally used for export purpose while box containing 210 (30×7) eggs used for shipment in domestic consumption.

Labelling

Labels are a source of important information for the wholesaler, retailer and consumer and not just pieces of paper stuck onto cartons or boxes. The important facts on the label contain information for buyers concerning the eggs, their size and weight and quality/grade description - AA, A or B. Labels may also indicate the producer, when the eggs were laid, how to store them and their expiration date. Persuading the buyer to purchase the product without tasting, smelling or touching is another function of labelling.

A sample label can be seen here below:

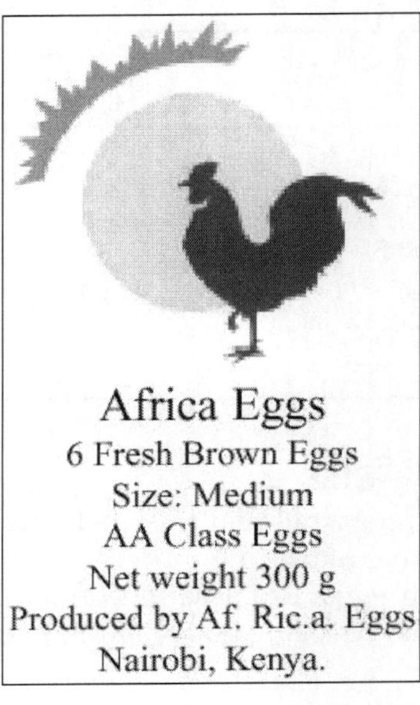

Labels can be either printed directly on cartons or attached to the cartons. The cost of labelling must be taken into consideration. Simple methods of labelling are available such as stencil or stamp as can be seen below.

Stencil and Stamp Labelling

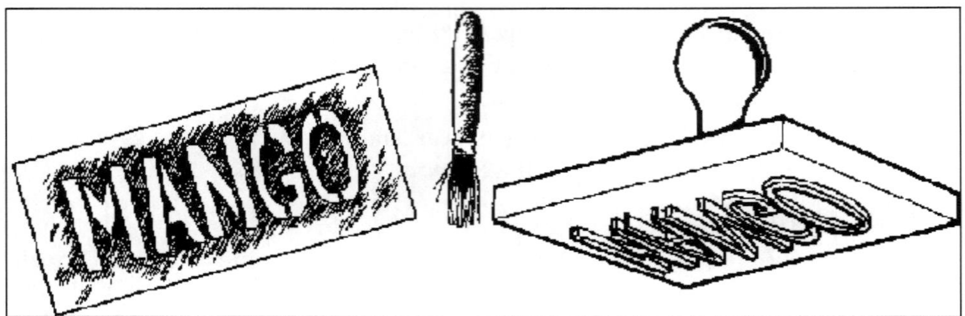

Source: Fellows and Axel, 1993

Costs of Packaging

When calculating the costs of packaging, expenses must be considered for:

- ☆ Packaging materials;
- ☆ Labelling;
- ☆ Labour;
- ☆ Additional working capital required;
- ☆ Changing existing facilities (if applicable); and
- ☆ Packaging machinery (if applicable).

Storage Condition	*Shelf Life (day5)*	
	Untreated	*Oil Treated*
100°F (37.7°C)	5	10
Dry bulb-100°F		
Wet bulb -82°F *i.e.* 65 per cent RH		
78°F, 72 per cent RH (25.5°C)	7	28
55°F, 85 per cent RH (12.8°C)	30	60
33° F, 90 per cent RH (0.5°C	6 months	8 months

Packaging of Liquid Eggs

1. *Frozen*-whole egg, egg white and yolk are frozen separately depending on the end use. The manufacturing process for frozen liquid egg consists of breaking of clean eggs, examination of contents, homogenization to pasteurization, blast freezing (-30 to -40°F) in bulk containers like metal

cans, drums, moulded plastic cartoons and flexible low density polyethylene film bags. Freezing of egg yolk, particularly below 21°F temperature it undergoes gelatinization which can be prevented by adding 0.02-0.03 per cent pepsin or 0.05 per cent trypsin.

2. Dehydrated eggs (egg powder and albumen flakes) - Albumen flakes are hygroscopic hence protection against moisture pick up is required. Whole egg and yolk powder also hygroscopic and sensitive to oxidation. The package should protect dehydrated whole egg and yolk against moisture pick up and ingress of O_2.

Packaging Materials

1. Metal cans/drums under inert gas (N_2)-Hermetically sealed container under N_2 the egg powder has shelf-life up to one year at room temperature.
2. Laminated pouches made up of paper/foil/PE flushed with nitrogen.

Pack within pack: unit packs (moderate barrier) kept in outer pack (bulk pack). The inner pack is good barrier to O, WV,Vacuum packed and outer pack is O+CO, N+O+CO or combination gas flushing.Slow diffusion of O from outer pack to inner pack. O tension is maintained for wholesale market. In retail market, outer pack is removed, unit pack is sold.

V. Quality Assurance and Marketing of Egg and Egg Products

The "quality" means meeting customer's expectations consistently with regard to pleasure, convenience, shelf life, freshness, naturalness, safety and price and to maintain these parameters is "quality control" (QC). In real sense, the QC system is designed to provide routine and consistent checks to ensure data integrity, correctness, and compactness; identify and address errors and omissions; and document and archive inventory material and record all QC activities. In order to achieve this purpose, processes are monitored and performance problems are solved. Quality exists, when price is long forgotten. Quality assurance (QA) is marketing tool to win the confidence of managers. Egg quality refers to the sum of characteristics of an egg which determine its degree of acceptance by the consumers. The main quality attributes of egg are size (weight), shape, cleanliness and soundness of shell, freshness, albumen and yolk quality, nutritive values wholesomeness and functional properties. Egg meant for consumption should have clean and intact shell, good internal quality and desirable taste and flavour. This can be achieved by adopting better methods of production, assembly, cleaning, grading, preservation, packaging, storage, transportation and distribution of eggs.

Organization and Functions of Quality Assurance Department

The organization of a quality assurance department depends highly on its duties and the size of the plant in which it operates. The quality assurance department should be to provide training, audits of records, specifications, as well as processes, inspections, technical support, and quality improvement. The QA manager and staff may share a variety of functions. The QA department, in general, should provide technical support, laboratory services and production or online services. The QA department should be involved in training production personnel, HACCP development, auditing and documentation of processes, specifications development, labouratory services, regulatory compliance, troubleshooting, product development, process improvement, and customer service.

The number of employees needed for the QA function will depend largely on the productive capacity of the plant and the number of products processed. A small single product operation might need only one individual having sound practical knowledge in labouratory and chemistry. On the other hand, large operations processing a variety of products and composed of multiple operations are likely to require a staff comprised of chemists, microbiologists, and supporting personnel. When large QA staffs are necessary, they are frequently structured to operate under the guidance of a technical director.

Quality Assurance

Technical Support	*Laboratory Services*	*On-line services*
1. Employee training	1. Micro testing and reporting	1. Audits and inspections
2. HACCP development	2. Environmental monitoring	2. In-process control
3. Documentation	3. Analytical testing and reporting	3. Documents audits
4. Specification evaluation and development	4. calibration	4. Sample collection
5. Research and development		5. Weights
		6. Packaging integrity
		7. Sanitation audits

Quality Management Systems

The appearance of diseases and contamination of egg products have led to rising public interest for food safety worldwide. The impact of these scars on consumers is a large concern for egg and egg products producers. In order to more prepared, the consumer strive to have more complete information on the sources of inputs in their products, because consumers are becoming more worried about this. Since 1955, a joint FAO/WHO expert committee started to bring awareness on the importance of quality standards. Result of that by the year 1993, there has been a rising interest in India on ISO 9000, particularly for companies seeking to expand into the European markets. ISO 9000 encompasses all of the activities of a company to ensure that it meets quality objectives and the HACCP system is directed towards ensuring the safety of food. ISO 9000 and HACCP are concerned with the quality and food safety management systems, respectively and have much in common. In fact, quality in a broader sense includes safety. Therefore, the best way is to use the ISO 9000 route to manage HACCP to ensure quality and safety of food. Both the systems are quality assurance systems designed to provide maximum confidence that a specified acceptance level of quality and safety are being achieved at an economic cost. HACCP is a technique, which involves examining the production process, identifying the critical areas of concerns (hazards) and putting measures in place to prevent potential problems from happening.

In 2001, in order to facilitate the implementation of HACCP and ISO 9001 in food organizations, the International Organization for Standardization (ISO) has published the guidelines on the application of ISO 9001:2000 for the food industry (ISO15161: 2000). This guideline gives an interpretation of how ISO 9001 could be applied on a food organization and are designed for organizations involved in all aspects of food industry. ISO15161: 2000 includes sourcing, processing and packaging food products and explain the possibility to link the commonalities and the communication between the two systems. It is important to considered, that ISO 15161 is not a HACCP standard and cannot be reference document at certification, but this guideline is intended to provide a clear management system supporting HACCP controls for an effective food safety system, under the recognized framework of an ISO 9000 Quality management System. ISO has advanced on its works for quality and safety of food products with the publication of ISO 15161:2000. Now ISO is published the standard ISO 22000 "Food safety Management System-Requirements". The two standards are quite different. ISO 15161 deals with all aspects of food quality and shows the HACCP system can be integrated in to the quality management system. On the other hand, ISO 22000 concentrates exclusively on food safety and that provides information to producer how they can build up the food safety system itself.

The other important quality management system includes total quality management (TQM) and ISO 14000 (Environmental Management System). TQM has long been considered an essential component of all production and service enterprises. It is essentially a problem detecting system, committed to continuous improvement and focusing on customer satisfaction. TQM employs data for progress and success, and it empowers personnel to be responsible and accountable for continuous improvement; in other words, it facilitates Good Manufacturing Practice (GMP). ISO 14000 deals with the surrounding environments in which organization operates, including air, water, land, natural resources, flora, fauna, humans and their interrelations.

Development and Maintaining a HACCP Programme

As a part of TQM, HACCP must be applied to all levels of processing. Using this approach, each process and product must be simplified to three levels of raw product, process and finished product. Critical control points can then be determined at each level. Each product must be considered separately. Quality or process attributes are determined based on safety, regulatory and customer specifications, and historical data. System capabilities and tolerances should be determined to place lower and upper limits on each quality attribute.

Implementation of HACCP Programme

Hazard analysis and critical control point (HACCP) is a team based programme which by identifying hazards and establishing monitoring systems and controls provides a means to build quality and wholesomeness into egg products. HACCP can be defined as a systemic approach to food safety, consisting of seven principles-

1. Assess hazards and risks associated with growing, harvesting, raw materials and ingredients, processing, manufacturing, distribution, marketing, preparation and consumption of food
2. Determination of critical control points required to control the identified hazard
3. Establishment of critical limits that must be met at each identified CCP
4. Establishment of procedures to monitoring CCP
5. Establishment of corrective action to be taken when there is a deviation identified by monitoring a CCP
6. Establishment of effective record keeping systems that document the HACCP plan
7. Establishment of procedures for verifications that HACCP system is working correctly.

Quality Relating to Microbial Safety

Microbiological safety of food and food borne Infections" include proper sanitary and phytosanitary measures; post harvest care of raw materials, reliable HACCP practices and serving freshly prepared food in community feeding.

Table 16.2: Microbiological Limits (Numbers) in different Egg Products

Sl.No.	*Bacteria*	*Products*	*USDA Standard*	*EEC standard*	*PFA standard*
1.	Aerobic plate counts	**Liquid eggs**			
		At production	$<10^3$	$<10^5$	–
		At expiration date	$<10^4$	$<10^5$	–
		Dried eggs	$<10^4$	$<10^5$	**<75,000**
		Frozen eggs	$<10^4$	$<10^5$	–
2.	Coliforms	**Liquid eggs**			
		At production	<10	–	–
		At expiration date	$<10^2$	$<10^2$	
		Dried eggs	$<10^2$	$<10^2$	$<10^2$
		Frozen eggs	$<10^2$	$<10^2$	–
		For all products			
3.	*Salmonella*		Absent in 100g	Absent in 25 g	Absent in 25g
4.	Yeast and mold		$<10^2$	–	<50
5.	*E. coli*		–ve/test		
6.	Coagulase positive *Staphylococcus aureus*		–ve/test	Absent in 1 g	–
7.	*Listeria monocytogenes*		–ve/25g	–	–

Eggs are good source of nutrients for microorganisms despite the presence of some inhibitory substances in the egg. Mostly freshly laid eggs are sterile, at least, inside, but the shell soon become contaminated by faecal matter from the hen, by the cage or nest, by wash water if the eggs are washed, by handling, and by the material in which eggs are packed. The total numbers of microorganisms per shell of hens egg vary from 10^2-10^7 with a mean of about 10^5. However some bacteria especially Salmonella can be transferred inside the egg when the egg is infected. Most common bacteria found on the eggshell are *Coliforms, Achromobacter, Pseudomonas, Serratia, Proteus, Alcaligenes, Citrobacter* etc. *Salmonella* organisms are the principal pathogens found in and on the eggs and are responsible for largest number of human disease outbreaks caused by eggs.

The shell acquires infection from all the surfaces with which it makes contact and the extent of infection is directly related to cleanliness of these surfaces. Under normal conditions of handling and storage, there are rare chances of growth of microorganisms because of low level of available water. Humid conditions in egg stores permit the growth of molds, and hype penetrates the pores thus infecting shell membranes and albumen. Bacteria remain localized at or near the surface of shell unless free water is present. They penetrate the shell along with water drawn into pores by capillary action or are sucked in when a warm egg contacts on cooling. Rubbing the shell with abrasive can increase the extent of penetration. The contaminants multiply in albumen and further when the yolk touches shell membranes or contaminants reach yolk.

Other Factors Affecting Egg Quality

These include production factors like *genetic factors, age, feed, medicament and chemicals, environmental temperature, management, frequency of gathering* (at least 3-4 times per day are recommended), *cooling, handling, grading, packaging and marketing* are important. In grading eggs are classified into different categories on the basis of their weight, and quality. Egg grading involves inspection of the shell for soundness, cleanliness, checking the internal quality like firmness of thick albumen, position of yolk, blood spot and size of air cell by candling as described earlier. Autoomatic egg candling machine with candling and sorting facilities has also been developed for commercial use. The AGMARK standard for table eggs is shown in the Table 16.3.

Table 16.3: The AGMARK Standard for Table Eggs

Grade	*Weight(g)*	*Shell*	*Air cell*	*White*	*Yolk*
A-Extra large A-Large A-Medium A-Small	60 and above 53 – 59 45 – 52 38 - 44	Clean and sound, shape normal	Up to 4 mm in depth, practically regular or better	Clear, reasonably firm	Fairly well centered, practically free from defects, outline distinct
B-Extra large B-Large B-Medium B-Small	60 and above 53 – 59 45 – 52 38 – 44	Clean to moderately stained, sound and slightly	8 mm in depth, may be free and slightly bubbly	Clean, may be slightly weak	May be slightly off-centered, outline slightly visible

The grade designation mark shall be attached by means of a lead seal bearing the word AGMARK to each container of table eggs and shall clearly show the following particulars: i) grade designation of table eggs; ii) Number of eggs; ii)Net weight of eggs; and iv)name of the grading station. The grade designation mark to each container of table eggs shall consists of a label specifying the grade and in the following colours- Extra large-White, Large- Red, Medium-Blue and Small- Yellow

Table 16.4: Storage Condition and Shelf-life (in days) of Untreated and Oil Coated Eggs

Storage Conditions	*Shelf-life (Untreated)*	*Shelf-life (Oil coated)*
100°F (37.7°C) (Dry bulb-100°F, Wet Bulb-82°F, R. H. 65 per cent)	5	10
78°F (25.5°C), R. H. 72 per cent	7	28
55°F (12.8°C), R. H. 85 per cent	30	60
33°F (0.5°C), R. H. 90 per cent	180	360

Marketing of Egg

Frequent marketing at least twice per week or more is essential to shorten time between production and final consumption. Before marketing proper grading and packaging is necessary. For export market 360 eggs are packed in bulk container (12×30).For rapid movement of egg in the market channel can be made by following ways-

1. Rapid and efficient handling in grading station with adequate refrigeration facilities.
2. Speedy transport through insulated or refrigerated track to retail or wholesale market.
3. Frequent delivery to retailer at least twice per week or possibly 3-5 times per week can be recommended.

Marketing of eggs is largely done in India in the unorganized sector with no control on the prices, even then while for any agricultural product, the producer gets only 30 per cent to 35 per cent of the consumer rupee while the egg producers in India obtain 70 per cent - 75 per cent of the consumer rupee as declared by National Egg Coordination Committee (NECC). NECC is an association of Poultry farmers and traders established in 1982.

NECC is a charitable trust with 24 zones and 118 local committees has about 25,000 farmers as its members spread out all over India in every production centre is helping the layer farmers obtain reasonable, remunerative, viable price for eggs based on demand and supply for a production centre and its connected consumption centers. To ensure traders do not exploit farmers, NECC undertakes Market Intervention Scheme as and where necessary by extension of subsidy or directly procuring eggs for cold storage in the domestic market. To enforce the price declared, NECC also has its market arm, Agrocorpex India Limited (ACIL), a Public Limited Company, entirely owned and managed by poultry farmers. NECC has also been instrumental, at the instance of poultry farmers, in incorporating Bharat Egg Producer's Association, which encourages export of shell eggs, promotion of eggs in electronic and print media and sponsors sports and related activities to promote consumption of poultry products. NECC is the only agency, well recognized by policy makers in State and Centre as representative body of poultry industry to represent the interests of poultry and has been effective to get its grievances addressed and remedial measures initiated.

However, eggs are largely marketed through a chain of wholesalers, the first of whom lifts eggs from the producer at a rate of fixed according to supply and demand. This rate has no connection with the cost of production of egg. The first wholesaler keeps a margin of 45 paise per egg. The product then goes through two to three sub-dealers before it reaches the consumer who pays roughly 15 paise more than what the farmer is paid for. Less than 5 percent of all eggs produced are retailed directly to consumers by the farmers. The rest go through a chain of middlemen before reaching the consumers. The following factors need consideration for improvement of egg marketing-

- ✰ The eggs are sold by number and not by weight, no grading rate mentioning is done, small pullet eggs are offered substantially lower rates, the egg rates paid to the farmer decided by wholesalers based on the supply and demand position and does not take care of cost of production into consideration, and the demand for eggs fluctuate with season.
- ✰ Formation of cooperatives at village or district levels and marketing federation at state level cloud more effectively handle the logistics of preservation, storage and transportation of eggs for which facilities are currently inadequate.
- ✰ The need for an effective cold chain infrastructure is imperative to regulate the supply in response to fluctuating demand.
- ✰ Overall efficiency depends on the speedy disposal of eggs from the producer to consumer at the lowest cost along with other facilities the consumer desires.
- ✰ Marketing cost and marketing margins vary depending on the set of conditions and circumstances under which the egg trade is done. About 30 percent of consumer price goes towards marketing costs.
- ✰ Factors such as quality of eggs, demand and supply position, intermediaries involved in the marketing channel and socioeconomic condition of the consumers and speed of disposal influence the marketing margin.

Marketing Challenges

In India, Eggs are still transported in open condition and in un-refrigerated vehicles. The entire chain of distribution and physical handling up to consumer is in open climate exposed to varying temperatures of seasons and agro climatic conditions. Shelf life of eggs is therefore restricted to 11-14 days in summer and 18-20 days in winter. The egg is still sold as a commodity in India and purchased by consumer mostly from shop next door for daily needs *i.e.* Pan shops, kirana stores, bakeries etc. India with a 11-12 crore daily egg production and with over its 70 per cent of human population living in villages each with 500 – 2000 population per hamlet is located across the length and breadth of country in over 6,27,000 villages. It is a marketer's nightmare to ensure sufficient availability of Eggs to consumers as it is a perishable product, to be made available in vast number of shops and stocked sufficient to meet daily needs of consumers.

Marketing Opportunities

Rural Market

Because of the location of farms in semi urban and urban centers and poultry traditionally developed in concentrated pockets in AP, TN, Punjab and Haryana and Maharashtra, the availability of eggs is high in few states in Urban and semi urban centers, but in rural centers and rest of the country, the availability is low. There is a vast scope to tap the rural markets and NE states where consumption is low because of poor availability. Sufficient number of sales outlets for eggs in interior villages will ensure in improving the per capita consumption of eggs. To tap the egg market potential in villages, more number of outlets by farmers needs to be opened in villages.

Even shell eggs free of antibiotics and pesticide residues could be exported to Japan, Fast East and Europe, which is currently sourcing at a high price from USA, Europe and other countries. India is exporting egg powders meeting strict quality norms of EU. While Egg powder from India is well accepted in EU, Japan and Far-East, the big layer farmers in India need to promote and tap the potential for shell eggs from India allaying the fears of pesticide and antibiotic residues.

Eggs in Mid-day Meal Scheme

Egg is a balanced food item that cannot be adulterated. The infertile egg produced in the modern farms is accepted as a part of vegetarian diet by a majority of population. The Supreme Court has advised all States to implement the mid day meals scheme which would improve the health status of the under privileged children, and improve the attendance in schools and academic standards, besides help in increasing the per capita egg consumption and maintaining remunerative price for eggs.

VI. Microbial Spoilage of Eggs

Eggs are good source of nutrients for microorganisms despite the presence of some inhibitory substances in the egg. Mostly freshly laid eggs are sterile, at least, inside, but the shell soon become contaminated by faecal matter from the hen, by the cage or nest, by wash water if the eggs are washed, by handling, and by the material in which eggs are packed. Most common bacteria found on the eggshell are *Coliforms, Achromobacter, Pseudomonas, Serratia, Proteus, Alcaligenes, Citrobacter* etc.

Changes of Eggs during Storage

The changes may be divided into-

a) Non-microbial Causes

1. Loss of moisture especially in untreated eggs (as evident from increase in the size of air cell).
2. Alkalinity of egg increase from 7.5 to 9.59 (due to escape of CO_2).
3. Weakening of vitelline membrane.
4. White of egg become thinner and more watery (due to decrease in interactions between Lysozyme and ovomucin with the increase in pH)

b) Microbial Causes

Bacteria cause more spoilage of eggs than molds.

Some of the important bacterial spoilage or rots are:

1. **Green rots:** Caused chiefly by *Pseudomonas fluorescens.*
2. **Colourless rots:** Caused by *Pseudomonas, Acinetobacter, Alcaligens,* certain Coliform spp. etc.
3. **Black rots:** Species of Proteus are usually involved, for example *Proteus melenovogenes.*
4. **Pink rots:** Caused by *P. fluorescens* and may at times later stage of some green rots.
5. **Yellow rots:** Caused by *Flavobacterium* and *Cytophaga* spp. In this rot yellow pigments are formed in shell membranes at the site of growth.

Spoilage of Eggs by Fungi

1. **Pin spot molding:** It is initial mold growth because there are small, compact colonies of molds appearing on shells or just inside it. The colour of pin spots varies with the mold *e.g. Penicillium* spp., *P. expansum, P. asperulum, P. oxalicum* causes Yellow/blue/green spots.

   Sporotrichum carnis-pink spot

   Cladosporium herbarum- dark green or black spots.
2. **Superficial fungal spoilage:** It is in form of fuzz or whiskers covering the shell. This occurs when eggs are stored at high relative humidity at low temperature.
3. **Fungal rottening:** This is the final stage of spoilage jelling of white takes place and coloured rots are produced.

   Red rots-*Sporotrichum* spp.

   Black rots- *Cladosporium herbarum*

Hyphae of molds may weaken yolk membrane enough to rupture. Sometimes off-flavours are also developed in eggs with little outward evidence of spoilage of *e.g.* Mustiness- caused by *Achromobacter prolens, Pseudomonas graveolens, Pseudomonas muciodolens,* Hay odour- caused by *Enterobacter cloacae* Fishy odour- caused by *E. coli.*

– Chapter 17 –

Quality Identification of Shell Eggs and Factors Influencing the Quality

Candling and Grading of Eggs

Quality of intact eggs can be correctly judged by candling. The practice of candling has been developed to enable the visualization of internal egg contents without breaking the shell. Candling not only helps in grading of eggs but detects cracked and abnormal eggs as well. The candlers are mainly of two types *viz.* hand candlers and automated candlers/mass scanning devices. However, hand candling is used very little in the present commercial grading operations but it is still considered an excellent method for teaching and demonstration of egg quality evaluation.

Requirements

1. Eggs
2. Egg Candler/candling lamp
3. Grader
4. Dark room

Procedure

1. Hold two eggs in each hand, supporting one egg by tips of thumb and first two fingers. The second egg should be held against the palm with other two fingers. The narrow ends of the eggs should point towards the palm of the hand.
2. Hold the first egg of right hand against the upper edge of aperture of Candler at an angle so that its long axis is almost perpendicular to the right.

3. Examine the all sides of egg with slow rotation
4. After the candling of the egg, it is shifted back in a rotating motion to the palm of the hand and the second egg is brought into candling position.
5. Examine the egg in the left hand while changing operation is done.

Air cell is normal: darker than rest egg, round and fixed on broad end side, Abnormal: bubbly, free, movable. Albumen is normal: clear white, free from shadows of foreign bodies and discolouration; Abnormal: foamy, blood stained, shadow of foreign body. Yolk is normal: when stable, well centered, outline well defined, Abnormal: off centered, stuck yolk, enlarged, flattened.

Common Defects Encountered during Candling

- ☆ **Blood Spots and Blood Streaks:** They appear as a bright red spots or streaks during candling. Generally, they are on surface of yolk and move with twirling. These may be due to fright, high perching, high egg production rate and vitamin K deficiency.
- ☆ **Bloody Egg:** It has red tint through out.
- ☆ **Meat Spot:** Any solid foreign material found between vitelline and shell membrane of egg. These may be found attached or floating in white of egg. Some time attached to chalaza. They are dark red, deep brown and brownish red.
- ☆ **Soft and thin shelled eggs:** These can be detected visually and during candling. This may occur may be due to high egg production and deficiency of calcium in diet.
- ☆ **Body Checks:** Sometime eggs become checked while egg is in formation and more calcium is deposited on it later on. So during candling appear as slight ridges or lines.
- ☆ **Double yolk eggs:** When two ova are released simultaneously, double yolk eggs occur. They are seen clearly in egg during candling.
- ☆ **Egg within egg:** Sometime due to reverse peristaltic movements egg is forced back in its initial position. Again it travels down and same procedure is followed. So egg within egg is formed.
- ☆ **Glossy egg:** They have glossy appearance and normal for sale.
- ☆ **Abnormal Shape:** These are due to peristaltic movements, shape of oviduct wall, foreign material and condition of glands etc.

Precautions

1. The temperature of egg to be candled should be between 50-70°F.
2. Candling light should not be too bright or too dim.
3. Candling must be done in a darkened room, which is comfortable, ventilated.
4. Candler should be kept clean to assure maximum light efficiency.

Grading of Eggs

Egg grading involves subjective classification of egg into categories according to their size, weight and other quality factors that ultimately determine its relative commercial value. This involves inspection of the shell for soundness, cleanliness, apparent strength and shape, checking the interior of egg by candling and sorting into sizes on the basis of weight. In India, the eggs are graded according to Egg Grading and Marketing rules, 1968.

The grade designation mark shall be attached by means of a lead seal bearing the word AGMARK to each container of table eggs and shall clearly show the following particulars: i) grade designation of table eggs; ii) Number of eggs; ii)Net weight of eggs; and iv)name of the grading station. The grade designation mark to each container of table eggs shall consists of a label specifying the grade and in the following colours.

- ☆ Extra large-White
- ☆ Large- Red
- ☆ Medium-Blue
- ☆ Small- Yellow

Procedure

1. Record the weight of the eggs.
2. Check the eggs for shell roundness and cleanliness.
3. Observe the interior of eggs with the help of Candler.
4. Grade the eggs based on observations as specified.

Precautions

1. Mark the eggs to avoid mixing.
2. Handle the eggs carefully to avoid breakage.
3. Record all the observations carefully.

Table 17.1: BIS Standards for Grading of Eggs

Grade	*Weight of egg (g)*	*Shell*	*Air cell*	*White*	*Yolk*
A Extra large A Large A Medium A Small	60 and above 53-59 45-52 38-44	Clean, unbroken, sound, normal shaped	Depth less than or equal to 4mm, practically regular	Clear and reasonably firm	Fairly well centred, practically free from defects, outline indistinct
B Extra large B Large B Medium B Small	60 and above 53-59 45-52 38-44	Clean to moderately stained and sound, slightly abnormal shape	5-8mm depth, may be free and slightly bubbly	Clear, may be slightly weak	May be slightly off centred, outline slightly visible

Eggs which do not qualify under the above two grades, may be debarred from entering trade channels for fresh shell eggs.

Table 17.2: USDA Standards for Grading of Eggs

Quality Factor	*AA Quality*	*A Quality*	*B Quality*	*C Quality*
Shell	Clean, unbroken, practically normal	Clean, unbroken, practically normal	Clean to very slightly stained, unbroken, may slightly be abnormal	Clean to moderately stained, unbroken, may be abnormal
Air Cell	1/8" or less in depth, practically regular	3/16" or less in depth, practically regular	3/8" or less in depth, may be free or bubbly	May be or over 3/8" depth may be free or bubbly
White	Clear, firm, H.U. 72 or more	Clear, may be reasonably firm, H.U.; 60-72	Clear, may be slightly weak firm, H.U 31-.60	May be weak watery, small blood clots or spots may be present H.U <31.
Yolk	Outline slightly defined, practically free from defects	Outline may be fairly defined, practically free from defects	Outline may be well defined, slightly enlarged, may show definite but not serious defects	Outline may be practically visible, may be enlarged, may show clear germ development but no blood, may show other serious defects

Evaluation of Egg Quality

Egg quality means the inherent properties present in an egg, which determines its degree of acceptability. Egg quality act as a marketing tool as well as provides valuable guidelines for the poultry farm managers to produce safe, wholesome and designer eggs with requisite nutritional and functional properties. Egg quality is broadly divided into two categories, *i.e.* external and internal quality.

I) Evaluation of Exterior Egg Quality

a) Soundness of Shell

Normal eggs: unbroken shell, normal shape and texture, Abnormal: Cracked but intact membranes, Blind cracks as hairline crack, leaker- shell and membranes both are broken

It is examined by visual inspection, belling and candling.

Classes of eggs based on soundness are as under:

- ☆ **Sound egg**: Shell intact and unbroken
- ☆ **Checked/cracked egg**: Shell cracked but intact shell membranes and contents do not leak.
- ☆ **Leaker egg**: Crack or rupture in shell and shell membranes and its contents are leaking.
- ☆ **Smashed egg**: Shell crushed or smashed.

b) Shape and Texture

Normal shape of an egg is oval. Abnormal shapes: round,spindle,pear etc. Maximum length: 5.6cm, Maximum width: 4.2cm. Inspect the eggs for their shape and texture. Shape index of an egg can be determined by measuring width and length with Vernier calliper as below:

Shape Index = (Width/Length) x 100

Good egg should have shape index between 70 to 75. Higher shape index indicates wider egg and lower index longer egg.

Classification of eggs with respect to shape and texture are as under:

- **Practically normal** – Usual shape and good even texture and strength, free from rough areas, ridges and thin spots.
- **Slightly abnormal** – Shell may be somewhat unusual in shape or slightly faulty in texture or strength. May show definite ridges but no pronounced thin spots or rough areas.
- **Abnormal** – Misshapen or faulty in texture or strength or that may show pronounced ridges, thin spots or rough areas.

c) Shell Cleanliness

Normal eggs: complete, clean, sound and desired strength and porosity, Abnormal: glassy,thin,soiled,cracked,soft,unsound.

Observe the eggs for shell cleanliness and classify as per specified below:

- **Clean** – Shell free from foreign material, stains, or discolorations that are readily visible.
- **Slightly stained** – Shell free from adhering dirt but shows presence of light stains on the surface covering upto $1/16^{th}$ of its surface.
- **Moderately stained** – Shell free from adhering dirt but has moderate degree of stains covering not more than $1/4^{th}$ of its surface.
- **Dirty** – Shell that has adhering dirt or stains covering more than $1/4^{th}$ of its total surface area.

d) Shell Thickness and per cent Shell

Weigh the egg accurately and break it with the help of glass rod. Remove the contents of egg completely. Take about 250 ml of NaOH solution in a beaker and boil it over hot plate. Add eggshell in the boiling solution and allow it to boil for 5 minutes to remove shell membranes. Remove the beaker from hot plate and take out the shell. Wash the shell with the tap water and dry in hot air oven at 100 °C for about 24 hours. Take out the shell from oven and allow it to cool. Record the thickness of shell with the help of screw gauge. The measurements of weight of the entire shell help to calculate the percent shell.

Per cent shell = (Weight of shell/Weight of egg) x 100

e) Shell Colour

Normal colour is characterstic of breed as White egg: leghorns, ancones; Brown shelled eggs: Rhode Island Red, New Hampshire, Plymouth Rocks, Cornish.

Grading parameters do not include shell colour, as shell colour is not at all related to egg quality.

f) Specific Gravity of Egg

Normal sp. Gravity of hen egg is 1.06 to 1.09, Higher sp. gr. is due to thick shell of eggs, Less sp. Gr. is due to thinner shells, Shell thickness affected by Inheritance, season, nutrition, stress, health. When dipping of eggs is done in water, eggs that sink are good and egg rising upright is of poor quality.

The specific gravity of egg is determined by Brine Floatation method developed by Tyler and Geake (1961). Solutions of known specific gravity ranging from 1.058-1.106 are prepared using different concentrations of sodium chloride as specified below. Egg is floated in each solution starting from the one with least specific gravity. The solution in which the egg just floats is the specific gravity of that egg.

Table 17.3: Specific Gravity of Salt Solutions

Quantity of Salt (g/l)	*Specific Gravity*
70.81	1.058
75.95	1.062
81.91	1.066
86.53	1.070
91.18	1.074
97.21	1.078
102.75	1.082
103.10	1.086
113.83	1.090
119.47	1.094
125.20	1.098
131.40	1.102
136.97	1.106

II) Interior Egg Quality

a) Albumen Index, Haugh Unit and Yolk Index

Albumen index measured by dividing height of thick albumen(cm) with spherometer by average width of thick albumen(cm) with vernier caliper.

Albumen index = Height of albumen/average Width of albumen

Fresh egg has albumen index value 0.1 or more

Normal albumen is clear, uniform in colour, free from blood spot, Abnormal: enlarged and flattened, blood and meat spot.

Yolk Index is ratio between height and width of yolk of egg

Yolk Index = Height of yolk/average Width of yolk

Good quality egg has yolk height not less than 1/3 of width.

Haugh unit = 100 log $(H+7.57-1.7\,W^{0.37})$

Where, H = Height of thick albumen in mm., W = Weight of egg in grams.

– Chapter 18 –

Pre-slaughter Care, Transportation, Resting, Fasting, Ante-mortem Examination

There is a substantial growth in poultry production and consumption in last few decades. The increasing emphasis on quality has led to remarkable advances in technological innovation in the poutry industry. Concern for animal welfare, too has produced fundamental changes in the approach to live bird collection, transportation unloading and slaughter.

Catching and Assembling of Birds

In general, broilers are caught at night for loading as at that time they are easier to catch, struggle less and settled down in the coops faster. Loading schedules should be arranged so that the birds arrive at the point within an hour before they are to be unloaded for slaughter. Turkey and fowl are caught and handled whenever they are needed for processing. This is normally the afternoon before slaughter since turkeys sometimes must be caught on open pasture and hens are moved from laying cages or laying houses. It is established that the majority of bruises resulting in downgrading occur during catching and transportation. Bruising occurs in 2 per cent or more of birds during harvesting and transport. The incidence of bruising is directly related to the length of the journey.

Manual Catching

Broilers are caught at night for loading. At that time they are easier to catch, Struggle less, settle down in the coops faster and in summer the weather is cooler at night. Loading schedules should be arranged so that the birds arrive at the plant within an hour before are to unloaded for slaughter Mountney and Gardner(1957) reported method of assembling broilers. A catching crew of 4 or 5 men are responsible for the loading. Before the birds are caught, all feeders, waterers and other equipment are removed to one corner of the house and the lights turned out or dimmed to prevent birds from becoming excitement. Then two men catch broilers by the shanks, four in each hand. The birds are then handed to two other men who carry them to truck outside the house, there the truck driver and the helper place them in coops and arrange them on the truck. The truck driver is responsible for seeing that the birds are properly crated and loaded and that they arrive at the plant on schedule and in good condition.

Poultry harvesting procedure can be divided in to four basic systems- *Loose crate system, Fixed crates, Modules, Novel mechanical methods* (Herding systems, Vacuum systems, Scooping systems, Mat systems).

1. **Loose crates:** earlier system, crates made of wood or wire, have now been replaced by plastic crates – advantages: lighter more robust, easier to clean, easy to handle. Empty crates from the lorry into the shed - a team of catchers fill the individual crates. The birds are caught by one leg and passed into the crate through a flapped opening at the top, which is sufficiently large to insert the bird. For unloading, there is often a larger aperture in the side or top of the crate; through which the birds can be extracted. To avoid injuries to the birds, the catchers must not use excessive force when placing them in crates. Low capital cost –but high labor requirement.
2. **Fixed crates:** The crates are constructed as fixtures on a lorry bed. A framework of about 96 crates is built on each side of a central ventilation tunnel. One side of the vehicle is loaded first and then the other. The catching crew pick up the birds by one leg and carry them out of the shed to the lorry, where the birds are inserted into one of the lower crates. After filling the crate, the hinged flap is fastened. This procedures continue until the lower crates have been filled. For loading the upper containers a loading flatform is attached. The amount of injury to the birds depend upon the care by the catchers. The capital cost in greater than loose crates. But labour requirements are marginally lower.
3. **Modules:** Modular systems were developed in response to the processors demand for improved carcass quality. The concepts involves a metal frame containing 4-16 crates or compartments. At catching, an empty module is taken into the house by a fork lift truck. The birds are caught by hand and put directly into the compartment, thus avoiding the need for multiple handling or carrying the birds for long distance before crating.

   Modules have the advantage not only of reducing injury to birds, but also in requiring fewer people to achieve catching rates comparable to those of loose or fixed crates.

   Different types of modules are:

   a) Multiple –floor modules.
   b) Metal drawer modules.
   c) Unrestrained plastic drawers.

4. **Novel mechanical methods:** can be divided into five groups according to the way they operate.
   (a) **Herding system:** series of conveyer belts.
   (b) **Sweeping systems:** The machine moves on tracks and has a central, retractable boom and sweeper arms fitted with rotating foam-rubber paddles which gently sweep the birds onto an inclined conveyer fitted with perches. A single machine with one operator is capable of catching and crating over 5000 boiler chickens.
   (c) **Vacuum system:** two systems.

   Boertien system: 60 meter long tubes through which the broilers are moved by gentle suction from the house floor to the crate filling device outside the house.

   Other system the Nicolai: suction power to pick the broilers from the floor. Immediately after being picked up, the birds are dropped onto a conveyer belt.
   (d) **Scooping system:** Scooping the birds mechanically from the floor and transporting them to a crating area for manual loading.
   (e) **Mat system:** 60 m long 1.4 m wide woven polypropylene mats, laid the full length of the house floor, 2h before harvesting a special device then rolls up the mats in sequence brings the birds to one end of the house – loaded into large open trays -stacked in tens, covered and loaded by means of a fork lift truck capacity 8000 birds/h, downgrading 50 per cent less.

Transportation

Transportation of poultry is carried out at cool hours of the day preferable at early morning just one hour before slaughter. Care should be taken from suffering of poultry from suffocation. By open sided vehicles- exposure to prevailing climate and to high wind speeds. Cages-on-rollers are tried in transportation of birds. Poultry transport trucks. Turkey handling trollers and trucks, Ducks/gease transport trucks, Pheasants, quails, guineafowls, pigeons-crates used.

Precautions: Protect from direct rays of sun, from adverse weather, provide adequate ventilation.

Reception and Unloading/Preslaughter Area

The reception area, often referred to, as the arrival area is where the birds are brought into the slaughterhouse for unloading. To comply with welfare requirements, the area should be under cover and of sufficient size to contain all the transport vehicles enter the building at one side and leave at the other after washing, thus avoiding cross contamination. In warm weather, ventilation fans are used to control R.H. 70 per cent and also to minimize bruising and broken bones. Unloading method depend upon transport system *i.e.* loose crates, fixed crates, modules. Preslaughter fasting and ante-mortem inspection of birds are conducted in the lairage penss of pre-slaughter area.

Weighing

Bulk weighing is now used almost exclusively in weighing birds. A truck loaded with empty crates is weighed at the public scale nearest the farm. Then the truck proceeds to the farm and the broilers are loaded into the crates, which are left on the truck.

Shrinkage

Contract hauling is practiced extensively in broiler areas. In some areas a shrinkage of 4 per cent during hauling is permitted, in other areas only 3 per cent is permitted. The pay price is determined by the weight of the birds when they are unloaded at the plant.

Pre-slaughter Resting and Fasting

After unloading in the slaughter house the birds must undergo a pre-slaughter resting and fasting of 12-16 hours in the poultry lairages. Preslaughter resting helps the birds to settle well and also the body physiologiological conditions become normal. Preslaughter fasting helps to empty the gastrointestinal tract and the microbial load of the intestine is greatly reduced to minimum. Fasting also helps in better bleeding and the colour, flavour, palatability and keeping quality of the meat is greatly improved.

Post Transport Antemortem (Preslaughter) Care

1. Animals should be cared for humanely during the post transport and/or antemortem period, generally defined as the 24 hours - 48 hours prior to slaughter. Humane treatment during this period should include:
   a. safe, careful unloading and movement into clean, uncrowded, dry holding areas. When unloading animals at a commercial abattoir (packing plant) attention should be paid to any animals that may have become downers (trampled) or non-ambulatory or injured during transport. In such cases the ante mortem inspector should be notified and proper segregation and care or euthanasia should be extended to these animals.
   b. reasonable protection from adverse weather, noise (such as exhaust fans or vehicles), noxious odours (such as exhaust from rendering or petrochemical sources)or views likely to upset the animals (such as people, vehicles, animals being stunned); and,
   c. access to clean water.
2. Proper ante mortem and/or post transport care will reduce weight loss, health problems and meat quality degradation.
3. Proper loading, unloading, care and management is important to the wellbeing of animals during the ante mortem period. Animals that will be kept for more than a few hours after transport should be provided with food, water and rest

Specific Considerations

1. All poultry do not have the same space requirements. Equipment specific to the species should be used. These guidelines emphasize the responsibilities of the poultry producer, the catching crew, and the transporter. They are intended to encourage humane, efficient, and considerate treatment of birds so that transport stress and injury are minimized at all stages of handling and transport.
2. Careless catching of birds is a common source of injury. Injured birds are particularly susceptible to transportation stress. This is inhumane and increases the loss of marketable product.
3. Piling of birds in corners can cause injury or mortality. Steps must be taken to prevent this from occurring.
4. The two most common procedures that facilitate easier catching of loose-housed birds are: lowering the light intensity in the pen or using blue bulbs to provide adequate llumination for humans but not for poultry; and corralling birds with a net or screen at the loading door.
5. Range birds can be loaded more easily by moving them in small groups.
6. Proper building design and accessibility to transport vehicles greatly improves the humane handling of loose-housed poultry. Owners and operators should ensure the following:
   a. appropriate access to loading and unloading areas of poultry barns is provided;
   b. loading and unloading areas and ramps are designed to permit proper bird handling;
   c. building design discourages needless transfer of birds between handlers;
   d. building design incorporates a door for every 15 m (49 ft) of building length, and doors on first, second, and third floors are not less than 120 cm wide (48 in) and not less than 200 cm (78 in) high; and,
   e. when birds have to be handed through floor openings, the openings are not less than 1 m^2 (10 sq.ft.) for broilers and not less than 1.2m^2 (13 sq.ft.) for turkeys, and no obstructions, such as floor joists, hinder the transfer of birds.
7. When birds are transported in crates or bins, the design, construction available space and state of repair should allow the birds to be loaded, conveyed, and removed without injury. Birds should be loaded only into clean transporting crates and clean vehicles.
8. Crate doors and panels on liner trucks should be large enough to permit easy passage of birds, thus avoiding injury.
9. Construction of crates and bins should provide adequate, uniform ventilation but prevent protrusion of the head, wings and legs of birds.

10. When loaded into bins or crates, birds must be positioned on their feet to avoid smothering.
11. The number of birds per crate or bin depends on available floor space, body size of birds, and prevailing environmental conditions at time of transport. Maximum density per crate or bin should permit all birds to rest on the floor at the same time if they are evenly distributed. Birds should be able to move their heads freely when sitting on the floor.
12. Covers should be used to protect birds in crates from wind, rain, and adverse weather conditions.
13. When birds are being transported in crates or bins, the driver should check the load and surrounding area for loose birds before departing.
14. Birds should be protected from getting wet. During loading they should be protected from sources of heat and steam to minimize the effect of exposure to a sudden drop in temperature.
15. Eaves troughs should be continuous across loading areas to prevent birds from getting wet during transfer from building to truck during a rainstorm.
16. Ideally, crates with live birds should be moved in a horizontal position. If a conveyor is used for loading crates of live birds, the conveyor angle should prevent tilting of crates that causes birds to pile up. Crates should not be thrown or dropped. They should be moved smoothly during loading, transport, and unloading.
17. One possible way to alleviate catching and loading problems and to avoid the potential for damage to the birds, is to collect the birds mechanically. Producers, catchers, and transporters should keep themselves informed of new technology. Only devices proven to be humane should be considered for use in gathering birds.
18. Loading of poultry is usually done by manual capture and lifting of the bird. This process happens under subdued lighting while the animals are at rest
19. Producers are responsible for ensuring proper interior and exterior design of buildings to facilitate loading and unloading of poultry.
20. In caged layer barns, cross conveyors should not be installed in such a way as to impede the flow of birds in carts travelling directly into or out of the barn via the proper loading doors. Where it is necessary to block the cage rows at the loading end, proper access must be given to the opposite end of the cage rows.
21. Weather conditions should be considered when determining load densities. For growing and adult birds, the recommended maximum live weight loading densities for crates and bins in cold weather are as follows:

    Chickens: 63 kg/m^2 (139 lbs/10 sq. ft.)

    Broiler Turkeys: 98 kg/m^2 (216 lbs/10 sq. ft.)

Heavy Hens: 98 kg/m^2 (216 lbs/10 sq. ft.)

Heavy Toms: 98 kg/m^2 (216 lbs/10 sq. ft.)

Source: Recommended Code of Practice for the Care and Handling of Poultry from Hatchery to Processing Plant (1989).

22. These maximum values are recommended for winter conditions and should be reduced during summer. On hot summer days, loading of turkeys at midday should be avoided. When temperature exceeds 32°C (90°F), birds should not be loaded unless they are scheduled for same-day delivery.
23. The driver of the vehicle is responsible for the care and welfare of all birds during transport. The driver should take into consideration climatic conditions and should adjust coverings to allow birds to warm up or cool off, as required.

Ante-mortem Inspection

Ante-mortem inspection of live poultry starts from farm to until slaughtering. It is essential to ensure that they are not affected with any disease or condition, which may render unwholesome meat production. The birds are carefully examined in poultry house, after transportation; during holding and finally just before slaughtering, and those are in good health and alert condition are declared fit for slaughter. AM inspection shall be made under adequate natural or artificial lighting.

It is performed on a group basis, while the birds are in coops or batteries before or after removal from trucks. When performing ante-mortem inspection, inspection program personnel are to observe the overall condition of the birds including the head, with attention to the eyes, legs, and the body of the birds; and whether there are any unusual swellings or other abnormalities on the birds.

Regulatory Requirements

- No poultry having been treated with antibiotics, coccidiostats or any other substance that may render the carcass, viscera or organs unfit for human consumption by reason of any residues remaining therein may be submitted for slaughter unless the withdrawal period prescribed to such substance has expired.
- No bird suffering from any disease or condition that may adversely affect the meat may be slaughtered.
- Ante-mortem inspections of poultry must be done by the authorised poultry meat inspector on the day of slaughter to ensure that the necessary arrangements can be made to accommodate suspect flocks or flocks that are suffering from a disease.
- The slaughtering of poultry, affected by a notifiable disease may not be carried out without the prior permission of the authorised person.
- Poultry affected by disease, excessive soiling, varying bird size, or any other condition that may lead to contamination of other birds must be slaughtered at the end of the shift.

- Poultry that died during transportation from the farm to the abattoir, must be placed in leak proof lockable containers with tight fitting lids, which are marked with the letters "CONDEMNED" in the case of low throughput abattoirs and in high throughput abattoirs in a room provided for storage awaiting disposal, if not removed on a continuous basis.
- No dead poultry may be presented for slaughter or brought into any area where approved poultry products are handled and must be regarded and handled as condemned.
- If post-mortem examinations are performed on D.O.A.'s (dead on arrivals) to establish the reason for death, it must be performed in a special room or area with adequate facilities.

Reasons for Ante-mortem Poultry Inspection

To ensure that:

- Only clean healthy birds are presented for slaughter and that contamination of healthy carcasses is prevented.
- Safe and wholesome meat for human consumption is made available to the consumer.
- To notify the abattoir manager in time about any disease/condition which will enable them to make the necessary arrangements to deal with the disease/condition.

Health Certification

1. No poultry may be slaughtered in an abattoir without a declaration of health status having been submitted:
   (*a*) in the case of a low throughput abattoir, on the day of slaughter;
   (*b*) in the case of a high throughput abattoir, 72 hours prior to slaughtering; and
   (*c*) the owner of the poultry must provide the above mentioned declaration.
2. Such health declaration must contain the following information
   (*a*) date of delivery;
   (*b*) name and address of owner/farm(s);
   (*c*) number of birds and specie(s);
   (*d*) average weight of birds;
   (*e*) health status of the flock(s) including mortality rate; and
   (*f*) medication, if given as well as withdrawal periods and dates;

Conditions Observed on the Farm and Response to it

The following disease conditions can already be observed in the broiler house on the farm and the necessary action taken:

- ☆ Obviously sick and injured poultry (to prevent cruelty to poultry) destroyed on the farm.
- ☆ Badly soiled poultry are cleaned satisfactorily before presented for slaughter.
- ☆ Diseases which are easier to observe (detect) in live poultry *e.g.* nerve problem cases, breathing (respiratory) diseases and fever be noted on the health certificate.
- ☆ Diseases, which pose a health, risk to humans and notifiable diseases must be reported to the state veterinarian of the province.
- ☆ Aesthetically unacceptable conditions *e.g.* pussy, gangrene-like lesions and cannibalism should be transported separately and handled and slaughtered at the end of the slaughtering shift.

Poultry Welfare

Animal welfare considerations are becoming increasingly more important.

Practices, which may once have been deemed acceptable, are now being reassessed and modified according to new knowledge and changing attitudes.

High standards of animal welfare are not only important legally, but also have direct economic benefits by enhancing productivity and helping to facilitate international market access.

Guidelines in Respect of Diseased Poultry Presented for Slaughter

- ☆ The abattoir management must inform, in advance, the Meat Inspector/ Meat Examiner of any abnormal conditions regarding consignments of live poultry from the farms (health certification).
- ☆ The inspector must, on reception of a load of suspected diseased poultry, carry out the necessary inspection to establish the nature and extent of the disease and to determine the immediate course of action.
- ☆ The inspector must bring his findings under the attention of the abattoir management or representatives and arrange procedures for the further handling of birds.
- ☆ If diseased birds are to be slaughtered, it has to be done at the end of the shift. A space has to be left on the hanging line between the healthy and suspected, diseased or contaminated chickens, in order to perform a thorough primary and secondary examination and to remove infected parts or remove the whole chicken from the line before it leaves the evisceration area.
- ☆ Equipment, which comes into contact with the suspected, diseased or contaminated chickens, must be cleaned thoroughly disinfected and sterilised to prevent possible transmission of the disease.
- ☆ Procedures for the handling of birds for emergency slaughter must be available although seldom used at poultry abattoirs.

Ante-mortem Dispositions

There are three possible outcomes, or dispositions, that follow observation of livestock or birds in ante-mortem inspection:

1. Passed for slaughter,
2. Suspect, and
3. Condemned

Let's discuss each of these outcomes in more detail. The animal or lot of birds can be passed for slaughter. This means that the animals or birds were determined to be fit for human food. Those animals that clearly exhibit signs of diseases and conditions listed in the regulations must be condemned. This means that they are clearly not fit for human food, and they must be destroyed and not allowed to enter commerce as human food.

Then there are those animals or birds that may exhibit signs of the diseases or conditions defined in the regulations, but further confirmation during post mortem inspection is needed before condemning the carcass or a part of the carcass. In each of these three cases, there are certain things that you must do.

Condemned

Birds plainly showing any disease or condition that would cause condemnation of the carcass on post mortem inspection are condemned on ante-mortem. They are not to be dressed, nor shall they be conveyed into any part of the official establishment where poultry are prepared or held. They must be disposed of appropriately. They include tanking, incineration, and denaturing. Dead-on-arrival (DOAs) are identified, counted, and weighed, and the number is recorded in the Public Health Information System (PHIS) Animal Disposition Reporting function.

Suspect

Birds that do not plainly show but are suspected of being affected by any disease or condition that would cause condemnation of the carcass or parts on post-mortem inspection are segregated and held for separate slaughter and examined under post-mortem. The establishment releases birds for treatment under the control of appropriate State of Federal officials. Public Health Veterinarians(PHV) are to notify the District Office and follow instructions as per regulations. Responsibilities Related to Foreign Animal Diseases and Reportable Conditions when he/she suspects a reportable or foreign animal disease according to the quarantine of diseased poultry are followed. It states that live poultry affected by a contagious disease transmissible to humans must be segregated and either:

- ✰ Slaughter separately if further handling does not create a health hazard, or
- ✰ Release for treatment if practicable (and if further handling is a hazard), or
- ✰ Condemn if treatment is not practicable (when further handling is determined to be hazardous)

Poultry suspected of having biological residues covers the requirements related to poultry suspected of having biological residues. There are three options. They can be returned to the grower if further holding is likely to result in their not being adulterated from the residue. They can be slaughtered and processed and retained for disposition. They also can be slaughtered and buried or incinerated.

Poultry used for research covers poultry that have been used for research. The establishment must have appropriate documentation that the biological product, drug, or chemical used in the research will not result in poultry products being adulterated – or it is condemned.

Abnormal Signs

Just as is true with livestock, there are signs that indicate poultry have a disease or condition outlined in the regulations making them unfit for human food. These diseases and conditions can sometimes be detected through observations of body position, body condition, and body surfaces of poultry.

Symptoms of disease that may be observed on ante-mortem inspection include the following:

- ☆ Swelling around the head and eyes
- ☆ Edema of the wattles
- ☆ Gasping and sneezing
- ☆ Off-colored diarrhea
- ☆ Skin lesions
- ☆ Lameness
- ☆ Torticollis or wry neck
- ☆ Bone or joint enlargement
- ☆ Dermatitis
- ☆ Emaciation

Different diseases, their ante-mortem and post-mortem findings with judgement will be given under poultry meat inspection in the separate chapter.

– Chapter 19 –

Methods of Slaughter and Slaughtering Procedure-Postmortem Inspection, Reasons for Condemnation of Carcass

Methods of Slaughter and Slaughtering Procedure

Ritual Methods of Slaughter

Ritual slaughter is the method of slaughter that is carried out as per religious rites of the particular community and is performed as specified in their religious books. Unfortunately stunning is not done in ritual methods. The method varies in different religions, mainly the following methods are used:

Halal method - for muslims

Kosher method - for jews

Jhatka method - for sikhs/hindus

Halal Method

Halal (Arabic:halâl; means *lawful* or *legal*) is a term designating any object or an action which is permissible to use or engage in, according to Islamic law. It is the opposite of *haraam*. The term is used to designate food seen as permissible according to Islamic law (Sharia).

The terms Halal and haram are both applied to many facets of life and one of the most useful uses of these terms is to refer to food items including meat products, food contact materials and pharmaceuticals. In Islam there are many things that are halal or haram, most of which are clear and obvious to all people. There are also items which are not clear as if they are halal or haram and in order to categorize them as halal or haram further information is needed. Items that are not clear are called mashbooh which means questionable. In Islam the general idea of food is halal except the following:

Pork and all its products, animals improperly slaughtered, alcoholic drinks including all forms of intoxicants, carnivorous animals, birds of prey and any food contaminated with any of these products.[1]

Islam has laws regarding which foods can and cannot be eaten and also on the proper method of slaughtering an animal for consumption, known as dhabihah.

A variety of substances are considered as harmful (haraam) for humans to consume and, therefore, forbidden as per various Quranic verses:

- Pork (*i.e.*, flesh of pig)[Qur'an 2:173]
- Blood[Qur'an 2:173]
- Animals slaughtered in the name of anyone but Allah. All that has been dedicated or offered in sacrifice to an idolatrous altar or saint or a person considered to be "divine"[Qur'an 2:173] [Qur'an 5:3]
- Carrion (carcasses of dead animals)[Qur'an 2:173]
- An animal that has been strangled, beaten (to death), killed by a fall, gored (to death), savaged by a beast of prey (except by a human)[Qur'an 5:3]
- Food over which Allah's name is not pronounced (or at least not in a name other than Allah)[Qur'an 6:121]
- Alcohol and other intoxicants[Qur'an 5:090]

Dhabiha: Method of Slaughter

Dhabiha (Arabic:), is the prescribed method of ritual slaughter of all animals excluding fish and most sea-life as per Islamic law. This method of slaughtering animals consists of a swift, deep transverse incision with a sharp knife across the neck, cutting through the windpipe, the food pipe, the vagus nerve jugular veins and carotid arteries of both sides but leaving the spinal cord intact. Furthermore it opens the circulatory system that is at high pressure to the air causing pressure to equalize and the blood pressure in the brain to fall to zero. As the brain requires a constant flow of blood under pressure for the animal to retain consciousness, anemia of the brain causes loss of awareness and perception. In this method the welfare of the animal is major consideration.In some countries it does not forbid stunning of animal prior to bleeding provided the stunning instruments have never been used for pigs. Eating of dead animals, consumption of blood and pork is not permitted. The slaughter is not permitted in production line where pig is slaughtered. Animals must not be slaughtered in the sight of other animals and those to be killed are fed and watered before death. Islamic laws prohibits slaughter of sick animals. Animals must be alive, healthy and free from injuries.

The butcher should be a muslim and mature. The site of cut is throat. the jugular veins and carotid arteries are cut by a sharp knife. The spinal cord is not cut hence, nerve centres controlling heart and lungs remain functional which ensures efficient bleeding. The head is not separated at the time of slaughter. Gods name is to be mentioned "in the name of allah and allah is great". Therefore machine slaughter is not permitted. The neck of animal should face kiblah (holy place for muslims) and the butcher should face kibla too if possible. The approved islamic organisation should certify halal slaughter. Although this method is not controlled by a central board but is overseen by local islamic authorities known as muftis. Mufti decides whether the slaughter related acts and thoughts confirm the islamic laws, shariah or not.

Jewish Slaughter Method

According to Jewish law an animal at the time of slaughter must be alive and healthy and must not have suffered from any injuries. This means that any form of prior stunning is prohibited. Regulations for Jewish method of slaughter have existed since 500 A.D. Even a blow on the head of an animal meant for Jewish consumption is forbidden, as perforation of the brain meninges occur which render the meat " terepha" or unfit for food.

Species

Cattle, calves, sheep, goats dear, all kinds of poultry.

The ancient prohibition against the consumption of pork may be due to the effect of the roundworm *Trichinella spiralis* and the tapeworm *Taenia solium.*

Slaughtered animals which are found on examination to be fit for Jewish consumption are described as "Kosher'.

Sticking Method

The neck of the animal is fully extended and the cut is made by one rapid thrust of a sharp knife which severs the skin, the muscles, esophagus, trachea, carotid arteries and jugular veins. This method of slaughter is known as "Schechita" and is carried out only by the " cutter" (Schochet) assisted by a "sealer" (shomer) who stamps kosher seal on each part of the carcass which is passed for Jewish food.

The five principles of Schechita are as follows

1. **Pause:** There must be no pause or interruption in the act of killing. Any slight pause renders the carcass unclean.
2. **Pressure:** No pressure may be used. This means that the knife used must be exceedingly sharp- a point which promotes humanity. For the same reason the animal must be on its back with the throat upwards, because if the throat is kept above the knife, the use of pressure will become necessary.
3. **Stabbing:** Stabbing is not permitted. Wool or hair must be removed first and the cut exposed through its entire length.
4. **Slanting:** The knife must not be held slanting to the skin. The cut must be at right angle to the surface.
5. **Tearing:** No tearing is allowed.

A razor sharp knife called chalef is used which is 15 inches long and 3 inches from back to edge and quadrilateral in sharp. The edge is like that of a razor and the schochet prepares it himself. He is not allowed to send it anywhere for grinding, and the schochet must examine the edge under a microscope before using it. If any dent is seen, the knife is discarded and not used as otherwise, the meat produced will become "Unclean" From the time of the application of the knife to the moment of unconsciousness, it takes about 5 to 6 'heart beats' period.

Certain continental countries have introduced legislation requirement that animals slaughtered for Jewish consumption shall be rendered unconscious by mechanical means before the throat-cut may be made. Legislation to this effect is in operation in Australia, Norway, Switzerland and Sweden.

The schochet and sealer are being trained and then licensed by rabbinical commission to perform slaughter. The meat fit for consumption is called as kosher meat and the carcass that is rendered unfit for consumption is called terepha. At slaughter the animal should be healthy, alive and without any injury. Stunning of the animal is not permitted. All the soft major blood vessels are severed and neck is kept stretched for thorough bleeding. The five rules for jewish slaughter are that the neck incision should be completed without pause, pressure, stabbing, slanting or tearing. If knife receives any nick during the act of schechita, meat is not permitted for jewish food.

After slaughter the schochet offers prayers and carry out a searching, postmortem examination by making an incision posterior to xiphoid process and inserting the arm to detect any adhesion posterior to xiphoid process and inserting the arm to detect any adhesion in thoracic cavity. Carcass approved for the consumption must have the meat porged to remove large blood vessels in forequarters. It is difficult to porge the vessels from hind quarters due to large number of blood vessels. Hence meat of hind quarters is not consumed by jews. Kosher meat is consumed within three days of slaughter if kept under chilling condition. Both in halal and jewish method of slaughter, anoxia makes animal unconcious and is therefore considered humane method, but the opponents say, as the vertebral artery and spinal canal remain intact which prolong the period of conciousness.

Jhatka Method

Jhatka is the official religious method of slaughtering food animals with the Sikhs, it is also used in religious ceremonial slaughtering of animals by the Hindus, In Jhatka the animal is made to stand in position, preferably with its neck in a forked stand, good aim is taken and head chopped off with one big blow of the axe or sword. It requires a certain amount of practices and bodily strength to work the method. Accuracy of the aim is of great importance, and Jhatkais should be quite adept in using the axe. But the method is not all together without danger to the operator, as his legs may be smashed by mishits. This method is liable to inflict the grossest cruelity by the hands of a novice. Head may be drawn on to one side to reduce dangers of mishits.

Since the medulla oblongata is practically destroyed, the method does not bring about complete bleeding, nor is the conscious and sensibility to pain deleterated. The

Jhatka meat cooks darker and decomposes sooner than halal, due to retention in it of a comparatively larger quantity of blood.

Slaughtering Techniques Used for Different Kinds of Birds

Now a day's various slaughtering technique have been developed in the world. But all the methods followed with same principles of stunning and bleeding, except religious slaughtering. Slaughtering and defeathering: consists of hanging, stunning, bleeding, scalding, picking and washing.

Receiving and Hanging

After weighing, the truck parks along sides the unloading dock where an overhead conveyor easier the shackles from the dressing room out into the duck. The loaded crates of broilers are removed from the truck and pushed to the processing line. There several men remove the birds from the crates and shackle them for slaughter.

Slaughtering: Involves stunning and bleeding.

Table 19.1: Recommendations or Requirements for Stunning and Slaughtering of Poultry

Species	*Recommendations or Requirements*
All species	Period between start of loading at the farm and end of unloading at the processing plant should not be exceed 12 hours
All species	Injured birds arriving at the plant must be slaughtered immediately.
All species	Birds must be slaughtered as soon as possible on arriving at the processing plant. Otherwise, they must be protected from direct sunlight and adverse weather and provided with adequate ventilation
All species	The relative humidity in the pre-slaughter holding accommodation should not be exceed 70 per cent
All species	Shackles must be of suitable size and type for the birds being processed
All species	Must not be suspended head-downwards for more than 3 min before being stunned
Chickens	Must not be suspended head-downwards for more that 6 min before being stunned
Turkeys	A stunning current of not less than 105 mA per bird should be used when applying 50Hz AC
Broiler chicken	Birds, which fail to be stunned by the water bath stunner, must either be killed by neck dislocation or stunned with hand held stunner
All species	Neck cutting should occur between 10 and 15 s after stunning
All species	Time between neck cutting and scalding must be less that 90 s.
Turkeys	Time between neck cutting and scalding must be less than 2 min
All species	Birds must be dead when they enter the scalding tank, as judged by the absence of the corneal reflex

Advantages of Stunning

1. Minimize the chance of birds feeling pain during and after neck cutting.
2. To minimize distress that could occur during bleeding out.

3. To minimize the bird to allow neck cutting to be performed easily and accurately.
4. To prevent convulsions which occur during bleeding out in unstained birds.

Stunning

Though to meet these above requirements various stunning methods are followed, electrical stunning is most commonly practiced. Stunning: with electric shocker frequently used to slaughter turkey to prevent struggling. Stunning also relax muscles which holds the feathers. Mountney Gardner and Gayvert (1956) have demonstrated that shocking reduces the rate of bleeding with turkeys but total amount of blood lost is same as other methods. Mountney and Parnell (1958) reported that shockers can be knife having electric current in the blade or an electric plate or wands which touches the heads of the birds as they more along the conveyor.

Five types of electrical stunning system can be used for poultry. These are water bath stunner, grid stunner, two type's electrified knife, and the v-shaped stunner. The water bath stunner is the preferred method in most plants/it consists of an open-top tank of water through which the birds are drawn as they are conveyed along the overhead line on the shank through shackle. The water acts as the live electrode, and the metal bar, which makes contact with the shackle usually, acts as the earth electrode. Thus current flows through the whole bird when it is being stunned. One of the weakness of this system is that it does not cater for all sizes of bird. Very small bird can miss the water altogether, whereas in large birds the current might bypass the brain and instead flows between the base of the wings and the legs.

Grid stunner usually consists of a dry, inclined metal plate placed across the path of the shackled birds. As the birds are conveyed along the overhead line, they are dragged over the plate, which because of its slop can be set so that it makes contact with all sizes of bird. In two –types of hand-held electrical stunning method, in one method-the head of the bird is restrained with one hand to bleed the bird out. In other system, the knife act as one electrode and is placed on the top or back of the bird's head. Current is pass through the birds to the shackle, which is earthed. The same knife is then used to cut the neck. In v-shaped stunning, it utilizes a set of wall-mounted v-shaped electrodes into which the birds head is pressed.

Carbon dioxide immobilization can be done. The concentration of the CO_2 must be carefully controlled. Otherwise the bird will be killed. Draewniak, Baush and Davis (1955) reported that practical limits for stunning turkeys varies from 73 to 75 per cent concentration but the optimum times for exposure varies for males, females and different verities. Kotula, Drewniak, and Davis (1957) have reported that carbon dioxide speeds up the rate of bleeding of chickens. Carbon dioxide immobilization is not generally practised in large scale. A concentration of 65-75 per cent carbon dioxide gas in air produced an effective stunning for poultry. The concentration of carbon dioxide required must be carefully controlled otherwise bird will be killed. Optimum times for exposure varies for males, females and different varieties. Carbon dioxide speeds up the rate of bleeding of chickens.

Piercing the cerebellum of the brain either by running a knife through eye or through the roof of the mouth was once most common method of stunning poultry, but now replaced with electrical stunning.

Bleeding

There are several ways of cutting poultry so that they can be bleed – i) 'Modified Kosher' killed birds are those where the jugular vein is served just below the jowls so that wind pipe and esophagus remain uncut, ii) manual cutting at one side of the neck usually cut one jugular vein plus one carotid artery, iii) 'Halal' slaughtered birds had all the tissues in the neck severed, except for a flap of skin and muscle at the back of the neck, iv) 'Schechita' slaughtered birds had a less extensive cut from the front of the neck which usually severe both carotid arteries plus one jugular vein, but in some instances missed one of the carotid arteries, v) a manual cut through the mouth usually sever the jugular vein, anastomosis at the top of the neck cutter which usually served the jugular veins only, vii) single bladed automatic neck cutter which usually cut one or both ventral arteries and sometimes an external carotid artery and the spinal cord, depending on the depth of the cut.

Decapitations: This method is seldom used.

Carcasses are pierced through the brain consists of severing the veins in the roof of the mouth.

Newell and shaffner (1950) reported that between 34 to 50 per cent of the total blood of the body of chicken is lost during the bleeding phase of the killing operation. They also reported that the birds which are decapitated lose less blood than those slaughtered by "Kosher" killing or those stuck and then pierced through the brain.

Davis and Coe (1954) reported that debraining before cutting the carotid arteries and jugular veins was of little value during the first 20 sec. of bleeding other than for inner bird. They also added that decapitating decreased the flow of blood.

Of the above methods of bleeding: 'Modified Kosher' slaughter is most widely used in modern processing operations because it is easier to obtain good bleeding (35-50 per cent of total blood) and leaves the neck intact for use in suspending the carcass for later eviscerating operation. "Modified Kosher" killed birds are those where the jugular vein is severed just below the jowls so that the windpipe and esophagus remains uncut. According to Jewis Law the wind pipe must pop out in true Kosher slaughtering.

Scalding

The birds are scalded by immersion in hot water or by spray scalding. Scald tanks are much more widely used than spray water systems. Spray scalding offers positive benefits for carcass hygiene. However, high water usages and the reported occurrence of quality defects have inhibited its wider adoption commercially. Spray scalding generally practiced at a water temperature of 65°C. Scalding of poultry can be categorized as:

1. Soft Scalding/Slack Scalding

Poultry immersed in water heated to 50-51.5°C for 2.5 min is considered to be soft and slack scalding. For fresh, chill market a soft scald at this temperature is required because this permits retention of cuticle which is essential if severe discolouration and drying of skin are to be avoided on air chilling. But its advantage is that it is harder to remove feathers and more hand pining is required or additional pickers must be installed on the processing line.

2. Semi Scalding

Temperature and time combination for this scalding method is 53-55°C for 1-2 min and most commonly used for scalding of broilers and heavy fowl.

3. Sub Scalding

Carcasses scalded in water of 56-60°C for 35-75 sec are generally considered as sub scalded. Such carcasses have the outer layer of skin broken down but the flesh is not affected. The main advantage of sub scalding is easy removal of fathers and uniform skin colour.

4. Hard Scalding

Spent hen and water fowl are generally hard scalded at 71-82°C for 30 to 60 sec because it is the only satisfactory way to release feathers. The flesh of the carcasses scalded in this manner expands and becomes slightly puffy the skin so that the carcass appears plump, doughy and lifeless and the skin becomes discoloured soon after processing. So carcass must be kept covered with a packaging material or moist with ice or water.

"Modified Kosher" killed birds are those where the jugular vein is severed just below the jowls so that the windpipe and esophagus remains uncut. According to Jewis Law the wind pipe most pop out in true Kosher slaughtering

The **U.S. Department of Agriculture (1953)** published a discussion of the considerations involved in the use of various methods of scalding poultry.

Hard-scalding: Poultry immersed in water heated to 160°-180°F for 30 to 60 sec. the flesh of carcasses scalded in this manner expands and becomes slightly puffy under the skin so that the carcass appears plump. Advantages: Feather removal easier.

Disadvantage: flesh becomes, "doughy" and lifeless skin becomes discoloured soon after processing. Hard scalding is followed mostly for water fowl.

Sub-scalding: Carcasses scalded in water of 138°-140°F for 30 to 75 sec. here the outer layer of skin broken down but the flesh is not affected.

Advantage: easy removal of feathers a uniform skin colour.

Semi-scalding: 123°-130°F for 90-120 secs.

Advantage: leaves the skin intact and so permits more diverse methods of chilling and packing.

Disadvantage: harder to remove feathers and more hand pinning is required or addition pickers must be installed on the processing line.

A new "Semi-scald" system was developed. Since the scalders are completely enclosed, blood and feathers are not splashed around the room and humidity, water sprays noise and odour levels are greatly reduced. The carcasses are showered hot water and then conveyed to humidity cabinets where they are sprayed with steam at 140°F.

Feather Release

Pool *et al.* (1954) observed that the force required to remove feathers from turkey carcasses decreased as the scalding temperature increased. The scalding temperature is of more importance than of scalding time. Klose, Meechi and Pool (1961) in work with chickens reported that scalding resulted in a reduction of feather pulling force to over 95 per cent at 140°F. Anaesthesizing the birds required more force to pull feathers from males than females and that fasting for 8 hours increased the force to remove feathers. Exercise 90 sec. also increased the force to remove feathers while tranquilizers and scalding time in most cases decreased the force required for removal of feathers.

Defeathering

Feathers are removed mechanically, immediately after scalding by a series of on line plucking machines (The numbers and types of machine used depend upon the species and size of the bird and the specific parts of carcass to be defeathered). The machines consists of banks of counter rotating stainless steel domes or disc with rubber fingers mounted on them. The machine should be positioned closed to the scald tank and adjacent to each other to avoid cooling of carcasses. However semi scalded birds require 50 per cent more defeathering capacity than sub scalded ones. A steady stream of water washes the feathers away and acts as lubricant. Sometimes pin feathers (protruding feathers) are observed in the carcasses should be removed by hand picking is known as pinning. The birds pass through an arc flame (1500-1600°C for 5-10 sec) to singe the remaining fine hairs (filoplumes) and pin feathers.

Wax Picking

It is used for water fowl. Water fowl carcasses after being scalded and rough picked they are usually dipped in wax to remove pin feathers. The carcasses are dropped into a tank of hot wax, while suspended on shackles removed and dipped a second time. Then they are immersed in cold water to harden the wax. When the wax is properly hardened it peels off the pin feathers thus leaving a clean carcass. The wax is reclaimed for further use.

Picking

Carcasses are carried in a conveyor line while hanging by the feet, through rubber-fingered pickers which beat and rich the feathers from the carcasses. A steady stream of water washes the feathers away and acts as lubricant.

Washing

Finally the carcasses are washed scrubbed by the rubber fingers at the same scrubbing loosens and removes the soiled area. It also reduces the number of microorganisms found on carcasses.

Removing Shank and Oil Glands

Shanks can be removed by knives, saws, manually operated shears or mechanized shears. The most efficient method to remove the oil gland was to suspend the carcass by the hocks rather than by the neck.

Evisceration

Positioning: Separate conveyor lines are used for dressed and evisceration.

Advantage of separate lines.

1. If one line stops the other operation can continue.
2. The evisceration line is not contaminnated with filth from the dressing line.

Most broiler carcasses are positioned for evisceration by hanging both hocks on a shackle. (two-point suspension). Turkeys are usually suspended by both the hocks and neck hanging on the shackle (three-point suspension).

Opening the Body cavity: done by knife with slicing motion or by a stabbing motion. The vent can be removed by cutting around it.

Removing the viscera: viscera should be removed carefully and kept intact to carcasses avoiding contamination and to facilitate inspection. For this, the viscera are generally left hanging outside the body but still attached to the carcasses.

Automatic eviscerations now available capacity of 40 carcasses/minute on a 2400 per hour line.

Inspection

for inspection the carcasses should be positioned in such a manner that the overhead light illuminates the body cavity. Guide rails help steady shackles and carcasses during inspection and SS hooks with swivels make it possible for the inspector to turn the carcass.

Processing Giblets

The heart and liver removed from the remaining viscera by cutting or pulling of them loose. The gall bladder is cut or pulled from the liver and the pericardial sac and the arteries are cut from the heart.

The gizzard is generally removed by first cutting it loose in front of the proventriculus and then cutting both incoming and outgoing tracts. Then it is spilt open with scissors, emptied, washed and the linning removed on a gizzard peeler.

Removing Lungs

Removed by a hand rake or a vacuum system. Vacuum system is most efficient method and used in large plant.

Decapitating

Heads can be removed manually with a V-shaped slot with tension obtained from the pull of the conveyor or with revolving from or other mechanical devices.

Removing Crop, Windpipe and Neck

Cut the neck from the back close to the body with a pair of shears then pulling and removing the crop and windpipe. The neck is then cut off with a knife.

Wrapping and Stuffing Giblets

Wrapped in 9X12 inch sheets of parchment paper, parchment bags or film and then stuffed into the body cavity. Stuff always before chilling the carcass.

Sorting Carcasses

After removing from eviscerating line the carcasses are hung on a sorter which passes over a row of chill tanks and drops the carcasses in the vat according to predesigned weight classification. You can refer BIS grades and USDA grades of dressed chicken carcasses described in other chapter of the book.

Chilling of Carcasses

According to USDA regulations carcasses must be chilled to at least 40°F internal temperature.

1. Cold running tap water is satisfactory for preliminary chilling but it generally not good enough to chill carcasses to 40°F and the amount of water required prohibits its use.
2. Crushed ice and water chill faster than crush ice alone because with water the carcasses are completely immersed in the cooling medium. By agitating water the rate of cooling is increased further.
3. Water can be agitated by placing a perforated galvanized pipe in the bottom of the chill vat and pumping air through the slush ice or by circulating the water from the bottom to the top of the vat with a pump.
4. On-the-line chillers used to eliminate batch operations, 4 types of chillers.
   (a) "drag" chillers
   (b) Paraller-flow tumble chillers
   (c) Counter flow tumble chillers
   (d) Oscillating vat chillers

Drag chillers consist of two vats in which carcasses, suspended on shackles are dragged through the cooling medium. The size of the vats depends on the rate at which carcasses are transported through the chiller. The first vat has a 50 ft. trough which contains water at about 41°F. The second vat contains slush ice at 32-33°F. The second vat is S- shaped and contains 200 lineal feet of cooling area.

Parallel-flow tumble systems for chilling also consist of two metal tanks about 26 ft. long depending on capacity. A cylindrical revolving drum tumbles the birds in the coolant and recirculated water provides a current to move the carcasses along the drum at a given rate of speed. The first tank uses tap water and the second tank contains slush ice.

Counter flow tumble chillers are essentially the same as the parallel-flow system except that the water circulates in the opposite direction of the carcasses. The carcasses are moved along the drum by a helical drive.

Oscillating vat chillers consist of two tanks. Tap water is used in the first one for precooling and water in the second tank is cooled to 33-35°F. with ice. The tanks are rocked from side to side on eccentric rollers to agitate the carcasses.

Ice Packing in Boxes

The ice-packing operation consists of receiving, storing, setting up, and distributing boxes. The operation also includes removing chilled carcasses from chill vats, packing them in containers, weighing the boxes of poultry and recording identifying information on the box lids, and stacking boxes preparatory to shipment. Generally 30-35 lb. of crushed ice areplaced on top of the birds in each box. In some operations after the ice has been placed on top of the poultry, the boxex are closed automatically.

Most processors supply carcasses iced or dry packed with CO_2.

Processing Water Fowl

Ducks

Ducks are delivered in open trucks in lots of 600 and processed at the rate of 600 per hr. after delivery they are weighted and then held for 1 or 2 hr carcasses are scalded twice in rocker scalders first at 140°F for 2 ½ min and then at 142°-145°F. next they are picked on batch type picker. After drying the carcasses are dipped in wax at 195°F and then cooled in water at 55°F. wax is removed by a wax stripping machine and the remainder by pinners. Next the ducks are eviscerated and chilled in a continuous chiller and then packaged in continues chillers and then packaged in cryovac and frozen at -28°F for 24 hr.

Geese

Birds are delivered to a holding corral. Then they are forced to swim through a canal to clean their feathers. After hanging on the conveyor line they are stunned and bled with an electric knife and then scalded at 150°-154°F in home made rocking scalders. Flight and shoulder feathers removed, the carcasses released from shackles and dropped into a hopper. The hopper drops groups of carcasses into a centrifuge type picker. The pinfeathers are removed by on-the-line picker – drying by a jet of compressed air – hung in a triangular suspense with the breast bone – dipped in molten wax at 220°F for 3 to 5 sec., cooled, redipped at 160°F for 3 to 5 sec and dipped in cold water to harden the wax. Head removed from the shackle. This breaks wax to stripe off in large pieces. The remaining wax is removed by a drum picker and then the carcasses are dipped in water at 180°F to tighten the skin. Tightening the skin makes it easy for pinners to remove the remaining pinfeathers. Carcasses are then eviscerated and inspected.

Geese are generally slaughtered at 17 wk of age at which time they generally average 6 to 7 lbs. live wt. Dressing yields generally are 70 per cent with a pickup of about 4.5 per cent during chilling.

Post-mortem Inspection

Guidelines in respect of diseased poultry presented for slaughter

- ☆ The abattoir management must inform, in advance, the Meat Inspector/ Meat Examiner of any abnormal conditions regarding consignments of live poultry from the farms (health certification).
- ☆ The inspector must, on reception of a load of suspected diseased poultry, carry out the necessary inspection to establish the nature and extent of the disease and to determine the immediate course of action.
- ☆ The inspector must bring his findings under the attention of the abattoir management or representatives and arrange procedures for the further handling of birds.
- ☆ If diseased birds are to be slaughtered, it has to be done at the end of the shift. A space has to be left on the hanging line between the healthy and suspected, diseased or contaminated chickens, in order to perform a thorough primary and secondary examination and to remove infected parts or remove the whole chicken from the line before it leaves the evisceration area.
- ☆ Equipment, which comes into contact with the suspected, diseased or contaminated chickens, must be cleaned thoroughly disinfected and sterilised to prevent possible transmission of the disease.
- ☆ Procedures for the handling of birds for emergency slaughter must be available although seldom used at poultry abattoirs.

Poultry Meat Inspection

General Regulatory Requirements

- ☆ All relevant information, including ante mortem and health records must be taken into consideration when doing meat inspection.
- ☆ No poultry, rough or red offal may be cut/sold/dispatched in an abattoir unless inspected and approved by a authorized person.
- ☆ No person may process a carcass or meat until it has been inspected and approved by the authorized person.
- ☆ No person may remove any sign/evidence of any disease/condition/ contamination/soiling in a carcass or its viscera before inspection.

☆ Evisceration must be such as to expose the organs and the body cavity for proper examination by the authorized person.

☆ No viscera or any part thereof may be removed from any dressed poultry, prior to inspection.

☆ The authorized person must inspect the carcass and viscera by viewing, palpation and, if necessary, incision.

☆ All viscera/organs must be correlated with the carcass of origin until the final inspection is completed.

Criteria for Meat Inspection and Judgements

If poultry, upon either ante- or post mortem inspection, is found on reasonable suspicion to be suffering from any notifiable diseases or conditions, referred to in the Animal Diseases Act, the local provincial state veterinarian must be notified immediately.

The Entire Carcass and Organs Must be Condemned if

1. Any disease is accompanied by emaciation, and/or dehydration;
2. Advanced pathological changes are observed;
3. a condition has so spread that affected portions or organs cannot easily be separated;
4. A disease is per-acute, acute, severe or advanced;
5. The conditions of the carcass, meat or viscera to be aesthetically unacceptable; or
6. Contaminated

Portions of the Carcass and Organs Must be Condemned if they are –

1. Affected by disease;
2. Contaminated;
3. Severely bruised;
4. In any other way rendered unsafe for human consumption; or
4. Soiled.

Portions of the poultry may be approved where removal and condemnation of affected parts or organs can be done. The abattoir owner must keep daily record of birds slaughtered and the amount of carcasses/portions condemned/or their condemned weight.

General Characteristics of Normal Poultry Carcasses

☆ The examination of poultry carcasses to determine whether they are normal or abnormal is accomplished by the use of the senses of sight, feeling and smell.

☆ Indications of abnormalities of carcasses, organs or parts may include differences in size, position, colour, shape, consistency, odour or a combination of these factors.

- The normal poultry carcass may vary in colour as a result of age, breed, sex, kind of feed, amount of exercise or scalding practices.
- The firmness of the flesh and the colour and sheen and the tissues will depend on the age of the bird.
- The head parts should not be enlarged nor should there be swellings around the eyes.
- The comb and wattles of normal commercial slaughtered birds may vary from bright red to pale red or even yellowish in colour.
- Fowls that may have been in heavy production may have shrunken combs and the normal yellow of the beaks and shanks will have diminished or disappeared.
- The skin of normal birds, which have white slate-coloured or black shanks, is usually lighter in colour than that of birds with yellow shanks. Certain breeds of birds, particularly Jersey Giants, have a greenish cast to the skin extending over the abdomen and thighs.
- The shanks and feet of older birds will be more angular and will not appear as rounded as those of younger birds.

Requirements for the Presentation of Carcasses for Inspection

Processing Requirements Key Points

- De-feathering: An occasional feather on the occasional bird can be described to human error, however, excessive occurrence of feathers after de-feathering, is unacceptable.
- To expose the carcass for inspection and to facilitate the inspection of the carcass removal/cutting off runners must take place through the hock joints. Joint surfaces and tendon sheath must be clearly visible for inspection.
- Exposure of the tendons and joint surfaces for inspection purpose.
- Removal/cutting off heads - The head is removed in the "dirty" area after defeathering. Heads are edible products for human consumption and must be subjected to meat inspection. Abdominal incision done either by hand or mechanically, and only sufficiently to ensure the viscera are exposed and easy to remove
- To avoid excessive water absorption and contamination, but still allowing for an adequate inspection
- Removal of viscera - Viscera are removed from the carcass but are identified with the proper carcass
- To provide the adequate view of all organs and surfaces for inspection
- Positioning all birds must come to the inspector in identical positions, including viscera, irection of hocks and direction of breasts.
- To permit the inspector to use of rhythmic, organised and efficient method of inspection, synchronising all hand and eye movements.

- ☆ Identification If an inspector is not responsible for all carcasses, the ones he is responsible for must be identifiable To prevent carcasses from slipping through not inspected
- ☆ Prevention of contamination of carcasses
- ☆ Care and skill must be employed in the opening of the carcass so that no contamination may occur through gall or intestinal contents
- ☆ To avoid contamination of wholesome, clean and healthy food for consumption by the Public

Meat Inspection Points

Meat inspection is divided into 6 inspection points, which takes place at different stages of the processing process:

- ☆ ANTE MORTEM which takes place in the dirty (pre-evisceration) area at the offloading and hanging areas.
- ☆ FIRST INSPECTION POINT which is in the "dirty" (pre-evisceration) area and situated directly after de-feathering
- ☆ SECOND INSPECTION POINT which is situated in the "clean" (post evisceration) area directly after evisceration when the carcass and organs are still corresponding with one another.
- ☆ RECOVERIES takes place in an area near to the second inspection point with it's own facilities where carcasses taken off the line at the second point, can be cut and the approved parts can be utilised as portions and the rest must be condemned.
- ☆ FINAL INSPECTION POINT which is situated before the final washing of the carcass is to be done
- ☆ RETURNS are inspected in a separate room near the dispatch and with it's own facilities.

The First Inspection Point

The First Carcass Inspection Point is situated just after defeathering and prior to removal of heads and feet and the pre-evisceration wash.

The purpose and function of the FIRST INSPECTION POINT

- ☆ Inspection of heads and feet, which are edible products
- ☆ Preventing the entering of obvious diseased poultry into the evisceration section and thus the spreading of contamination by means of septic and disease contaminated parts.
- ☆ Re-hanging of carcasses which have not been properly de-feathered for re-de-feathering.
- ☆ Application of quality standards in respect of carcass selection.
- ☆ Quality control over the de-feathering- and slaughtering processes in general.

- ☆ To effectively record deficiencies for *e.g.* Poorly bled carcasses, machine damage, overscalded carcasses, injuries and bruising.
- ☆ To monitor the occurrence of contamination.
- ☆ To monitor the standard of hygiene during slaughtering.

Conditions recognizable at the FIRST INSPECTION POINT and action to be taken

Condition Description Action

Ammonia Burns

- ☆ Small to large brown discolouration of skin over breast, hocks and footpads due to wet litter.
- ☆ Can become infected in which case the area will be swollen and crusty and inflamed tissue will be visible when cutting into the lesion.
- ☆ May lead to "bumble feet"
  1. Carcass – no action at 1st inspection point. 2nd inspection point take off the line and partially condemn affected area in recovery area.
  2. Feet – even severe ammonia burns on footpads are acceptable as long as no secondary infection is present.
  3. If infected condemn feet.

Ascites (Water Belly)

- ☆ Excessive accumulation of abdominal and pericardial fluid.
- ☆ Carcass condition varies from normal to pot-bellied with darkened colour.
  1. Remove from line at 1st inspection point and condemn carcass.

Arthritis/Synovitis/Tendosynovitis

- ☆ Inflammation and swelling of joints and sheaths of legs and feet.
- ☆ Mostly the hock joint is involved.
- ☆ White/yellow puss may be present.
  1. Take off the line at the 2nd inspection point.
  2. Take to recovery for partial condemnation.

Breast Blisters

- ☆ Small to large pressure blisters on breastbone.
- ☆ Visible as soft swelling on front end of the breastbone.

  Prone to become infected.
- ☆ Small - (less than 1cm diameter)
- ☆ Large - (more than 1cm diameter)
  1. Leave carcass on line at 1st inspection point.
  2. Carcass must be taken off the line at the 2nd inspection point partial condemnation at the recovery area.

Bruises/Haemorrhages/Fractures

- ☆ Yellow, green to purplish discolouration: during the growing stage and before the catchers arrive at the chicken houses (24 hours or longer before slaughter).
- ☆ Deep red or purple discoloration: during catching, loading and transport of poultry (4 to 6 hours before slaughter).
- ☆ Pink or bright red discoloration: during off-loading and hanging of poultry onto the slaughter line (2 to 15 min. before slaughter).
    1. Remove from the line at 1st inspection point and condemn the carcass if more than 50 per cent is affected.
    2. If less than 50 per cent is affected, leave on the line for 2nd inspection point and partial condemnation at recovery area.

Contamination

- ☆ Crop content contamination
- ☆ Faecal contamination
- ☆ Bile contamination
- ☆ Pus contaminationg.
- ☆ Oil contamination
    1. Poultry falling off shackle lines onto the floor in the de-feathering area may be rinsed in running chlorinated water to a concentration of 50 parts per million available chlorine, or water with bactericidal levels of another approved chemical, and put back onto the line.
    2. In smaller abattoirs, carcasses may be rinsed in a drum for 30 seconds with 100 parts per million available chlorine concentration. The water in the drum must be replaced regularly to avoid contamination but running water is recommended.
    3. When birds fall onto or in the drainage channel under the plucker machines, they must be condemned because the water used for washing the feathers away is re-circulated water and therefore contaminated with dirt, feacal material etc.
    4. If the carcass merely dropped on the floor it may be placed in the spin chiller at the bird entering point.

Torn Skin Syndrome/Dermatitis/Cellulitis

- ☆ Localised to extensive areas of inflammation on the skin (easily damaged by pluckers).
- ☆ Becomes red, thickened and crusting of the skin appears as a result of physical, chemical and/or microbiological factors
- ☆ Generalised if more than 50 per cent of carcass is affected.

1. If less than 50 per cent affected take off the line at 2nd inspection point and do partial condemnation in recovery area.
2. Condemn carcasses with generalized dermatitis.

Emaction (as a result of not enough food or due to illness) and dehydrated carcass

- ☆ Carcass could be of normal colour to dark red-blue colour.
- ☆ Muscles have wasted away and the breastbone and other bones are very prominent.
  1. Remove from the line at 1st inspection point and totally condemn.

Fevered Carcass

- ☆ Carcass of normal or abnormal conformation but with dark red colour caused by acute infectious diseases.
  1. Remove from the line at 1st inspection point and totally condemn.

Overscalding

- ☆ Carcass has a boiled or par-boiled appearance depending on time and temperature of exposure.
- ☆ Breast muscle has a deep white appearance.
- ☆ Skin is pliable and damage is often seen caused by the pluckers.
- ☆ Occurs normally after the line has stopped.
  1. If severely overscalded remove from the line and condemn.
  2. If scalding is done by hand, - partially condemn at recovery.
  3. Test at 2nd inspection point by cutting into meat – 2 mm
  4. If deeper than 2 mm – totally condemn
  5. If less than 2 mm – partially condemn.

Plucker Damage (Machine damage)

- ☆ Damage caused by improper plucker setting, rubber finger maintenance, abnormal sized birds, skin weaknesses caused on farm and overscalding.
- ☆ Visible as the skin tears and fractures and dislocation of joints especially wing joints without bleeding into surrounding tissues.
  1. If more than 50 per cent, take off at 1st inspection point and totally condemn.
  2. If less than 50 per cent is affected leave on line for 2nd inspection point and total condemnation or partial condemnation at recovery area.

Poor Defeathering

- ☆ Carcasses with feathers that could not be readily removed by pinners
  1. Remove from the line at 1st inspection point and rehang before pluckers if possible
  2. If not possible total condemnation.

Poorly Bled

- ☆ Bright red discolouration of whole carcass.
- ☆ Neck flap shows bright to dark red
- ☆ Wingtips shows bright to dark red.
  1. Remove from the line at 1st inspection point and totally condemn the carcass.
  2. Leave on line if only neck flap displays a bright red discoloration.

Small Carcass

- ☆ Small but normal conformation and colour.
- ☆ Must not be confused with emaciated diseased carcasses.
  1. Approve.

Inspection procedures in Respect of the First Inspection Point

1. The whole carcass, including the head and feet, must be inspected;
2. Only carcasses that will be totally condemned must be removed from the line, trimming of carcasses must not be done at the First Inspection Point;
3. Where trimming has to be done, carcasses must remain on the line and trimming to be done at the detention and recovery area;
4. Carcasses coming into contact with re-circulated, contaminated water used for the conveyance of feathers, are unsafe for human consumption and must be totally condemned; and
5. Carcasses accidentally coming into contact with the floor may be recovered by rinsing the carcass under running potable water containing bactericidal levels of a chemical approved by the National Executive Officer for the use on foodstuffs.

   The meat examiner/inspector must, when inspecting a carcass and its organs, give special attention to –

   1. State of nutrition;
   2. Completeness of bleeding;
   3. Trauma;
   4. Evidence of disease/condition;
   5. Colour;
   6. Odour;
   7. Consistency;
   8. Conformation; and
   9. Any other abnormalities.

Duties of the meat examiner at the FIRST INSPECTION POINT

Manning the first carcass inspection point and performing meat inspection.

Second Inspection Point

The Second Inspection Point is situated after evisceration and the pack is asociable with the carcass.

The purpose and function of the SECOND INSPECTION POINT

- ✰ The inspection of the carcass and its intestines.
- ✰ The removal from the line for total or partial condemnation.

Conditions recognisable at the SECOND INSPECTION POINT and action to be taken

Poultry Meat Inspection

(Some conditions recognizable at the SECOND INSPECTION POINT)

(Post evisceration)

Airsaculitis

- ✰ Inflammation of airsacs in the chest and abdomen visible as white/yellow cheesy deposit on the membranes in the chest and abdomen due to bacterial infection.
- ✰ Lumps of cheesy material are often the only visible sign.
  1. Take carcass to recovery.
  2. Condemn the organs that are affected.

Breast Blisters

- ✰ Small to large pressure blisters on breastbone.
- ✰ Visible as soft swelling on front end of the breastbone. Prone to become infected.
- ✰ Small - (less than 1cm diameter)
- ✰ Large - (more than 1cm diameter)
  1. Leave carcass on line at 1st inspection point.
  2. Carcass must be taken off the line at the 2nd inspection point for recovery.

Fatty Live Syndrome

- ✰ Occurs in laying hens.
- ✰ The liver appears pale and friable due to the accumulation of fat in the liver cells.
- ✰ Haemorrhages in the liver could occur.
- ✰ Liver may rapture, with the accumulation of blood in the intestinal cavity and death of the bird.
  1. Partial or total condemnation of the liver depending on the extent of the fat deposit

HEPATITIS

- Normal to enlarged liver with haemorrhages or abnormal discolouration and spots due to various infectious and non-infectious causes.
- Not to be mistaken for light brown liver due to excess fat accumulation.
  1. Take off line at 2nd inspection point and take carcass to recovery.
  2. Condemn affected organs.

Pericarditis

- This is an inflammation of the heartsac.
- It can be thickened or covered with a cream coloured fibrous membrane.
- In severe cases the membrane might be attached to the heart and may affect the function of the heart.
  1. Take off line at 2nd inspection point and take carcass to recovery.
  2. Condemn affected organs.

Perihepatitis (Inflammation of liver membranes)

- Normal to enlarged liver with white/yellow cheesy deposition outer surface due to bacterial infection.
  1. Take off line at 2nd inspection point and take carcass to recovery.
  2. Condemn liver.

Penumonia/Pleuritis

- Inflammation of lung or lung membrane visible as white/yellow cheesy material in or around the lung.
  1. Take off line at 2nd inspection point and take to recovery.
  2. Condemn affected organs.

Poli-Serocitis/Colisepticaemia

- Septicaemia is associated with the accumulation of yellowish-white exudate in the airsacs.
- May have enlargement of the liver, spleen and kidneys.
- Visceral serositis (inflammation of serous membranes), airsacculitis, tracheitis, pericarditis, tenosynovitis (inflammation of the tendons).
- Pericarditis
- Peritonitis
  1. Total condemnation of carcass and organs.

Arthritis/Synovitis/Tendosynovitis

- Inflammation and swelling of joints and sheaths of legs and feet.
- Mostly the hock joint is involved.

- White/yellow puss may be present.
  1. Take off the line at the 2nd inspection point.
  2. Take to recovery for partial condemnation.

Gumboro

- Bursa of Fabricius: yellowish transudate, increase in size and weight and could be haemorrhagic.
- Dehydration, accompanied by kidney lesions
- Haemorrhages in leg and pectoral muscles
  1. Total condemnation in acute stage (feverish carcass).
  2. After acute phase only partial condemnations may be made depending on secondary *E. coli* infection.

Peritonitis

- Inflammation of the peritonium.
  1. Take to recovery for partial condemnation.

Torn Skin Syndrome

Dermatitis/Cellulitis

- Localised to extensive areas of inflammation on the skin (easily damaged by pluckers).
- Becomes red, thickened and crusting of the skin appears as a result of physical, chemical and/or microbiological factors
- Generalised if more than 50 per cent of carcass is affected.
  1. If less than 50 per cent affected take off the line at 2nd inspection point and do partial condemnation in recovery area. 2. Condemn carcasses with generalised dermatitis.

Contamination

- Crop content contamination
- Faecal contamination
- Bile contamination
- Pus contamination
- Oil contamination
  1. If any contamination is visible at the second inspection point, the carcass must be removed and trimmed at recovery.
  2. If more than 50 per cent of the carcass is affected, the carcass must be condemned.

Inspection Procedures in Respect of the SECOND INSPECTION POINT

Inspection procedures at the Second Inspection Point:

1. Hock joints and skin surface must be observed;

2. Observe the back of the carcass;
3. Observe the wings, legs, thighs and breast;
4. Inspect by observation the body cavity, air sacs, lungs, heart, liver, spleen, gizzard, intestines, cloaca and bursa; and Depending on the judgement, the following may be done with the carcass, organ or meat:
   (*a*) Approved for human or animal consumption;
   (*b*) Partially approved;
   (*c*) Conditionally approved; or
   (*d*) Condemned totally.

Duties of the Meat Examiner at the SECOND INSPECTION POINT

Manning of the "second" carcass inspection point and doing physical inspection of the poultry carcasses and organs.

Recovery

Where carcasses require partial condemnation as a result of a minor localised lesion and this condition is of such a nature that it holds no meat safety risk the quality controller may do the necessary trimmings and partial condemnation at the portioning section and approve of the rest of the carcass or viscera.

Carcasses that require removal from the line, due to conditions that hold a meat safety risk and renders it unsafe for human or animal consumption, such detained carcasses must be kept apart from healthy carcasses.

Trimming and recovery of portions that can be approved for human and animal consumption, must be:

1. Done in a separate room/area as prescribed;
2. Done by an authorised meat examiner;
3. Washed under running chlorinated water;
4. Chilled; and
5. Utilised as a frozen product only.

Final Inspection

The purpose and function of the FINAL INSPECTION POINT

- ☆ The inspection of the carcass for contamination after harvesting.
- ☆ The removal from the line for total or partial condemnation.

Conditions recognisable at the FINAL INSPECTION POINT and action to be taken

Poultry Meat Insepction

(Some conditions recognisable at the FINAL INSPECTION POINT)

(Post harvesting)

Contamination

Poor Pack Harvesting

- ☆ Crop content contamination
- ☆ Faecal contamination
- ☆ Bile contamination
- ☆ Pus contamination
- ☆ Oil contamination
- ☆ Part of intestines
    1. If any contamination is visible at the final inspection point, the carcass must be removed and trimmed at recovery.
    2. If more than 50 per cent of the carcass is affected, the carcass must be condemned
    3. Re-hanging for effective removal of organs or intestines.

Inspection Procedures in Respect of the FINAL INSPECTION POINT

Inspection procedures at the Final Inspection Point:

1. Hock joints and skin surface must be observed;
2. Observe the back of the carcass;
3. Observe the wings, legs, thighs and breast;
4. Inspect by observation the body cavity, air sacs, lungs, heart, liver, spleen, gizzard, intestines, cloaca and bursa; and

   Depending on the judgement, the following may be done with the carcass or meat:

   (*a*) Approved for human or animal consumption;

   (*b*) Partially approved;

   (*c*) Conditionally approved; or

   (*d*) Condemned totally.

Duties of the Meat Examiner at the FINAL INSPECTION POINT

Manning of the "final" carcass inspection point and doing physical inspection of the poultry carcasses.

Inspection of Returns

The handling of "returns" often is a critical process because, the product being handled will already be in a sensitive state either because of expired sell by dates, breaking of the cold chain or the exposure to contaminant situations.

To minimise the possibility of contaminating the processing areas, these products must be handled in a secured manner before the recovered portions can be re-introduced into the process to be frozen after de-contamination (washed in chlorinated or Trisodium Phosphate treated water or water with bactericidal levels of an approved chemical).

Regulatory Requirements

Inspected and approved poultry carcasses that have left the abattoir may be returned to the abattoir for re-inspection and re-packing, provided:

- ☆ An area/room or approved facility is available for the handling of "returns";
- ☆ It may only be wrapped and packed whole carcasses
- ☆ It may not be frozen blocks of :mala" including intestines, gallbladders, heads and feet
- ☆ The re-introduced product is examined by the authorised person on arrival, and found to be free of any signs of contamination or spoiling and to be unconditionally fit for human consumption;
- ☆ Any poultry carcasses, parts thereof or offal brought into an abattoir and found to be contaminated, spoiled or unsafe for human consumption, must be condemned;
- ☆ The wrapping still bears the original marking of the abattoir of origin, no unmarked products may be accepted.
- ☆ On receipt the temperature of products is between minus 1 and 7 °C. Any product above this temperature may not be accepted. Proof of maintaining the cold chain must be provided (Thermographs etc).
- ☆ The director may impose any additional hygiene requirements in respect of facilities and procedures of cutting-up, packing, cooling, storage and transportation.
- ☆ No imported poultry meat may be handled in an abattoir without the written approval of the provincial Director Veterinary Services.
- ☆ It is only utilised for frozen products
- ☆ No offal is accepted
- ☆ Movement or re-introduction of poultry meat, carcasses, parts thereof and red offal between an abattoir and further processing plants is permitted, provided that the requirements for transport of meat are adhered to.
- ☆ No poultry meat from foreign countries may be handled in an abattoir a room for the recovery of returns should comply to the following minimum standards:
    - Such a room must comply with the normal structural requirements of abattoirs.
    - The receiving area for these "returned" products must have a pre-receiving area where obvious contaminated/adulterated products can be sorted and removed.
    - The receiving area must be connected to the recovery area via a hatch only.

Facilities Needed in this Room

- ☆ Hand wash facilities and washing facilities with hot and cold water for the washing of equipment must be provided.

- ☆ Sterilisers for sterilising equipment and hand tools used in this area at a temp of 82 °C.
- ☆ Acceptable equipment for the purpose of re-inspection and salvaging of the returned carcasses.
- ☆ Lockable, properly marked containers for condemned material.
- ☆ A small spin chiller at < 7°C with a constant replacement of chilled water with a chlorine content of 50 p.p.m. free chlorine or bactericidal levels of an approved chemical.
- ☆ Adequate lighting is essential, minimum of 540 Lux is required.
- ☆ Bins for disposal of packing and wrapping material must be available.

Returns may include:

- ☆ Fresh products which "Sell-By" or "Use-By" -date have expired.
- ☆ Products of which the wrapping or packing was damaged during transport.
- ☆ Cancelled orders due to over supply, etc.

Products originating from further processing plants and other slaughtering facilities

- ☆ Movement and re-introduction of poultry meat, carcasses and giblets between an abattoir and its further processing plant belonging to the same owner and/or company is permitted, provided that:
  - (a) A veterinary public health officer or designated official is stationed at the plant concerned
  - (b) Regulations for transport are adhered to.
- ☆ Products from another abattoir although belonging to the same owner or company are not permissible. Each abattoir must have its own area for the handling of returns.

Control over the re-inspection area

- ☆ This is considered a high-risk area. A qualified poultry meat inspector must examine the reintroduced product.
- ☆ Record keeping of numbers/weights of carcasses/portions to be kept of all returns.
- ☆ Record keeping of recovered and re-approved carcasses and portions.
- ☆ Record keeping of disposal of condemned products.
- ☆ All giblet and red offal returns will be considered as unfit for human consumption and must be condemned and destroyed.
- ☆ Temperature control of less than 12°C in the receiving and re-packing area.

Poultry Meat Inspection Component

Duties of a Poultry Meat Inspector

Work Area

The whole abattoir and processing plant, including any other activities that might take place including farm visits.

Duties

- ☆ Monitoring the security system of approval and packaging material stickers.
- ☆ See that compliance with the Registration Certificate is carried out.
- ☆ See that compliance with the Meat Safety Act, Act 40 of 2 000 is carried out.
- ☆ Monitoring the poultry meat examiners manning the first and second carcass inspection points.
- ☆ Other aspects of HMS as decided by management.

Proposed Recommended Meat Inspection Component for Poultry Abattoirs

The number of inspectors will be determined by the line speed and health status of the livestock being slaughtered,

High Throughput poultry abattoirs

Involvement of a veterinarian

It is the prerogative of the abattoir owner to employ a veterinarian on a full-time or on ad hoc basis.

A designated veterinarian should however be available for/to do:

- ☆ Ante- mortem inspection, liaison with farm managers and the issuing of health Certificates.
- ☆ Interpretation of laboratory test results
- ☆ Post-mortems on DOA's, mortalities and poultry not fit for slaughter with written reports to the abattoir manager/processing manager.
- ☆ Notify authorities of outbreaks of notifiable diseases.

Provincial Veterinary Government

The Veterinary Authorities of a province may specify the maximum rate at which poultry in an abattoir may be slaughtered if insufficient meat examiners are available.

The Veterinary Authority of a province may require additional meat inspectors/ examiners after having considered:

- ☆ The abattoir design
- ☆ Number of inspection stations
- ☆ Line-speed
- ☆ Different type of poultry
- ☆ Structural and managerial aspects.

Low Throughput poultry abattoirs

Involvement of veterinarian

Ad hoc veterinarian involvement is to be encourage

Table 19.2: Guideline for the Determination of the Minimum Number of Meat Examiners Required

Grade	*First Inspection Point*	*Second Inspection Point*	*Recovery*	*Final Inspection Point*	*Total*
A	1 + R	1 + R	1 + R	1+R	8
B	1 + R	1 + R	1 + R	1+R	8
C	1	1	1	3	
D *	1	1			2
E *	1				1

The figures mentioned are per line per shift. The supervisory meat inspector can however supervise more than one line. The recovery area needs a minimum of one examiner but may require more depending on the quantity of recoveries. The meat examiners may only do meat inspection under the supervision of the meat inspector.

(* In the D and E grade abattoir, one examiner can do meat inspection at both the inspection points if these functions are carried out at different times.)

Post-Mortem Examination of Poultry

Post-mortem inspection is critical and systemic examination of a carcass by systematic dissection. Post-mortem inspection is essential to detect diseased poultry, which is unfit for human consumption. Post-mortem examination ensures hygienic and wholesome meat production.

Requirements

1. Light source of 540 lux – light should be non diffusing and simulated to natural light
2. Dissection knife
3. Cleavers
4. Hot water – 80 °C ± 2 °C, Water for cleaning
5. Gelatin strips or edible marking ink.

Procedure

Outer Inspection

1. Thorough physical examination of dorsal, lateral and ventral surfaces of the body along with head, tail, wings and legs of a de-skinned carcass is carried out.
2. Attention should be specially directed towards the diseases like eczymatous disease, wounds, lesions, staining, inadequate bleeding, haemorrhages in skin or subcutaneous tissue or muscles or joints and tendon sheath, heavy

Table 19.3: Post-mortem Judgements of Dressed Poultry

Sl.No.	*Disease*	*Cause/Causative Organism*	*Description of the Lesions*	*Judgement*
1.	Abscesses	Breast blisters, wounds and canibalism	Abscesses do not show thick capsules, pus appears often dry and odourless.	Local trimming and passing of the carcass
2.	Ascities	Diseases of viscera, liver and tumour.	Accumulation of excess fluids in the body cavity and becomes prominent when it is suspended by the head and neck.	Totally reject the carcass
3.	Avin Leukosis	Virus Complex	Nodular lymphoid tumours in the bursa fabricus, spleen, kidney; enlarged liver, cherry red in colour	Totally reject the carcass
4.	Black Head	*Histomonas meleagridis*	Cynosis and blackening of wattles and skin of the head, enlarged liver with focal necrosis of liver, haemorrhagic ulcers in the caeca.	Reject the carcass depending on the severity of the lesion
5.	Botulism	*Clostridium botulinum*	Paralysis of legs and wings, extended neck and head along the ground in a limping manner or may be over the shoulder, distended and catarrhal enteritis, with few intense haemorrhagic areas.	Totally reject the carcass
6.	Bumble foot	Injury or penetration of foreign body	Non infectious, localized lesion of foot.	Local trimming is sufficient
7.	Cannibalism	Overcrowding and use of fluorescent light without red filters	Mild skin discolouration to extensive wounds in the region of vent, head, back and wings of the birds.	Decision is to be taken depending on the severity of the lesion
8.	Coccidiosis	*Eimeria spp.*	Pataechial to severe haemorrhagic lesions in the intestines, caceca often filled with coagulated blood and necrotic material.	Decision depends on the state of the carcass. Reject severely emaciated and oedematous carcass
9.	Egg Peritonitis	–	Viscera get covered with yellow yolk like material, oviduct impacted with solidified yolk of varying size.	Totally reject the carcass

Contd...

Table 19.3–*Contd...*

Sl.No.	*Disease*	*Cause/Causative Organism*	*Description of the Lesions*	*Judgement*
10.	Erysipelas	*Erysipelothrix rhusiopathie*	Septicaemic haemorrhages in the skin, head, heart and breast muscles. Enlarged liver and spleen, lungs appear brown. In chronic form head and skin appear leather like. Endocarditis and purulent synovitis may be seen.	Totally reject the carcass
11.	Fatty liver syndrome	–	Enlarged liver, friable, yellow in colour and greasy to touch.	Reject liver. For rest of the carcass decide as per its state.
12.	Fowl cholera	*Pasteurella multocida*	Purplish comb and waste less, pin point haemorrhages on the heart, liver, gizzard, proventriculus and intestines. Streaked liver with light areas mingled with tiny haemorrhages and greyish dots.	Decide as per the state of the carcass. If localized reject the part and pass the rest, if not then reject the whole carcass.
13.	Fowl paralysis (Marek's disease)	Virus	Bronchial and sciatic nerves appear enlarged and yellow instead of grey. Diffuse enlargement of bursa fabricus and thymus. Skin tumours are associated with feather follicles. Muscle and skin lesions are noticed when defeathered.	Reject the carcass totally.
14.	Fowl pox	Virus	Dry or moist wart like growth on the unfeathered part of the head, face, eyelids, comb, wattles, legs and feet, warts are raised hard brown nodular-rounded scabs. Dull to pale yellow firmly attached plaque in the mouth and pharynx. Discharge from eyes and nostrils.	Totally reject the carcass
15.	Fowl typhoid	*Salmonella gallinarum*	Carcass appears pale. Congestion and enlargement of liver and spleen. Lungs and liver give a typical bronzed appearance. Degenerative changes in ovary.	Totally reject the carcass
16.	Gout	Systemic physiological disturbances	Deposition of salt and uric acid in the joints, feet, legs and surface of heart and liver	Reject the locally affected parts (joint, feet and legs). In case of visceral gout involving organs reject the whole carcass.

Contd...

Table 19.3–*Contd...*

Sl.No.	*Disease*	*Cause/Causative Organism*	*Description of the Lesions*	*Judgement*
17.	Gumboro disease	Virus	Inflammation of bursa fabricus that adjoins cloaea, appears swollen, gelatinous and haemorrhagic. Kidneys look swollen with degenerative changes.	Decide as per thestate of the carcass.
18.	Pullorum disease	*Salmonella pullorum*	Enlarged liver with multiple necrotic foci and fibrinous exudates, heart and kidney are enlarged and the former may give a defective appearance. Ova are discoloured, shrunken or cystic.	Totally reject the carcass
19.	Ranikhet	Virus	Excess of mucous in windpipe. Air sacs give cloudy to yellowish appearance. Haemorrhagic areas in the proventiculus, gizzard and intestines. Ulcerations of the intestine.	Totally reject the carcass
20.	Rickets	Vitamin D deficiency	Joints are enlarged, deformity in bones. Beak, bone and claw bones appear soft.	Totally reject the carcass
21.	Salmonellosis	*Salmonella spp.*	Enlarged liver and spleen, Inflammation of heart with yellowish fluid as in pullorum disease.	Totally reject the carcass
22.	Synovitis	Multiple Etiology	Joints and tendon sheaths are swollen and appear filled with exudates.	Decide as per the state of the carcass.
23.	Tapeworms	*Davinia proglottina, Railletina echinobothridia, Raillietine tetragona*	Presence of nodules in the intestine.	Decide as per the state of the carcass.
24.	Thrush (Moniliasis)	*Candida albicans*	Crop appears empty with mucous membrane appearing slimy, thickened with whitish raised circular ulcers which flake off leaving aside raw areas. Similar lesions can also be seen in the esophagus and mouth.	Decide as per the state of the carcass.
25.	Tuberculosis	*Mycobacterium avium*	Irregular, greyish yellow to white nodules appear in liver, spleen, intestine and bone marrow.	Reject the carcass totally.

contamination of intestinal contents, emaciation, fractures, muscular atrophy, prestromal bursitis, abscesses, tumours, inflammation, etc. Affected birds are segregated or condemned.

3. Give a transverse incision and gently pull out all the visceral organs.
4. All the visceral organs should be inspected for inflammatory processes or other pathological conditions. The connective tissue and musculature on the medial surface is inspected for major haemorrhages, inflammatory changes, contamination through bile or faecal material etc. Contaminated birds shall be segregated.

Inner Inspection

1. Abdominal and thoracic organs.
2. Serous membranes.
3. Air sacs.
4. Collection of blood, exudates or transudate in the body cavity.
5. Wash the carcass and edible organs after examination.

– *Chapter 20* –

Yield And Loss in Poultry Carcass Component Parts, Deboned Meat Quality and Grading of Dressed Chicken

Introduction

Yields of poultry vary considerably among lots even at the same stage of processing. At the present time, many measurements, especially on methods of taking yields of cut-up parts, cooking yields, and meat yields have not been standardized. Shrinkages during processing are influenced by the kinds and classes of poultry, the age, sex, size and breeding. In general, shrinkage is greater in young birds and light weight ones than in older or heavier birds. Blood generally amounts to form 3.3 to 4.8 per cent and feathers from 4.8 to 8.5 per cent of the total carcass weight. Because of lack of standardization in obtaining yields and individual carcass variations, average values serve only as rough guides.

Proportions of different Carcasses Component Parts

The increased use of poultry parts sold in separate packages of a given weight, the use of certain parts for ready-to-serve convenience items, and the problem of portion control when poultry is served in large quantities has created a need for more information for use in quality control methods in poultry processing and marketing. The results of such information are valuable for uniform portion and weight control and for predicting the yields and proportions of various parts of carcasses to the whole weight. The yield can also be predicted within various tolerances.

Table 20.1: Weights of the Several Parts of Various Kinds of Poultry

Kind	Sex	Age Weeks	No. of Birds	Live	Hot Dressed	Heads	Legs	Carcass and Neck	Giblets				Total[1] Ready-to-Cook	Chilled[2] Carcass and Neck	Water Uptake in Cooling
									Hearts	Liver	Gizzard	Total			
Chicken-broilers	Male	8.5	105	3.8	3.5	0.1	0.2	2.7	0.02	0.08	0.07	0.17	2.9	2.7	0.02
	Female	8.5	105	3.0	2.8	0.1	0.1	2.1	0.02	0.07	0.07	0.15	2.3	2.2	0.04
Capons		18.7	104	8.7	7.8	0.2	0.3	6.2	0.03	0.14	0.17	0.35	6.5	6.3	0.10
Turkeys B.B.W	Male	26.0	100	27.0	25.0	0.5	0.4	20.8	0.11	0.51	0.34	0.96	21.7	21.6	0.80
	Female	23.0	100	16.2	14.9	0.3	0.4	12.3	0.06	0.27	0.25	0.59	12.9	12.8	0.50
Pekin ducks	Male	7.6	100	5.8	5.0	0.2	0.1	3.8	0.04	0.19	0.10	0.33	4.1	4.0	0.20
	Female	7.6	100	5.5	4.7	0.2	0.1	3.6	0.04	0.17	0.10	0.31	3.9	3.7	0.10
Pheasants	Male	21.0	79	3.1	2.8	0.1	0.1	2.3	0.01	0.05	0.05	0.13	2.5	2.4	0.10
	Female	21.0	75	2.4	2.1	0.1	0.05	1.8	0.01	0.04	0.05	0.10	1.9	1.9	0.10

Snyder and Orr (1964), Ontario Agr. College.

1. Ready-to-cook = carcass + neck + giblets. 2. Cooled by procedure prevailing in each other. 3. Under supervision of authors. 4. Hearts and livers

Table 20.2: Weight of the Several Parts and Dressing Percentages of Poultry

Kind	*Sex*	*Age, Weeks*	*No. of Birds*	*Average Weight of, Lb*				*As a Percentage of Life Weight*			*As a Percentage of Dressed Weight*	
				Live	*Hot Dressed*	*Carcass*[1]	*Total*[2] *Ready-to-Cook*	*Hot Dressed*	*Carcass*[1]	*Total*[2] *Ready-to-Cook*	*Carcass*[1]	*Total*[2] *Ready-to-Cook*
Roasters	Male	16	29	8.2	7.3	5.4	6.0	89.5	66.3	73.2	74.1	81.7
White RockFowl	Female	49	100	7.2	6.7	4.9	5.3	92.2	67.3	73.2	73.0	79.4
White Leghornfowl	Female	50	100	3.5	3.1	2.2	2.3	89.9	62.6	66.4	69.6	73.8
Cross turkeys	Female	22	33	15.3	14.2	11.3	12.4	92.5	73.7	81.1	79.7	87.7

Synder and Orr (1964), Ontario Agri. College.

1. Carcass only (giblets and neck not included except W.L. fowl which includes carcass and neck)

2. Includes carcass, neck, and giblets (before chilling)

Table 20.3: Dressing Percentages of the Several Kinds of Poultry Processed

Kind	*Sex*	*Hot Dressed*	*Heads*	*Legs*	*Carcass and Neck*	*Giblets*				*Total Ready-to-Cook*	*As a Percentage of Dressed Weight*				
						Hearts	*Liver*	*Gizzard*	*Total*		*Chilled Carcass and Neck*	*Carcass and Neck*	*Total Giblets*	*Total Ready-to-Cook*	*Chilled Carcass*
Chicken broilers	Male	92.1	2.7	5.3	72.2	0.5	2.1	1.9	4.6	76.7	72.8	78.3	4.9	83.3	79.0
	Female	91.8	2.9	4.8	71.5	0.5	2.2	2.3	5.1	76.7	72.9	77.9	5.6	83.5	79.5
	Male	94.5	2.6	4.7	74.2	0.4	1.9	1.6	3.9	78.2	76.4	78.5	4.2	82.7	80.9
	Female	92.6	2.5	3.9	73.8	0.4	1.9	2.3	4.7	78.5	74.8	79.7	5.1	84.8	80.7
Capons		90.3	2.4	3.9	68.9	0.4	1.7	2.0	4.0	75.7	71.5	79.3	4.5	83.8	79.1
Turkeys B.B.W	Male	92.6	1.8	1.7	77.0	0.4	1.9	1.2	3.6	80.6	80.1	83.2	3.8	87.1	86.6
	Female	92.0	1.5	2.7	75.8	0.4	1.7	1.6	3.6	79.4	78.7	82.4	4.0	86.3	85.5
Turkey broilers B.B.W.	Male	89.9	3.7	3.1	75.8	0.4	1.3	1.4	3.2	79.0	81.5	84.3	3.5	87.8	89.5
	Female	92.8	2.8	2.6	77.0	1.7[2]	1.5	3.2	80.1	80.5	83.0	3.4	86.3	86.8	
Pekin ducks	Male	85.8	4.3	2.1	64.4	0.7	3.3	1.8	5.7	70.1	67.9	75.1	6.6	81.7	79.1
	Female	84.8	4.0	2.0	64.7	0.6	3.0	1.9	5.5	70.3	64.7	76.3	6.5	82.9	76.3
Pheasants	Male	91.7	3.0	2.4	76.8	0.5	1.9	1.8	4.3	81.1	78.9	83.7	4.7	88.4	86.0
	Female	90.8	2.8	2.1	75.1	0.5	1.8	2.2	4.5	79.6	78.8	82.7	4.9	87.6	86.8

Snyder and Orr (1964),Ontario Agr. College.

1. Refer to Table 1 for any explanations. 2. Hearts and livers.

Table 20.4: Average Weight of Live, Ready-toCcook[1]; Cooked Edible Portion, Parts and Bones of Poultry

Kind	Sex	No. of Birds	Average Weight of, Lb										Cooking Loss		
			Live	Ready-to-cook Carcass	Cooked Carcass	White Meat	Dark Meat	Skin	Separable Fate	Total Edible Meat	Carcass Bones	Loss in[3] Deboning	Dripping	Evaporation	Total
Roasters	Male	10	8.6	5.8	4.0	1.3	1.2	0.4	–	3.0	0.7	0.3	0.3	1.6	1.8
White Rock Fowl	Female	10	7.0	5.1[2]	3.3[2]	1.1	0.9	0.3	–	2.5[2]	0.5	0.1	0.9	0.9	1.9
White Leghorn Fowl	Female	10	3.5	2.3[2]	1.3[2]	0.5	0.3	0.1	–	0.9[2]	0.2	0.1	0.2	0.8	0.9
Turkeys Broilers (smallwhite)	Male	18	15.7	11.2	8.1	3.3	1.8	0.6	–	5.7	1.7	0.7	0.7	2.4	3.1
	Female	30	10.7	7.6	5.5	2.3	1.3	0.4	–	4.0	1.0	0.4	0.5	1.5	2.1
Large white X	Male	08	25.7	19.5	13.3	5.8	2.9	1.2	0.7	10.7	1.8	0.7	2.4	3.7	6.1
Small white turkeys	Female	11	14.6	11.1	7.4	3.2	1.8	0.7	0.3	5.8	1.0	0.5	1.6	2.0	3.5
Large white X	Male	08	28.6	21.4	14.4	5.9	3.4	1.3	0.9	11.5	2.1	0.8	3.1	3.7	6.9
Bourbon Red Turkeys	Female	04	15.4	11.4	7.6	3.2	1.9	0.7	0.3	6.0	1.1	0.5	1.7	2.2	3.8
Bourbon Red X	Male	08	24.8	18.5	12.8	5.3	3.1	1.1	0.7	10.2	1.8	0.7	2.2	3.4	5.6
Small white turkeys	Female	08	13.8	10.2	7.0	2.9	1.7	0.7	0.3	5.5	1.0	0.6	1.4	3.2	3.2
Bourbon Red turkeys	Male	19	22.9	16.6	11.6	4.5	2.9	1.1	0.5	8.9	1.9	0.7	2.0	3.0	5.0
	Female	07	13.3	9.7	6.5	2.5	1.7	0.6	0.2	5.0	1.0	0.5	1.5	1.6	3.1
Color-strain	Male	19	24.0	18.1	12.8	5.4	3.3	0.8	–	9.5	2.3	1.0	2.2	3.0	5.2
Cross turkeys	Female	33	15.3	11.7	8.0	3.4	2.2	0.6	–	6.1	1.3	0.6	1.7	1.9	3.6

Snyder and Orr (1964),Ontario Agr. College.

1. Defrosted weight; 2. Neck included; 3. Includes waste + evaporation.

A processor can predict with a fair degree of accuracy, the relation of the total carcass weight of broilers to the weight of size of any part of the total carcass commonly removed in a cut-up operation. With this method not only the average weight of all the parts can be predicted, but also the number of parts which will fall into certain ranges. Another method sometimes used is the range between the high and low values. Since there is often quite a difference between these extremes, the range serves only as a guide.

Table 20.5: Weight Range and Variation of Broiler Parts from 32-36 Ounce Carcass

Part	*Weight Range for 95 per cent of the Parts, Oz.*	*Weight Variation for 95 per cent of the Parts, Oz.*	*Average Part Weight, Oz.*
Wing	2.0 - 2.9	0.9	2.5
Drumstick	2.3-3.3	1.0	2.8
Thigh	2.9-4.4	1.5	3.7
Back	3.7-5.7	2.0	4.7
Breast	9.3-12.8	3.5	11.1

Source: Walters, May and Rodgers (1963)

A comparative study of the distribution of cut-up parts for broilers, turkeys, ducks, and geese was done. Breast meat made up the largest portion of large turkeys, ducks, and geese and the legs and thighs the largest portion of broilers and small turkeys. Giblets amounted to four per cent of the weight of large turkeys and 10.7 per cent of the weight of 11- lb. geese.

Moisture Absorption During Washing and Chilling

The losses in weight and variations in the rate in which moisture is released from poultry carcass chilled in a slush ice mixture and then stored in crushed ice are problems of considerable magnitude in the poultry industry. Not only is there considerable variation in the amount of water absorbed during washing and chilling, but it is also difficult to predict the amount and the rate of loss during the period the carcass are stored in crushed ice. In an attempt to standardize the amounts of moisture absorbed during the essential washing and chilling operations, the U.S. Department of Agriculture has set up regulations which limit the weight increases permitted during these operations for carcasses packed for consumer use or freezing. They are:

Ready-to-cook Weight

Turkeys –20 lb. or Over	4.5 per cent
Turkeys –10-20 lb.	6.0 per cent
Turkeys –under 10 lb.	8.0 per cent
Chickens -5 lb. and under	8.0 per cent
All other kinds and weight of poultry	6.0 per cent

Table 20.6: Percentage Distribution of Cut-Up Parts in different Species of Ready-to-Cook Poultry

Kinds	*Number of Birds*	*Average Age, Weeks*	*Average Live Wt. Lb.*	*Legs and Thighs, per cent*	*Breast per cent*	*Back and Ribs[1], per cent*	*Wings, per cent*	*Neck, per cent*	*Gizzard, per cent*	*Liver, per cent*	*Heart, per cent*
Broilers											
Male	10	10	3-9	34.1	25.4	17.0	13.3	3.5	3.5	2.6	0.6
Female	10	10	3.0	32.4	25.7	16.6	13.6	4.1	4.1	2.8	0.7
Turkeys											
Small											
Male	10	16	10.0	29.3	28.3	19.9	13.0	3.3	3.8	2.3	1.0
Female	10	16	7.0	29.0	29.9	20.0	12.0	3.7	3.8	2.1	0.4
Large											
Male	10	28	22.0	24.1	41.3	18.4	9.5	3.4	1.8	1.1	0.4
Female	10	28	14.0	25.5	35.5	20.6	11.3	2.4	2.8	1.6	0.3
Ducks											
Male	10	7.5	7.1	23.4	29.7	23.0	10.6	5.4	4.3	2.7	0.9
Female	10	7.5	6.3	23.5	30.1	23.6	10.8	4.7	3.9	2.5	0.9
Geese	20	10-12	10.8	21.9	23.8	21.3	16.0	6.3	6.3	3.5	0.9

Winter and Clements (1957)

1 Ribs separated from breast and attached to back, pelvic meat attached to thighs.

If the poultry is to be ice, packed, the maximum weight increase is 12 per cent. The losses in weight during the period after chilling and before actual retail sale are sufficient to compensate for the additional moisture absorption a processor could only receive 3 to 12 cents per hundred pounds additional income by excessive water chilling.

Carcasses absorb from 2.00-3.25 per cent moisture during washing. The period of time carcasses are left in the chilling influences the amount of water absorbed. The longer the immersion period the greater the increase in moisture. The rate of absorption is fastest during the first few hours but carcasses can continue to absorb moisture for as long as seven days. Agitation of the slush/ice water mixture has little if any effect no moisture absorption but movement of the carcasses has a pronounced effect. Absorption of as much as 22.7 per cent moisture in 30 min. using a tumbling type chiller has been reported. The temperature of the chilling mixture appears to have some effect on moisture absorption but reports are conflicting to whether it causes a gain or loss.

Polyphosphates added to the chilling solution, generally at a level of six percent, influence the amount of moisture absorption and the rate of loss. In general, moisture absorption is not as great during chilling when polyphosphates are added and moisture losses are less than with untreated groups during storage in crushed ice. Cooking losses have been reported to decrease slightly in some cases and not at all in others. However, carcasses treated with polyphosphates have a bluish color, a slippery texture and a slightly different flavour and texture upon cooking.

Draining after chilling causes a rapid loss of moisture for the first few hours. After 18 hr. in cellophane bags at 34°F., moisture losses in one experiment amounted to four percent. However, it appears that in most cases an equilibrium is reached when the absorbed moisture content reaches sx per cent.

Absorption of moisture is greatest in the skin, muscle, bone, and fatty tissue in that order. Carcasses high in fat absorb less moisture than those containing less fat.

With the exception of phosphate-treated carcasses, moisture absorption appears to have effect on cooking losses or the quality of the cooked meat.

In a review of chilling poultry meat, it is reported that, compared with immersion chilling, spray chilling results in a 1-3 per cent moisture uptake with considerable variability and dry chilling under experimental conditions results in a 1 per cent loss and under commercial conditions, from 5-8 per cent. On the other hand, immersion chilled broilers lost more weight from cooking than dry chilled ones.

Cooking Losses and Cooked Edible Meat Yields

A number of factors influence cooking losses. They are the degree of fatness, distribution, post-mortem stage, age, size, and cooking times. Other factors which is important are covered vs. uncovered pans, basting, breast up or down, double vs. single cooking periods, time and temperature of cooking and the stage of doneness.

Table 20.7: Percentage of Edible Meat Yields of Poultry Cooked by different Methods[1]

Cooking Method	*Average*	*Range*
Chicken		
Fricassee	66	69-63 with skin, without giblets
Roasted	62	69-58 without skin or giblets
Breast	86	92-71 fricassee with skin
Drumstick	68	74-58 fricassee with skin
Thigh	79	82-74 fricassee with skin
Wing	56	71-44 fricassee with skin
Back	58	67-48 fricassee with skin
Ribs	47	55-39 fricassee with skin
Neck	59	73-44 fricassee with skin
Turkey		
Roasted	71	88-57 with skin, without giblets
Boiled or Stewed	65	72-60 without skin, with neck and giblets
Pressure cooked	55	56-54 without skin, with neck without giblets
Breast	89	92-86 with skin
Drumstick	69	73-63 with skin
Thigh	81	84-76 with skin
Wing	63	69-55 with skin
Foreback	59	67-48 with skin
Rearback	64	77-54 with skin

Compiled from Agriculture Handbook 102, Food Yields, U.S. Dept. Agr.

1 Complied from cooked weighs.

From an edible yield standpoint the best yields come from large turkeys with 1.76 lb. of ready-to-cook meat required for each pound of cooked edible meat, followed by small turkeys which require 1.85 lb., chicken broilers, 1.94 lb., chicken breasts, 1.58 lb., giblets., 1.71 lb. and the legs and thighs of turkeys and chicken 1.75 and1.88 lb., respectively.

In a study of the quality of Leghorn hens, it is reported that before cooking 27 to 30-month old hens had a higher prepared carcass yields than 18 to 20-month old ones but after cooking the older hens had lower carcass yields. Grade A carcasses had the lowest percentage cooked carcass yields and Grade C ones the highest.

Deboned Meat

Muscle, bone and fat are the gross components of dressed carcass. Their properties and proportions are responsible for the quality and leanness of meat. Meat bone ratio can be defined as ratio between weights of separated lean meat and bones of carcass/cut up parts. It is considered as important criteria to evaluate the carcass. Meat bone ratio influenced by various factors, which include species, breed, age, sex,

Table 20.8: Percentage Relationship of Cooked Edible Portion, Parts and Bones to Live Weight of various kinds of Poultry

Kind	*Sex*	*Method of Cooking per cent*	*Cooked Carcass[1] and Neck per cent*	*White Meat, per cent*	*Dark Meat, per cent*	*Skin, per cent*	*Neck Meat, per cent*	*Total Edible Meat, per cent*	*Carcass Bones, per cent*	*Neck Bones, per cent*	*Total Bones, per cent*	*Total Loss[2] in Deboning, per cent*
Chicken broilers	Male	Combined	51.9	15.3	13.5	4.2	1.3	36.8	10.9	0.7	11.6	3.5
	Female	Combined	52.7	17.0	13.8	5.1	1.4	37.4	11.0	0.8	11.7	3.6
Chicken broilers	Male	Combined	51.8	16.9	14.4	4.1	1.2	36.6	11.0	0.7	11.8	3.4
	Female	Combined	51.2	17.2	13.6	4.5	1.4	36.8	10.2	0.7	10.8	2.7
Capons		Combined	47.9	17.6	14.7	3.5	—	35.8	8.7	—	—	3.4
Turkey broilers	Male	Roasted	54.8	21.8	14.1	3.4	1.4	40.6	11.0	0.7	11.7	2.5
	Female	Roasted	57.7	22.3	15.1	3.5	1.3	42.2	10.7	0.7	11.4	3.6
Pekinducks	Male	Roasted	34.2	10.7[3]	9.0	4.3	—	24.1	7.8	—	—	2.6
	Female	Roasted	33.2	10.1	8.7	4.2	—	23.0	7.1	—	—	3.0
Pheasants	Male	Roasted	57.7	26.0	13.7	3.2	1.2	44.1	7.9	0.5	8.4	5.1
	Female	Roasted	52.7	24.0	12.3	3.0	1.0	40.4	6.8	0.4	7.2	5.0

Snyder and Orr. (1964), Ontario Agr. College.

1. For capons and ducks—carcass only, necks not included.
2. Includes waste + evaporation
3. Breast meat.

Table 20.9: Percentage Relationship of Cooked Edible Portion, Parts and Bones to Ready-to-Cook[1] Weight of Various Kinds of Poultry

Kind	Sex	Method of Cooking	Cooked Carcass[2] and Neck, per cent	White Meat, per cent	Dark Meat, per cent	Skin, per cent	Neck Meat, per cent	Total Edible Meat, per cent	Carcass Bones, per cent	Neck Bones, per cent	Total Bones, per cent	Loss in[3] Deboning, per cent	Cooking Loss		
													Drippings, per cent	Evaporation, per cent	Total, per cent
Chicken broilers	Male	Rotisserie	73.2	20.0	18.3	7.4	1.8	53.6	15.7	0.9	16.6	3.0	—	—	26.7
		Roasted	76.2	23.7	20.3	5.0	2.1	52.8	15.7	1.1	16.8	6.6	5.3	18.4	23.7
		Combined	75.0	22.1	19.4	6.0	1.9	53.1	15.7	1.0	16.7	5.1	—	—	25.0
	Female	Rotisserie	76.2	25.4	20.5	8.0	2.1	56.0	15.4	1.1	16.5	3.7	—	—	23.8
		Roasted	74.2	23.2	18.9	6.6	1.9	50.6	15.8	1.1	16.9	6.7	8.3	17.5	25.8
		Combined	75.2	24.3	19.7	7.3	2.0	53.3	15.6	1.1	16.7	5.2	—	—	24.8
Chicken broilers	Male	Rotisserie	72.4	23.9	20.1	6.1	1.7	51.9	15.5	1.0	16.5	3.9	—	—	27.6
		Roasted	69.1	21.9	19.0	4.4	1.7	47.0	14.5	1.0	15.5	6.6	13.4	17.4	30.8
		Combined	71.4	23.3	19.8	5.6	1.7	50.4	15.2	1.0	16.2	4.7	—	—	28.6
	Female	Rotisserie	71.7	24.6	20.1	8.5	1.9	55.1	14.5	0.8	15.2	1.3	—	—	28.3
		Roasted	72.1	24.0	18.8	5.4	2.1	50.3	14.2	1.0	15.2	4.8	12.3	15.6	27.9
		Combined	72.0	24.2	19.2	6.3	2.0	51.8	14.3	1.0	15.2	3.7	—	—	28.0
Capons		Rotisserie	74.4	27.0	22.9	5.9	–	55.8	13.4	–	–	5.1	–	–	25.6
		Roasted	66.7	24.7	20.4	4.6	–	49.7	12.1	–	–	4.9	9.4	23.9	33.3
		Combined	70.4	25.8	21.6	5.2	–	52.6	12.7	–	–	5.0	–	–	29.6
Turkey	Male	Roasted	72.0	28.6	18.5	4.5	1.8	53.3	14.4	1.0	15.4	3.3	5.4	22.6	28.0
broiler	Female	Roasted	75.0	28.9	19.6	4.5	1.7	54.8	13.9	1.0	14.8	4.7	6.2	18.8	25.0
Pekin	Male	Roasted	60.7	18.5[4]	15.6	7.4	–	41.5	13.4	–	–	4.4	21.7	17.6	39.3
ducks	Female	Roasted	57.8	17.7	15.2	7.3	–	40.1	12.5	–	–	5.2	24.4	17.7	42.1
Pheasants	Male	Roasted	72.9	32.9	17.4	4.0	1.5	55.8	10.0	0.6	10.6	6.5	12.9	14.1	27.0
	Female	Roasted	68.1	31.1	15.9	3.9	1.3	52.3	8.8	0.6	9.3	6.5	20.3	11.6	31.9

Snyder and Orr. (1964), Ontario Agr. College.

1. Ready-to-Cook = defrosted drained weight of carcass and neck, with exception of capons and ducks in which necks are not included; 2. Necks not included in capons and ducks; 3. Includes waste + evaporation; 4. Breast meat.

Table 20.10: Percentage Relationship of Deboning and Cooking Losses to Ready-to-cook[1] Weight and per cent Jelly and Fat in Drippings of Various Kinds of Poultry

Kind	Sex	Deboning Loss, per cent			Cooking Loss, per cent			Percentage in Drippings	
		Waste	Evaporation	Total	Drippings	Evaporation	Total	Jelly	Fat
Roasters	Male	1.1	3.4	4.5	5.1	26.6	31.7	53.1	46.9
White Rock Fowl	Female	0.8	1.4	2.2	17.6	18.5	36.1	27.3	72.7
White Leghorn Fowl	Female	0.6	3.8	4.4	7.6	34.1	41.7	37.4	62.6
Turkeys Broilers (small white)	Male	1.1	4.9	6.0	6.1	21.7	27.8	82.1	17.9
	Female	1.2	3.9	5.1	7.3	19.9	27.2	74.1	25.9
Large white X	Male	0.5	3.3	3.8	12.2	19.2	31.4	37.0	63.0
Small white turkeys	Female	0.3	4.1	4.4	14.7	18.2	32.9	19.1	80.9
Large white X	Male	0.4	3.6	4.0	14.7	17.6	32.5	35.1	64.9
Bourbon Red Turkeys	Female	0.3	3.7	4.0	14.6	18.9	33.5	14.9	85.1
Bourbon Red X	Male	0.3	3.7	4.0	11.9	18.4	30.3	33.0	67.0
Small white turkeys	Female	0.2	5.2	5.5	14.0	17.1	31.2	20.9	79.1
Bourbon Red turkeys	Male	0.1	4.4	4.5	12.2	17.9	30.2	28.8	71.2
	Female	0.3	5.0	5.3	15.6	16.5	32.1	22.9	77.1
Color-strain	Male	1.1	4.3	5.4	12.4	16.7	29.1	59.6	40.4
Cross turkeys	Female	1.0	4.1	5.1	14.7	16.4	31.2	34.1	65.9

Snyder and Orr (1964), Ontario Agr. College

Defrosted ready-to-cook weight as in Table (5.4).

deboning methods, state of carcass etc. The poultry has higher meat bone ratio than ruminants and other simple stomach animals. Meat breed yield better meat bone ratio than others.

Methods of Deboning

Two types, Manual method and Mechanical method. Manual deboning requires great expertise and skilful operations.

Requirements

Knives, dressed poultry birds, weighing balance, stainless steel top table, meat cutting board etc.

Procedure

1. Take dressed poultry carcass.
2. Weigh the carcass
3. Manually deboned the carcass and separate out bones and meat.
4. Trimmed out separable fat, tendon, ligaments etc from the muscles to get lean meat.
5. Weighed the meat and bone separately and calculate the meat bone ratio.

Precaution

1. Deboning should be done carefully by expert persons ensuring maximum possible recovery of meat from bone.
2. Meat should be separated from separable fat, ligament, tendons etc before weighing.

Manual deboning can be performed either before chilling (hot deboning/hot processing) of after chilling (cold deboning/cold processing) of the carcass. There are several advantages or disadvantages in hot deboning/hot processing:

Advantages	*Disadvantages*
1. Greater meat yield	1. Greater hygiene and temp control required.
2. Less drip in vacuum packs	2. Difficulty of boning on rail
3. Less unsightly staining of fat	3. Less easy to cut, trim and vacuum packaging
4. More uniform color	4. Unconventional shape of cut
5. Saving refrigeration cost	5. Difficulty in synchronizing slaughter, boning and manufacturer line
6. Saving labor	6. Difficulty in introducing into conventional plants
7. Greater WHC	–
8. Shorter processing times	–

Table 20.11: Percent Yield of Saleable Meat, Bone and Trim from Hot and Cold Deboned Sides

Sl.No.	Particulars	Hot Deboned (per cent)	Cold Deboned (per cent)
1.	Total saleable meat	76.1	73.6
2.	Fat trim	5.6	8.2
3.	Bone	17.6	16.3
4.	Evaporative loss during disjointing, boning and packing	0.6	0.2
5.	Evaporative loss during chilling	0	1.7

Mechanical Deboning

Mechanical deboning was first introduced in Japan, in 1940 for the deboning of fish, However, now it is used for low priced cuts of other species such as neck of poultry, rib plates, bone extremities and head meat of beef etc. This meat has higher pigment and mineral content. It is dark in colour so its use is restricted in some meat products. Mechanical deboning is of following types:

1. Belt-Drum System

Equipment: Paoli separator

Tissue: Primarily fish, some poultry and in few cases red meat

Operation: Tissue passed between a rubber belt and a micro grooved steel drum.

2. Rotating Auger

Equipment: Beehive

Tissue: Fish, poultry and red meat

Operation: Pressure from an auger force coarsely grounded soft tissue through approximately 0.5mm orifices.

3. Hydraulic Press Batch System

Equipment: Protecon, Inject star

Tissue: Fish, poultry and red meat

Operation: Bones are forced in a batch chamber against a stationary slotted surface in the chamber.

Specification for Mechanically Deboned Meat

1. Bone particle should be less than 0.5mm (98 per cent) and none larger than 0.85mm.
2. Maximum calcium 0.75 per cent (3 per cent of bone solids).
3. Minimum proteins-14 per cent

4. Maximum fat-30 per cent
5. Minimum protein efficiency ratio 2.5 (Minimum 33 per cent essential amino acids of total amino acids).
6. Maximum permissible limits in products-20 per cent

"Can not be used in baby foods, ground beef, hamburger, fabricated steak, some cured pork items, and meat pieces".

Mechanically Deboned Poultry Meat

1. Maximum bone 1 per cent in finished products.
2. Need to be labeled in ingredient section of chicken and turkey ("contain MDP meat").
3. Can be used up to 100 per cent in bologna and frankfurters.
4. A maximum of 15 per cent in red meat.

Grading of Dressed Chicken

Table 20.12: Tale BIS Grades for Dressed Chicken

Sl.No.	Characteristics	Grade 1	Grade 2
1.	Conformation	Free of deformities that detract from its appearance or that affect the normal distribution of flesh. Slight deformities, such as slightly curved or dented breast-bones and slightly curved backs may be present.	Slight abnormalities, such as dented, curved or crooked breastbone, crooked back or misshapen legs or wings, which do not materially affect the distribution of flesh or the appearance of the carcass or part.
2.	Fleshing	The breast is moderately long and deep and has sufficient flesh to give it a rounded appearance with the flesh carrying well up to the crest of the breastbone along its entire length.	The breast has a substantial covering of flesh with the flesh carrying up to the crest of the breastbone sufficiently to prevent a thin appearance.
3.	Fat covering	The fat is well distributed so that there is a noticeable amount of fat in the skin in the areas between the heavy feather tracts.	The fat under the skin is sufficient to prevent a distinct appearance of the flesh through the skin, especially on the breast and legs.
4.	Defeathering	Free of pinfeathers, diminutive feathers and hair, which are visible to the inspector or grader?	Not more than an occasional protruding pinfeathers or diminutive feathers shall be in evidence under a careful examination
5.	Cuts and Tears	Free of cuts and tears on the breast and legs.	The carcass may have very few cuts and tears.

Contd...

Table 20.12–*Contd...*

Sl.No.	*Characteristics*	*Grade 1*	*Grade 2*
6.	Discolouration	Discoloration due to bruising shall be free of clots. Flesh bruises and discoloration of the skin, such as 'blue black' are not permitted on the breast or legs of the carcass or on these individual parts and only lightly shaded discoloration are permitted elsewhere.	Discoloration due to bruising shall be free of clots. Moderate areas of discoloration due to bruises in the skin or flesh and moderately shaded discoloration of the skin or flesh, such as 'blue black' are permitted.
7.	Freezer burn	May have an occasional pock-mark due to drying of the inner layer of skin (derma), provided that none exceeds the area of a circle 0.5 cm in diameter.	May have a few pockmarks due to drying of the inner layer of skin (derma), provided that no single area exceeds that of a circle 1.5 cm in diameter.

USDA Grades of Dressed Chicken

Please refer Chapter 14 Quality Identification of Poultry.

– *Chapter 21* –

Structure, Nutritive Value, Compositional Chemistry, Microbiology and Functional Properties of Eggs

Structure of Egg

Size

Several factors influence the size of an egg. The major factor is the age of the hen. As the hen ages, her eggs increase in size.The breed of hen from which the egg comes is a second factor. Weight of the bird is another. Pullets significantly underweight at sexual maturity will produce small eggs.Environmental factors that lower egg weights are heat, stress, overcrowding and poor nutrition.All of these variables are of great importance to the egg producer. Even a slight shift in egg weight influences size classification and size is one of the factors considered when eggs are priced. Careful flock management benefits both the hens and the producer.Egg sizes are Jumbo, Extra Large, Large, Medium, Small and Peewee. Medium, Large and Extra Large are the sizes most commonly available.Sizes are classified according to minimum net weight expressed in ounces per dozen.

Structure of the Egg

It is generally accepted that a hen forms an egg in about two weeks. It is assumed that at the time of hatching, the ovary of the female chick has many small ova. The number has been estimated to be over 3,000. The yolk is formed during last 10-12 days prior to laying of the egg. Its structure consists of the latebra, germinal disc or blastodisc, a concentric layer of white and yellow yolk surrounded by vitteline membrane, albumen, shell membranes and egg shell.

Germinal Disc/Blastodisc

The entrance of the latebra, the channel leading to the center of the yolk. The germinal disc is barely noticeable as a slight depression on the surface of the yolk. When the egg is fertilized, sperm enter by way of the germinal disc, travel to the center and a chick embryo starts to form.

It is an opaque, circular, white spot usually visible on the surface of the yolk. In unfertilized egg is called the blastodisc or cicatricula. If fertilized egg, it is known as blastoderm. It is 3 to 4 mm in diam. Its central portion or the germinal area is encircled by a more opaque collar, the periblast. Inner periblastic ring divides these two regions. The blastodisc's periphery or outer periblastic ring merge with the surrounding yolk. The periblast with a mottled appearance due to the presence of vacuoles called lacunae- the characteristic of the infertile egg. Unfertilized egg – small circular area and fertilized egg – large, oval, homogenous area.

Yolk

The yolk is formed from one of many hundreds of oocytes, small cellular structures on the surface of the ovary. The oocytes develop sequentially. Early development is quite slow, but for a period of 6-10 days before ovulation (the process whereby the newly formed yolk is detached from the ovary) the yolk accumulates its rich content of fats and proteins. These are laid down in layers corresponding to days of development. The germ cell is located on the surface of the ovum and remains there, awaiting fertilization, which, in the case of commercial eggs, seldom if ever happens. The ovum or yolk is contained within a transparent membrane which remains intact when it is released from the ovary and is important in preventing the yolk material from escaping into the rest of the egg contents.

Gross Organization of Yolk

Latebra is an approximately spherical core about 6mm in diameter located in the center of the yolk. It contains white vitellin, a fluid constitute 0.6 per cent of the entire yolk. Extending from the latebra, toward the blastodisc is a vase shaped accumulation of white yolk, the neck of the latebra whose outer portion bells out beneath the blastodisc, to form the nucleus of Pander or nucleus cicatriculae.

Stratification of Yolk

A concentric layer of yellow yolk in the form of a spheroid encloses the latebra. About the spheroid of yellow yolk is a very thin layer of white yolk. The entire yolk mass outside the latebra and neck is composed of similarly alternating yellow and white layers. An extremely thin white stratum immediately underlies the envelope that invests the vitellus.The layers in the interior of yolk are interrupted and deformed by the neck of the latebra, as are the outer strata by the nucleus of Pander and the blastodisc. There are usually about 6 layers each of yellow and white yolk in eggs produced by hen. More strata are found when the rate of ovulation is lower. The white yolk constitute only 3 to 4 per cent of total yolk. It contains less fat and pigment than yellow yolk.

When the fat and pigment content of the hen's diet does not vary throughout the day, no stratification is visible in the yolk. It is only when, pigment containing feeds are restricted to a short period in the day, or when the feeds regularly given every day are low in pigments, that strata of white yolk are laid down during the dark hours of early morning. At that time, the blood of the hen is depleted of the materials necessary for yellow yolk formation.

Vitelline Membrane

The yolk of the newly laid egg is enclosed in a thin, pliable envelope, known as the membrana vitellina or yolk membrane which consists of 3 layers, the middle layer is composed of keratin and the others of mucin (Moran and Hale, 1936). Only two strata, a thin collagen layer within a much thicker mucin layer (Mc Nally, 1943).

The Albumen

The albumen is laid down over a period of 3-4 hours while the developing egg passes through the magnum region of the hen's oviduct. There are two distinct layers, the inner thick and outer thin layers. The egg white is mostly water and protein. In addition to the thick and thin layers, the chalazae also form part of the egg white. The chalazae are twisted strands of thickened protein that are arranged so as to hold the yolk in its central position within the egg.

Sorrounding the yolk and enclosed by the external coverings of the egg, is a clear material of yellowish tint, constituting 6 per cent of the weight of egg. This is called albumen (albus = white) or egg white, because of its appearance after coagulation. The yellowish cast is due to a pigment, ovoflavin. Occasionally, egg albumen may be pink or slightly green. Certain ingredients of the diet may cause the unusual tint.

Gross organization: About 40 per cent of the albumen is a viscous liquid, the remainder is gelatinous and semisolid. The whole is organized in the definite manner.

Chalaza

Along the egg's long axis, a roapy structure of cloudy appearance spirals from the yolk into the albumen at either end of the egg. These two structures are called chalazae (means 'tubercles'from Greek) or 'hailstones' according to Bartelnez(1918), compose of numerous mucin like fibers. At the proximal end, the fibers are firmly attached over the surface of the yolk in its equatorial region. At the distal end, the fibers are interlaced with similar fibers in the albumen. The cloacal chalaza (which extends towards the sharp end of the egg) is the longer and larger, fibers are disposed into two heavy strands, twisted counter clockwise on each other. The infundibular chalaza at the blunt end of the egg, consists of a single strand of fibers, twisted clockwise and less firmly moored in the albumen than those of the cloacal chalaza.

The chalazae serve to stabilize the position of the yolk, because when the egg is turned the yolk rotates until the blastodisc is uppermost. The chalazae become twisted and their tension pulls the yolk nearer to the geometric center of the egg.

Four Layers of Albumen

Disposed in four concentric layers.

(1) Chalaziferous Layer

The fibers of the chalazae continue in a slightly spiral course over the surface of yolk. They form a matted fibrous capsule, inseparable from and embedded in a thin layer of dense albumen immediately about the vitelline membrane and sometimes closely united with it. Together, the fibrous capsule and the envelope of dense albumen constitute the chalaziferous layer or the membrane chalazifera. This constitute 2.7 per cent of the total volume of albumen and weighs less than 1 gm. The weight of two chalazae alone is 0.15gm.

(2) Inner Liquid Layer

The yolk and the chalaziferous layer moored in the approximate ceter of the egg by the chalazae, float in a fluid, viscous albumen. This is the inner liquid layer of the albumen. It constitutes 16.8 per cent of the total albumen. Mucin fibers are almost totally absent from this layer.

(3) Middle Dense Layer

Often termed as albuminous sac, sorrounds the inner liquid albumen, constitutes 57.3 per cent of total volume of albumen; a heavy plastic envelope capable of maintaining of its shape to some degree. The numerous semisolid mucin fibers found in this layer provide a structural framework which contains liquid albumen dispersed in its interstices. This layer forms a cushion for the protection of yolk, sufficiently firm to provide anchorage to chalazae, whose ends are embedded in it. The albuminous sac is attached to the inner shell membrane at each extremity of the egg by a ligamentum albuminis. The two ligaments are formed by the penetration of numerous mucin fibers of the albumen into the membrane. Av. Area of attachment at cloacal end is 2.54 sq.cm. and its infundibular end is 10.2 sq.cm.

(4) Outer Liquid Layer

Sorrounding the albuminoud sac, except where the ligaments are attached, lies the outer liquid layer of albumen. Like inner liquid layer, the outer liquid layer is a viscous fluid containing few mucin fibers.

Shell Membranes

The next layers of the egg are the inner and outer shell membranes. These relatively thin keratin like membranes are one of the egg's chief defenses against bacterial invasion. The inner membrane is thinner than outer membrane, but together they are only 0.01-0.02 mm thick. The inner or egg membrane, the membrane putaminis (putamen, latin for pod or husk) sorrounds the albumen. The membrane is in contact with the outer liquid albumen in all but the polar regions of the egg, where some of the mucin fibers of the albuminous sac penetrate the membrane to form ligamenta albuminis. The outer surface of the inner membrane is firmly cemented to the inside of the outer membrane, except in a small area, usually at the blunt end of the egg. In

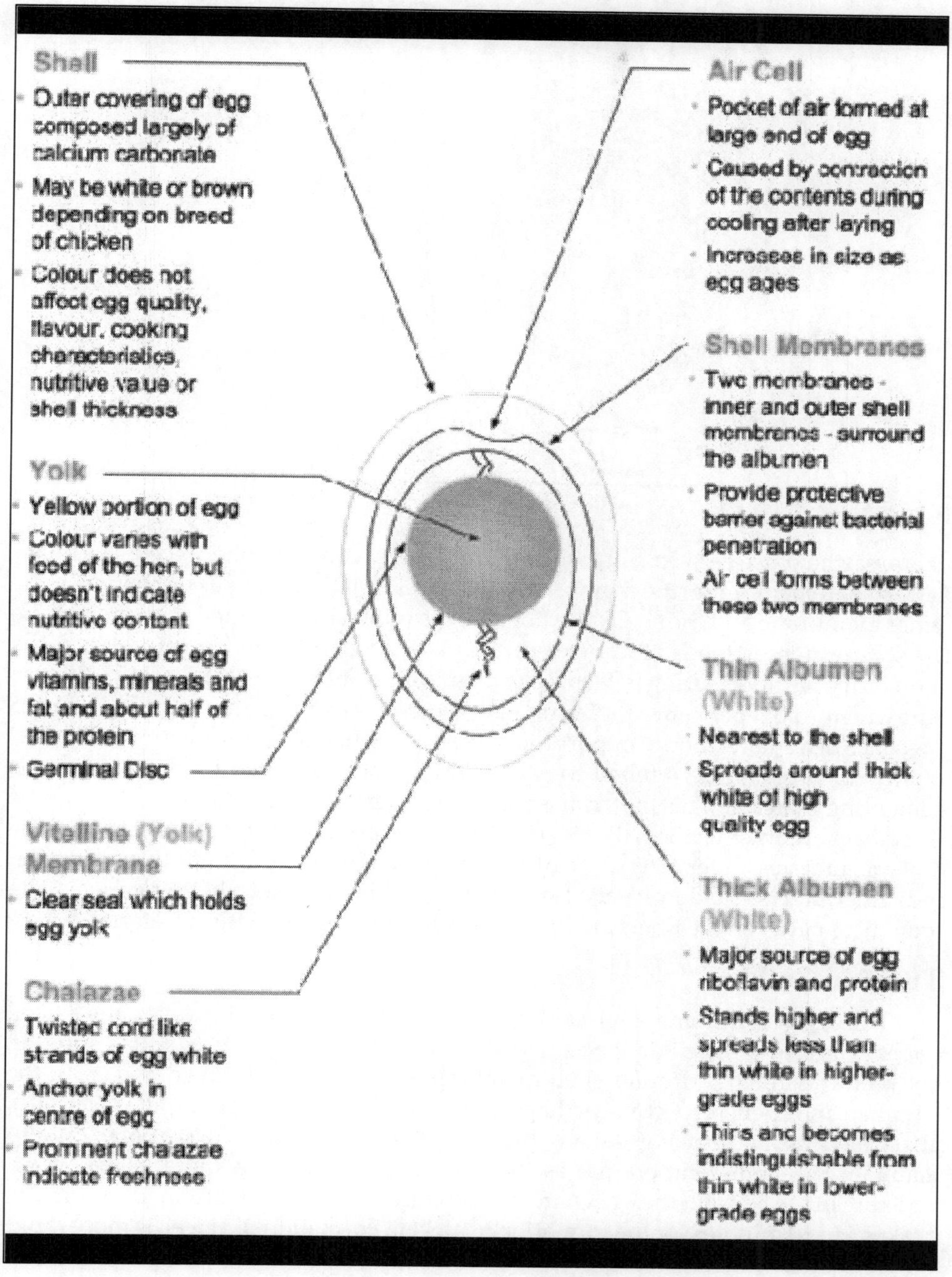

Shell

- Outer covering of egg composed largely of calcium carbonate
- May be white or brown depending on breed of chicken
- Colour does not affect egg quality, flavour, cooking characteristics, nutritive value or shell thickness

Yolk

- Yellow portion of egg
- Colour varies with food of the hen, but doesn't indicate nutritive content
- Major source of egg vitamins, minerals and fat and about half of the protein
- Germinal Disc

Vitelline (Yolk) Membrane

- Clear seal which holds egg yolk

Chalazae

- Twisted cord like strands of egg white
- Anchor yolk in centre of egg
- Prominent chalazae indicate freshness

Air Cell

- Pocket of air formed at large end of egg
- Caused by contraction of the contents during cooling after laying
- Increases in size as egg ages

Shell Membranes

- Two membranes - inner and outer shell membranes - surround the albumen
- Provide protective barrier against bacterial penetration
- Air cell forms between these two membranes

Thin Albumen (White)

- Nearest to the shell
- Spreads around thick white of high quality egg

Thick Albumen (White)

- Major source of egg riboflavin and protein
- Stands higher and spreads less than thin white in higher-grade eggs
- Thins and becomes indistinguishable from thin white in lower-grade eggs

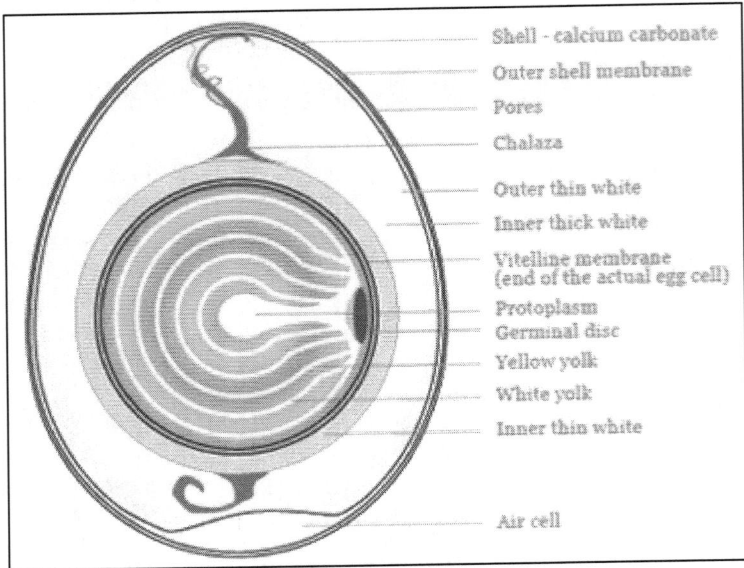

this area, the space between the two membranes is occupied by the air cell. The outer, or the shell membrane, the membrane testae (testa, latin for shell) lies between the inner membrane and the shell. The fibers of the outer surface of the shell membrane are so firmly embedded in the inner surface of the shell that it is difficult to detach the membrane without tearing it. Hen's egg membranes are chalk white, weigh 0.36 gm., equivalent to 0.6 per cent of a 58 gm egg. On closer examination – pinkish due to presence of a small amount of porphyrin pigment. Microscopic structure composed mainly of protein fibers felted together and are strengthened by an albuminous cementing material. This material is found between the two membranes and in the interstices among the fibers. Pores present in both membranes, but numerous in the inner membrane. Outer membrane has 3 major layers, inner membrane two somewhat indistinct layers. Made of very fine branching fibers of keratin and mucin. The interstices between the fibers are filled with albuminous cementing material.

The Air Cell

The egg at the moment it is laid, contains no air cell. Soon, however, the air cell appears as a small circular space, usually at the blunt end of the egg. It is situated between the inner and outer shell membranes, which remain in contact with the albumen and shell, respectively. Shape of the air cell is double convex lens. Air cell is also called the air space or the air chamber. After the egg is laid, it cools down to maintain the same temperature as the surrounding air. Thus there is loss of air, moisture of the egg and the egg contents also contract, so air cell is formed.In chicken, it takes 6 to 60 minutes for the formation of air cell. Formation of air cell is more rapid in cool air than with high temperature and humidity. Air cell supplies air to embryo when pulmonary respiration is initiated, otherwise the embryo shall be died. After the formation, the air cell increases in size as the evaporation of moisture causes the volume of the egg contents to decrease.

Egg Shell

The outer covering of the egg, the shell, comprises of 9-12 per cent of total weight. It consists largely of calcium carbonate (94 per cent), with some magnesium carbonate (1 per cent), and calcium phosphate (1 per cent), and organic matter chiefly protein (4 per cent). In coloured eggs, the colour is due to pigments (ooporphins) deposited on shell surface. The shell is formed in distinct pattern with pores for gas exchange (no. varies 7,000-17,000). Even though the pores are partially sealed by protein (keratin), thereby still permit the escape of carbon dioxide and moisture from the egg. The air cell developed by a separation of two-shell membrane, usually at larger end of the egg, as the egg contents shrink during cooling.

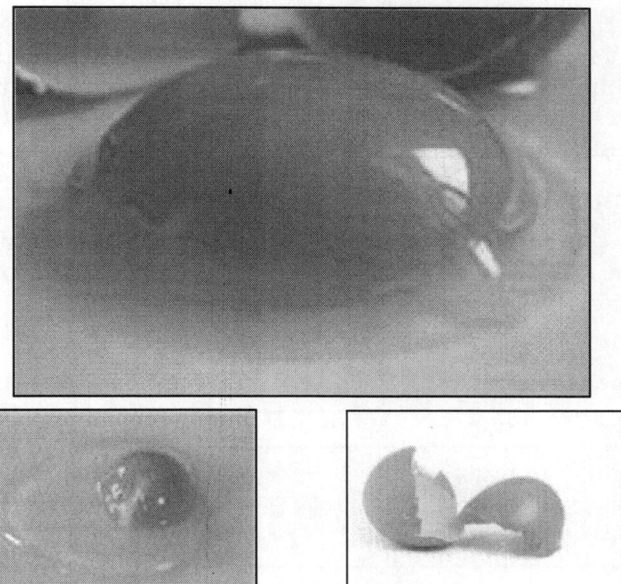

The egg shell is formed in the last 20-22 hours before the egg is laid. The eggshell has a protective function, maintaining the embryo within a carefully controlled environment. In eggs destined for human consumption, the shell protects the contents from damage or spoilage. The shell consists of about 97 per cent calcium carbonate. However, the remaining 3 per cent, which is mostly protein, has a major effect on the structure of the shell.

Gross Organization of Egg Shell

The bird's egg shell is not a homogenous structure. It is compounded of two widely different materials: an organic matrix or framework of delicate, interwoven fibers and an interstitial substance composed of a mixture of inorganic salt. The organic matrix is a collagen like protein. The minerals mainly carbonates and phosphates of calcium and magnesium ; calcium carbonate is by far the most plentiful. The matrix is a meshwork of fine fibers and granules and the minerals are laid down in its interstices. There are two main layers in the shell proper. These are the inner or mammilary layer and the outer or spongy layer. Mammilary layer constitutes the lesser portion of the shell, rests on the outer surface of the shell membrane and is partially embedded in it. It is composed of numerous roughly conical knobs or mammillae. A mamilla consists of noncrystalline minerals concentrically aggregated about granular matrix material. Spongy layer is superimposed on the mammilary layer and is firmly cemented to its uneven surface, constitute the greater part of the shell. Contrary to its name, this layer is very compact although numerous microscopic canals traverse to its entire depth at irregular intervals. Its deposition about the fragile mamillary layer confirms the shape of the egg and gives rigidity and strength to the shell. There is no visible indication of stratification in its mineral structure.

The Cuticle

On the external surface of eggs, there is an extremely thin, transparent coating of protein, probably mucin. This outermost covering of the egg is cuticle. It is very securely attached to the shell and is continuous over the entire surface, including the mouths of the pores. But it is permeable to gases.

Gross Composition of the Egg

The gross composition of the egg is given in Table 21.1. These data can serve as a good estimate for large-scale calculations. However, composition of eggs does vary with breed, age of layer, and even nutrition, within certain limits that will be discussed later.

Table 21.1: Gross Composition of an Egg

Per cent	*Water*	*Protein*	*Fat*	*Ash*
Whole egg	74	13	11	1
White	88	11	0	0
Yolk	48	17	13	1

Table 21.2: Composition of Egg Component

Component	*Per cent*	*Component*	*Per cent*
Shell	9	Yolk	29
Albumen	62	Fat/complete yolk	33.0
Protein/complete yolk	15.7	Yolk solids	51.0
Albumen protein	10.5	Albumen solids	11.8

Adapted from Tharrington *et al*, 1999. Poultry Science, 79, 591-594

The edible portion of the egg, *i.e.* the white and the yolk, have very different analyses. All of the fat and the fat- soluble vitamins are contained in the yolk, while the white is composed of a large amount of water, plus protein. In addition to fat and protein, eggs contain all of the known vitamins with the exception of Vitamin C. Table 21.3 shows the major nutrients in one 60g egg, and Table 21.4 shows the micro-nutrient content. These may vary slightly depending on the age, nutrition and environment of the hen, but can be used with confidence in most circumstances.

Table 21.3: Major Nutrients in 1 Egg (weighing 60g)

Nutrient	*Quantity*	*Per cent RDA**
Protein (g)	6.7	12
Energy (kcal)	78	11
Energy (kjoules)	324	11
Fat	6	n/a
PUFA (g)	1.17	12
MUFA (g)	2.46	20
Saturated fat	2	n/a

*: RDA: Recommended Daily Allowance; PUFA: Polyunsaturated fatty acids; MUFA: Mono-unsaturated fatty acids.

Contents of these may vary considerably depending on the diet of the hen, and may be deliberately altered by feeding specific diets.

Table 21.4: Average Amount of Chemical Components of Entire Chicken Egg

Particulars	*Amount (grams)*
Total	58.0
Water	38.1
Solids	19.9
Organic matter	13.6 (range in per cent)
Proteins	7.0 (12.8-13.4)
Lipids	6.1 (10.5-11.8)
Carbohydrates	0.5 (0.3-1.0)
Inorganic matter	6.3 (0.8-1.0)

Table 21.5: Elemental Composition of Egg

Particulars	*Per cent*
Carbon	53
Oxygen	20
Nitrogen	15
Hydrogen	7
Phosphorus	4
Sulfur	1

Table 21.6: Proportional Amounts of Major Chemical Constituents in the Egg Contents of Various Birds

Chemical Constituents	*Land Birds: Gallifermes*		*Water Fowl: Anseriformes*	
	Chicken	*Turkey*	*Duck*	*Goose*
Av. Wt. (gms)	51.6	71.6	66.6	177.0
Water	73.6	73.7	69.7	70.6
Solids	26.4	26.3	30.3	29.4
Organic matter	25.6	25.5	29.3	28.2
Proteins	12.8	13.1	13.7	14.0
Fats (lipids)	11.8	11.7	14.4	13.0
Carbohydrates	1.0	0.7	1.2	1.2
Inorganic matter	0.8	0.8	1.0	1.2

Composition of Egg Shell, Egg Shell Membrane, and Albumen and Yolk

The egg's outer covering, accounting for about 9 to 12 per cent of its total weight depending on egg size. The shell is the egg's first line of defense against bacterial contamination. The shell is largely composed of calcium carbonate (about 94 per cent) with small amounts of magnesium carbonate, calcium phosphate and other organic matter including protein. Shell strength is greatly influenced by the minerals and vitamins in the hen's diet, particularly calcium, phosphorus, manganese and Vitamin D. If the diet is deficient in calcium, for instance, the hen will produce a thin or soft-shelled egg or possibly an egg with no shell at all. Occasionally an egg may be prematurely expelled from the uterus due to injury or excitement. In this case, the shell has not had time to be completely formed. Shell thickness is also related to egg size which, in turn, is related to the hen's age. As the hen ages, egg size increases. The same amount of shell material which covers a smaller egg must be "stretched" to cover a larger one, hence the shell is thinner.

Seven to 17 thousand tiny pores are distributed over the shell surface, a greater number at the large end. As the egg ages, these tiny holes permit moisture and carbon dioxide to move out and air to move in to form the air cell. The shell is covered with a protective coating called the cuticle or bloom. By blocking the pores, the cuticle helps to preserve freshness and prevent microbial contamination of the contents. Uses for eggshells vary from the thrifty (compost) to the creative (decorating).

In the egg shell matrix calcite crystal represent in the proportion of 1: 50. The matrix consists of two regions, the mammilary matrix and spongy matrix, which differ in their staining capacity of polysaccharides. The elemental composition of eggshell has been reported to be 98.2 per cent calcium, 0.9 per cent magnesium, and 0.9 per cent phosphorus. The proteins in shell membranes have a high content of arginine, glutamic acid, methionine, histidine, cystine, and prolein, but compared to cuticle or matrix proteins, the membrane proteins are relatively low in glycine.

The composition of the shell is important from the viewpoint of food safety, sanitation, and esthetics. It contains calcium carbonate (94 per cent), magnesium carbonate (1 per cent), calcium phosphate (1 per cent), and 4 per cent organic matter. The egg shell including the gelatinous covering or cuticle, contains a large proportions of inorganic salts, some organic material and very little water.

Table 21.7: Composition of Egg Shell

Composition	Per cent
Total	100
Water	1.6
Solids	98.4
Organic matter	3.3
Proteins	3.3
Lipids	0.03
Inorganic matter	95.1

Shell Membrane

The shell membrane constitutes 4 or 5 per cent of the entire egg covering, consist almost wholly of protein, except for very small amount of water and traces of mineral.

Table 21.8: Composition of Shell Membrane

Composition	Per cent
Total	100
Water	20.0
Solids	80.0
Organic matter	70.0
Proteins	70.0
Inorganic matter	10.0

Egg Albumen

Albumen also known as egg white. Albumen accounts for most of an egg's liquid weight, about 67 per cent. It contains more than half the egg's total protein, niacin, riboflavin, chlorine, magnesium, potassium, sodium and sulfur. The albumen consists of 4 alternating layers of thick and thin consistencies. From the yolk outward, they are designated as the inner thick or chalaziferous white, the inner thin white, the outer thick white and the outer thin white. Egg white tends to thin out as an egg ages because its protein changes in character. That's why fresh eggs sit up tall and firm in the pan while older ones tend to spread out.Albumen is more opalescent than truly white. The cloudy appearance comes from carbon dioxide. As the egg ages, carbon dioxide escapes, so the albumen of older eggs is more transparent than that of fresher eggs.When egg albumen is beaten vigorously, it foams and increases in volume 6 to 8 times. Egg foams are essential for making souffles, meringues, puffy omelets, and angel food and sponge cakes.

Water is the major constituent of albumen and is generally decrease from outer to inner albumen layers. The total solid content of albumen as a whole ranges from 11 to 13 per cent, however, varied depending on strain and age of the hens, size of the egg etc. Carbohydrate of albumen exists in both free (0.4 per cent) and combined forms (0.5 per cent) in protein. Free carbohydrate mainly glucose (98 per cent) and bounds carbohydrate as glycoprotein are mannose and galactose. The elemental composition of albumen is extremely variable as depends on hens diet. The pH of freshly laid egg albumen is in the range of 7.6-8.5, but increase during storage up to a value of 9.7.

Egg albumen is the principal reservoir of water for the developing embryo. Its main organic constituents is protein, small amount of carbohydrates and minerals and negligible amounts of lipids.

Table 21.9: Chemical Composition of Egg Albumen

Chemical Constituents	*Galliformes*		*Anseriformes*	
	Chicken	*Turkey*	*Duck*	*Goose*
Av. Wt. of egg albumen(gms)	32.9	44.2	40.4	110.2
Water, per cent	87.9	86.5	86.8	86.7
Solids, per cent	12.	13.5	13.2	13.3
Organic matter, per cent	11.5	12.8	12.4	12.5
Proteins, per cent	10.6	11.5	11.3	11.3
Lipids, per cent	0.03	0.03	0.08	0.04
Carbohydrates, per cent	0.9	1.3	1.0	1.2
Inorganic matter, per cent	0.6	0.7	0.8	0.8

Egg Yolk

The yolk or yellow portion makes up about 33 per cent of the liquid weight of the egg. It contains all of the fat in the egg and a little less than half of the protein. With the exception of riboflavin and niacin, the yolk contains a higher proportion of the egg's vitamins than the white. All of the egg's vitamins A, D and E are in the yolk. Egg yolks are one of the few foods naturally containing vitamin D. The yolk also contains more phosphorus, manganese, iron, iodine, copper, and calcium than the white, and it contains all of the zinc. The yolk of a Large egg contains about 59 calories. Double-yolked eggs are often produced by young hens whose egg production cycles are not yet completely synchronized. They're often produced, too, by hens who are old enough to produce Extra Large eggs. Genetics is a factor, also. Occasionally a hen will produce double-yolked eggs throughout her egg-laying career. It is rare, but not unusual, for a young hen to produce an egg with no yolk at all.In fertilized eggs, the yolk is the site of embryo formation.

It is the yolk which is responsible for the egg's emulsifying properties.

The total solid content of yolk is generally 52 per cent, whereas moisture contents 48 per cent. Yolk solid comprises of lipid (31.8-35.5 per cent), protein (15.7-16.6 per cent), carbohydrate (0.2-1.0 per cent) and ash (1.1). One yolk on the average contained about 226 mg of cholesterol. The pH of freshly laid egg yolk is around 6.0, but this value increase even up to a pH of 6.4 to 6.9 during storage.

Table 21.10: Composition of Egg Yolk

Chemical Components (%)	*Galliformes*		*Anseriformes*	
	Chicken	*Turkey*	*Duck*	*Goose*
Av. Wt. of yolk(gm)	18.7	27.4	26.2	66.8
Water	48.7	48.3	44.8	43.3
Solids	51.3	51.7	55.2	56.7
Organic matter	50.2	50.4	54.0	55.1
Proteins	16.6	16.3	17.7	18.0
Lipids	32.6	33.2	35.2	36.0
Carbohydrates	1.0	0.9	1.1	1.1
Inorganic matter	1.1	1.3	1.2	1.6

Table 21.11: Modified from "USDA Egg Grading Manual" 1969. Agriculture Handbook No. 75. per cent Composition Whole Egg

Composition	*Per cent*
Water	65.5
Protein	11.8
Fat	11.0
Ash	11.7

Colour

Egg shell and yolk color may vary, but color has nothing to do with egg quality, flavour, nutritive value, cooking characteristics or shell thickness.

Shell

The color comes from pigments in the outer layer of the shell and may range in various breeds from white to deep brown. The breed of hen determines the color of the shell. Breeds with white feathers and ear lobes lay white eggs; breeds with red feathers and ear lobes lay brown eggs. White eggs are most in demand among American buyers. In some parts of the country, however, particularly in New England, brown shells are preferred. The Rhode Island Red, New Hampshire and Plymouth Rock are breeds that lay brown eggs. Since brown-egg layers are slightly larger birds and require more food, brown eggs are usually more expensive than white.

White

Egg albumen in raw eggs is opalescent and does not appear white until it is beaten or cooked. A yellow or greenish cast in raw white may indicate the presence of riboflavin. Cloudiness of the raw white is due to the presence of carbon dioxide which has not had time to escape through the shell and thus indicates a very fresh egg.On very rare occasions, a hard-cooked egg white may darken to a caramel shade due to a high amount of iron in the cooking water or to a carbonylamine-type reaction. Using fresh eggs and cooling them quickly after cooking helps to prevent this darkening.

Yolk

Yolk color depends on the diet of the hen. If she gets plenty of yellow-orange plant pigments known as xanthophylls, they will be deposited in the yolk. Hens fed mashes containing yellow corn and alfalfa meal lay eggs with medium yellow yolks, while those eating wheat or barley yield lighter-colored yolks. A colorless diet, such as white cornmeal produces almost colorless yolks. Natural yellow-orange substances such as marigold petals may be added to light-colored feeds to enhance yolk color. Artificial color additives are not permitted. Gold or lemon-colored yolks are preferred by most buyers in this country. Yolk pigments are relatively stable and are not lost or changed in cooking.Sometimes there is a greenish ring around hard-cooked egg yolks. It is the result of sulfur and iron compounds in the egg reacting at the surface of the yolk. It may occur when eggs are overcooked or when there is a high amount of iron in the cooking water. Although the color may be a bit unappealing, the eggs are still wholesome and nutritious and their flavour is unaffected. Greenish yolks can best be avoided by using the proper cooking time and temperature and by rapidly cooling the cooked eggs.Occasionally several concentric green rings may be seen in hard-cooked egg yolks. A yolk develops within the hen in rings. Iron in the hen's feed or water as the rings are formed may cause this coloring.Sometimes a large batch of scrambled eggs may turn green. Although not pretty, the color change is harmless. It is due to a chemical change brought on by heat and occurs when eggs are cooked at too high a temperature, held for too long or both. Using stainless steel equipment and low cooking temperature, cooking in small batches and serving as soon as possible after cooking will help to prevent this. If it is necessary to hold scrambled eggs for a short time before serving, it helps to avoid direct heat. Place a pan of hot water between the pan of eggs and the heat source.

Air Cell

The empty space between the white and shell at the large end of the egg.When an egg is first laid, it is warm. As it cools, the contents contract and the inner shell membrane separates from the outer shell membrane to form the air cell. The candler uses the size of the air cell as one basis for determining grade. In Grade AA eggs, the air cell may not exceed 1/8-inch in depth and is about the size of a dime. The air cell of Grade A eggs may exceed 3/16-inch in depth. For Grade B eggs, there is no limit on air cell size.As the egg ages, moisture and carbon dioxide leave through the pores of the shell, air enters to replace them and the air cell becomes larger. Although the air cell usually forms in the large end of the egg, it occasionally moves freely toward the uppermost point of the egg as the egg is rotated. It is then called a free or floating air cell. If the main air cell ruptures, resulting in one or more small separate air bubbles floating beneath the main air cell, it is known as a bubbly air cell. You can see the air cell in the flattened end of a peeled, hard-cooked egg.

Fertile Eggs

Eggs which can be incubated and developed into chicks. Fertile eggs are not more nutritious than nonfertile eggs, do not keep as well as nonfertile eggs and are more expensive to produce. Fertile eggs may contain a small amount of male hormone, but there are no known advantages.

Free-Range Eggs

True free-range eggs are those produced by hens raised outdoors or that have daily access to the outdoors. Due to seasonal conditions, however, few hens are actually raised outdoors. Some egg farms are indoor floor operations and these are sometimes erroneously referred to as free-range operations. Due to higher production costs and lower volume per farm,free-range eggs are generally more expensive. The nutrient content of eggs is not affected by whether hens are raised free-range or in floor or cage operations.

Chemistry of Eggs and Egg products

Knowledge of the chemical composition and physico-chemical properties of native albumen and yolk should be useful for interpreting the changes which occur during shell egg storage and during pasteurizing, drying and freezing. Alteration in the egg components will be reflected as a loss of functionality of albumen (foaming power) and yolk (emulsifying ability).

Proteins in Egg Albumen

Albumen may be regarded as a protein system consisting of ovomucin fibers in an aqueous solution of numerous globular proteins. The protein composition of the thin and thick layers of albumen are different only in the ovomucin content. The principal protein fractions of albumen have been separated by the stepwise addition of ammonium sulphate. The ion-exchange technique using carboxymethyl cellulose (CMC) and diethylaminoethyl cellulose (DEAE) have been used for fractionation and purification of albumen proteins. The major proteins are ovalbumin, conalbumin, ovomucoid, lysozyme and globulins. The albumen proteins and their characteristics are presented in the Table 21.12.

Several electrophoretic methods have been used to separate the proteins of albumen and of albumen fractions. The proteins of albumen were resolved by moving-boundary electrophoresis into 7 major peaks, including ovalbumin A_1 and A_2, globulins G_2 and G_3, ovomucoid and conalbumin. Using paper electrophoresis, obtained distinct bands of ovalbumin, ovomucoid plus ovoglobulin, conalbumin and lysozyme. With starch-gel electrophoresis, the proteins of albumen was separated into as many as 19 bands. Genetic polymorphism studied on variation of the nos. of bands for albumen from various strains and inbred lines. Globulins in particular were found to be genetically controlled. Polyacrylamide disc-gel electrophoresis was capable of resolving albumen proteins into 12 bands.

Table 21.12: The Albumen Proteins and their Characteristics

Sl.No.	Protein	Relative Amount in Albumen Per cent	Isolelectric Point	Molecular Weight	Characteristics
1.	Ovalbumin	54	4.6	45,000	Phosphoglycoprotein
2.	Conalbumin	13	6.6	80,000	Binds metals especially iron
3.	Ovomucoid	11	3.9-4.3	28,000	Inhibits trypsin
4.	Lysozyme(G_1-globulin)	3.5	10.7	14,600	Lyses some bacteria
5.	G_2 globulin	4.0	5.5	30,000 to 45,000	—
6.	G_3 globulin	4.0	5.8	—	—
7.	Ovomucin	1.5	—	—	Sialoprotein
8.	Flavoprotein	0.8	4.1	35,000	Binds rivoflavin
9.	Ovoglycoprotein	0.5	3.9	24,000	Sioaloprotein
10.	Ovomacroglobulin	0.5	4.5-4.7	760,000 to 900,000	—
11.	Ovoinhibitor	0.1	5.2	44,000	Inhibits several proteases
12.	Avidin	0.05	9.5	53,000	Binds biotin

Ovalbumin

It is the predominant protein in albumen, a phosphoglycoprotein, since carbohydrate and phosphate moities are attached to the polypeptide. Ovalbumin can be obtained by fractionation with ammonium sulphate or sodium sulphate and by chromatography. Mol.wt. about 45,000; has 3 components A_1, A_2, and A_3 which differ in phosphorus content. A_1 has 2 phophates per molecule, A_2 has 1 and A_3 has none. The relative proportion of A_1, A_2, and A_3 = 85:12:3. Recent studies indicated 4-SH groups in ovalbumin molecule, 3 of which are reactive to p-chloromercuribenzoate in native protein and the fourth in the denatured protein. Besides 4-SH groups ovalbuumin contained two disulfide groups per molecule.

Carbohydrate in ovalbumin – 2 per cent D-mannose and 1.2 per cent 2-amino-2-deoxy-D-glucose or an average of 5 and 3 residues, respectively of these sugars per molecule of protein. One carbohydrate group is attached to a polypeptide chain through asparagine. The carbohydrate moiety has not wt. between 1560 and 1580.

Ovalbumin is converted to S-ovalbumin, a more heat-stable protein, during the storage of eggs. Since the physical and chemical properties of ovalbomin and S-ovalbumin are comparable sulfhydryl-disulfide interchange is a plausible explanation for the conversion.

Ovalbmin in solution is readily denatured and coagulated by exposure to new surfaces (eg: shaking) but it is resistant to thermal denaturation. Heatingof albumen at pH 9 to 62^{0}C for 3.5 minutes altered only 3 to 5 per cent of the ovalbumin, whereas negligible amounts of this protein were changed by heating albumin with a pH of 7.

Conalbumin

It is a glycoprotein, easily prepared by fractional precipitation with ammonium sulphate or seprated from ovalbumin by shaking the protein solution until the ovalbumin coagulates. Starch-gel electrophoresis showed two forms of conalbumin in the ratio of 4:1. Again two conalbumin fractions from egg albumen was separated by ion-exchange chromatography. The fraction with mol.wt. about 80,000, contains no phosphorus and free sulfhydryl groups. Wallians(1962 A) has shown that the protein moieties of conalbumin and transferrin of chicken blood serum are identical, but the carbohydrate prosthetic groups are different.Conalbumin contains about 0.8 per cent hexose and 1.4 per cent hexosamine. The isoelectric point of purified conalbumin is about 6.6.

Conalbumin is more heat-sensitive than ovalbumin but less susceptible to surface denaturation. Conalbumin in phosphate- bicarbonate buffer at the 1 per cent level had minimum heat stability near pH 6. At pH 6 conalbumin in buffer was altered to the extent of about 40 per cent upon heating to 57^{0}C for 10 minute. At pH 9, if heated under the same conditions, the protein was not altered significantly. The heat stability of conalbumin in albumen was similar to that purified conalbumin in buffer.

Di- and trivalent metallic ions are bound firmly by conalbumin. Two atoms of Fe(III), Al(III), Cu(II) and Zn(II) per molecule of protein form stable complexes with conalbumin abve pH 6. These complexes are red, colourless, yellow and colourless, respectively. When conalbumin is complexed with metallic ions, the complexes are resistant to the denaturation and proteolytic attack. Iron is bound by 3 phenolic hydroxyl groups of protein as well as by 1 carbonate ion; 2 nitrogen groups may also be involved in the chelation.

Ovomucoid

Ovomucoid is a heat-resistant 11 per cent glycoprotein, prepared by first precipitating out the other albumen proteins with trichloroacetic acid at pH 3.5 and then precipitating ovomucoid with acetone. Ovomucoid can be precipitated out of the solution upon saturation with ammonium sulphate. Mol.wt is approx.28000, I.P. between 3.9 and 4.3. Ovomucoid is found to be trypsin inhibitor. less than I molecules of ovomucoid is required to reduce the activity of 1 molecule of trypsin by 50 per cent.

Moving-boundary electrophoresis separated two forms of ovomucoid. Column chromatography with buffers of different pH values showed 3 forms of ovomucoid. Starch-gel electrophoresis – 3 discrete bands of ovomucoid. In addition to the 3 forms of ovomucoid the TCA precipitated ovomucoid fraction contains ovoinhibitor which can be purified by column chromatography.

Carbohydrates of ovomucoids are :- D-galactose 1.0 to 1.5 per cent, D-mannose 4.3 to 4.7 per cent ; 2-amino-2deoxy-D-glucose 12.5 to15.4 per cent, sialic acid 0.4 to 4 per cent, total hexoses 6 to 9 per cent

The carbohydrate is present as 3 oligosaccharides each joined to the polypeptide chain through an asparaginyl residue.

This glycoprotein has a single polypeptide chain with helical portions(about 22 per cent) and random coils. Every 11th amino residue in ovomucoid is on the average an end of a disulfide linkage; 8disulfied linkages are present in each chain. In acidic solutions, ovomucoid is very resistant to heat denaturation, but in the alkaline region (pH 9) this protein is altered rapidly at 80°C· The criteria for thermal denaturation of ovomucoid were a loss of antitryptic activity and an increase in rate of hydrolysis by chymotrypsin. Presumably the helical structure is changed during heat treatment.

Lysozyme

It is reported that the G_1 globulin of Longsworth et al (1940) was lysozyme, the albumen enzyme which has a lytic action on bacterial cell walls; consists of 2 or 3 components which can be separated by cation exchange chromatography and moving- boundany eletropheresis. Lysozyme has mol.wt.approx.14,300 to 14,600, I.P. 10.7.

The enzyme contains 129 amino acids residues and 4 disulfide bonds. No free sulfhydryl groups have been found. This is according to primary structure. X-ray diffraction analysis has been used to obtain an insight into the secondary and tertiany structure.

Lysozyme is capable of hydrolyzing the β (1,4)linkages between N-acetyl meuraminic acid and N-acetyl glucosamine in bacterial cell walls.

Thermal inactivation of lysozyme is dependent on pH and temperature. At 149°F(65°C), the activity of lysozyme in phosphate buffer at PH 9 was reduced to about 70 per cent during a 10 min. period. Lysozyme is about 50 times never heat sensitive in egg albumen than in phosphate buffer. Egg white heated to 145°F(62.5°C) for 10 mins. lysozyme inactivated to a greater degree as the pH increased above 7.

Ovomucin

It is a glycoprotein, may contribute to the gel like structure of thick white in the form of flexible, microscopic fibers. The amount of ovomucin in the thick white is about 4 times greater than that in thin white. Ovomucin has the ability to inhibit viral heamagglutination.

Ovomucin can be precipitated from solution by diluting albumen with 2 or 3 volumes of water (pH 6 to 8), or by lowering the pH of albumen to pH 4. The ovomucin precipitate is soluble in dilute salt solution at about pH 7. or in alkalin solutions.

Ovomucin fraction can be separated into 3 parts by moving-boundary electrophoresis. Water- precipitated ovomucin is not resolved effectively by starch-gel electrophoresis. Only one band moving in the ovalbumin region, is formed in the starch-gel. When the solubility of ovomucin was increased by reduction with mercaptoethanol, the protein did not migrate on paper or starch gel, but did move as a single component on polyacrylamide gel during eletrophoresis. It has carbohydrate contents about 33 per cent. The unfractionated ovomucin consists of 10 to 20 per cent hexosamine, 15 per cent hexose, 2.6 to 8 per cent sialic acid. The purified mercaptoethanol- reduced ovomucin had the carbohydrates- 9.3 per cent galactose, 1.4 per cent mannose, 9.1 per cent glucosamine, 4.8 per cent galactosamine and 8.7 per cent sialic acid.

The ovomucin in solution is resistant to heat alterations. The solution of ovomucin between pH 7.1 and 9.4 did not change in viscosity or optical density during heating at about 194°F (90°C) for 2 hrs. Ovomucin and lysozyme in solution can interact through electrostatic bonds to form a water insoluble complex. Over the pH range of 7.2 to 10.4, the interaction of these proteins decreases as the pH increases. In egg albumen, the amount of complex formation decreased as the pH approached the isolectric point (10.7) of lysozyme. This complex plays an important role in the thinning of egg white during storage of eggs, but contradictory hypotheses have been advanced. The thinning of thick albumen is caused, partly at least by the interaction of ovomucin with lysozyme when the pH rises to around 9 during the normal loss of CO_2 from the egg upon storage.

The lysozyme activity loss of about 20 to 25 per cent during storage of eggs at 36°F(2°C) for 45 days may be caused by the formation of an insoluble ovomucin-lysozyme complex. Cotteril and Winter (1955) have suggested that thinning is caused by a reduction in the amount of naturally occurring ovomucin-lysozyme complex at pH about 9 to 9.5.

Avidin

Avidin is the albumen protein which binds biotin. About 3 moles of biotin are bound to 1 mole of Avidin. Purfication procedure include ammonium sulphate precipitation, absorption on bentonite and ion exchange cellulose. The heterogenous avidin fraction has 3 components A, B and C. Avidin has mol. wt. = 53,000 and I.P. = 9.5

Ovoglobulin

Demonstrated by moving-boundary electrophoresis that the globulin fraction consisted of 3 proteins G_1, G_2 and G_3. G_1 was considered to be lysozyme. The G_2 and G_3 components have been separated by starch-gel electrophoresis and by ion-exchange chromatography. G_2 component was isolated by chromatography on DEAE and CM cellulose, along with precipitation with ammonium sulphate. G_2 isolate has mol.wt. = 35,000 and I.P. = 5.5.

Ovoglobulins have been found to be excellent forming agents.

Ovoinhibitors

Demonstrated by paper electrophoresis that the ovoinhibitor is a homogeneous protein with negligible sialic acid. Purification of ovoinhibitor can be achieved by chromatography of TCA precipitated ovomucoid. Ovoinhibitor is capable of inhibiting trypsin and chymotrypsin as well as fungal and bacterial proteases.

Flavoprotein

All the riboflavin in egg albumen is bound as flavoprotein. Chicken albumen contains about equal amounts of flavoprotein and the apoprotein (none-riboflavin containing protein). According to Winter et al (1967), the apoprotein binds riboflavin very tightly. The major function of the ribo-flavin-binding apoprotein is presumably to ensure transfer of riboflavin from the blood serum to the albumen.

With paper and starch gel electrophoresis, the flavoprotein migrates slightly in front of the ovalbumin A band. The apoprotein migrated at the same rate as the flavoprotein in starch gel electrophoresis. Two fractions of apoprotein separated on cellulose columns by eluting at pH 4.5 and 4.3, had 7 and 8 phosphate groups per mole, respectively. Mol.wt. of apoprotein is between 32,000 and 36,000 and I.P.= between 3.9 and 4.1.

Microstructure of Yolk Particles

Yolk may be classified as a complex system containing a variety of particles suspended in a protein (livetin) solution. The main types of particles are:

1. Yolk spheres
2. Free floating drops or granules
3. Profiles or low-density lipoprotein
4. Nyelin figures

1. Yolk Spheres

In optical microscope, round masses with diam. ranging from 25 to 150μ could be observed(Moran 1925). Diam. of spheres in yellow yolk were much larger (25 to 150μ) than the diam. of white yolk spheres (4 to 75)(Romanoff and Romanoff 1949). Yellow yolk spheres had numerous tightly packed droplets within them; whereas white yolk spheres had only a few droplets in a protein fluid (Grodzinski 1946). Numerous spheres about (20μ) were found in white yolk but very few spheres (about 40μ) were present in yellow yolk (Chang 1969). Grodzinski (1946, 1951) considered spheres as osmometers since each has presumably a semipermeable membrane.

Bellairs (1961) noted 3 types of sphere surfaces in electron micrographs: lamellated capsule (several layers of membrane), unit membrane like structure and naked surface.

2. Free-Floating Drops or Granules

These are smaller and more numerous than yolk spheres. Granules tended to be circular and ranged in diameter from 0.3 to 1.6μ. Most of the granules had diameters in the vicinity of 0.5μ. Bellairs (1961) reported that granules (lipid drops) had diameters of about 2μ. The majority of the hydrated granules had diameters between 0 and 1.7μ. Electron micrographs of Bellairs (1961) indicated that granules had high and low density patches with diameters between 30 and 60A^0. Chang(1969) suggested that granules are made up of electron- dense subunits.

When isolated granules were treated with 1.71M NaCl, large and small globules (300 to 1000A^0) and myelin figures (560 to 1300A^0 in length) as well as electron dense masses were evident in the micrographs. Centrifugation of the dispersion of granules in 1.71M. NaCl yielded 2 floating and 3 sedimenting fractions. As shown by electron microscopy, the floating fractions contained small and large globules as well as myelin figures. Fractions III and V consisted predominantly of fluffy masses (made up of entangled strands to which electron- dense microparticles were attached). The microparticles which were roughly circular had a mean diameter of about 100A^{0}. In fraction IV numerous electron-dense masses interspersed with small globules occurred. Change (1969) has hypothesized that the strands of the fluffy masses are phosvitin complexes and the attached microparticles are lipovitellin. Radmonski and Cook (1964A, 1964B) showed that lipovitellins and phosvitin had an affinity for each other and suggested that a phosvitin-lipovitellin complex is a basic unit of the granule.

Bellairs (1961) noted that small (diam 250A^{0}) round profiles were present in the electron micrographs of egg yolk. Chang (1969) confirmed the presence of these particles in yolk. These profiles can be considered as low density lipoprotein (LDL). Diam. of LDL ranges from 117 to 480A^{0}.

Proteins and Lipoproteins in the Granules and Plasma

Schmidt *et al.* (1956) reported that yolk can be separated by high speed centrifugation into sedimented granules and a clear fluid supernatant called plasma. The granules make up about 19 to 23 per cent of the solids in yolk and about 11.5 per cent of the liquid yolk. Moisture content of granules (unwashed) = 44 per cent. Granules on moisture free basis contains lipid 34 per cent, protein 60 per cent and ash 6 per cent including 0.5 per cent divalent cations such as calcium. Phospholipid fractions – represent 37 per cent of the total lipid consists phosphatidyl choline (82 per cent) and phosphatidyl ethanolamine(15 per cent). The major portion of the yolk is plasma (about 78 per cent of the total liquid yolk). The moisture content of plasma is about 49 per cent. On a dry weight basis, plasma consists of lipid 77 to 81 per cent, ash 2.2 per cent, and non-lipid residue mostly protein about 18 per cent.

Separation of yolk proteins and lipoproteins have been achieved by using paper and gel electrophoresis. Paper electrophoresis showed yolk lipovitellins remained at the origin, whereas lowdensity lipoproteins livetins and phosvitin migrated. Disc–gel electrophoresis showed 19 bands including livetins, phosvitin(when EDAT was added to yolk) and lipovitellins were formed but no low density lipoproteins.

Proteins and Lipoproteins in Granules

Burley and Cook (1961)-granules are composed of α- and β- lipovitelins= 70 per cent, phosvitin= 16 per cent, low density lipoproteins= 12 per cent. Phosvitin is a non-lipid phosphoprotein. The lipovitellins and low-density lipoproteins are lipid protein complexes.

Phosvitin

Phosvitin was isolated by diluting yolk with a magnesium sulphate solution to form an insoluble complex. The phosvitin contains 12 to 13 per cent nitrogen and about 10 per cent phosphorus, which represents about 80 per cent of the yolk protein phosphorus. It can be isolated by chromatography. Phosvitin was separated into 2 components by chromatography on a DEAE cellulose column. When isolated phosvitin was used for gel electrophehesis, obtained 2 diffuse bands.

Phosvitin is homogeneous when analyzed by ultracentrifugation. Amino acid analysis showed no cysteine, cystine, methionine, tryptophan or tyrosin. About 31 per cent of the total amino acid residues are serine. The phosphorus in phosvitin is presumably present as phosphoserine. At least 6 phosphoserine residues are grouped together in the polypeptide. Phosvitin has a mol.wt. between 36,000 and 40,000. It is an elongated molecule with dimension of about 14 A^0 by 280A^0.

Phovitin is the iron carrier in yolk. Ferric ions are bound tightly to phosvitin, yet the phosvitin-iron complex is in solution except when the iron is in excess(P/Fe ratio is about 2). Macromolecules can also interact with phosvitin. There is demonstration of lipovitellin-phosvitin complex.

Lipovitellins

A crude lipovitellin fraction can be prepared from yolk by centrifuging water-diluted yolk, whereupon a high density fraction was sedimented. This high density mass is lipovitellin. In reality such a fraction in made up of granules. Add 10 per cent or 2M NaCl to yolk, granules are dispersed. NaCl-yolk dispersion is centrifuged, then 2 floating fractions and 2 subnatant layers are formed. The floating fractions contain low-density lipoprotein (LDL) whereas the subnatant layer is called high density fraction at the bottom of the tube contain lipovitellins, phosvitin and livetins.

Lipovitellin has 2 components - α and β lipovitellin by moving-boundary electrophoresis. By chromatography = 2 components successfully separated.

Lipid and protein phosphorus contents of α- and β- lipovitellins(LV) isolated by Column Chromatography.

Chromatography Column	Lipid Content (per cent)		Protein Phosphorus (per cent)	
	α - LV	β -LV	α - LV	β -LV
Hydroxyapatite (HA)	20	20	1.20	0.45
Dowen I, then HA	22	22	0.50	0.27
TEAE cellulose	14.6	16.5	0.54	0.28

The protein phosphorus values for α- and β- lipoproteins were about 0.50 and 0.27 per cent, respectively. At pH below 7.0, the lepoproteins existed in the dimer form, but monomers were created when the pH was raised. The mol.wt. of the dimmers of α- and β- lipovitellins are in the vicinity of 400,000.

The lipid content of the lipovitellins depend upon the method of preparation. However it can be stated that the lipid content of both α- and β- lipovitellins is in the vicinity of 20 per cent (40 per cent neutral lipid + 60 per cent phospholipid). Neutral lipid includes 4.1 per cent free cholesterol and 0.14 to 0.2 per cent of the ester. Each phospholipid fraction consists of about 75 per cent phosphatidylcholine, 18 per cent phosphatidyl ethanolamine and 7 per cent sphingomyelin and lysophospholipids.

Proteins and Lipoproteins in Plasma

Plasma is composed of livetins which are lipid-free globular proteins and low density lipoproteins (LDL). The livetins and low density lipoproteins represent about 10.6 and 66 per cent, respectively,of the total yolk solids.

Livetins

Livetins fraction was first isolated in the undenatured state with the procedure of removing lipoproteins precipitating the livetins by half saturation with ammonium sulphate and extracting with an alcohol-ether mixture of 5°F (-15°C). Three components of the livetin fraction could be resolved by moving- boundary electrophoresis. Martin *et al.* (1959, 1962) confirmed the presence of α-, β- and γ-livetins in yolk of egg.

Table 21.13: Composition of Livetins

Composition	*α-livetins*	*β-livetins*	*γ-livetins*
Nitrogen, per cent	14.3	14.3	15.6
Hexose, per cent	–	7	2.6
Hexosamine, per cent	–	–	1.8

The mean mol.wt. of α-, β- and γ- livetins were reported to be 80,000, 45,000 and 150,000, respectively. The isoelectric point of livetin is about 4.8 to 5.0. The relative amounts of α-, β- and γ- livetins in yolk have been reported as 2:3:5 by Shepard and Hottle and as 2:5:3 by Bernadi and Cook. Using immunological technique, it is stated that livetins were indeed blood serum proteins of the chicken. Williams (1962b) identified α-livetin are serum albumin, β- livetin as α_s-glycoprotein and γ-livetin as γ-globulin.

Low Density Lipoprotein

Since density of LDL is 0.98, this fraction is successfully isolated by floatation. Nichol et al (1954) isolated LDL from egg yolk by a floatation procedure and found the fraction to have a lipid content of 89 per cent. Turner and Cook reported lipid content as 80 per cent, Martin et al. (1963) as 89 per cent, Sugano and Watanabe (1961) as 84 per cent. Martin et al (1963) reported that lipid in LDL consists of neutral lipid 74 per cent (free cholesterol 4 per cent and ester 0.2 per cent) and phospholipid 26 per cent (phosphatidyl choline 71 to 76 per cent, phosphatidyl ethanolamine 16 to 20 per cent sphingomyelin and lysophospholipids 8 to 9 per cent).

There are two ultrafugally distinguishable fractions LDL_1 and LDL_2. The composition of these LDL fractions were similar. The total lipid for LDL_1 = 87-89 per cent whereas LDL_2 has 83 to 86 per cent. The lipid from LDL fractions consisted of : phospholipid 25 to 28 per cent, cholesterol 3.3 per cent, free fatty acid 5 per cent, triglycerides rest. Av. Mol.wt. of LDL_1 = 10 million and LDL_2 = 3 million.

Table 21.14: Composition of Low-density Lipoproteins

Composition	LDL_1	LDL_2
Total lipids	89	86
Lipid phosphorus	1.0	1.14
Lipid molar N/P ratio	1.04	1.14
Cholesterol, per cent of lipid	3.3	3.4
Free fatty acid, per cent of lipid	5	4.5
Phopholipid composition, per cent		
Phosphatidyl choline	84	83
Phosphatidyl ethanolamine	13	14
Non-lipid residue, per cent	11	14
Nitrogen, per cent of non-lipid residue	14.8	13.7
Phosphorus, per cent of non-lipid residue	0.15	0.16

Source: Saari *et al.* (1964).

Cook and Martin (1962) have visualized low-density lipoproteins as spheres, each with a triglyceride core upon which phospholipids and proteins are layered. Presumably proteins with their hydrophilic groups are located on the outer surfaces. Papain hydrolyzes the protein of LDL_1 and LDL_2. About 2/3rd of the surface of a LDL micelle could be covered by protein if the thickness of the protein molecules is assumed to be 8 A^0. Presumably phosphate groups on phospholipids are exposed at the micellar surfaces, as it was found that 95 per cent of the phospholipid in LDL was hydrolyzed by phospholipase D. Recently it is estimated that at least 100 cationic sites are located on the surface of each LDL micelle.

Freshness and Nutritive Value of Egg

Freshness

How recently an egg was laid has a bearing on its freshness but is onlyone of many factors. The temperature at which it is held, the humidityand the handling all play their part. These variables are so importantthat an egg one week old, held under ideal conditions, can be fresherthan an egg left at room temperature for one day. The ideal conditions are temperatures that don't go above 40°F. (4°C.) and a relative humidity of 70 to 80 per cent.Proper handling means prompt gathering, washing and oiling of the eggs within a few hours after laying. Most commercially produced eggs reach supermarkets within a few days of leaving the laying house. If the market and the buyer handle them properly, they will still be fresh whenthey reach the table. It is not true that freshness can be judged by placing an egg in salt water. A carefully controlled brine test is sometimes used to judge shell thickness of eggs for hatching purposes but has no application to freshness of table eggs.

How important is "freshness"? As an egg ages, the white becomes thinner and the yolk becomes flatter. These changes do not have any great effect on the nutritional quality of the egg or its functional cooking properties in recipes. Appearance may be affected, though. When poached or fried, the fresher the egg, the more it will hold its shape rather than spread out in the pan. On the other hand, if you hard cook eggs that are at least a week old, you'll find them easier to peel after cooking and cooling than fresher eggs.

Organic Eggs

Eggs from hens fed rations having ingredients that were grown without pesticides, fungicides, herbicides or commercial fertilizers. No commercial laying hen rations ever contain hormones. Due to higher production costs and lower volume per farm, organic eggs are more expensive than eggs from hens fed conventional feed. The nutrient content of eggs is not affected by whether or not the ration is organic.

Nutritive Value of Egg

Table 21.15: Values of Nutrient Composition per Egg Edible Portion (50 g)

Nutrients Unit	*Whole Egg*	*White*	*Yolk*
Proximate			
Solids, g	13.47	4.6	8.8
Water (per cent)	73.7	87.6	48
Calories	84.0		
		19.0	
			64
Proteins, g	6.60	3.88	2.74
Total lipids, g	6.00	–	5.80
Ash, g	0.55	0.26	0.29

Eggs are rich source of protein that is of high biological value. The protein quality of the egg is often the standard for the measuring the quality of all other food proteins. Eggs are also an important source of essential unsaturated fatty acids linoleic 18:2 n6, oleic acid a monounsaturated fatty acid, iron phosphorus, trace minerals, the fat-soluble vitamins A, D, E and K and many of the water-soluble B vitamins. The egg is potent source of vitamin D but it is low in calcium and devoid of vitamin C.

Protein

An egg contains 6 to 7 gm protein. Egg protein is one of the highest quality proteins known for human food. The various parts of average chicken egg contain the following amount of proteins – yolk 44.3, albumen 50.0, shell 2.1 and shell membrane 3.6, total being 100.

In egg albumen the protein is present in dissolved state and in yolk as coplex combination with fats. The major yolk protein, ovovitellin is high in glutamic acid, leucine, arginine and lysine. The major albumen protein, ovalbumin has predominantly glutamic acid, leucine, alanine and aspartic acid. Egg is popularly rich in arginine and other sulfur containing amino acids. Besides this. Protein present in hen's egg are of higher biological value when compared with proteins of milk,

Egg proteins contain all the essential amino acids, those amino acids required in the diet of man and are of such high quality that nutritionists use the egg as standard of reference against which other protein foods are evaluated.

Table 21.16: Amino Acids Essential for Growth of Children and their Availability from Eggs

Amino Acids	*Availability in Egg*	*Essential for Growth of Children*	*Esential for Growth of Adults*
Histidine	*	*	*
Isoleucine	*	*	*
Leucine	*	*	*
Lysine	*	*	*
Methionine	*	*	*
Phenyl alanine	*	*	*
Threonine	*	*	*
Tryptophan	*	*	*
Valine	*	*	*

* Positive Holt *et al.* (1960).

Table 21.17: Amino Acid make up of Egg in Relation to Cow and Human Milk (Amino acid per 100gm of protein)

Amino Acid	*Provisional Pattern of 'Ref. Protein'*	*Egg*	*Human Milk*	*Cow Milk*
Isoleucine	4.2	6.8	6.4	6.4
Leucine	4.8	9.0	8.9	9.9
Lysine	4.2	6.3	6.3	7.8
Phenyl alanine	2.8	6.0	4.6	4.9
Tyrosine	2.8	4.4	5.5	5.1
Methionine	2.2	3.1	2.2	2.4
Threonine	2.8	5.0	4.6	4.6
Tryptophan	1.4	1.7	1.6	1.4
Valine	4.2	7.4	6.6	6.9

One egg provides almost an equivalent amount of essential amino acids available from 200gm of milk.

Lipids

An egg contains 5 to 6 gm of fat which is readily digestible and includes both saturated (33 per cent) and unsaturated(66 per cent) fatty acids(FA). The amount of desirable FA are more than are found in most other animal products. Lipids are predominantly present in yolk. The most abundant fatty acids in the egg are palmitic, oleic and linoleic acid.

Table 21.18: Nutritive Value of Egg in Comparison to Certain other Protein Foods

Item	*Biological Value (per cent)*	*Coefficient of Digestibility (per cent)*	*Protein Efficiency Ratio*
Egg (whole)	97.0	96.0	3.8
Milk (whole)	89.0	93.7	1.3
Beef (raw)	67.0	97.6	2.6
Meat (goat)	60.	-	-
Soybean	54.0	76.0	1.3
Wheat	54.0	76.0	0.8 to 1.3
Groundnut(raw)	57.8	97.4	1.7 to 1.8
Fish(fresh water)	72.1to 86.8	84 to 97.1	1.4 to 2.0

Talble 21.19: Lipid per Egg Edible Portion 50g

	Whole Egg		*White Yolk*
Fatty acids, g			
SFA	2.01	-	1.95
USFA	3.26	-	3.22
Cholesterol (mg)	226	-	226
Lecithin, g	1.27	-	1.22
Cephalin, g	0.253	-	0.241

Carbohydrates

An egg contains about 0.5 gm of carbohydrate. It is low in calories. So included in low calorie diet. Carbohydrates are found in the free form and in chemical combination with proteins and fats. Freeform as glucose and combined form as mannose and galactose. Carbohydrates are present in the phosphoproteins, phospholipids and cerebrosides bof yolk and in the glycoproteins and other simple proteins of albumen.

Vitamins

Eggs contain generous quantities of all the essential vitamins, except vitamin C. The fat soluble vitamins (A,D,E and K) and water soluble vitamins (the B-complex; thimine, riboflavin pantothenic acid, niacin, folic acid and vit. B_{12}) and other related growth factors are present.

Table 21.20: Vitamin Content of an Egg

Vitamins	*Quantity per 100g of Edible Portion*
Vitamin A	1180 I.U.
Vitamin D	170 I.U.
Vitamin E	2.0 mg
Vitamin K	Traces
Biotin	22μg
Choline	504 mg
Folic acid	5.1μg
Nicotinic acid	0.10 mg
Pantothenic acid	1.5 mg
Pyridoxine	0.25 mg
Riboflavin	0.30 mg
Thiamine	0.10 mg
Vitamin B_{12}	0.7 μg
Vitamin C	

Egg is a good source of riboflavin, pantothenic acid, niacin, vitamin B_6 and vitamin B_{12}.

Minerals

Table 21.21: Mineral Content of an Egg (fresh whole egg/100 gm)

Minerals	*Quantity in mg*
Calcium	54
Phosphorus	205
Magnesium	11.0
Copper	0.03
Iron	2.3
Manganese	0.005-0.025
Potassium	129
Sodium	122
Chlorine	149
Sulphur	173

Egg contain rich amount of iron and phosphorus.

Microbiology of Egg

Microbial Spoilage of Egg and Egg Products

The interior of the new-laid eggs is usually free of microorganisms because of the natural protection provided by the eggs physical structure and by the chemical constitution of the albumen. Contamination of the egg contents occurs either before the egg is laid or shortly thereafter. As a result the egg may eventually decompose or it may be responsible for the dissemination of disease among poultry or human beings.

Microbial Contamination

1. Congenital
2. Extragenital

Congenital

Contamination is more frequent in yolk than in the albumen. It may be due to the entry of bacteria into the yolk before it leaves the ovary. It has been observed that *Salmonella pullorum*may enter the yolk in the ovary. The bird becomes infected by way of the digestive tract and the organisms are carried to the ovary by the blood stream. Other organisms found in the ovary are *Sal. Anatum, Sal. typhimurium, Sal. enteritidis* and *Mycobacterium avium*. Egg may acquires bacteria as it passes through the oviduct – antiperistalsis can impel bacteria upward from the cloaca.

Extragenital

Potentially pores are the avenues for the entrance of bacteria and fungi into the egg's interior. The egg shell is pervious to the following organisms (experimentally).

- ☆ *Escherichia coli*, fluorescent organisms, *Eberthella typhi, Serratia marcescens, Sal. paratyphi, Pseudomonas aeruginosa, Staph. aurius, Proteus vulgaris.*

The presence of moisture on the exterior of the egg is conducive to bacterial invasion. Rapid changes in environmental temperature favour the microbial invasion of the egg. Dirty and soiled eggs – entrance of bacteria through shell. Washing of eggs – cold water, bacteria drawn in, Enlargement of the pores by the hyphae of molds may facilitate the entrance of bacteria. Motile rods and spirilla are able to pass through the shell. As the new-laid egg cools, bacteria are possibly drawn in with the air that forms the air cell.

Types of Microorganisms Present on the Shell of Hen's Egg

Streptococcus	Alcaligenes
Staphylococcus	Flavobacterium
Micrococcus	Cytophaga
Sarcinia	Escherichia
Arthrobacter	Aerobacter
Bacillus	Aeromonas
Pseudomonas	Proteus
Achromobacter	Serratia

Types of Bacteria Found in Rotten Eggs

Pseudo. aeruginosa
Pseudo. fluorescens
Pseudo. putida
Pseudo. maltophilia
Flavobacterium
Alcaligenes
Achromobacter
Cytophaga
Aeromonas
Proteus
Escherichia
Hafnia
Citrobacter
Bacillus
Micrococcus
Streptococcus
Arthrobacter

Antimicrobial Defense

1. Physical defense
2. Chemical defense

Physical Defense

- Cuticle covering the egg pores does not permit microbial penetration.
- Shell membrances, formed of inlacing fibers act as a filter for the removal of the microorganisms that succeed in penetrating the egg pores.
- Albumen is the third successive barrier to microflora. Microorganisms which pass through the shell membranes are often killed in the albumen before they can reach the yolk.

Chemical Defense

- The eggs chemical defenses against bacteria are conrained in the albumen. It is due to the inability of many bacteria to utilize native proteins of albumen.
- The high alkalinily of the albumen causes inhibition to bacterial growth.
- Presence of germicidal substances such as Lysozyme.
- Avidin aids in inhibiting bacterial growth in egg albumen by depriving microorganism of biotin.
- Ovoconalbumin can completely inhibit various species of beacteria by making iron unavailable.

Spoilage Changes Caused by Microorganisms

To cause spoilage of an undamaged shell egg the causal organisms must do the following:

1. Contaminate the shell
2. Penetrate the pores to reach the shell memberance
3. Go through the shell membrance to reach the egg white or yolk.

4. Grow in the white, reach the yolk where they can grow readily and complete spoilage of the egg. Bacteria unable to grow in the white can reach the yolk and flourish there only when the yolk touches the inner shell membrane. In general more spoilage of eggs is caused by bacteria than by moulds. The types of bacterial spoilage or rots of eggs go by different names as follows.

A. Bacterial Rots

1. Green Rot

Caused by *Pseudomonas fluorescense*, grows at 0ºC, bright-green colour of the white during the early stages of development. Later the yolk may disintegrate and blend with the white so as to mask the green colour. Odour is lacking or is fruily or "sweetish". The contents of eggs so rotted fluoresce strongly under ultraviolet light.

2. Colourless Rot

Caused by *Pseudomonas* and *Alcaligenes,* coliform bacteria or other types of bactria. These rots are detected readily by candling for the yolk usually is involved, except in very early stages and disintegrates or at least shows a white incrustation. The odour varies from a scarely detectable one to fruity to highly offensive.

3. Black Rots

The eggs are almost opaque to the candling lamp, because the yolks become blackened and breakdown to give rise the whole egg contents a muddy-brown colour. The odour is putrid, with hydrogen sulfide evident and gas pressure may develop in the egg. Caused by the organisms – Proteus, Pseudomonas, Areromonas, *Proteus melanovogenes*. This happen at higher storage temperature. Haines (1939) divided black rots into two types. Type 1 caused by Proteus spp such as *Proteus melanovogenes* to give a gas, a hard, black, solid yolk and liquified. White that may be murky or greenish-brown. Type II caused primarily by *Pseudomonas spp* where the white is lliquified and is fluorescent-green or greenish-brown in colour and the yolk is a soft, greenish-black mass. Type-I has a faecal odour and Type II a "cabbage-water" smell.

4. Pink Rots/Red Rots

Occur less frequently, pink rots are caused by Pseudomonas, may at times be a latter stage of some of the green rots; resemble the colorless rots, except for a pinkish precipitate on the yolk and a pink colour in the white. Red rots are caused by *Serratia Spp.*, are mild in odour and not offensive.

B. Spoilage due to Moulds and Fungi

The spoilage of eggs by fungi goes through stages of mould growth that give the defects their names. Very early mould growth is termed.

1. Pin-Spot Moulding

Because of the shell and colonies of moulds appearing on the shell and usually just inside it. The colour of these pin-spots varies with the kind of mould, *Penicillium spp.* – yellow or blue or green spots inside the shell. *Cladosporium spp.* – dark green or black spots and *Sporotrichum spp* – pink spots. In storage atmosphere of very high humidity a variety of moulds may cause spoilage.

2. Superficial Fungal Spoilage

First in the form of a fuzz or whiskers covering the shell and later more luxuriant growth. Moulds causing spoilage of eggs include species of *Penicillium, Cladosporium, Sporotrichum, Mucor, Thamnidium, Botrytis, Alternaria,* and other genera. The final stage of spoilage by moulds is

3. Fungal Rotting

The mycelium of the mould has grown through the pores or cracks in the egg. Jellying of the white may result and coloured rots may be produced. *e.g.* Fungal red rot by *Sporotrichum* and a black colour by *Cladosporium*, the cause of black spot of eggs. The hyphae of the mould may weaken the vitelline membrane enough to cause its rupture after which the growth of the mould is stimulated greatly by the food released from the yolk.

Off-flavour sometimes are developed in eggs with little outward evidence of spoilage. Thus mustiness may be caused by bacteria such as *Achromobacter perolens, Pseudomonas graveolens* and *Pseudomonas mucidolens*. The growth of *Streptomyces* may produce earthy or musty flavours that are absorbed by the egg. Moulds growing on the shell also give musty odour and tastes. A hay odour is caused by *Enterobacter cloacae* while fishy flavours are produced by Escherichia coli. Off-flavour such as the cold-storage taste may be absorbed from packaging materials.

Functional Properties of Egg

The term "functional properties" refers to the attributes of egg which make them a useful ingredient in foods such as noodles, mayonnaises, cakes and candy (Forsythe 1963). These functional properties are classified as:

1. Coagulating – custards, pie fillings
2. Foaming – for cakes, confectionery
3. Emulsifying – mayonnaise, shortened cakes
4. Colouring and flavouring ingredients.

1. Coagulation

Changes in the structure of the egg protein molecules resulting in the loss of solubility and thickening or change from the fluid (sol) to the solid or semisolid (gel) state, may be brought about by heat mechnical means salts, acids, alkalies and other reagents such as urea. Coagulation designates a loss of sulubility whereas gelation refers to thickning and loss of fluidity (Lowe 1955). Lepeschkin (1922) considered coagulation as synonyms with agglutination. Over coagulation squeezes liquid out and separates into liquid and curd phases, the phenemonon is called "syneresis"

Mechanism of Coagulation

1. Chick and Martin (1910) – heat coagulation is a reaction between the proteins and water followed by separation or agglutination of the protein.

2. Smith (1964) – investigated the influence of urea on ovalbumin and found first an unfolding of the molecule followed by aggregation. Secondly unfolding may occur during or after aggregation.
3. Kauzmann (1959) – suggested that formation of intermolecular hydrophobic bonds - hydrogen bonds and disulfide bonds causes the protein to become insoluble.
4. Ferry (1948) – the higher the concentration of unfolded molecules and the faster the rate of unfolding, the finer the gel network.
5. A strong electrostatic force plays a role in keeping proteins in solution. When the coulombic repulsion is lessened by the presence of a neutral salt, the polypeptide chains tend to associate and form a gel network (Ferry 1948).

Coagulable Components

Feeney (1964) – listed proteins as per cent of egg white solids are – ovalbumin 54 per cent conalbumin 13 per cent, ovomucoid 11 per cent, lysozyme 3.5 per cent, Ovomucin 1.5 per cent, Flavoprotein – apoprotein 0.8 per cent proteinase inhibitor 0.1 per cent, avidin 0.05 per cent and unidentified proteins 8 per cent. Parkinson (1966) – ovomucoid is non-coagulable by heat. Azari and Feeney 1958 Cunningham and Lineweaver (1965) – conalbumin is especially heat sensitive unless it is complexed with a metal ion such as iron or aluminium. In yolk – properties of the yolk livetin, phosphoprotein and lipoprotein are subject to heat coagulation but phosvitin is not heat coagulable.

Factor Influencing Coagulation of Eggs

Factor	*Influence*
✩ Temperature	white beings to coagulate at 62°C (144°F). yolk beings to coagulate at 65°C overcoagulated with extended time of heating, cooking at high temperature reduces the difference between temperature at which optimum and overcoagulation occur.
✩ Dilution	Raises temperature required for coagulation
✩ Salts	Naturally occuring salts essential to coagulation added salts promotes coagulation.
✩ Sugar	Raises tempeature of coagulation
✩ Acid	Lowers temperature of initial coagulation
✩ Alkali	Translucent gel formed above pH 11.9

1. Temperature

Chick and Martin (1910) – heat coagulation is a time process in which heat is the accelerator. The average speed of coagulation of albumen is increased 191 times with a rise in temperature of 1°C (1.8°F) and approximately 635 times with a 10°C (18°F) increase in temperature. Lowe (1955) – at high temp. coagulation occur almost instantaneously. Coagulation begins at about 62°C (144°F) and the albumen ceases to flow when it reaches a temperature of about 65°C (149°F). at 70°C (158°F) – coagulation is fairly firm but tender and becomes very firm at higher temperature. Microwave heating – albumen coagulate at 57.2°C. the white from duck egg coagulats at 55°C (131°F) if held at this temperature for 10 min. Egg yolk begins to coagulate at 65°C (149°F) and ceases to flow when it reahes at about 70°C (158°F). The coagulation reaction is endothermic *i.e.* heat is absorbed. The composition of the food product determines the temperature at which thickening occurs.

2. Dilution

raises the temp. of coagulation of egg. The amount of liquid combined with eggs for scrambling determines whether a small firm mass or a large soft one is obtained. Excess liquid – curd like consistency separate during cooking. Too little liquid added – worked too long and a rubbery mass results 10 to 25ml milk per egg suitable for scrambled eggs of optimum consistency. Final temperature of the coagula exposed to microwaves is lower when the amount of dilution is increased as compared to conventional heating.

3. Salts

Removal of natural occuring salts from egg white impairs its ability to coagulate. This property can be restored by adding back the salts in optimum amounts (Lepeschkin 1922). Lactates, chlorides, sulfates, phosphates and combinations of $MgCl_2$ and NaSCN and NaCl Na_2SO_4 and $CaCl_2$ promote coagulation. The gel strength is the functional of the cation and amino activity of the salt. Curdling is caused by high salt conc. Decreasing amounts of salts are required to promote coagulation amounts as the valence of the cation increases (Lowe, 1955). Addition of NaCl to the water in which eggs are poached improves the appearance of the finished products due to its tendency to promote coagulation (Adross 1940; St. John and Flor 1931)

4. Sugar

Sucrose increases the temperature required to cause coagulation in proportion to the amount added (Lowe 1955). This effect is greater when the pH of the albumen is above 8.5 (Siedeman *et al.*, 1963). Barmore (1936) – sugar elevates the temperature of coagulation of egg white in the presence and in the absence of acid. The acid lowers the temperature of initial coagulation both in the presence and absence of sugar.Addition of sugar and potassium acid tartrate to egg white in the proportion used in cake batter results in elevation of the initial coagulation temperature.

5. Acidity or Alkalinity

The efect of acid or alkali on albumen depends upon the pH and its relation to the isoelectric points of the proteins. Coagulation is favoured and the shape of poached eggs improved by adding acid to the water in which they are cooked. (Andross, 1940). Also soft gel can be attained in custards. Coagula more tender when acidified. When the pH of albumen is adjuested to 11.9 or more it forms a translucent gel which in time under goes self-liquefaction. The time required for gelation depends upon the strength of the alkali, the rate at which it is added to the albumen, the volume ratio of the two and the temperature (Cunningham and Coterill 1962).

Foaming Property of Egg

A foam is a colloidal dispersion in which a gas phase is dispersed in a liquid phase when egg white is beaten, air bubbles are trapped in the liquid albumen and a foam is formed. During the beating of egg, the air bubbles decrease in size and increase in number and the translucent albumen takes on an opaque but moist appearance. As increased amount of air are incorporated, the foam becomes stiff and looses its flow properties. If beating is continued, the foam becomes friable and looses its moist, glossy appearance (Lowe 1955). Uses of foaming property – carrier of air for leavening; contributes lightness to certain food products *e.g.* merringues – are highly aerated egg white containing sugar; Angel cakes, souffles, foamy omelets; sponge cakes.

Mechanism of Foam Formation

1. Griswold (1962) – unfolding of the protein molecules so that polypeptide chains exist with the long axes parallel to the surface. This results in loss of solubility or coagulation of some of the albumen which collects at the liquid – air interface. This adsorption film is essential to this stabiliy of the foam.
2. Also essential to the formation of a stable foam is a liquid with high tensile strength or elasticity. Elasticity is lost if too much air is beaten into the foam and the albumen is stretched to such an extent that it can expand no further. Foams subjected to heat, air inside the cell expands albumen surrounding it stretch or break – if latter occurs the foam cannot contribute maximum leavening to the food.
3. Foaming power is often attributed to low surface tension. Also high viscosity and low vapour pressure are more important. A viscous liquid has little tendency to drain away from the air cells and a liquid low vapour pressure has little tendency to evaporate from around the bubbles.

Foaming Components

Ovomucin is the component of egg white that forms a film of insoluble material which stabilities the foam. Over whipping insolubilizes too much of this fraction and lowers the elasticity of the bubbles. (Mac Donnell *et al.*, 1955). If the first foam is beaten for a long period, the drainage liquid exhibits poor whipping properties. Globulin – contribute to high viscocity and decrease the tendency for liquid to drain away from the air bubbles, also lowers surface tension. So formation of small air bubbles and smooth texture. Ovalbumin is unaltererd by whipping but the cake batter without ovalbumin, collapse after rising during the baking period.

Factors Affecting Foam Formation

Egg foams are influenced by method and extent of beating pretreatments, added ingredients and chemical additives or stabilizers.

1. Methods of Beating

When specific gravity of foams were above.170 – insufficient air for adequate leavening of cakes. When sp.gr. were below 0.150 lacked sufficient stability for suitable leavening. The stage of maximum stability for egg white foams is reached before maximum volume is attained. With whole eggs, increasing the time of beating caused improved volume in foams but did not influence the volume of the batter or of the sponge cakes made with the foams. St. John and Flor (1931) – using a hand beater obtained greater volume with thin than with thick egg white. The same result when electric mixer was used. Bailey (1935) – larger more stable foams with thick white than with thin white when using a mixer with a hypocycloidal motion. Air can be incorporated into thin egg white more quickly than in thick (Herry and Barbour 1933).

2. Blending or Homogenizing

Blending caused a decrease in ovomucin fiber length, increases in beating rate of egg and volume of cakes when ovomucin fibers were 300μ in length. Homogenization caused reduced whip time and lower volume in cakes containing homogenized albumen.

3. Temperature

Elevation of temperature results in a lowering of surface tension. Albumen foams more easily and attains greater volume at room temperature than at refrigerator temperature. Barmore (1934) – egg white could be heated to 50°C for 30 min without inhibiting foaming properties but heating for 15 min at 65°C caused decreased stability of foams from the heat-treated material.

4. Acidity or Alkalinity

When the pH of egg white was adjusted to 8.75 improved performance reflected by volume of cakes and whip time resulted from heating albumen for 3 min at 58°C. Slosberg *et al.* (1948) – an increase in stability of egg white to heat, when pH was as low as 6.5 and when the acidulant was lactic or hydrochloric acid or potassium acid tartrate. By adjusting pH, the ovalbumin, lysozyme and ovomucoid can be protected against heat damage during pastaurization, conalbumin can be protected by addition of aluminum. Recently heat damage can be protected by treating albumen with 3-3 dimethyl glutaric anhydride. Rhodes *et al.* (1960) – whipping properties improved in albumen from duck eggs by adding lemon juice – influence on ovomcin, reduced whipping time. Barmore (1934) - $Ca(OH)_2$, NaCl, or Na_2SO_4 had litle if any effect on albumen foams.

5. Dilution

Henry and Barbour (1933) – the volume of foams could be increased by adding water to the albumen before beating. Addition of 5ml of water per 10 gm of agg white increased vol. of foam, imparted a fluffy, less pasty quality.

6. Sodium Chloride

Hanning (1945) – stability of foam affected adversely when foams beaten 6 min and contained 2gm of Nacl per 80gm of egg white. Smith (1960) – NaCl increased whip time, but exerted a protective effect against high humidity and low baking temperature on angel cakes. However products containing NaCl exhibited on "Open" grain. Addiing NaCl to whole eggs before beating causes soft foams which are small in volume.

7. Sugar

Delay of foam formation. Hanning (1945) - with 50 per cent sugar, more than 9 min of heating was necessary to incorporate all liquid into the foam whereas only 3 to 4 min when no sugar was present. Slosberg (1948) - when sugar was added prior to heating and subsequent whipping reported beneficial effects on rate of beating. The favourable effects resulted from addition of sucrose, lactose, dextrose and maltose especially the last three.

8. Egg Yolk

St. John and Flor (1931) – one drop of yolk caused a reduction from 135 to 40 ml in volume of egg white foam. Smith (1959) – triglyceride fraction of egg yolk was more detrimental to foaming of egg white than cholesterol and phospholipids. Cunningham and Cotterill (1964) – detrimental effect of yolk is due to complexing of a yolk component with ovomucin, this complex may dissociate on heat treatment.

9. Oil

Henry and Barbour (1933) – adding 0.01 to 1.0 per cent refined cottonseed oil reduced volume of egg white foam. Stability of the beaten foam was not affected unless the amount of oil was 0.5 per cent Dizmang and Sunderlin (1933) – corn and coconut oil, butter fat, cream or unhomogenized raw whole milk have pronouced inhibiting effcets. Also olive oil is detrimental.

10. Chemical Additives or Stabilizers

Cotterill *et al.* (1963 b) – improved volume of angel cakes was obtained with both yolk – free and yolk containing foams when an anionic surfactant was added to the albumen. Yolk lipid was retained in the foam by anionic surfactant, but not by cationic surfactant. Cationic surfactant – only in yolk free system. Nonionic surfactant – increase in lipid content of albumen foam, but detrimental for angel cakes. **Triethyl citrate** – counteracts the detrimental effects of yolk on egg white foams. **Sodium lauryl sulfate** – lower the surface tension, increase the foaming efficiency of egg white. It also complexes with lysozyme. **Hydrocolloid stabilizers** – for merringues at a level of 1 per cent by wt. or 3 per cent based on the amount of water added. **Sea plant extractives** – act directly with the protein of egg white in such a way that loss of liquid from the merringues is prevented.

Guar gum – (0.06 per cent based on wt. of egg white) - effective in improving the quality of merringues cooked by microwaves.

Carboxy methyl cellulose – prevent collapse of frozen souffle's and merringues.

Table 21.22: Influence of Chemical Additives and Stabilizers on Egg Foam

Additive or Stabilizer	*Influence*
Anionic surfactant	Improved performance of egg white with and without added yollk
Carboxy methyl cellulose	Improved stability of souffles and merringues during frozen storage
Cationic surfactant	Improved performance in egg white with yolk added

Contd...

Table 21.22–*Contd...*

Additive or Stabilizer	*Influence*
Guar gum	Improved merringues cooked by microwaves
Nonionic surfectant	Detrimental to performance of egg white with and without added yolk
Sodium lauryl sulfate	Increased foaming efficiency and volume of angel cakes, coarse texture
Triethyl citrate	Reduced whip time in egg white with and without added yolk improved volume in cakes made with system containing yolk

Table 21.23: Influence or Method of Beating and Pretreatments on Egg Foams

Variable	*Influence*
Method of Beating	Maximum stability attained before maximum volume in egg white foam. Increased time of beating improved volume of whole egg foams but volume of cakes made from these foams is not increased. Foam immobilized around beaters operating on stationary axes. Greater volume with thin than with thick white when hand operated beater used. greater volume with thin than thick white when beaten with electric beater but loss of volume with continued beating. greater volume with thick than with thin white when beaten with hypocycloidal action.
Blending	Blending (until ovomucin fibers were 300 microns in length) increased beating rate and volume of cakes made with blended whites.
Homogenizing	Reduced whip time and volume of cakes made with homogenized egg white
Temperature	Quicker foaming at room temperature than at refrigerator temperature. Stability of egg white foam similar at 20°C (38°F) and 34°C (39°F). Holding albumen at 58°C (136°F) detrimental to foaming properties. Improved foaming albumen heated at 58°C (136°F) for 3 min if pH adjusted to 8.75. Improved stability of egg white foams due to potassium acid tartrate or acetic or citric acid. Increased stability to heat in egg white adjusted to pH 6.5. Improved foaming of white from duck eggs if lemon juice added.
Water	Increased volume in foams from diluted white, decreased stability dilution of 40 per cent or more
NaCl	Decreased stability in egg white foams. Increased whip time in egg white contributes to soft whole egg foams
Sugar	Delay in foam formation and decreased expansion. Functional properties of albumen protected again detrimental effects of heat if sucrose, lactose, dextrose or maltose added prior to heating.
Egg yolk	Reduced volume in egg white foams. Decreased whip time but detrimental to volume of cakes
Cotton seed oil	Reduced volume in egg white foams and decreased stability if present in excess of 0.5 per cent. did not prevent stiff egg white foams
Corn or coconut oil	Did not prevent stiff egg white foams
Butter fat, cream, raw whole milk	Inhibitory effects on stability of egg white foams

Emulsification Property of Egg

Egg yolk is itself an emulsion, a dispersion of oil droplets in a continuous phase of aqueous components. Also egg yolk is an efficient emulsifying agent. So essential ingredients for mayonnaises, cake batter containing shortening, cream puffs and Hollandoise sauce.

Mechanism of Emulsion Formation

1. Vincent *et al.* (1966) – reduction of interfacial tension is the first step in emulsion formation and surface active agents in egg yolk are essential to its function in emulsification.
2. The surface active agents form a film around the oil globules and prevent their coalescence. In sorrounding the oil droplets, the emulsifier orients itsef with the non-polar part of the molecule extending into the oil and the polar portion into the aqueous phase.
3. Corran and Lewis (1924) – Lecithin favours formation of an oil-in-water emulsion whereas cholesterol tends to form a water-in-oil emulsion. An emulsifier which is more attracted to one phase than the other lowers the surface tension in the liquid in which it is more soluble. Thus, this liquid forms the continuous phase of the emulsion.

Components Involved in Emulsification

Lecithin, cholesterol, lipoproteins and proteins are the emulsifying components of egg yolk. Chapin (1951) – identified the ether-insoluble portion of egg (protein and lipoprotein) as the most important emulsifying substances in whole egg. Griswold (1962) – the emulsifying ability of the white is considerably less than that of the yolk.

Factors Affecting Emulsions

1. Yeadon *et al.* (1958) – surface active agents are essential to formation of emulsions.
2. Emulsions stabilized by egg yolk tend to be viscous, promotes stability of emulsions because it impedes movement and coalescence of dispersed oil droplets (King and Mukherjee 1940)
3. King (1941) – an excess of aqueous phase is not conductive to a good emulsion. Since sugar and spices tend to hold water, thus preventing excessive free water, they promote emulsion formation (kiglore 1933, 1935)
4. Capin (1951) – the emulsifying ability of whole egg was reduced by addition of phospholipids. Sell *et al.* (1935) – addition of lecithin or cephalin lowered the efficency of the "lecitho-protein" as an emulsifer.
5. Yeadon *et al.* (1958) – good emulsifiers are mixtures or complexes.
6. Becher (1957) – In a system containing half water and half oil, a lecithin; cholesterol ratio below 8:1 favours a water-in-oil emulsion, since the lecithin: cholesterol ratio in fresh yolk is 6.7:1 the finely divided solid, mustard probably contributes measurably to the success of the oil-in-water wmulsion in mayownaise.

7. Hanson and Fletcher (1961) increased the egg yolk level and found increased stability of salad dressing in frozen storage. Use of 8 per cent fresh yolk prevented oil separation for 3 months in salad dressing stored at -7°C to -34°C (+20°F to -3°F)

Control of Crystalization

The influence of egg white on the characteristics of candy were classified by cotterill *et al.* (1963 a) – (i) controlling growth of sugar crystals by "cutting the grain" or serving as "doctors". (ii) Contributing lightness or aerating (iii) imparting a short or friable quality (iv) binding water and preventing syneresis (v) improving the ability to hold shape or to be cast. Swanson (1929) – long time was required for crystal formation when sugar and water syrup was incorporated with stiffly beaten egg white. Smaller crystals could be attained in candy by adding both egg white and corn syrup than adding only corn syrup. For this 1.3 oz egg white per pound of sugar is recommended. Too little egg white allows growth of large sugar crystals and too much results in a fluffy product which becomes powdery. Crystal size was not influenced by pH of the egg white. Addition of yolk (upto 0.4 per cent) to the egg white result in increased crystal size and a cationic surfactant caused a reduction in crystal size.

Divinity made with egg white adjusted to the pH range 4.0 to 5.5 exhibited greater specific volume and greater solubility than that prepared with egg white adjusted to pH levels 8.0 to 10.0. also more beating was required and crystalization and "set-up" occurred faster in candy prepared from albumen adjusted to the low pH range (Cotterill *et al.*, 1963A). It was suggested that since both egg white and corn syrup function as "doctors" and exert some control over crystal growth, the role of egg white might be delineated more clearly by altering the formula for candy by reducing the level of corn syrup. In this way increased stress would be placed on the role of egg white.

Colour as Functional Property of Egg

Natural colouring pigments in egg yolk are – alcohol soluble xanthophylls, luten and zeaxanthin. Very little β-carotene and cryptoxanthin are present. The visual impression of egg yolk colour determines acceptability. Preference has been shown for gold-or lemon-coloured yolks (Schroeder 1933).

Contribution of Colour to Foods

Egg yolk pigments contribute a pleasing yellow colour to many foods especially baked products, noodles, ice-creams, custards, sauces and omelets. By controlling the diet of the hens, eggs were obtained in which the yolks ranged from a light yellow to a deep orange colour. Yolks from eggs laid by hens fed a diet high in canthaxanthin caused an undesirable pink colour in cakes. In general cakes made with light coloured yolks were preferred. In sponge cakes – dark coloured yolks - more moist, higher sp.gr. than light-coloured ones.

Colour Changes Due to Food Preparation

Xanthophylls, the major pigment tend to be stable. Hard-cooked eggs – greenish black discolouration on the surface of yolk and a carbonyl amine browing is observed in the albumen. This greenish black discolouration is due to formation of FeS. It is due to H_2S from albumen react with Fe of yolk. The enzyme cystine desulfhydrase may be responsible for the occurence of H_2S in egg white. Duck eggs are less subjected to this type of discoluration. The longer the eggs are held in boiling water during cooking the greater the discoluration. Cooling and peeling the eggs as soon as possible after cooking tends to retard green colour formation. During heating the outward pressure of gases tends to prevent the reaction between H_2S from the albumen and the iron from the yolk. However while egg cools it contracts and the H_2S moves towards yolk. If the eggs are held for a period of time after cooking the discolouration lessens due to the oxidation of FeS. Increased alkalinity in the egg yolk favours Fes formation.

The albumen of hard cooked eggs occasionally is camel brown in colour. This colour is due to carbonyl-amine type browing. To minimize this discolouration, fresh eggs should be taken for hard-cooking and cooling them immediately after cooking. Hard-cooked eggs rolls exposed to UV radiation brownish discolouration – due to hydrolysis of peptide chains increase availability of tryptophan and lastly oxidation of tryptophan. Conalbumin – iron complex gives red coloour. It is possible in acidic products high in content of egg white and if it is prepared in an iron container.

Flavour as Functional Property of Egg

One of the most important factors influencing acceptability of eggs is flavour. Recommendations to evaluate egg flavour (Sharp 1937) - (i) Egg yolks with a minimum of flavour should be used as standards. To develop a series of samples with a range of flavours, pure chemicals should be added to the yolks selected for minimum flavour. (ii) Judges should evaluate eggs with a range of flavour from time to time; and after agreeing on the flavour in the samples, should attempt to memorize the standards.

Table 21.24: Use and Function of Eggs in Foods

Food Product	*Functional Property*
Cakes, angel	Foaming and coagulation, foaming and coagulation of duck egg white, flavour
Cakes, sponge	Foaming and coagulation of whole egg, colour of egg yolk
Candy, divinity	Inhibition of crystals
Candy, fundant	Inhibition of crystals
Custards	Coagulation, flavour
Egg white	Coagulation
Eggs cooked in shell, fried, scrambled or poached	Coagulation, flavour
Mayonnaise	Emulsifying
Merringues	Foaming, foaming and coagulation
Salad dressing	Emulsifying

Falvour Components

Adjective to flavour – fresh, mild, sweet. Sulfury and hydrolyzed protein flavour in stored eggs fishy flavour – by some taste panelist bitter flavour if the cooked eggs were held at elevated temperature 80°C upto 25 hours.

Flavour Changes during Cooking

Off-flavours were most apparent in the soft-cooked eggs and least in angel cakes. Fat used in cooking may have some influence on the flavour components.

Industrial Uses of Eggs

1. Baby foods – Fresh/stored whole, liquid/frozen whole and yolk
2. Biscuits and cookies – Fresh/stored whole, liquid/Frozen albumen and yolk
3. Cakes (dark) – Fresh/stored whole liquid, whole albumen and frozen whole yolk. Cakes (white) – do – liquid/frozen albumen
4. Candies and confectionaries – Liquid/frozen/dried albumen
5. Custards – Fresh/stored whole, liquid frozen yolk
6. Doughnuts – do – liquid/frozen/dried albumen
7. Drinks – do – liquid/frozen whole albumen and yolk.
8. Food Beverages – do – lliquid/frozen whole and albumen, dried whole and yolk
9. Ice cream – do – liquid/frozen all parts, dried whole and yolk
10. Icing – do – Liquid/dried, albumen, frozen whole and albumen
11. Macaroni – do – Liquid/frozen/dried yolk
12. Mayonaises – do – Liquid/frozen/dried whole and yolk
13. Noodles – do – do –
14. Pudding – Liquid/frozen whole and albumen, dried whole
15. Pies – fresh/stored whole, liquid/frozen/dried whole egg
16. Salad dressing – do – Liquid/frozen/Dried yolk only

Other Uses

17. Animal food – fresh/stored whole, liquid/forzen/dried whole
18. Adhesives – liquid/frozen/dried albumen
19. Cosmetics – fresh/stored/liquid/frozen/dried all parts
20. Leather industry – liquid albumen/yolk, frozen/dried albumen
21. Lithographing – liquid/frozen/dried albumen
22. Pet foods – fresh/stored whole, liquid/dried whole and yolk
23. Pharmaceuticals – do – Liquid, frozen whole and albumen, dried whole

References

Stadelman, W.J. and Coterill, O.J.. Egg Science and Technology. AVI Publishing Co., Inc.

Romanoff, A.L. and Romanoff, A.J. The Avian Egg. John Wiley and Sons, Inc, New York.

Mountney, G.J. Poultry Products Technology. Second Edition. The AVI Publishing Company, Inc.

Panda, P.C. Worth of an egg. Poultry Advisor. Aug 1976, page 25-29

Panda, P.C. An egg- your childs breakfast. Poultry Guide. Nov. 1979, pp. 107-110.

http://www.isapoultry.com/en/support/publications/at-isa-our-business-is-eggs/structure-and-composition/

http://www.tonis.at/en/das-ei/interesting-facts/the-structure-of-a-chicken-egg.html

– Chapter 22 –

Low Cholesterol-cum-Designer Eggs

Introduction

Current discussions concerning factors which determine our health started long ago. During the last decade it has become clear that our lifestyle, which includes diet, stress, smoking, medical attention, exercise and genetics is a major determinant of our health status and resistance to different diseases. In this context diet plays the most important role.SoTraditionally,food products like egg have been developed for taste, appearance, value, and convenience for the consumer. An egg is one of the most nutritious food items in our diet. Egg is a nature's original functional food packed with 13 important vitamins,minerals and high quality protein,all of which are easily absorbed by the body.It is most inexpensive as compared to other animal protein sources (Hasler, 2000). Eggs are a good source of essential minerals such as calcium, iron, phosphorus, zinc and iodine. When it comes to calories, a médium sized egg has about 75-76 kcal,rich in vitamin B, especially vitamin B12, vitamin A, vitamin D, vitamin E and vitamin K except vitamin C.It is composed of about 11 per cent proteins,that contains all the essential amino acids necessary for body metabolism. This makes eggs an essential part of the diet of those who wish to increase weight and build muscles.Eggs contain only traces of carbohydrate and no dietary fiber.Fat content of egg is 10.8 per cent.The fat of an egg is found almost entirely in the yolk and there is less than 0.05 per cent in the albumen. Approximately 11 per cent of an egg'sfattyacids are polyunsaturated, 44 per cent monounsaturated and only 29 per cent saturated fat.Egg yolk is considered one of the richest sources of cholesterol in human diet. Cholesterol content of eggs is about 200-220 mg/egg.So the major problems with egg consumption in recent years is cholesterol content of eggs.It was initially believed that egg consumption was associated with a rise in bloodcholesterol levels and as a consequence was deleterious to health and life expectancy. In the wake of health fears per capita consumption of eggs is declined in whole world over the past 50 years and it is one of more challenging problem in the egg industry and facing today.So scientist develop designer egg by altering their compositional and nutritive values.

DESIGNER EGG is the egg whose nutrient contents have been modified from the standard egg. The designer egg contains low cholesterol, omega-3 fatty acid rich, high in Vitamins, mineral enriched, Fairly high in antioxidant and Pigment rich egg.

Different Trade Names for Designer Eggs

- ✰ Everyday Egg
- ✰ Egg+ plus
- ✰ Bio- Omega 3 Egg
- ✰ Super Egg
- ✰ England's Best.
- ✰ DHA Enriched Egg

In India there are:

- ✰ Diet Eggs (Bangalore.)
- ✰ Smart Egg (Punjab.)
- ✰ HEDE- Herbal Enriched Designer Egg (Chennai)

Disadvantage of Designer Egg

1. Cost of production is high.
2. Limited supply as production units are very few.
3. More expensive as compared to normal egg.

History of Designer Eggs

Fatty acid composition modification by dietary manipulation (Cruickshank, 1934). In late 80s Sim Jiang and their associates in the University of Alberta, Canada developed a designer egg rich in ω-3 fatty acid and antioxidants by feeding diets having flax seeds. Farell (1998) enriched the egg with folic acid and iron which are good for anemic patients. Leeson (2004) produced Lutein-enriched egg- retinal tonic.

Narahari (2004) developed Herbal enriched designer eggs (HEDE) rich in ω-3 PUFA, vit-E, Se, carotenoids, certain B-complex vitamins and trace minerals, but also rich in herbal active principle like allicin, betaine, euginal, lumiflavin, luetin, sulphoraphane, taurine and many more active principle depending on herbs fed to hen.

Modifications

(1) Vitamin Content

Designer eggs have been produced that contain higher concentrations of several vitamins. Two vitamins, A and E, are receiving the most interest as components of designer eggs. The vitamin content of the egg is variable and is somewhat dependent on the dietary concentration of any specific vitamin. In addition, the hen does not transfer different vitamins into the egg with equal efficiency. Because of this, the vitamin transfer efficiency and cost of the vitamin must be taken into consideration when determining the economic feasibility of marketing such eggs. Eggs higher in Vitamin E are currently available in stores.Vit-E levels seven times higher than traditional eggs if vitamin-E is added to chicken feed.

Efforts of Fortification of other vitamins like A, D_3, E, K, B_1, B_2, B_6 Biotin, Folic acid, Niacin, Pantothenic acid, B_{12} were made but only five vitamins *i.e.* E (25 per cent), K (108 per cent), Biotin (60 per cent), Pantothenic acid (24 per cent) and B_{12} (139 per cent) deposited in the egg in sufficient quantities to exceed 20 per cent of the recommended daily intake (Leeson and Caston, 2003).

It Reduces free radicals in blood, Decreases risk of cancer,Delay ageing process and Reduces the risk of heart disease since it is an antioxidant.

(2) Lowered Cholesterol

In order for a company to claim a reduce amount of a nutrient the product must have 25 percent less than the normal product standards for that nutrient. A large egg contains approximately 200 - 220 mg of cholesterol.

Genetic selection of hens for lowered cholesterol has not been successful in lowering the egg cholesterol content. There have been claims that eggs from the Araucana chicken contain less cholesterol when compared to eggs of other breeds. Dozens of Araucana eggs have been sold in health food stores for exorbitant prices promoting them as "health eggs." There is no scientific evidence to support this claim. There have been numerous well-designed scientific studies that have compared the cholesterol content of Araucana eggs to eggs from other breeds, especially the White Leghorn, a breed that dominates the Amercian commercial egg market. In these comparisons the egg content was corrected for egg size. The Araucana eggs consistently contain higher concentrations of yolk cholesterol than White Leghorns. Egg cholesterol is found only in the yolk. Arauanca chickens simply lay a smaller egg so that cholesterol content, on a per egg basis is lower.

Research into lowering egg cholesterol has centered mostly around diet and pharamcological intervention (drugs). Drugs have been successful in lowering egg cholesterol by as much as 50 per cent. Drugs lower cholesterol in the egg by either inhibiting the synthesis of cholesterol in the hen or by inhibiting the transfer of cholesterol from the blood to the developing yolk on the ovary. Today, the drugs which have shown promise in lowering cholesterol are not yet approved by the FDA for commercial use.

Chromium supplementation to laying hen diets at concentrations of less than 1 ppm have been shown to lower egg cholesterol and also improve egg interior quality.

Research has also shown that the most effective way to lower egg cholesterol content is to lower the energy consumption of the hen. Tampa Farm Services (Florida) markets an egg with reduced cholesterol content (185 mg). The eggs are produced by feeding a special all-vegetarian diet that is higher in protein and fiber, and enriched in vitamin E.

(3) Fat and Fatty Acid Content

Altering the total fat content in the diet of the hen has little effect on the total fat content of the egg yolk. However, the fatty acid profile (or the ratios of the different types of fatty acids) of egg yolk lipid can easily be changed, simply by changing the type of fat used in the diet.

Consumption of polyunsaturated fatty acids has been reported to reduce the risk of atherosclerosis and stroke. Consumption of these fatty acids has also been shown to promote infant growth.Different feeds, such as flaxseed (linseed), safflower oil, perilla oils3, chia4, marine algae, fish, fish oil, and vegetable oil have been added to chicken feeds to increase the omega-3 fatty acid content in the egg yolk. Omega-3 fatty acid-rich eggs may provide an alternative food source for enhancing consumer intake of these 'healthy' fatty acids. Evaluation of the eggs during storage indicates that the shelf life of the enriched eggs was comparable to that of typical eggs.

Many omega-3 fatty acid-enhanced eggs are available in the U.S. market under various brand names such as Gold Circle Farms, EggPlus, and the Country Hen Better Eggs. Omega-3 fatty acid-enriched eggs taste and cook like any other chicken eggs available in the grocery store. However, they typically have a darker yellow yolk.There are also designer eggs on the market that contain a lowered saturated to unsaturated fatty acid ratio. Canola oil is commonly used to alter the ratio of saturated to unsaturated fatty acids. Tampa Farm Services produces an egg said to contain 25 per cent less saturated fat than regular eggs.

(4) Anti Oxidants

Egg is a rich source of natural antioxidants like vitamin-E, selenium, carotenoid pigments, flavinoid compounds, lecithin and phosvitin. These compounds will protect the fat-soluble vitamins and other yolk lipids from oxidative rancidity. However, these levels are not sufficient to protect the designer eggs rich in N-3 PUFA. Hence it is essential to increase the anti-oxidant levels in the designer eggs. The designer egg not only contain high levels of the above anti-oxidants; but also contain synthetic anti-oxidants like Ethoxyquin and anti-oxidants of herbal origin such as Lycopene, Curcumin, Sulforaphene, Carnosine, Quercetin, depending upon the herbs used in hens' diet. Supplementation of these anti-oxidants in hens' diet will increase their levels in the egg.

The advantages of enrichment of the egg with anti oxidants include:

- ☆ Decreased susceptibility to lipid peroxidation
- ☆ Prevention of fishy odour to the product
- ☆ Designer foods could be a good source of antioxidants in human diet
- ☆ Prevents destruction of fat-soluble vitamins
- ☆ Prevents denaturation of natural fat-soluble pigments
- ☆ Promotes the overall health of the consumers

For designer egg/meat production, vitamin E and organic selenium (Selplex) are added as anti-oxidants at levels of 200-400mg/kg and 0.1-0.3ppm, respectively. Besides these, other anti-oxidants as chemicals and herbs may be added, to prevent oxidative rancidity. The vitamin E and Selenium levels, as well as the anti-oxidant properties of the regular and designer eggs.

(5) Mineral Content

The shell contains the majority of the minerals in an egg. There are approximately 2,200 mg of calcium and 20 mg of phosphorus in the shell. There has been very little success in changing the calcium and phosphorus content of the albumen and yolk. It is possible, however, to increase the content of selenium, iodine and chromium. This has been done through dietary supplementation of the hen. These three minerals are important in human health. There has been some interest, therefore, in promoting these eggs as designer eggs. Such products, however, have not yet appeared on the U.S. market.

(6) Iodine Enriched

A hen egg normally contain about 53 µg iodine/100 gm edible portion, which is about 33 per cent of recommended dietary intake. Supplementation of a hen diet with 5 mg of KI/kg of feed does not affect the bird's performance but increase the iodine content of a 60 gm egg from 26-88 µg which is more than 50 per cent of an adult dietary intake (Rottger *et al.*, 2008). It reduces plasma cholesterol in humans and laboratory animals (Kaufmann *et al.*, 1998). Reduces lipid peroxide level in the brain (Katamine *et al.*, 1987), still birth and mental retardation in infants and the rate of goiter mainly in adults.

(7) Selenium Enriched

Introduction of organic selenium in the form of Se-enriched yeast into poultry diets was a revolutionary decision, making it possible to produce egg with an increased Se concentration. Main form of selenium in the egg is Selano-methionin (Se-met) (Surai, 2000).

Benefits of Se-enriched egg on Human Health:

- ☆ Decreases risk of DNA damage associated with cancer
- ☆ Reduces arthritis, C.V.D., cataract, cholestasis, maculardegeneration, muscular dystrophy (Surai, 2001)
- ☆ Beneficial in asthma and rheumatoid arthritis
- ☆ Se status has been associated with a reduced risk of osteoporotic hip fracture in elder subjects (Zhong et al, 2006)
- ☆ Cancer protecting effect (Pappo et al, 2007)
- ☆ Improves blood fluidity by metabolic modification of lipoproteins (Abdulah *et al.*, 2006)

(8) Pigment content

The colour of the yolk is a reflection of its pigment content. In addition, the type of pigment in the egg and its concentration are directly influenced by the dietary concentration of any particular pigment. Consumer preferences vary greatly on yolk colour, even in the same country. Colour is described on the basis of the Roche Colour Fan (RCF). Yolk colours from 6 to 15 can be achieved by using only natural pigmenters obtained from natural raw materials. Natural sources can be from plants such as marigold, chili, or corn. The high protein blue-green algae known as Spirulina has also been shown to be a very efficient pigment source for poultry skin and egg yolk. Recent research has shown that eggs may be beneficial in preventing macular degeneration, a major cause of blindness in the elderly.

A recent study indicated that higher intake of carotenoids reduced the risk of age-related macular degeneration. Most of the carotenoids in egg yolk are hydroxy compounds called xanthophylls. Lutein and zeaxanthin are two of the most common xanthophylls found in eggyolk, that is high in pigmented feed ingredients such as yellow corn, alfalfa meal, corn gluten meal, dried algae meal, and marigold-petal meal. Fortunately, both lutein and zeaxanthin are efficiently transferred to the yolk when these various feed ingredients are fed to laying hens.

The egg processing industry has routinely produced highly pigmented yolks for use in bakery products, pasta and mayonnaise. Perhaps there would be a market for eggs having a higher level of lutein and zeaxanthin. Unfortunately, American consumers prefer a lighter coloured yolk and eggs from hens fed these xanthophylls will have more highly pigmented yolks. Perhaps the consumer can be educated to accept a darker yolk colour. But with a growing problem of macular degeneration in the elderly, the egg industry may want to seize this opportunity.

(9) Immunomodulating Egg Production

Chicken egg is abundant in antibodies like "IgY"; which is cheaper and better than mammalian immunoglobulin "IgG". In a 6-week period, a hen produces about 298mg of specific antibodies, compared with only 17mg from a rabbit. This "IgY" can be used to treat human rotavirus, E.coli, Streptococcus, Pseudomonas, Staphylococcus and Salmonella infections. The lysozyme (G1-globulin), G2 and G3 globulins, ovomacroglobulin, antibody - "IgY" and other natural antimicrobials and immune stimulants in the egg, prolong the life of AIDS patients, by their high nutritional value, as well as immune stimulant and anti-viral properties. The IgY level in the egg can be increased by dietary manipulations. The functional feed rich in omega - 3 fatty acids and anti-oxidants it self will increase the IgY level in the egg. Herbal supplementation will further boost the IgY level in the egg. Among the herbs, Basil leaves (Tulasi) at 0.3-0.5 per cent dietary level is having the highest ability to boost the IgY level in the egg. Other herbs like Rosemary, Turmeric, Garlic, Fenugreek, Spirulina, Aswagandha, Arogyapacha etc.are also possessing immune modulating properties.

(10) Pharmaceuticals

New biotechnology is being used to develop genetically modified chickens that produce compounds that can be harvested from the eggs. These compounds include insulin for the treatment of diabetes. The hen, like all animals, produces antibodies to neutralize the antigens (viruses, bacteria, etc.) to which she is exposed to each day. These antibodies circulate throughout her body and are transferred to her egg as protection to the developing chick. Immunologists are taking advantage of the fact that the hen can develop antibodies against a large array of antigens and concentrate them in the egg. Specific antigens are now being selected and injected into the hen who develops antibodies against them. As new biotechnology knowledge is gained in this area, designer eggs in the future may be produced that result in a range of antibodies for treatment against snake venoms to the countering of microorganisms which cause tooth decay.

Table 22.1: Comparative Nutrient Differences/60 g of Egg

Nutrient	*Regular Egg*	*Designer Egg*
Energy	70 kcal.	75 kcal.
Protein	6.3 gm.	6.3 gm.
Fat	5.0 gm	5.0 gm
Cholesterol	200-240 mg	160-180 mg
Omega 6	800 mg	750 mg
Vitamin E	0.7 mg	1.4 mg
Omega 3	60 mg	350 mg
LNA C18:3	40 mg	250 mg
DHA C22:6	20 mg	100 mg
n-6:n3	13.0	2.6

Availability of Designer Egg in India

M/s Kool Komestibles Bangalore, Karnataka

The eggs have been sent to an independent testing laboratory in Bangalore for final tests before the department goes in for marketing tieups or transfer of technology.

BANGALORE-BASED KoolKomestibles Private Ltd (KKPL) has launched designer eggs, branded 'Diet Eggs', supposed to have beneficial nutritional properties.

According to Mr Naveed, the Chairman and Managing Director of KKPL, KoolKomestibles is the exclusive licensee for marketing the patented designer eggs in India, Pakistan, Sri Lanka and the Middle East. The eggs are the result of layer birds being fed with special feed formulation developed by Dr Jeong S. Sim, a Professor at the University of Alberta, Canada.

Dr Sim is the principal patent holder for the designer eggs and KKPL has entered into a royalty-based agreement with him. When compared to normal eggs, 'Diet Eggs' have 19 times more poly unsaturated fatty acids (600 mg omega-3 fatty acids which is equivalent to 100 g of fish), and twice the quantity of vitamin E.

Experimental studies have indicated beneficial impact of diet eggs on cholesterol and its ratio, and blood pressure, according to Mr Naveed, apart from these beneficial properties, 'Diet Eggs' did not have the strong odour of traditional eggs. However, it was identical in taste and flavour, and could be cooked like the traditional egg without loss of its positive features.

The eggs, produced at three poultry farms located in Karnataka, were at present being marketed in Bangalore, Mysore, Belgaum and Kochi. These markets had absorbed 45,000 eggs per day, and Chennai was expected to consume about 50,000-75,000 eggs. Priced at Rs. 8, they were available in packs of six in special containers. The company had invested Rs. 2.5 crore in the farms, and there were plans to export 'Diet Eggs' shortly. KKPL would set up farms in the north once it entered the markets there.

Future Designer Eggs

- ☆ Vitamin-C enriched designer egg
- ☆ Fiber enriched designer egg
- ☆ Choline enriched designer egg

Conclusion

Designer egg is an attempt of improving the nutrient intake of consumer.Feeding chickens a percentage of flax or other alternatives, having a higher than normal level of Omega 3 and Vitamin E and Se. Future of designer egg with regard to lutein enrichment and immune modulation will be more fruitful. The cost justification for this added expenditure depends on the public's perception of value for nutritive enhancement of egg.Finally Designer Egg is only one approach for differentiation of the product in the market place

This approach for branding and creating the perception of a unique product must be weighed against the public's perception for specialty egg products.

References

American egg board www.aeb.org

Cang, D. K., Kim, S. I., CHO, C. H., Yim, Y. H. and Kim, H. S. 2003. Use of lycopene, and antioxidant carotenoids, in laying hen for egg yolk pigmentation. Asian-Australian Journal of Animal Scinece.16(12):1799-1803.

Caston, L. and Leeson, S. 1990. Research note: Dietary flax seed and egg composition. Poultry Sci. 69:1617-1620.

Chowdhary, S. R., Sarker, D. K., Chowdhary, S. D., Smith, T. K., Roy, P. K. and Wahid, M. A. 2005. Effect of dietary tamarind on cholesterol metabolism in laying hen. Poultry Science 84(1):56-60.

Cruickshank, E. M., 1934. Studies in fat metabolism in the fowl. In: The composition of the egg fat and depot fat of the fowl as affected by the ingestion of large amount of fat.Biochem. J. 28:965-971.

Dietary manipulation for enhancing nutritive quality of egg. http://fao.org.htm

Egg Nutrition Centre www.enc-online.org

Farrell, D. J. 1998. enrichment of hen eggs with n-3 long chain fatty acid and evaluation of enriched egg in human. American Journal of Clinical Nutrition.68:538-544

Grashorn, M. A. and Steinberg, W. 2002.Deposition rate of canthaxanthin in egg yolk. Archiv fur Gefliigelakunde. 66(6): 258-262.

Hasler, C. M. 2000.The changing face of functional foods.Jornal of American college of Nutrition. 19:499S-506S.

Jacqueline Jacob and Richard Miles,2000 Designer and Specialty Eggs. website at http://edis.ifas.ufl.edu.

Jeongseok.Sim and Hoon.H.Sunwoo,1998. Designer egg: Nutritional and functional significance http://www.ansci.umn.edu.

Kim, J. H., Hong, S. T., Lee, H. S. and Kim, H. J. 2004. Oral administration of pravastatin reduces egg cholesterol but not plasma cholesterol in laying hen. Poultry Science. 83(9):1539-1543.

Mahdavi,A.H., Rahmani H.R. and Pourreza, J. 2005. Effect of Probiotic Supplements on Egg Quality and Laying Hen's Performance. Poultry Science 4 (7): 488-492.

Maurice, D.V.1998. Personal Communication

Naber, E.C. 1993. Vitamin profile of eggs as indicators of nutritional status in laying hen. Poultry Sci.72:1046-1056

Narhari, D. 2006. Nutritional manipulation for value added egg and meat production. ClAFA of India vol.03 No.1,April-May 2006

Rottger, A. S., Halle, I., Danicke, S., Wagner, H., Reeves, G. and Flachowsky, G. 2008. Long term effect of varying nutrient iodine on the performance of laying hen and the carry over into egg.Proceeding of the XIII World Poultry Congress, Brisbane, Queensland, Australia. 29 June.

United egg producers www.unitedegg.com

Venardos, K. M. and Kaye, D. M. 2007. Myocardial ischemia-reperfusion injury antioxidant enzyme system, and selenium: a review. Current Medical Chemistry 14:1539-1549.

Yannakopoulos, A. 2005. Enhanced Egg Production in Practice: The Case of Bio-Omega-3 Egg Poultry Science 4 (8): 531-535, 2005.

Zhang, J., Munger, R. G., West, N. A., Cutler, D. R., Wengreen, H. J. and Corcoran, C. D. 2006. Antioxidnat intake and risk of osteoporotic hip fracture in Utah: and effect modified by smoking status. American Journal of Epidemiology 163:9-17.

– Chapter 23 –

GMP, HACCP Procedures for Food Safety, Codex Regulation for Food Products Safety, WTO/ GOI Regulations for Import and Export of Poultry Products

I. Good Manufacturing Practices (GMP)

Good Manufacturing Practices (GMPs) as defined by the Food and Drug Administration in 21 CFR part 110 are the minimum sanitary and processing requirements for food companies. GMPs are fairly broad and general and can be used to help guide the development of Standard Operating Procedures (SOPs) which are very specific.

GMP guidelines are not prescriptive instructions on how to manufacture products. They are a series of general principles that must be observed during manufacturing. When a company is setting up its quality program and manufacturing process, there may be many ways it can fulfill GMP requirements. It is the company's responsibility to determine the most effective and efficient quality process.

Although there are a number of them, all guidelines follow a few basic principles.

- ✰ Manufacturing processes are clearly defined and controlled. All critical processes are validated to ensure consistency and compliance with specifications.

- Manufacturing processes are controlled, and any changes to the process are evaluated. Changes that have an impact on the quality of the drug are validated as necessary.
- Instructions and procedures are written in clear and unambiguous language. (Good Documentation Practices)
- Operators are trained to carry out and document procedures.
- Records are made, manually or by instruments, during manufacture that demonstrate that all the steps required by the defined procedures and instructions were in fact taken and that the quantity and quality of the drug was as expected. Deviations are investigated and documented.
- Records of manufacture (including distribution) that enable the complete history of a batch to be traced are retained in a comprehensible and accessible form.
- The distribution of the drugs minimizes any risk to their quality.
- A system is available for recalling any batch of drug from sale or supply.
- Complaints about marketed drugs are examined, the causes of quality defects are investigated, and appropriate measures are taken with respect to the defective drugs and to prevent recurrence.

GLP: Good Laboratory Practice

GLP is an FDA regulation.

Definition

An internationally recognized definition of GLP can be found on the website for the Medicines and Healthcare products Regulatory Agency-UK which defines GLP as:

Good Laboratory Practice (GLP) embodies a set of principles that provides a framework within which laboratory studies are planned, performed, monitored, recorded, reported and archived. These studies are undertaken to generate data by which the hazards and risks to users, consumers and third parties, including the environment, can be assessed for pharmaceuticals (only preclinical studies), agrochemicals, cosmetics, food additives, feed additives and contaminants, novel foods, biocides, detergents etc. GLP helps assure regulatory authorities that the data submitted are a true reflection of the results obtained during the study and can therefore be relied upon when making risk/safety assessments.

GLP is sometimes confused with the standards of laboratory safety like wearing safety goggles.

Mission of GLP

- Test systems.
- Archiving of records and materials.

- ✫ Apparatus, material and reagent facilities.
- ✫ Quality assurance programs.
- ✫ Performance of the study.
- ✫ Reporting of study results.
- ✫ Standard operating procedures (SOP)
- ✫ Personnel and test facility organization

II. Hazard Analysis Critical Control Points (HACCP) for Meat Sector

The share of livestock product is estimated as 35.95 per cent of total agricultural sector which contributes to 25.95 per cent of GDP in our country. On the other hand the plan investments in Animal Husbandry sector are only about 5 per cent of agriculture. This speaks of political negligence to livestock sector. Moreover, India has a vast livestock population of 220, 94, 18, 58, 124 and 413 millions of cattle, buffalo, pig, sheep, goat and poultry producing 1.46, 1.43, 0.23, 0.47, 0.6 and 0.6 million tones of beef, carabeef, mutton, chevron, pork and poultry meat, respectively.

In the decade (1991-2001) total meat production increased by 27.8 per cent reaching to 4.92 million tones in the year 2001 from 3.85 million tones in 1991. The value of exports from the meat sector had been increased from Rs 894.98 crores in 1997-98 to Rs 1553.26 crores in 2000-01. On comparing the annual export performance of Indian meat industry in 2001-02 and 2002-03, a clear growth of approx. 12.4 per cent (Economic Division, Ministry of Commerce) was witnessed. Now the foreign exchange revenue from the export of meat is around Rs. 20,000/- crores and from that of by products, skin, hides and leather products is Rs. 10,000 crores.

Demand of Quality Meat and Safety Aspects

Meat consumption is increasing day by day. Per capita availability of meat is 4.7 kg/annum and eggs 34/annum, whereas milk is 224 ml/day. The per capita animal protein consumption is 10 g in India, whereas the world average is 25 g. Based on targeted minimum requirement of 20 g per capita per day for animal protein (from milk 10 g, meat 4 g, fish 4 g, eggs 2 g), the estimated demand for the present population would be milk 104 MT, Meat 7.7 MT, fish 7.7 MT and eggs 4.6 MT (104 billion number) as against the present production of milk 78 MT, Meat 4.6 MT, fish 5.6 MT and eggs 30 billion. It is certain that there is good demand of meat, but now-a-days not only quantity of meat production is important but also quality of meat and meat products is more important. Meat based fast foods are receiving greater attention in metro cities and other urban areas.

Consumers world over are becoming quality conscious. Growing consumer awareness regarding safety and quality of food product, changing patterns of life style, markets, etc. mandates producers to achieve food safety standards to international level. Problems in food safety in recent past like incidence of BSE (Bovine Spongiform Encephalitis), outbreaks of E. coli 0157: H7, *Listeria monocytogenes,*

Campylobacter, Salmonella; problems of insecticide, pesticide and drug residues in meat products have had greater impact on prioritizing food safety as important quality assessment. Trend towards processed and further processed meat products to compete internationally mandates adherence to food safety standards for all producers in production drain.

Impact of the WTO Agreement

Consequent to the establishment of WTO regime liberalizing the trade, its member countries have been called upon to conform their production systems to the food safety standards as given in *Codex Alimentarius Commission* (CAC) and the International Office of Epizootics (OIE) so as to prevent the spread of diseases on account of international movement of plants, animals and their products (SPS Agreement). From the point of view of international trade the diseases from which the member countries of WTO are required to be declared free are placed in List A of OIE. According to a report, United Arab Emirates (UAE) in the year 2000, banned the import of meat from 10 Indian companies from Delhi, Mumbai and Hyderabad, as they failed to adhere to the sanitary and phytosanitary measures. Thus, on account of laxity in compliance of SPS Provisions, Indian Livestock products do not find much favor for export.

Quality regulating system throughout meat production chain is essential to ensure the quality and safety of product. To achieve an acceptable level of confidence we need programs that undertake risk assessment and preventive measures. Hazard Analysis Critical Control Point (HACCP) is one such program proposed by US Department of Agriculture (USDA) as final rule for pathogen reduction, HACCP 9 CFR part, 304 in 1996 often referred as 'Mega Reg' HACCP system a well established concept in food safety identifies specific hazards.

To avoid the production of defective items and to ensure that the quality of the products is within the limits specified, all aspects of production from raw materials and ingredients to processing stages, storage, sale, distribution and retailing, right through to the potential for consumer abuse, have to be considered.

Origin and Development of HACCP

The concept and practice of Hazard Analysis Critical Control Point (HACCP) system is directly related to The Pillsbury Company projects in food production and research for the United States space programme. The basics were developed by The Pillsbury company with the cooperation and participation of the National Aeronautics and Space Administration (NASA), The Natik Laboratories of US Armed Forces, and the US Air Force Space Laboratory Project Group.

The beginning of HACCP system occurred in 1959 when the Quartermaster Food and Container Institute, now known as the Natik Laboratories asked whether Pillsbury would produce a food that could be used under zero gravity conditions by astronauts. The initial conservative approach to solving this problem was to produce bite sized foods covered with a flexible edible coating to prevent crumbling and consequent atmospheric contamination. The main problem was to give 100 per cent assurance that the food for space use would not be contaminated with pathogens, toxins, chemicals or physical hazards that could cause an illness.

In search for answers, the zero defects programme utilized by NASA was examined and was found to be designed for hardware, but were not suitable for food testing. In looking for a better system, it was concluded after extensive evaluation that the only way to succeed would be to develop a preventive system. This would require control over the raw materials the process, the environment, personnel, storage and distribution. Pillsbury were required by NASA contract to keep records of all stages of food production starting from production of raw ingredients till consumption of finished food items with an aim **for tracing problems back to the source**. It is still a basic part of the HACCP system as ity now exists.

The HACCP system was first formally presented to the general public in the 1971 National Conference of Food Protection. At this stage it was proposed to follow three principles

1. Identification and assessment of hazards associated with growing/ harvesting to marketing/preparation.
2. Determination of critical control points to control any identifiable hazards.
3. Establishment of systems to monitor critical control points.

During 1970s and early 1980s a number of companies were given information and help in establishing their own HACCP programme. In 1985 the HACCP system was seriously considered for broad application nationally in the food industry. 1985 National academy of Sciences (NAS) Report.

- ☆ Rekindled HACCP
- ☆ Report asserted HACCP as most effective and efficient means of food safety.

Now it is mandatory for all food processors in USA to have a HACCP plan since January, 2000.

Hazard Analysis involves investigations intended to disclose (through examination), identify, estimate and calculate the risks of all factors associated with the processing and marketing of a given product *i.e.* materials and sensitive ingredients, processes, practices, products, premises, equipment, utensils and personnel, as they affect product quality. In other words, it is necessary to asses all possible hazards and the likelihood of their occurrence.

Control Points

Can be defined as those points in a process where hazards or risks exist concerning aspects of the quality of the product (for example, in relation to product compliance with the requirements of inspection regulations) and therefore, the system must be maintained under strict control. It must be certain that no hazardous sites are neglected. The points involved can include almost everything:

Suppliers	*Food Received*
Raw materials	Specifications, storage
Facilities maintenance	
Equipments/utensils	Operation procedures, sanitation
Personnel	Food handling practices, hygiene/sanitation, personnel habits
Process steps	Time/temperature relationships (chilling, chilled or frozen storage) procedures.
Recipe formulations	–
But also	Management risk

Critical Control Points

All avoidable hazards can be removed from control points. The remaining control points are called 'critical control points' and these are those processing determinants for which loss of control would result in an unacceptable food quality risk. Such risks can be microbiological or physical in nature.

Principles of HACCP

- Identify the potential hazards (Physical, chemical, biological) associated with food production at all stages from growth, processing, manufacture and distribution of occurrence of hazards and identify the preventive measures for their control.
- Determine the points, procedures, operational steps that can be controlled to eliminate the hazards or minimize the likelihood of critical control point. Step means any stage in food production including raw materials, their receipt, harvesting, transport, formulation, processing, storage etc.
- Establish critical limits, which must be met to ensure CCP under control.
- Establish a system to monitor control of CCP by scheduled testing or observation.
- Establish the corrective action to be taken when monitoring indicates that a particular CCP is not under control.
- Establish procedures for verification including supplementary tests and procedures to confirm that the HACCP system is working effectively.
- Establish documentation concerning all procedures and records appropriate to these and their application.

A significant feature of HACCP is that it involves proactive risk assessment. It still requires end product testing but it is able to identify areas of concern where a process failure has yet to take place and implement the necessary monitoring and control procedures to hopefully prevent a problem arising. Hitherto much of meat industry has regarded HACCP applicable only to processing step not implement concept further upstream. The result is that the burden of hazard coming to processing plant is far too high and represents significant risk to consumers. Application of

HACCP regulations begins with identification of various hazards possible in production chain.

Sources of Hazards

Physical Hazards

Entry of deleterious extraneous elements in production chain *e.g.* insect, thorns, wood splinters, hair, mould, rodent droppings, cigarette butts, buttons, tags, metal, glass etc. either naturally or deliberately, injuries caused/occurred to meat and other products.

Detection and removal of these matter is through magnet, Metal Detector Screen or sifter aspirator, Riffle Board and Bone Separator.

Prevention of Physical Hazards

- ☆ Complying Good Manufacturing Practices (GMP)
- ☆ Using appropriate specifications for ingredients and supplies
- ☆ Obtaining letters of guarantee from suppliers
- ☆ Utilizing vendor certification
- ☆ Identifying types and sources of physical hazards
- ☆ Determining critical control points
- ☆ Installing instruments that can detect and/or remove the physical hazards.
- ☆ Monitoring the critical control points and demonstrating control performance
- ☆ Training the employees.

Chemical Hazards

- ☆ Agricultural chemicals used on crops which flow into food chain as livestock feed.
- ☆ Chemicals used directly on the animals or used in diet for some therapeutic use.
- ☆ Industrial chemicals like sanitizers cleaning compounds, lubricants, paints and coatings.
- ☆ Naturally occurring toxicants *viz.*, products of plants, animals or microbial metabolites such as aflatoxins may be toxic or mutagenic.
- ☆ Food chemicals such as preservatives, acids, food additives, colouring matter etc.
- ☆ Migration of polymer from plastic material, which may not be of food grade.
- ☆ Environmental pollutants such as air born lead.
- ☆ Water as carrier of dissolved chemicals and other impurities such as arsenic, lead, tin and other chemicals.

CCPs for Chemical Hazards

- Prior to receipt of food ingredients and packaging materials
- Upon receipt of these materials
- During processing at the point where these chemicals are used
- During storage of food ingredients packaging materials and hazardous chemicals
- During the use of cleaning agents, sanitizers, lubricants and other sanitation and maintenance chemicals.
- Prior to shipment of finished goods

Biological Hazards

Microbiological hazard is major among biological hazard. These include fecal source, water, raw materials, environmental hygiene, personal hygiene, cleaning equipment and food contact surface. Prevention of these hazards needs regular audit of each step involved at respective hazard entry point creating regular network of assessment for reducing the risk of hazards to as low as possible. Regular monitoring of critical standard limit with reference to chemical and microbial load in production chain.

Common CCPs for Biological Hazards

- Microbiological criteria for raw materials
- Preventive factors for food (pH, a_w etc.)
- Prevention of cross-contamination
- Time/temperature applications
- Food handling practices
- Employee hygiene
- Packaging integrity
- Storage, distribution and display practices
- Consumer directions for use (prevent abuse)

Success of HACCP application depends on effective monitoring system and proper corrective actions undertaken wherever critical limits have been breached HACCP risk assessment can be applied to most activities in food chain that impact on food safety including hygiene, cleaning, pest control, product and chemical, storage, drug administration etc.

Further steps involved in Hazard Analysis are as follows:

- Identification of potential hazard
- Determination of probability of occurrence and severity of identified hazards.
- Establish preventive measures for each hazard.

- ☆ Determination of significance of hazard.
- ☆ Tabulation of results of hazard analysis.

Conclusion

Compromising on food safety will not risk the consumer alone but whole meat industry will be at stake. Implementation of global standard quality management system like HACCP would ensure the confidence in both producer and consumer. Meat industry has to successfully implement HACCP regulations to go in line with the globalization of market.

ISI and Legal Standards for Poultry Products

Table 23.1: BIS Grades for Dressed Chicken

Sl.No.	Characteristics	Grade 1	Grade 2
1.	Conformation	Free of deformities that detract from its appearance or that affect the normal distribution of flesh. Slight deformities, such as slightly curved or dented breast bones and slightly curved backs may be present.	Slight abnormalities, such as dented, curved or crooked breastbone, crooked back or misshapen legs or wings, which do not materially affect the distribution of flesh or the appearance of the carcass or part.
2.	Fleshing	The breast is moderately long and deep and has sufficient flesh to give it a rounded appearance with the flesh carrying well up to the crest of the breastbone along its entire length.	The breast has a substantial covering of flesh with the flesh carrying up to the crest of the breastbone sufficiently to prevent a thin appearance.
3.	Fat covering	The fat is well distributed so that there is a noticeable amount of fat in the skin in the areas between the heavy feather tracts.	The fat under the skin is sufficient to prevent a distinct appearance of the flesh through the skin, especially on the breast and legs.
4.	Defeathering	Free of pinfeathers, diminutive feathers and hair, which are visible to the inspector or grader?	Not more than an occasional protruding pinfeathers or diminutive feathers shall be in evidence under a careful examination
5.	Cuts and Tears	Free of cuts and tears on the breast and legs.	The carcass may have very few cuts and tears.
6.	Discolouration	Discoloration due to bruising shall be free of clots. Flesh bruises and discoloration of the skin, such as 'blue black' are not permitted on the breast or legs of the carcass or on these individual parts and only lightly shaded discoloration are permitted elsewhere.	Discoloration due to bruising shall be free of clots. Moderate areas of discoloration due to bruises in the skin or flesh and moderately shaded discoloration of the skin or flesh, such as 'blue black' are permitted.
7.	Freezer burn	May have an occasional pockmark due to drying of the inner layer of skin (derma), provided that none exceeds the area of a circle 0.5 cm in diameter.	May have a few pockmarks due to drying of the inner layer of skin (derma), provided that no single area exceeds that of a circle 1.5 cm in diameter.

Table 23.2: BIS Standards for Grading of Eggs

Grade	*Weight of egg (g)*	*Shell*	*Air cell*	*White*	*Yolk*
A Extra large A Large A Medium A Small	60 and above 53-59 45-52 38-44	Clean, unbroken, sound, normal shaped	Depth less than or equal to 4mm, practically regular	Clear and reasonably firm	Fairly well centred, practically free from defects, outline indistinct
B Extra large B Large B Medium B Small	60 and above 53-59 45-52 38-44	Clean to moderately stained and sound, slightly abnormal shape	5-8mm depth, may be free and slightly bubbly	Clear, may be slightly weak	May be slightly off centred, outline slightly visible

III. Codex Regulation for Food Products Safety vis-a-vis Poultry Products Export

Introduction

What is Codex Alimentarius Commission?

The Codex Alimentarius (meaning 'Food Code' or 'Food Law' in Latin) is a collection of food standards, Codes of Practices and other recommendations presented in a uniform way. Codex standards, guidelines and other recommendations ensure that food products are not harmful to the consumer and can be traded safely between countries.

- ☆ The ***United Nations*** (UN) established *the* **Codex Alimentarius Commission** (often shortened *to* **'Codex'**) in ***1963*** through two of its own organs, the ***Food and Agriculture Organization*** (FAO) and the ***World Health Organization*** (WHO), jointly to promote consumer food safety and fair practice in the global food trading.
- ☆ The Codex Alimentarius Commission is an inter-governmental body with around **170 member countries**. The Commission co-ordinates work undertaken by international governmental and non-governmental organisations (NGOs) on food guidelines and standards.
- ☆ *Codex* has become the primary international standard-setting body for the global food trade and is comprised of a *secretariat* based at the FAO's ***HQ in Rome***. There are around *30 committees* and intergovernmental task forces hosted by different countries around of the world; each dealing with specific aspects of the food chain, on issues ranging from dairy to cereals, pulses to meats, organic foods, genetically modified (GM) foods, food additives, food supplements, pesticide residues and food hygiene.
- ☆ ***Approximately 300 Codex guidelines and standards*** are used by its member countries as the basis for their regional and national laws, as well as by the **World Trade Organization** (WTO) as the basis for dealing with international trade disputes.

☆ Decisions at Codex are based on consensus voting by the government delegates present at a given meeting. The Chair can overule any decision and NGOs can influence discussion but have no voting rights. Much of the decision-making among the most powerful and influential countries in Codex meetings has been made prior to the start of each meeting.

Purpose of CAC

(a) Protecting the health of consumers and ensuring fair practices in the food trade;

(b) Promoting coordination of all food stan-dards work undertaken by international governmental and non-governmental organizations;

(c) Determining priorities and initiating and guiding the preparation of draft standards through and with the aid of appropriate organizations;

(d) Finalizing standards elaborated under (c) above and, after acceptance by governments, publishing them in a Codex Alimentarius either as regional or world wide standards, together with international standards already finalized by other bodies under (b) above, wherever this is practicable;

(e) Amending published standards, after appropriate survey in the light of developments.

General Principles of the Codex

1. No food should be in international trade which:
   - has any substance which is poisonous, harmful or injurious to health;
   - consists of any filthy, putrid, rotten, decomposed substance;
   - is adulterated;
   - is sold, prepared, packaged, stored or transported for sale under insanitary conditions.
2. **Food additives:** Should be in accordance with the General Principles for the Use of Food Additives.
3. **Pesticide residues:** Limits for pesticide residues in food should be in accordance with the international maximum limits recommended for pesticide residues.
4. **Microbiological contaminants:** All food should be free from micro-organisms and parasites in amounts harmful to man and should not contain any substance originating from micro-organisms or parasites.
5. **Food standards:** Appropriate and adequate national food standards should be established through the acceptance of food standards of the Codex Alimentarius.
6. **Food hygiene:** Food should be subject at all times to hygienic practices.
7. **Labeling:** All food should be accompanied by accurate and adequate descriptive information.

8. **Irradiated food:** Irradiated food should be produced and controlled in accordance with provisions and standards.
9. Foods for infants, children and other vulnerable groups:

   Food for infants, children and other vulnerable groups should be in accordance with specific standards.
10. Nutritional aspects concerning in particular vulnerable groups and regions where malnutrition exists:

    No claims in any form should be made about food with minimal nutritive value stating that the food can make a valuable contribution to the diet.
11. **Implementation:** Food that is exported should conform to regulations in force in the importing country.

Guidlines for Import and Export of Poultry Products

- The exporting countries must have a competent **veterinary authority** to implement effective inspection and guarantee certification of the relevant veterinary and general hygiene conditions.
- The country should be a member of the World Organisation for Animal Health **(OIE)** and should meet the organisation's standards and reporting obligations.
- Approved countries have to **notify** within 24 hours **outbreaks** of avian influenza and Newcastle disease, including also important changes in their health situation.
- Countries wishing to export live poultry must have in place adequate **avian influenza surveillance** programmes.
- Adequate veterinary services must ensure effective enforcement of all necessary **health controls**.
- Imports are only authorised from approved establishments (*e.g.* breeding establishments, other holdings, **hatcheries**), which have been inspected by the competent authority of the exporting country.
- The veterinary authorities must have at its disposal one or more laboratories that comply with certain minimum requirements, ensuring sufficient capability for **disease diagnosis.**
- The national authorities must also guarantee that the relevant animal and **public health**, hygiene requirements are met.
- A **monitoring system** must be in place to verify residues of veterinary medicines, pesticides and contaminants.
- A **Salmonella control** programme must be in place to comply with EU requirements to provide equivalent guarantees for imports of certain poultry commodities.

Indian Poultry Industry

Poultry is one of the fastest growing segments of the agricultural sector in India today. While the production of agricultural crops has been rising at a rate of 1.5 to 2 percent per annum, that of eggs and broilers has been rising at a rate of **8 to 10 percent per annum**. As a result, India is now the world's **fifth largest egg producer** and the **eighteenth largest** producer of **broilers**. The Potential in the sector is due to a combination of factors - growth in per capita income, a growing urban population and falling real poultry prices.

Poultry meat is the fastest growing component of global meat demand, and India, the world's second largest developing country, is experiencing rapid growth in its poultry sector. In India, poultry sector growth is being driven by rising incomes and a rapidly expanding middle class, together with the emergence of vertically integrated poultry producers that have reduced consumer prices by lowering production and marketing costs.

Integrated production, market transition from live birds to chilled and frozen products, and policies that ensure supplies of competitively priced corn and soybeans are keys to future poultry industry growth in India. There are number of small poultry dressing plants in the country. These plants are producing dressed chickens. In addition to these plants, there are five modern integrated poultry processing plants producing dressed chicken, chicken cut parts and other chicken products.

Areas of Production

Over all, Tamil Nadu counts for maximum egg production. In Andhra Pradesh, Hyderabad is the city with maximum poultry and hatcheries. Besides the state of Andhra Pradesh, Vishakhapatnam, Chittoor, Karnataka, Tamil Nadu, Maharashtra, Gujarat, Madhya Pradesh, Orissa and North Eastern States are the major egg contributors.

India Facts and Figures

India's Export of Poultry Products has reached to **Rs 422.06 Crores in 2008-09.**

Table 23.3: India's Poultry Export

Hatching Eggs	UAE (38.0 per cent)
	Oman (26.8 per cent)
	Kuwait (5.4 per cent)
Table Eggs	UAE (72.8 per cent)
	Kuwait (8.3 per cent)
	Oman (8.3 per cent)
Egg powder	Japan (16.0 per cent)
	Poland (14.5 per cent)
	UAE (8.9 per cent)
Frozen Eggs	UAE (83.0 per cent)
	Oman (5.0 per cent)
	Kuwait (3.9 per cent)

Table 23.4: India's Major Poultry Export Destinations

Qty in MT. **Value in Mill. Rs.**

Country	2008-2009		2009-2010	
	Qty	Value	Qty	Value
Afghanistan	336,516.81	712.34	376,051.10	881.60
Oman	27,921.62	81.09	177,340.18	369.46
Germany	1,647.57	391.47	2,395.12	335.28
Angola	151,465.60	298.93	132,732.22	326.17
Indonesia	1,038.73	240.39	1,071.66	247.38
Liberia	76,285.18	169.87	65,077.19	171.26
Denmark	1,389.26	341.50	753.04	162.62
Bahrain	44,374.42	149.41	47,440.61	135.50
Japan	749.09	229.97	551.72	114.38
Netherland	7,006.96	66.67	1,011.75	109.42

References

http://www.apeda.com/apedawebsite/SubHead_Products/Poultry_Products.htm

http://bis.org.in

http://mofpi.nic.in/ContentPage.aspx?CategoryId=173

http://www.ers.usda.gov/publications/WRS0403/WRS0403f.pdf

http://www.iiml.ac.in/events/C13_02_Amerender_Reddy.pdf

http://www.thepoultrysite.com/articles.

www.codexalimentarius.net

www.fao.org

www.who.int/foodsafety/codex/trustfund/en/

www.standardsfacility.org

www.wto.org

www.foodsafetyforum.org

http://ec.europa.eu/food/international/trade/poultry_en.htm

Quality Standards and Regulations of Foods of Animal Origin with Special Emphasis to Codex Alimentarius Commission (CAC).

Safety of food is a basic requirement of food quality. "Food safety" implies absence or acceptable and safe levels of contaminants, adulterants, naturally occurring toxins or any HAZARD that may make food injurious to health on an acute or chronic basis.

Food quality can be considered as a complex characteristic of food that determines its value or acceptability to consumers. Besides safety, quality attributes include: nutritional value and organoleptic properties such as appearance, colour, texture, taste etc.

The Importance of Food Quality and Safety for Developing Countries

- For domestic and international trade.
- Building up the trust and confidence of importers in the quality and safety of food supply systems.
- Improving Food Quality and Safety makes economic sense also.

Standards

- A standard is a document established by consensus, approved by recognized body, who issues rules, guidelines etc. for achieving optimum order.
- Standards are authoritative statements of criteria necessary to ensure that the material, product or procedure is fit for its intended purpose.

Advantages

- Increased mechanization.
- Longer runs of Production.
- Easier training of operatives.
- Simpler Inspection techniques.
- Uniform conformity assessment procedures.
- Improved Service.
- Lesser trade disputes.

International Regulatory Agencies

- Codex Alimentarius Commission (CAC).
- Office International des Epizooties (OIE).
- FAO/WHO.
- International Commission on Microbiological Specifications for Foods (ICMSF).
- British Standards Institute (BIS).
- World Trade Organization (WTO).
- USDA/FDA.
- International Organization of Standardization (ISO).
- Commission of European Union.

National Regulatory Agencies

- Bureau of Indian Standards (BIS).

- Meat Food Products Order (MFPO), 1973.
- The Prevention of Food Adulteration Act, (PFA) 1954.
- Agricultural and Processed Food Products Export Development Authority (APEDA).
- AGMARK Grading.

Codex Alimentarius Commission

- The term Codex Alimentarius is taken from Latin and means food code.
- Codex Alimentarius brings together all the interested parties -scientists, technical experts, governments, consumers and industry representatives to help develop standards for food manufacturing and trade.
- These standards are more and more being used in international trade negotiations and also for setting of disputes by WTO.
- The Codex Alimentarius Commission was created in 1963 by FAO and WHO to develop food standards, guidelines and related texts such as codes of practice under the Joint FAO/WHO Food Standards Programme.
- The main purposes of this Programme are:
  1. Protecting health of the consumers
  2. Ensuring fair trade practices in the food trade,
  3. Promoting coordination of all food standards work undertaken by international governmental and non-governmental organizations.

Organization of CAC

- Executive Committee,
- 5 Regional Committees,
- 9 Horizontal Committees,
- 11 Product Committees,
- 3 Ad-hoc Intergovernmental Task Working Groups

CAC Supports

- Scientists and researchers,
- Scientific and research laboratories,
- Scientific and research institutes,
- Joint FAO/WHO Expert Committees

Achievements of CAC

- 237 Food Standards,
- 3274 Limits for pesticides residues,
- 1300 Food additives evaluated,
- 289 Limits of veterinary drug residues,
- 197 Pesticides evaluated,

- 43 Code of Practice,
- 33 Guidelines.

Codex Alimentarius is composed of 14 volumes distributed in 17 books. Each book contains standards, guidelines and recommendations.

- CODEX established standards for food additives, food hygiene, veterinary drugs, pesticide residues, contaminants, methods of analysis, sampling etc.
- CODEX standards are considered scientifically justified and are accepted as bench marks against which national measures are evaluated.
- Food standards contain provisions for protecting consumers health and ensuring fair practices in food trade.

OIE

- An intergovernmental organisation created by an international agreement in 1924 for addressing issues relating to animal health.
- An International Committee (IC) comprising permanent delegates appointed by the governments of the member countries- is the apex decision making body in OIE.
- International Committee,
- Central Bureau,
- Working Groups,
- 5 Regional Commissions,
- 4 Specialist Technical Commissions

Achievements

- The Code - provides international standards,
- The Manual - gives the diagnostic techniques and vaccine control methods,
- A Code and Manual for aquatic animals.
- To guarantee the transparency of animal disease status world wide.
- To collect, analyze and disseminate veterinary scientific information.
- To provide expertise and promote international consensus for the control of animal diseases.
- OIE has four committees to develop standards *viz.*, International Animal Healthcare Commission, The Standards Commission, The Foot and Mouth Disease (FMD) and other Epizootics and Fish Diseases Commission.

WTO

- International body dealing with Rules of trade between countries.
- 153 (till 23-07-2008) member countries.
- Provides permanent institutional framework for the multilateral trading system.
- Provides Rule based dispute settlement mechanism.

Main Objectives

- ☆ Help trade flow as freely as possible.
- ☆ Help achieve further liberalization through negotiations.
- ☆ Dispute settlement.

Agreement on Agriculture

Define the rules for trade of food and agricultural products.

- ☆ Agreement on SPS.
- ☆ Agreement on TBT.

Agreement on SPS Measure

- ☆ Was signed during the Uruguay round of trade negotiations.
- ☆ Primary objective: safeguard health or life of humans, plants and animals.
- ☆ Approach route: ensuring food safety.
- ☆ Encourage member countries to follow international standards developed by CODEX and OIE.

TBT

- ☆ The Technical Barriers to Trade Agreement (TBT) tries to ensure that regulations, standards, testing and certification procedures do not create unnecessary hurdles in international trade.

British Standard Institute

- ☆ UK's national standards organization.
- ☆ Its role is to produce and publish British Standards and information products that promote and share best practice.
- ☆ BSI serves the interests of a wide range of industry sectors as well as governments, consumers, employees and society overall, to make sure that BS British standards, EN European standards and ISO international standards are useful, relevant and authoritative.

MFPO

- ☆ To regulate production and sale of meat food products through licensing of manufacturers, enforce sanitary and hygienic conditions prescribed for production of wholesome meat food products.
- ☆ To exercise strict quality control at all stages of production of meat food products, fish products including chilled poultry etc.
- ☆ Under the provision of MFPO all manufacturers of meat food products engaged in the business of manufacturing, packing, repacking, relabeling meat food products meant for sale are licensed but excluding those manufacturers who manufactures such products for consumption on the spot like a restaurant, hotel, boarding house, snack bar, eating house or any other similar establishment.

Existing Acts, Rules and Orders

Health and Food Processing

- ☆ The Prevention of Food Adulteration Act, (PFA) 1954.
- ☆ Meat Food Products Order (MFPO) 1973.

Consumer Affairs, Food and Public Distribution

- ☆ Essential Commodities Act, 1955
- ☆ Bureau of Indian Standards Act, 1986
- ☆ Standards of Weights and Measures Act, 1976
- ☆ The Consumer Protection Act, 1986
- ☆ Standards of Weights and Measures (Enforcement) Act, 1985

Commerce and Industry

- ☆ Marine Products Export Development Authority Act, 1972.
- ☆ Export (Quality Control and Inspection) Act, 1963.
- ☆ Foreign Trade (Development and Regulation) Act, 1992.
- ☆ The Agricultural and Processed Food Products Export Development Authority Act, 1985.

Agriculture and Marketing

- ☆ Agriculture Produce (Grading and Marking)Act,1937.
- ☆ General Grading and Marking Rules 1988.
- ☆ Insecticides Act,1968.
- ☆ Milk and Milk Products Control Order (MMPO), 1992.

Bureau of Indian Standards

- ☆ Bureau of Indian Standards (BIS), erstwhile ISI, works under the aegis of Ministry of Consumer Affairs, Food and Public Distribution, Govt. of India.
- ☆ It is governed by Bureau of Indian Standards Act, 1986 and Rules and Regulations framed there under.
- ☆ BIS has been entrusted the job of formulation of National Standards under an Act of Parliament.

Objectives of BIS

- ☆ Harmonious development of activities of standardization, marking and quality certification.
- ☆ To provide new thrust to standardization and quality control.
- ☆ To evolve a national strategy for according recognition to standards and integrating them with growth and development of industrial production and exports.

BIS resolves to be the leader in all matters concerning Standardization, Certification and Quality. In order to attain this, the Bureau would strive:

- To provide efficient timely service.
- To satisfy the customer's need for quality and safety of goods and services, and
- To work and act in such a way that each task performed as individuals or as corporate entity, leads to excellence and enhances the credibility and image of the organization.

ICMSF

- Significance of microbes and their toxins in food and their enumeration.
- Sampling for microbiological analysis.
- Microbial ecology of foods.
- Application of HACCP.
- Microbiological testing in food safety management.
- Microbial ecology of food commodities.
- Characterisation of microbial pathogens.

PFA

- Covers food standards, general procedures for sampling, analysis of food, powers of authorized officers, nature of penalties and other parameters related to food.
- It deals with parameters relating to food additives, preservative, colouring matters, packing and labelling of foods, prohibition and regulations of sales etc.
- Prevention of Food Adulteration Act, 1954 will be repealed from the date to be notified by the Central Government as per the Food Safety and Standards Act,2006.
- Till that date new standards are specified, the requirement and other provisions of the PFA Act, 1954 and Rules, 1955 shall continue to be in force as a transitory provision for food standards.

Food Safety Issues

Residues of Pesticides

- Pesticides used to control fungal diseases, pests, weeds etc.
- Difference in International and National standards.
- MRLs being harmonised with Codex.
- IPM being implemented to reduce chemical pesticides.
- Organic farming is the best option.

Food Safety and laws implementing and controlling authorities in India:

Mandatory Standards/Compulsory Legislation

- Food Safety Authority of India

a) Prevention of Food Adulteration Act-1954.

b) Essential Commodity Act-1954. It includes various organization and quality standards or laws or acts, which "Implement and control" food laws and acts.

Voluntary Standards

- Bureau of Indian Standards (B.I.S)
- Directorate of Marketing and Inspection (D.M.I)- "Agmark"
- Eco-Mark.
- I.S.O Standards.
- Recently the government of India has constituted a committee to harmonized all the food laws under one umbrella so that only one Authority or Ministry shall look after all food related issues which are concerned with formulation of quality standards and food safety issues.
- A "Food Safety and Standards Bill 2005" has already been prepared by the government of India and has been put up in the Parliament for its implementation in the country.
- The "National Codex Alimentarius Contact Point" in India is the Directorate General of Health Services (DGHS) in the Ministry of Health.
- The Ministry of Food Processing Industries is closely associated with the activities of Codex Alimentarius. It coordinates and promotes Codex activities in India in association with the National Codex Committee and facilitates India's input to the work of Codex through an established consultation process.

Problems faced in implementing SPS Measures

- Inadequate advance warning about the new Measures.
- Lack of adequate time to adapt to SPS Measures.
- High cost of adaptation.
- Unwillingness on the part of the developed countries to accept equivalent measures of developing countries.
- Lack of adequate infrastructure required for conformity assessment procedures.
- Ineffective participation in activities of international standardizing bodies.

Strategies/Action Plans for SPS Management

1. Participate in International standard-setting process.
2. Develop appropriate legislation and standards.
3. Conduct basic research, diagnosis and analysis.
4. Develop/apply quarantine procedures, including those for emergency situations.

5. Accredit food and pesticide residue testing laboratories.
6. Develop/maintain pest or disease free areas.
7. Notify WTO/trading partners on new SPS measures.
8. Apply GAP, GMP, HACCP and QM at farm and enterprise level.

Good Manufacturing Practices/Good Hygiene Practices

- ☆ Produce Cleaning and Treatment.
- ☆ Sanitizing Agents.
- ☆ Use of Sanitizers to Reduce Microbial Pathogens on Fresh Produce.
- ☆ Technologies to Treat Fresh Produce (Irradiation, Pulsed Light etc).
- ☆ Hurdle Technology.

Introduction to Hazard Analysis and Critical Control Point (HACCP) Systems

Prerequisites to HACCP

- ☆ Good Manufacturing Practices and Sanitation (US).
- ☆ Good Hygiene Practices (Codex).
- ☆ Other Prerequisite Programs.
- ☆ Relationship of Prerequisite Programs to HACCP Program.

Preliminary Steps in Developing a HACCP Program

- ☆ Assemble the HACCP Team.
- ☆ Food Product Description and Distribution.
- ☆ Describe Intended Use and Consumers of Food Product.
- ☆ Develop a Flow Diagram Which Describes the Process.
- ☆ Verify the Flow Diagram.

Food Safety and Standards Act, 2006

- ☆ The Food Safety and Standards Act, 2006 (the Act) has 12 chapters containing 101 sections and two schedules.
- ☆ The Act incorporates the salient provisions of the Prevention of Food Adulteration Act 1954, and is based on international legislations, instrumentalities and Codex Alimentarius Commission.
- ☆ This Act with its three tier structure (an apex food safety and standards authority, a central advisory committee and various scientific panels and committees) is expected to lay more emphasis on science based and participatory decisions while adopting the contemporary approach in both standard setting and implementation.

Salient Features of the Act

- ☆ Food additives/processing aids are to be added only in accordance with provisions/regulations under the Act.

- Foods are not to contain any insecticides or pesticides residues, veterinary drugs residues, antibiotic residues, solvent residues, pharmacological active substances and micro-biological contaminants in excess of limits prescribed under the regulation.
- Regulations to be made for the manufacture, distribution or trade of any novel foods, genetically modified foods,irradiated foods, organic foods, foods for special dietary uses, functional foods, nutraceuticals, health supplements, proprietary foods, etc.
- The Act provides the general administrative principles to be followed by the Central Government, State Governments, and FSSAI while implementing the provisions of this Act.
- The Act prohibits advertisements which are misleading or deceiving or contravenes the provisions of this Act, and prohibits unfair trade practices.
- No person shall import any unsafe or misbranded or sub-standard food or food containing extraneous matter.
- The Act impose the responsibility on the food business operator to ensure that the articles of food satisfy the requirements of this Act at all stages of production, processing, import and distribution.
- The Act also imposes certain liabilities on the manufacturers, packers, wholesalers, distributors and sellers if an article of food fails to meet the requirements of this Act.
- The Act compels the establishment of food recall procedures.
- The FSSAI and the State Food Safety Authorities are responsible for the enforcement of this Act.
- The Act compel licensing and registration of food business. Small business operators and temporary stall holders are exempted from the license but need to get their businesses registered with the local municipality.
- The Act makes provision for graded penalties where offenses like manufacturing, storing or selling misbranded or sub-standard food is punished with a fine, and more serious offences with imprisonment.

Conclusions

- Specify standards and guidelines in relation to food items, limits for food additives, labelling and quality control.
- Rules and regulation for enforcement activities and analysis of food; Enforcement Model for States.
- Designate and finalise upgradation plans for Referral labs and food laboratory infrastructure.
- Safety Standards in Milk.
- Standards for Meat Industry.

References

www.icmsf.org

www.standardsuk.com

www.codexindia.nic.in

http://mofpi.nic.in/foodsfty.p

www.fssai.gov.in

Luning, P.A., Devlieghere, F. and Verhe, R. 2006. In : Safety in the agri-food chain. Wageningen Academic Publishers, The Netherlands. pp 249-298.

Jay, J.M., Martin, J.L. and Golden, D.A. 2005. In : Modern Food Microbiology. Springer Private Limited, New York. Pp 471-512.

IV. Quality Assurance and Traceability of Health Hazards in Livestock Products During Processing, Preservation and Storage

Quality Assurance

Introduction

- ☆ Good Manufacturing Practice (GMP) is the part of Quality Assurance that ensures that products are produced and controlled consistently and reliably. This consistency of production and control is essential. It can only come about by having clear descriptions of the way in which the work will be done.
- ☆ GMP specifically addresses risks of cross-contamination and mix-up that cannot be fully controlled by testing of the final product.
- ☆ These risks can best be controlled by having a properly managed system of working that takes them into account. This means that the quality checking system must be designed with these risks in mind and set out to find whether any errors have occurred.
- ☆ EU is establishing a variety of measures to protect quality, safety, authenticity and the rights of all parties in the food chain, between a farm and a consumer table
- ☆ Regulation 178/2002 introduced several procedures in matters of food safety. For example a European Food Safety Authority (EFSA) shall:
  - provide scientific advice and technical support, independent information on all matters
  - establish monitoring procedures for searching for, collating and analyzing information and data with a view to the identification of risk and rapid alert system

Quality Assurance

- ☆ All the planned and systematic activities implemented within the quality system that can be demonstrated to provide confidence a product or service will fulfill requirements for quality. **Or** The promise we make to consumers that the food that comes from our livestock will be of the highest possible quality and we will do everything we can to make those products safe to eat.

Why Quality Assurance?

- QA is the **heart and soul** of quality control.

  QA = QC + GMP
- Improves food quality
- Improves care and management
- Avoids drug residues
- Increases product value

Variety of the Food Related Risks

- Pathogenic microorganism, their metabolites, viruses, parasites, toxins etc.
- Natural toxic substances normally present in foodstuffs or raw materials, various chemicals (pesticides, herbicides, antibiotics, detergents, heavy metals) which remain from the various earlier treatments or were added by chance or on purpose (terrorism),
- Particles of metals, glass, plastics, dust and other unwanted physical matter.

The Best Defence

- Good risk assessment analysis (within HACCP implementation),
- Immediate response to signals,
- Honest explanation of issue,
- Undertaken measures to localize treats,
- Advertising if a product recall is necessary,
- Good co-operation with important clients,
- Reassurance that the incident is being handled in a controlled manner.

Objectives

- To understand key elements in quality control.
- To understand specific requirements on organization, procedures, processes and resources.

Scope

- Quality control involved sampling, inspecting and testing of starting materials, in process, intermediate, bulk and finished products.
- It also includes where applicable, environment monitoring program, review of batch documentation, sample retention programs, stability studies and maintaining correct specification of materials and products.

General Principles

- ☆ Each holder of a manufacturing authorization should have a QC Department
- ☆ Independence from production and other departments is considered to be fundamental
- ☆ Under the authority of an appropriately qualified and experienced person with one or several control laboratories at his or her disposal.
- ☆ If do not have any facility, it can be managed by appointed respective external laboratory institution(s).

Basic Requirements

Quality Control department should have

Resources

- ☆ Adequate facilities
- ☆ Qualified personnel
- ☆ Approved written procedures
- ☆ Tasks
- ☆ Sampling, inspecting, testing,
- ☆ Releasing or rejecting
- ☆ Monitoring

Objects

- ☆ Starting materials, intermediates, bulk, and finished products
- ☆ Returned products
- ☆ Environmental conditions

Responsibilities

- ☆ Examines, approves or rejects incoming materials, intermediates, bulk, the finished products, and returned products.
- ☆ Does the inspection during production (in-process control)
- ☆ Establishes, standardizes, and implements all QC procedures, and also establish the specification of each incoming materials.
- ☆ Establishes specification of intermediates, bulk and finished goods together with head of Production.
- ☆ Approves reprocessing instruction and rework instruction
- ☆ Reviews production records to determine errors and ensures that investigations have been conducted and corrective action taken
- ☆ Involves in all decisions concern with the product quality

Other Responsibilities

- ☆ Establishing, verification, and implementing all QC procedures

- ☆ Evaluating, maintaining, storing, and monitoring all reference standards and retained samples
- ☆ Reviewing batch documentation
- ☆ Maintaining correct specification of materials and finished products
- ☆ Stability testing of each finished product
- ☆ Participating in:
  - Complaint investigations
  - Environmental monitoring
  - GMP training

Need Of Quality Assurance

- ☆ The consumer's confidence in the safety of food is decreasing.
- ☆ Modern agriculture is contributing to the increase of drug-resistant pathogens in humans.
- ☆ The consumer tendency to ask for more and more fresh and naturally raised products.
- ☆ The traditional mandatory meat inspection still is indispensable.

HACCP and Food Safety

- ☆ A system used in meat packing plants to prevent food safety problems
- ☆ Regulated by the USDA Food Safety and Inspection Service (FSIS)

HACCP: Five Preliminary Steps

- ☆ Bring together your HACCP resources .. assemble the HACCP team.
- ☆ Describe the product and method of Distribution.
- ☆ Identify the intended use and consumers of the product.
- ☆ Develop a process flow diagram.
  - Verify the diagram
- ☆ Meet the requirements for Sanitation SOPs and Good Management/ Production Practices (GMP/GPP)

Seven Specific HACCP Steps

- ☆ Identify potential hazards: B-C-P
- ☆ Identify critical control points
- ☆ Establish critical limits for CCPs
- ☆ Establish CCP monitor procedure
- ☆ Establish corrective actions
- ☆ Establish record keeping procedure
- ☆ Establish verification procedures

Difference between QA and QC

- **Quality control:** is evaluation of a final product prior to its marketing, *i.e.* it is based on quality checks at the end of a production chain aiming at assigning the final product to quality categories such as "high quality", "regular quality", "low quality" and "non-marketable".
- **Quality Assurance:** is the implementation of quality checks and procedures to immediately correct any failure and mistake that is able to reduce the quality of the interim products at every production step.

Examples for Quality Control versus Quality Assurance

- The testing of carcasses for residues is quality control, the implementation of residue avoiding production procedures at farm level is quality assurance.
- The testing of meat products for salmonella prior to their marketing and consumption is quality control, the implementation of on- and off-farm salmonella-reducing measures as standard operating procedures is quality assurance.

The Targets for Intervention Measures in the Food Chain

- On-farm residue avoidance programs with consistent record keeping, proper drug use, storage and extended withdrawal times.
- On- and off-farm programs to develop Trichinella-and Toxoplasma-free herds.
- On-farm salmonella reduction programs.
- On-farm programs to reduce the introduction of Yersinia enterocolitica, Campylobacter jejuni and Listeria monocytogenes.

Pre-harvest Food Safety Programs

- Implementation of GMP and HACCP programs aiming at reducing food-borne risks to human health at farm level.
- Implementation of monitoring and surveillance programs at slaughter to determine the frequency of the introduction of food-borne health risks into the food chain.
- Implementation of a certification procedure involving independent agencies and persons such as accredited veterinarians and quality consultants.

The Steps in Quality Monitoring

Step One: Decide what information you need

- Select services to be monitored
- Describe the process of care
- Draw a systems view of the services
- Make critical standards explicit
- Develop performance indicators

Step Two: Collect the Data

- ☆ Choose appropriate data collection methods
- ☆ Design the monitoring tools.
- ☆ Test the monitoring tools
- ☆ Select the monitoring strategy
- ☆ Collect data

Step Three: Use the Information and Results

- ☆ Tabulate results
- ☆ Analyze the information
- ☆ Interpret and use results
- ☆ Design a data storage and retrieval system
- ☆ Disseminate information

Processed Meat Products

- ☆ Two types of danger exist:
    1. Infections from the living animal that are carried by the meat or infectious organisms such as parasites that grow in the meat.
    2. Infections caused by contamination of the meat after slaughter.
- ☆ The risk associated with the particular product, is assessed by hazard analysis using the HACCP
- ☆ The level of quality assurance in meat processing depends on the risk associated with the particular product.
- ☆ Meat products are analysed as:
    - Low-risk meat products: None.
    - Medium-risk meat products: Biltong and similar cured, dried meats, smoked meats, bacon.
    - High-risk meat products: Sausages and other ground meat products, cooked hams.

New Times – New Methods

- ☆ New methods are frequently time saving, but are more expensive when used.
- ☆ Their application require a well-trained staff, availability of reference materials, proficiency testing, establishing a net of reference laboratories in each country and other features.
- ☆ Quality assurance systems implemented in a form of HACCP and in addition tracking and tracing system will call for easy and clear analytical methods for examination of parameters at CCP (critical control points).

Antibiotics in Food – Important Field

- Antibiotics are often used as feed additives to increase weight gain, to improve the efficiency of the feed conversion and mainly as prophylactic treatment to avoid sickness.
- The EU Directive 70/524/EEC or Council Regulation EEC 2377/90 regulates the use of antibiotics. Their residues present a potential hazard for a human health. Most commonly used test to determine antibacterial substances is a traditional microbiological test, but the need for more efficient method is obvious.

New four-step strategy

- Identification of broad category (e. g. sulphonamides, beta-lactams, tetracydines, amino glycosides, macrolides, phenicoles etc.)
- Detailed chemical identification using GC, GC/MS, HPLC/UV, LC/MS or other.
- The instrumental method must be tested and validated in relation to maximum residue limit (MRL), allowed by EU standards.

Traceability

Introduction

- Traceability is increasingly becoming standard across the agri-food industry, largely driven by recent food crises and the consequent demands for transparency within the food chain.
- Traceability in the food industry must aim to create a link between the various steps in the entire food chain, so-called "from farm to fork".
- Traceability provides the ability to identify and track a product or a component to its point of origin.
- Traceability provides a means of identifying the units for recall.

Traceability

- EU General Food Law Regulation defines traceability as "the ability to trace and follow a food, feed, food-producing animal or substance. through all stages of production, processing and distribution".
- **ISO 22005:2007** established the principles and requirements for the design and implementation of a feed and food traceability system.

EU General Food (ISO 22005:2007)

- The identification of the origin of feed and food ingredients and food sources is of prime importance for the protection of consumers.
- Traceability facilitates the withdrawal of foods by providing targeted and accurate information on the implicated products.
- From the EU's legal point of view, the requirement for traceability is limited to ensuring that businesses are *at least* able to identify the immediate supplier of the product in question and the immediate subsequent recipient.

- ☆ EU importers often demand trading partners to apply traceability systems beyond the legal requirements.
- ☆ The identification of the origin of feed and food ingredients and food sources is of prime importance for the protection of consumers, particularly when products are found to be faulty.
- ☆ Traceability facilitates the withdrawal of foods and enables consumers to be provided with targeted and accurate information concerning implicated products.

General Food Law – Implementation Guidelines (EU)

- ☆ **Article 11:** import of food and feed
- ☆ **Article 12:** export of food and feed
- ☆ **Article 17:** responsibilities of member states
- ☆ **Article 18:** traceability
- ☆ **Article 19:** withdrawal,recall and notification by food business operators
- ☆ **Article 20:** withdrawal, recall and notification by feed business operators

Article 18 : Traceability

Implementation of Traceability Requirement

1. **Identification of suppliers and customers by food business operators.**

   A food business operator should be able to identify any "person" from whom it received its food/raw materials. This person can be an individual (for example a hunter or a mushroom collector) or a legal person.

2. **Internal traceability**

   - Food business operators should be encouraged to develop systems ofinternal traceability designed in relation to the nature of their activities (food processing, storage, distribution etc).
   - An internal traceability system will benefit the operator by contributing to more targeted and accurate withdrawals (avoid unnecessary wider disruption).

3. Types of information to be kept:

   (a) The first category which shall be made available to the competent Authorities in all cases:

   - Name, address of supplier, nature of products which were supplied from him.
   - Name, address of customer, nature of products that were delivered to that customer.
   - Date of transaction/delivery.

   (b) The second category includes additional information which is highly recommended to be kept:

   - Volume or quantity

- Batch number, if any.
- More detailed description of the product (pre-packed or bulk product, raw or processed product).

4. Time of records keeping
   - For products without a specified shelf life, the general rule of 5 years applies;
   - For products with a shelf life above 5 years, records should be kept for the period of the shelf-life plus 6 months.
   - For highly perishable products, which have a "use by" date less than 3 months or without a specified date, destined directly to final consumer, records should be kept for the period of 6 months after date of manufacturing or delivery.

Article 19: Withdrawal, Recall and Notification by Food Business Operators

1. If a food business operator considers has reason to believe that a food which it has imported, produced, processed, manufactured or distributed is not in compliance with the food safety requirements, it shall immediately initiate procedures to withdraw the food in question from the market and inform the competent authorities thereof.
2. Food business operator in retail or distribution activities which do not affect the packaging, labeling, safety or integrity of the food shall, within the limits of its respective activities, initiate procedures to withdraw from the market products not in compliance with the food-safety requirements.
3. A food business operator shall immediately inform the competent authorities if it considers or has reason to believe that a food which it has placed on the market may be injurious to human health.
4. Food business operators shall collaborate with the competent authorities on action taken to avoid or reduce risks posed by a food which they supply or have supplied.

Characteristics of Traceability Systems

The basic characteristics of traceability systems are:

- ☆ Identification of units/batches of all ingredients and products,
- ☆ Information on when and where they are moved or transformed,
- ☆ A system linking these data.

Implementation

- ☆ Simply conduct one-up and one-back traceability (*i.e.*, the ability to determine the supplier of a raw ingredient or the destination of a finished good) may no longer be sufficient to operate in today's market.
- ☆ Consumers today demand much higher assurances of safety and quality.
- ☆ Machine-readable identification, *e.g.* bar codes and radio frequency tags, has been rapidly replacing or supplementing simple hand-written or labels.

Tracking and Tracing

- ☆ Tracking can be defined as the retrieval of the actual status of a shipment, a package, etc. while 'tracing' can be defined as the retrieval of information to reconstruct the history of a shipment, package etc.
- ☆ They are used to locate defective or unsafe foods, so that they can be removed quickly from retailers' shelves.
- ☆ It is a tool in fighting product counterfeiting and protecting brands.

Tracing Methods

- ☆ The basic characteristics of traceability systems are similar, requiring product identification, product tracking and maintenance of information relating to products and its movement.
    - Ear tags and tattoos-live animals
    - Radio Frequency Identification (RFID) tags and transponders.
    - Paper bar codes-simple and cheap
    - DNA based methods

1. Radio Frequency Identification (RFID)

- ☆ Robust and potentially more cost effective solution than barcodes for tracking meat.
- ☆ Unaffected by contamination and withstand both the temperatures and chemicals used in cleaning and disinfection.
- ☆ An RFID system consists of an antenna and a transceiver, which read the radio frequency and transfer the information to a processing device, and a transponder, or tag, which is an integrated circuit containing the RF circuitry and information to be transmitted.

2. DNA – Based Traceability

- ☆ The basic principle of DNA – based traceability is that each animal is genetically unique and that the animal's own DNA code can be used to identify it and products derived from it.
- ☆ Advantages: The code is permanent, unique to the individual and remains intact throughout the life history of the animal or product.
- ☆ DNA can be detected in the raw as well as cooked meat.

3. DNA – Based Traceability

- ☆ The basic principle of DNA – based traceability is that each animal is genetically unique and that the animal's own DNA code can be used to identify it and products derived from it.
- ☆ Advantages: The code is permanent, unique to the individual and remains intact throughout the life history of the animal or product.
- ☆ DNA can be detected in the raw as well as cooked meat.

4. EAN UCC Numbering System

- ✰ The European Parliament has adapted a regulation on compulsory labeling of beef (EC) 1760/2000.
- ✰ This regulation aims to ensure a link between, on one hand, the identification of the carcass, quarter or pieces of beef and on the other hand individual animal or the group of animals from which they are derived.

Conclusions

- ✰ The 'farm to fork' approach to food safety can only be successful if the whole process is transparent, with every stage monitored to ensure the maximum degree of traceability.
- ✰ The suppliers unable to meet these concerns may be denied access, irrespective of quality or price competitiveness.
- ✰ Technologies exist to maintain the identity of animals and animal products from birth to consumption. Public and private groups should avail themselves of these opportunities to improve public health and quality parameters for animal products.

References

Luning P.A.,Devlieghere F., Verhe R.,2006,Wageningen Academic Publishers,Safety in the agri-food chain,Quality assurance systems and food safety,PP.249-298,Traceability in food supply chain,PP.439-469

http://ec.europa.eu/food/food/foodlaw/traceability/factsheet_trace_2007_en.pdf

http://www.ers.usda.gov

http://www.ipccnggip.iges.or.jp

www.icdonline.org

http://www.ciesnet.com

http://members.ift.org

http://www.foodlabelcompliance.com

http://www.discoverrfid.org

http://www.diagnosisp.com/

http://www.oie.int/boutique/extrait/29butlerang.pdf

www.library.cmu.ac.th

http://www.ciesnet.com/

– Chapter 24 –

National and International Rgulations, Standards, Quality Control and Marketing of Fish and Fish Products

Introduction

Fishing fleets have moved away from home and deeper into the ocean in search of new Resources. Tragedy of diminishing marine resources has to be overcome on time. The international scope of fisheries and their markets needs regulation at a global level. Total global fish production is 145.1MT including capture and culture fisheries. The top producer is China (47.5MT),followed by Peru, then India (78.510lakh tones)

National Regulations

- The Indian ports act, 1963
- Wildlife act, 1972
- Water act, 1974
- Environment protection act, 1986
- General standards act for discharge of wastewaters in marine and costal areas, 1993
- Notification declaring certain costal areas as marine sanctuary or marine national park
- The Indian fisheries act, 1897

- ✰ The marine products export development authority act, 1972
- ✰ The marine products export development authority rules, 1972
- ✰ The marine fishing policy, 2004
- ✰ The coastal aquaculture authority act, 2005
- ✰ Model bill on inland fisheries and aquaculture

1. The Indian Fisheries Act, 1897

Under this act there is prohibition of use of destructive methods of fishing such as dynamiting in inland and coastal waters, Poisoning of water with noxious material. The Provincial governments to frame rules for catching fish, put limit on mesh size, and to ban on fishing in certain seasons and places for 2 years(declaration of closed season and sanctuaries)

2. CRZ (Coastal Regulation Zone) notification in February 1991

This notification is issued by MOEF(Ministry of environment and forests).The Coastal stretches influenced by tidal action up to 500m from high tidal line shall be treated as CRZ,where setting new industries is prohibited.

3. The Indian Wildlife Protection Act,1972

To protect endangered species of turtles, dolphins. India is member of CITES(prohibits trade in turtle products),Bonn convention(conservation of migratory species).

4. The Marine Products Export Development Authority Act, 1972 (MPEDA)

Under Ministry of Commerce,GOI. Its various functions are to Promote such measures for development of marine products industry. Regulating, conservation and management offshore and deep sea fishing. Registering fishing vessels, processing plants or storage premises, conveyances for marine products, Fixing standards and specifications for export of products, Inspection authority: inspection and collection of statistics.

5. The Marine Products Export Development Authority Rules, 1972

It made in exercise of powers conferred under section 33 of MPEDA. The jurisdiction of rules is throughout India.

6. The Marine Fishing Policy, 2004

It was developed for deep sea fishery in country. It was Introduced after the expiry of charter policy(1981) to rectify the deficiencies noticed. Its main functions were: To augment marine fish production and suitable development and to ensure socio economic security for artisanal fisherman.

7. The Coastal Aquaculture Act, 2005

Its main aim are: to Prevent construction of shrimp farms in mangrove areas, agricultural lands, Fixing Wastewater quality standards, Effluent treatment plant, to prevent Use of chemicals and drugs, registration of shrimp farms for a period of 5yrs which may be renewed form time to time.

8. Model Bill on Inland Fisheries and Aquaculture

Its main aim is better management of inland fishery resources to ensure sustainability and increased productivity, to ban on destructive fishing craft gears and crafts, Conservation of fish stocks and resources and Leasing/opening of fishing areas.

International Regulations

More than 90 per cent of marine fisheries take place in Exclusive Economic Zones.(EEZs) of 200 nautical miles (nm) outside a nation's coastline and coastal state has the sovereignty to execute its national policies in its own EEZ. These are of **three types:** Regional Fisheries Management Organizations (RFMOs), Bilateral agreements between a fishing industry and a coastal state and Illegal, Unreported and Unregulated (IUU) fishing

1. *IUU Fishing*: IUU fishing includes a wide range of unscrupulous fishing activities,in areas where fishing is not permitted. Banned technologies, outlawed net types, or flaunt fishing regulations in other ways. Others under-report their catches–or they simply don't report them at all. The FAO fights a continuing battle pushing its member nations to take action. Its major instrument is the **International Plan of Action against IUU fishing** (FAO, 2003). *e.g.* The Japanese tuna industry has developed a long list of vessels that are known to have fished illegally and should therefore be banned from ports.
2. *Bilateral Fisheries Agreements*: It arranges for mutual access of two neighboring countries' fleets in each other's waters. This essay is limited to agreements in which an access fee is paid to obtain a fishing license. It can be done as a:private agreement (company to government),a bilateral agreement (government to government) or Joint venture (company to company). A foreign company needs to seek a minority stake in a local company. It comprise 1–5 years. There is no clear overview of all bilateral fisheries agreements that are currently in force. The European agreements are all published online (EC, 2004), hence allowing more scrutiny than those of the other fishing nations.
3. *Regional Fisheries Regulation (RFMO's)*: Fish do not know international borders. When a common objective is to manage fisheries in a sustainable manner, it is widely acknowledged that regulation needs to cover the full distribution area of the targeted fish. This may involve two, three or more countries and often regional fisheries management organizations (RFMOs). RFMOs address shared stocks, in particular **highly migratory species like tuna and salmon.** Extra complication of these species they spend part of their life in international waters, where there is no recognized jurisdiction of any government.

The United Nations adopted a legislative instrument, as part of the 1982 Law of the Sea, for the conservation and management of straddling Stocks (UN, 1995). The 'UN fish stock' agreement came into force in late 2001, and by December 2003 over 50 nations had ratified the agreement (UN,2004).

Quality

Definition: confirmance to standards or specifications. (Kramer and Twigg, 1970) and with reference to fish: quality embraces intrinsic composition, nutritive value, degree of contamination with undesirable materials, degree of spoilage, damage, deterioration during processing, storage, distribution, sale and presentation to consumers, hazards to health, satisfaction on buying and eating, aesthetic appeal, yield and profitability to the producer and middleman.

Quality Control

Definition: Maintenance of quality at levels and tolerances acceptable to the buyer while minimizing costs for the vendor(Kramer and Twigg,1970). Concerned with: raw materials, control of actual processing of food and final product to ensure that they match with standards lay down. It is **replaced by TQM system**-encompasses to all aspects of product and conditions under which product is processed, packaged and stored.

Quality Assurance

Evaluation of raw material and final product, standards, Design of factory: design is according to specifications, Process line layout, Design of machinery Packaging, storage of raw and final product, distribution and retailing of final product

Quality Management

This includes GMP.HACCP,ISO 9000 Series of standards.

GMP (Good Manufacturing Practices)

It was developed by USFDA. It includes General provision: regulations concerning personnel, cleanliness, health. Building facility: cleanliness, pest control, sufficient storage spaces. Equipments: Production and process control: inspection, cleaning, storage of raw material, packaging process.

HACCP

In 1973, USFDA adopted HACCP low acid canned food processing plants to prevent *C. botulinum* contamination. IN 1975: meat processing plants adopted HACCP. In 1980: WHO/ICMSF adopted it for food safety. EC: made HACCP based quality management system to export in shrimps/fish.

ISO 9000 Series of Standards

Worldwide federation of national standard bodies consisting of **127 members** including India and develops standards required by the market. ISO/TC 176(ISO technical committee 176)-develops and maintains ISO 9000 family of standard. Different countries have adopted this voluntary standard *e.g.* EC-EN 29000(European countries),US-ANSI/ASQC 9000(USA), BIS-IS14000(India).

Table 24.1: Series of Standards

ISO Standard	*Title*
ISO 9000	Quality management and quality assurance standards-guidelines and selection for use
ISO 9001	Quality systems-model for quality assurance in design/development, production, installation and servicing
ISO 9002	Quality systems-model for quality assurance in production and installation
ISO 9003	Quality systems-model for quality assurance in final inspection and test
ISO 9004	Quality management and quality systems elements-guidelines

Fisheries Access and the Markets

The fisheries market amongst the most international ones-much of the production in developing countries is shipped to the **three main markets in the north, US, Japan** and the EU-responsible for **75 per cent** of the global import value of fish product. Shipments of fish products were stopped in the EU entrance ports due to **antibiotics or other traces** that are considered damaging to human health. In 2003, the FAO joined with world experts to produce a draft set of guidelines aimed at helping ensure that ecolabels used by different countries and companies adhere to a common set of science-based standards. (guidelines match very well standard of the Marine Stewardship Council).

Fish Marketing In India

It involves different intermediaries, these rare:

Auctioneer

It is the First intermediary and auctions fish to traders at landing centers there is Virtual barrier to enter this profession because of local fisherman community or associations (Kumar *et al.*).

Wholesaler

He buys fish in bulk from auctioneers and sell to retailers. Some value addition: sorting, grading, cleaning, icing, packing done by wholesaler. Ice and transportation-major costs to wholesaler

Retailer

He sells fish to consumers and have assessment of local demand and limitations of their purchasing power maximum value addition and keep a market margin of 20 per cent.Labour-are largest share of retailer

Vendor

Being mobile sell fish directly at the consumer doorstep. Ice and transportation –major costs

Marine Fisherman Cooperatives

Mostly small and incur losses due to poor management, lack of marketing strategy and well defined policy. *e.g.*, **Matsyafed**-kerela state cooperative federation for fisheries development ltd an exception and ensures better price and immediate payment to fisherman (Gupta, 1984).

Freshwater Fisherman Cooperatives

The fishers dispose catch through cooperative or contractor.

Different Policies for Fish Marketing

West Bengal Fish Dealer's Licensing Order, 1975

Control the process of supply of fish to other states from West Bengal. Every fisherman has to pay annual fee to get a license.

There are several organizations for promoting fisheries: NCDC: creation of infrastructural facility for fish marketing, ice plants, cold storages, retail outlets.

FISHCOPFED

It promotes fishery cooperatives and sell fisherman produce to metropolitan cities and thus providing good prices to them

NFDB

It promotes domestic fish marketing through modernization of wholesale market and establishment of cold chains, technology up gradation etc.

Marine Stewardship Council (MSC)

It is a private initiative that was originally started by Unilever, (big buyer of frozen fish) and the WWF an internationally respected conservation organization. It became fully independent in 1998. Its main functions are: The MSC has a transparent process involving all interest groups on a voluntary basis, including industries and civil society groups and sustainable fisheries.

Conclusion

The current state of marine fisheries in the world shows that drastic changes are needed in international policies and management for sizeable exploitation of natural marine resources over time. An estimated 75 per cent of the major commercial marine fish species is currently being overfished, recovering from overfishing or exploited at their maximum capacity. It is a shared responsibility for coastal states and distant water fishing fleets to avoid further collapses of fish stocks and to let depleted resources recover to healthy levels. Domestic fish marketing holds huge potential, but it is still unorganized and unregulated in India and hygienic conditions of marketing to be improved tremendously. There is need to formulate a uniform market policy for fishery so that becomes easier in operation and regulation.

References

Websites:FAO. (2004). [Online]. Available: www.fao.org

FFA. (2004). Forum Fisheries Agency [Online]Available: www.ffa.int

Kees Lankester, Scomber International Regulation and Market Tools for Sustainable Fisheries, Amsterdam, The Netherlands,Version of record first published:02 Feb 2010 pp. 307–320. http://dx.doi.org/10.1080/15693430412331304251.

M.K. Mukundan. Solutions for Hazards and Quality Defects in Fish Processing Industry 2007

Google Wikipedia fishery regulations

K.Gopakkumar Textbook of fish processing technology chapter 17 Pg. no 368-372.

II. National and International Regulations and Standards for Fish and Fish Products

Introduction

Leading Fish Exporting Nations

Led by the People's Republic, the following nations generate about 50 per cent of seafood shipments worldwide.

- China ...US$6.6 billion (9.2 per cent of total exports)
- Norway ...$4.1 billion (5.7 per cent)
- Thailand ...$4 billion (5.6 per cent)
- United States ..$3.9 billion (5.5 per cent)
- Denmark ..$3.6 billion (5 per cent)
- Canada ..$3.5 billion (4.9 per cent)
- Spain ...$2.6 billion (3.6 per cent)
- Chile ..$2.5 billion (3.5 per cent)
- Netherlands ..$2.5 billion (3.5 per cent)
- Vietnam ..$2.4 billion (3.4 per cent)
- Leading Fish Importing Nations
- Japan ..$14.6 billion (19.5 per cent of total imports)
- United States ..$12 billion (16 per cent)
- Spain ...$5.2 billion (6.9 per cent)
- France ..$4.2 billion (5.6 per cent)
- Italy ..$3.9 billion (5.2 per cent)
- United Kingdom ..$2.8 billion (3.7 per cent)
- Germany ..$2.8 billion (3.7 per cent).

Export and Import Policy of India

The domestic institutional framework is geared towards the EXIM Policy statements issued from time to time. This policy statement is issued by the Ministry of commerce. Notably, the international stipulations following WTO Agreement is coordinated by this Ministry for the country.The Export and Import Policy (EXIM) of India is drawn up for a period of five years, with some changes being effected in an annual review in April and some other changes as and when necessitated. There are many export promotion measures built into the EXIM Policy, including the grant of special import licenses for firms having ISO certification. At present, the imports of all commodities can be carried out under Open General License (OGL) or 'free' list. The latest EXIM policy announced in April 2002 also outline import policies regarding food safety standards, etc.

Rules and Regulations on Product Standards

The Ministry of Food and Consumer Affairs is the main Government agency dealing with product standards for consumption in the domestic market, although each Ministry/Department also has its own system of framing and notifying product standards. State Governments also have their own systems of adoption of standards, notably in the area of weights and measures. For the products under consideration in this research study, the main Rules and Regulations are contained in The Prevention of Food Adulteration Act, The Export Quality Control and Inspection Act and the regulations for spice quality. A notable point in the product standardisation in India is that while the enforcement agencies have establishments to enforce these rules in domestic units, effective or not, there is little possibility of enforcing them on imported goods. One reason could be that the Indian consumer market was comparatively closed till recently, and very little imported goods came in. With the passage of time, it would be advisable for the concerned agencies to devise systems to enforce these rules on imported goods. Today, the imported goods seem to get even better than national treatment as they are seldom subjected to the same enforcement procedures as the domestic units producing like goods. It is understood that an exercise to review the packaging rules has been initiated by the Ministry of Food and Consumer Affairs in order to apply the same rules to imported goods as are applied to domestic goods.

Standard Setting Bodies

The Bureau of Indian Standards (BIS)

It is the main Standard Setting body in India for all domestic market requirements. It sets voluntary standards that can be acquired to indicate the quality of the product by the use of "ISI" mark. However, BIS is also the guiding organisation behind most of the mandatory standards set by Government agencies. Notably, BIS is also the enquiry point of India under the WTO Agreement on Technical Barriers to Trade.

Enforcement Bodies

The Export Inspection Council (EIC)

It is the Chief enforcement body for exports. The EIC was set up by the Government of India in order to ensure sound development of export trade of India through quality control and inspection. EIC, as the official export certification body of India, has initiated dialogue with several of India's trading partners seeking recognition of its certification.

Presently, EIC's certification is recognized in the following areas:

(a) Fish and Fishery Products by European Commission (as per which, the processing units are specifically approved for export to European Union and the names of approved units sent to the European Commission for formal notification, after which they can export to EU countries).

(b) Fish and Fishery Products by Australian Quarantine and Inspection Service (AQIS) Australia's official import control agency (as per which seafood consignments from India accompanied by EIC's certificates will undergo only random verification sampling not exceeding 5 per cent of the consignments and health certificates issued by EIC will be accepted).

Purpose of Developing Standards

To assist fish processors in meeting their food safety obligations, the Ministry of Natural Resources, in collaboration with the Ontario Ministry of Agriculture, Food and Rural Affairs, developed Standards of Compliance for Fish Processors based on Fish Inspection Act, 1990 and Quality Control Regulation (Reg. 456). These standards incorporate internationally and nationally accepted practices for food safety.

The standards are intended to achieve the following food safety goals:

- ✰ Minimize the risk of introducing chemical, physical or biological hazards to food fish during handling, processing, packaging, storage and transport
- ✰ Ensure that the design, construction and operating practices of fish processing plants are consistent with requirements of the Fish Inspection Act and the production of safe fish and fish products
- ✰ Ensure that fish and fish products produced are wholesome and suitable for human consumption.

International Standards

International Standards Organization (ISO)

ISO is the most important of international standard setting organizations. It is a world federation of 123 national standards bodies, an international non-governmental organization with, however, a majority of its members coming from the public sector. Its core business is the development, approval and promulgation of consensus based international standards. Unlike WTO, however, majority vote is practiced in this organization.

ISO develops standards through 200 technical committees split into about 650 sub-committees and 2000 working groups. It also develops guide for standard setting. In preparing these, ISO interfaces with specific users of standards including those in the private sector. All its standards and guides are voluntary in nature. However, given its credibility as the most internationally accepted organization, ISO standards have considerable trade affects due to their wide use in international trade. Therefore, those who can afford do apply for ISO certification. ISO certification is a costly process by Indian standards. It may take anything between rupees 100,000 to 500,000 to get certified, apart from the cost of maintaining the certificate. While ISO 9000 series is the general quality certification standard of ISO, there is an environmental management standard also, *viz.* ISO 14000 series. India has about 5000 ISO 9000 companies. About 100 companies have taken ISO 14000 certification.

Codex Alimentarius Commission

The Codex Alimentarius Commission, a UN body, compiles agreed-upon standards, guidelines and other recommendations into the Codex Alimentarius (the Codex Food Code). The CFC attempts to create harmonized standards. Prior to the SPS Agreement, the CFC could be adopted, applied and/or ignored at the discretion of a government. However, the CFC has now been adopted within the SPS Agreement as the benchmark. Thus, countries, not imposing standards higher than CFC standards have right to seek these standards for their imports. Codex Alimentarius has incorporated HACCP plans and principles as an integral part of the CFC. Volume V of the Food Code sets standards for number of specific fish and fish products.

HACCP

The Hazard Analysis Critical Control Point (HACCP) system is being increasingly used as a food safety system all over the developed world. HACCP is not the magic bullet that solves all food safety problems. It is, when properly applied, a set of preliminary steps and principles that gives a systematic method for identifying significant hazards and properly applying preventive measures so that food borne hazards are prevented, eliminated or reduced to an acceptable level. With emerging international and national agreement on HACCP principles, their application would create commonality of understanding of the development, implementation and maintenance of a food safety system. Having these commonly understood principles, many food processors, for example, require their suppliers to have a HACCP system for production of ingredients that they supply. Knowing that a source of food borne hazards can be from a particular point there will be more attention given to that for implementation of effective, documented systems that eliminate or reduce the likely occurrence of food borne hazards. Application of HACCP offers widely understood principles for identifying significant risks and their control.

HACCP does not cover only pathogenic bacteria. In applying HACCP, all food borne hazards are to be considered. There are a number of hazards that can originate during production. Some examples of food borne hazards that can originate during production include Biological -Salmonella, Campylobacter jejuni, E.coli, Listeria monocytogenes, Yersinia enterocolitica, Cryptosporidium parvum, and Trichinella; and some chemicals, particularly pesticides and drugs.

An important definition in HACCP is the one for Critical Control Point (CCP): a point, step or procedure at which control can be applied and a food safety hazard can be prevented, eliminated, or reduced to an acceptable level. Therefore, if the identified food safety hazards are to be controlled through a HACCP system, there must be a step or steps in production where control can be applied and there must be an associated preventive measure. It is essential that there be scientifically documented steps and preventive measures. If this criterion cannot be met, then a HACCP system cannot be developed. A HACCP system can only be developed through proper application of the preliminary steps and principles of HACCP. An essential prerequisite to HACCP is the adoption of Good Manufacturing Practices (GMPs).

Table 24.2: Microbiological Standard for Sea Foods in Japan

Food Category	*TPC*	*Coliforms*	*V. parahaemolyticus*
Fish fillet, shucked shellfish, frozen fish/shellfish intended for consumption (Raw)	10^5/g	Negative	<100 MNP count/g
Oyster (Raw)	5X$10^{4/g}$	*E. coli* (<230/100g)	<100 MNP count/g

Table 24.3: Microbiological Standard for Sea Foods in Canada

Food Category	*Microbes*	*Sampling Methods*			*M*
		n	*c*	*m*	
Cooked/ready-to-eat products	*E. coli*	5	1	40cfu/10g	400cfu/10g
	Coagulase +ve	5	1	1000cfu/g	10000cfu/g
	S. aureus	5	0	Absent in 25g	
	Salmonella	5	0	Absent in 25g	
	V. parahaemolyticus	5	0	Absent in 25g	
	L. monocytogenes				
All types of products	*E. coli* (except ready-to-eat)	5	1	40cfu/10g	400cfu/10g
	Coagulase +ve	5	1	1000cfu/g	10000cfu/g
	S. aureus	5	0	Absent in 25g	
	Salmonella	5	0	Absent in 25g	
	V. parahaemolyticus	5	0	Absent in 25g	
	L. monocytogenes				

Indian Standards

Table 24.4: PFA (India) Standard for Compositional Requirements in Fish and Fish Products

Food Category	*Moisture*	*Sod. Chloride*	*Ash (Acid Insoluble)*	*Y and M Counts*
Dried shark fins	<10.0	–	<1.0	Absent in 25g
Salted fish/dried salted fish	<16.0	10.0>15.0	<1.0	Absent in 25g

Table 24.5: PFA (India) Standard for Quality Requirement in Fish and Fish Products

Food Category	*Total Volatile Bases (TVB)*	*Histamine*
Frozen shrimp or Prawns, Lobster, Squid (Raw)	<30mg/100g	
Frozen shrimp or Prawns, Lobster (cooked)	Absent in 25g	
Frozen finfish, fish fillet. Minced fish flesh	<30mg/100g	<20mg/100g
Canned finfish, canned shrimp, canned tuna and Bonito	<30mg/100g	<20mg/100g
Canned salmon, canned shrimp, canned crab meat	<30mg/100g	

Table 24.6: Microbiological Requirements for Sea Foods (PFA Standard, India)

Food Category	*Standard*	*TPC/g*	*E.coli/g*	*S. aureus/g 25g*	*Salmonella 25g*	*V. Cholerae 25g*	*V.parahae-molyticus*
Fresh fish	EU25	<5X10^5 <1X10^5/g	<20 <20	100 100	Absent Absent	Absent Absent	
Fresh shrimp		<5X10^5 <5X10^5	<20 <20	100 100	Absent Absent	Absent Absent	
Frozen shrimp, Prawns, Lobster, Squid, finfish (Raw)	EU15	<5x10^5	<20	100	Absent	Absent	Absent Absent
Frozen shrimp or Prawns, Lobster (cooked)	25	<1X10$^{5/g}$	Absent	100	Absent	Absent	Absent Absent
Frozen fish fillets or fish or minced fish, dried shark fins, salted fish	15	<5X10^5/g	<20	100	Absent	Absent	Absent
Canned finfish, canned shrimp and canned sardines	15	Nil	Absent	Absent	Absent	Absent	Absent

Fish Inspection Act: Regulation 456

1. " No person who,

   (a) is known to be suffering from a communicable disease;

   (b) is a known carrier of a communicable disease; or

   (c) has an infected wound or open lesion on any part of his or her body, shall be employed in any working area of an establishment"

   Rationale

1. Employees who are suffering from communicable diseases, or are known to be carriers of communicable diseases are a potential source of microbial contamination, and must not be permitted to handle food in any capacity. Infected wounds or open lesions on the body can also become a source of microbial contamination, and persons having such wounds or lesions must not be allowed to work in any food handling areas, unless the injury is treated and completely protected by a secure, waterproof covering.
2. "No person in an establishment shall smoke or spit in a working area"

   Rationale: Humans are an important source of food contamination through the handling of food. Personal behaviour that could result in the contamination of fish, such as smoking, use of tobacco, eating or drinking any substance other than water from a drinking fountain, or chewing gum are prohibited in any area of an establishment where food is handled. Tags, pins, cords, or other objects that will subsequently be handled by a plant employee or directly or indirectly contact fish or fish products should not be held in the mouths of plant personnel.
3. "Every person engaged in handling or processing fish in an establishment shall wash his or her hands thoroughly with warm water and liquid or powdered soap immediately before commencing each work shift and after each absence from duty."

   Rationale: It is essential that employees engaged in handling or processing fish practice good hygiene and do not let their hands become a source of contamination. All persons entering a room where fish is being handled must be required to thoroughly wash their hands with warm water and soap. Hands must be washed before commencing each work shift, and when returning from each absence from duty (using the toilet or leaving the processing area for any reason). Hands must also be washed after handling contaminated material, and in-between the handling of incompatible fish and fish products. Unhygienic practices, such as spitting, scratching the head, placing the fingers in or about the mouth or nose, or indiscriminate and unprotected sneezing or coughing, should also be prohibited in any part of the plant where food is handled. Employee training and supervision to ensure people wash their hands after touching the face, sneezing or coughing. Training to cough or sneeze into the shoulder is helpful in minimizing contamination.
4. "No employee who handles fish with his or her bare hands in an establishment shall wear finger-nail polish."

Rationale: Employees who handle fish with their bare hands must not be permitted to wear fingernail polish, because it can chip and become incorporated into food, and contaminate food products. Plant employees engaged in the handling of fish or fish products should not be permitted to wear jewellery, because it has the potential to cause physical and microbial contamination of food products. Jewellery items that cannot be removed (medic alert devices) may be worn, but must be adequately covered. Earrings or other facial adornments may fall into food products. Simple covering with a hairnet is not sufficient to ensure security. Covering rings and bracelets with tape may add to the potential for contamination.

Other items that could fall into food products such as pens, pencils and thermometers must not be kept in areas where they are likely to fall out such as coat and shirt pockets. Fingernail polish, jewellery, pens and others present not only the potential for physical contamination or adulteration of food, but also have the potential of carrying microbial contamination from people into food products.

5. "Except for a filleter, skinner, scaler, handler of round or dressed fish or a worker in a frozen storage room in a fresh-fish, freezing or semi-preserving establishment, every employee engaged in a fish processing operation in a cannery or a fresh-fish, freezing or semi-preserving establishment shall wear a clean coverall, smock or coat and headgear that completely covers the hair."

   "All protective outer garments worn by an employee in a fish processing operation in a cannery shall be kept thoroughly cleaned."

   "A worker in a frozen storage room in a fresh-fish, freezing or semi-preserving establishment shall wear clean outer garments."

   Rationale: Employee/visitor clothing and hair must not be allowed to become a potential source of contamination. Where appropriate, employees/visitors should wear protective clothing, head covering, gloves, footwear or aprons while working in/visiting rooms where fish and fish products are handled. Protective clothing must be cleanable, unless designed to be disposable. For hygienic reasons, coveralls are discouraged. Protective clothing should be removed immediately after leaving a processing area, and should be cleaned and stored under sanitary conditions. Storage of protective clothing should be separate from employee street clothing. Protective clothing must be kept in a good state of repair.

6. "All waterproof garments in an establishment shall be thoroughly cleaned after each work shift."

   Rationale: Employees engaged in food handling must maintain a high degree of personal cleanliness. All waterproof garments must be able to be effectively cleaned. Waterproof garments worn during each work shift must be thoroughly cleaned after each shift, in order to prevent dirt from drying and caking on. Appropriate equipment to clean and disinfect waterproof garments must be provided, including hand dips and foot dips to clean waterproof gloves and boots. Waterproof garments must be stored under sanitary conditions.

7. "Every cannery and every fresh-fish, freezing or semi-preserving establishment shall be provided with facilities for disinfecting the protective hand coverings used in processing areas".

   "All protective hand coverings worn by employees in any processing area in a cannery or a fresh-fish, freezing or semi-preserving establishment shall be disinfected immediately after each break in a work shift and at the end of every work shift".

   Rationale: Gloves are worn for many purposes in a processing plant. Workers may require them for safety, to protect themselves from knife cuts or other injuries, cold conditions or fish, or to facilitate the grip on slippery products. Gloves are also useful barriers for personal protection against food borne pathogens. If used correctly, they are useful in preserving the integrity and safety of the food product.

   Gloves, when misused, can be a source of contamination, if they are soiled by contact with contaminated surfaces. If workers who wear gloves do not also wash their hands, they can be a source of contamination when punctured or cut. Even though hands may be washed, resident skin bacteria will multiply in the warm, moist environment inside a glove, and contamination may be spread when the glove is punctured, or removed and placed on a product or product contact surface. Gloves must always be clean and sanitized when used for handling fish products, and facilities must be available to ensure that they can be frequently washed and cleaned.

   Gloves can become a source of cross-contamination, and employees must be trained to wash or change gloves when in contact with contaminated material.

8. "The surface of a floor in a wet working area of an establishment shall be sloped for drainage purposes and shall be constructed of durable and impervious material that permits rapid disposal of waste and that can be readily cleaned."

   Rationale: It is essential that all floors in wet working areas (processing, receiving and holding) be constructed of materials that are smooth, impervious to moisture, non-absorbent and non-toxic such as dense, acid resisting, non-dusting and water-proof concrete, masonry floor tile, vitrified bricks or approved synthetic materials. Linoleum and other similar floor coverings are not acceptable, as they offer significant cleaning and sanitizing challenges.

   Floors must be durable for the activities that are carried out within the establishment, and must be easy to clean and disinfect.

9. It is essential that floors in wet working areas (processing, receiving and holding) be sloped sufficiently to facilitate drainage. A slope of 1 per cent to 2 per cent (1 – 2 cm/meter) should be adequate. Floors should slope uniformly to drains so that liquids do not accumulate.

10. "Drains in an establishment shall be of a type and size sufficient to carry off process effluents and water from cleaning operations and shall be equipped with traps or other devices to prevent the entry of gases or vermin into the establishment through the drains."

Rationale: It is essential that all rooms, processing and storage areas be provided with drains to facilitate continued disposal of process effluents and cleaning water in those areas.

Drains must be of sufficient size and quantity to carry off any processing effluent without overflowing. A floor plan must be designed to determine the drainage required the size of the drains, and appropriate location and number of drain inlets.

It is recommended that all drain lines be sloped at least 2 cm per meter and have not less than 10 cm inside diameter, be deep-seal trapped, properly vented to the outside air, and equipped with effective rodent screens. Drain inlets should be at least 30 x 30 cm or equivalent, with a minimum free area of 30 per cent of the total. Drain covers shall be provided with apertures having a minimum size of 4 cm^2.

11. "The inside surfaces of walls in a wet working area of an establishment shall be constructed of smooth, durable, waterproof and light-colored material that can be thoroughly cleaned up to a height of not less than four feet"

    Rationale: Walls in wet working areas (processing, receiving and holding) must be constructed of materials that are impervious to moisture, non-absorbent and non-toxic such as prefabricated panels, glazed tile, smooth steel, trowelled cement plaster or other approved materials. Up to a height that is appropriate for the operation but no less than four feet, walls should be smooth, easy to clean and disinfect, and light-colored to promote sanitation and increase light levels within the establishment. Doors and door frames are a significant part of the structure, and must meet the same standards of construction. Doors and fittings (hinges, handles and latches) must be made of approved materials, designed and installed so that they can be easily cleaned and sanitized. Where possible, door handles should be eliminated, so that doors can be pushed open with minimal or no hand contact. Where door handles are needed, they should be one piece construction. Door knobs and similar devices are difficult to clean and maintain.

12. "Ceilings shall be constructed of smooth, non-absorbent, durable and non-toxic materials that are light-colored, washable, of a height acceptable to the president of the agency and maintained in a sound condition for ease of cleaning and disinfection".

    Rationale: It is essential that ceilings in fish processing establishments be of sufficient height to accommodate the operations carried out within the area. A ceiling height of about 3 meters (10 feet) or greater has been found to be suitable because it allows for ease of operation, movement of equipment, and allows the installation of equipment that requires elevated ceilings. A high ceiling also helps the establishment to be well lit and ventilated. Where ceiling heights are lower than recommended, ventilation, lighting and sanitation must be maintained to ensure a safe food processing environment.

13. "Every establishment shall be equipped with a natural or mechanical ventilation system that will provide clean air, remove undesirable odors, steam and smoke and prevent condensation in rooms where work is performed."

Rationale: It is essential that the ventilation system within an establishment be designed and constructed to provide air exchange sufficient to remove undesirable odours, dust, smoke and contaminated air from the establishment. The ventilation system must also remove moisture from the air to prevent condensation from contaminating walls and equipment. Any openings for ventilation should be covered with animal and insect-proof screens or similar devices, to prevent the ventilation system from becoming a point of entry for small animals and insects. Screens should be easily removable for cleaning purposes.

It is essential that air not be allowed to flow from contaminated areas to clean areas. Air should flow from the cleanest area to less clean areas.

14. "Every working surface in a processing room in an establishment shall be provided with an illumination having a minimum intensity of twenty foot-candles."

    Rationale: Lighting (natural or artificial) of adequate intensity must be provided in processing areas to enable activities to be hygienically performed. In processing and support areas, a minimum intensity of twenty foot-candles (220 lux) must be provided. In areas where inspection is taking place, an illumination of at least 75 foot candles (800 lux) is required.

    Non working areas such as maintenance, utility room and storage rooms can have a minimum intensity of ten-foot candles (110 lux). It is recommended that light approximate natural daylight.

15. "Fish that is intended for human consumption shall be adequately iced or chilled while being held or transported and shall be protected from contamination and the weather

    Rationale: Light bulbs and ceilings fixtures may become sources for contamination due to falling debris, dust and in case of breakage and faulty maintenance in the area where fish, ingredients and packaging materials are exposed to the environment. Therefore it is critical that all lighting fixtures be protected with acceptable covers to prevent contamination of food upon breakage. Light bulb, tube lights and fixtures in all fish handling and processing environments and support areas such as transportation vehicle where there is exposed fish, ingredients, or packaging materials must be adequately covered or be coated with a shatterproof materials in case of breakage and also be maintained in good condition

16. "Every establishment shall contain toilet facilities that are constructed and located in such a manner as to prevent the contamination of the establishment or the water supply of the establishment."

    "The room in which a toilet facility in an establishment is located shall,

    (a) have self-closing doors;

    (b) be ventilated to the outside;

(c) have walls and a ceiling that are smooth, light in colour and that can be readily cleaned; and

(d) have a floor that is constructed of impervious material and that can be readily cleaned."

Rationale: It is essential that welfare and toilet facilities do not become a source of contamination. Toilet facilities should be conveniently located and easily accessible, but must not open directly into food handling areas. "Flush toilets shall be:

(a) present in adequate numbers for both sexes;

(b) conveniently located adjacent to processing areas;

(c) designed so that areas do not lead directly into processing area; and

(d) equipped with floor drains that will prevent any overflow of water or sewage from entering or contaminating a processing area

Rationale: It is essential that an adequate number of toilets be available to meet the needs of employees. As a guideline, a minimum number of toilets must be provided for the following numbers of employees:

1 to 9 employees – 1 toilet

10 to 24 employees – 2 toilets

25 to 49 employees – 3 toilets

50 to 100 employees – 5 toilets

Every 30 employees over 100 – 1 toilet

17. "Every establishment shall be provided with sanitary washbasins in locations that are visible from the working area, equipped with hot and cold running water, liquid or powdered soap and air dryers or single service towels."

    Rationale: The temperature of water used in hand-washing is critical. All hand washing facilities must be equipped with hot and cold running water of potable quality. Washbasin must have combination faucets that enable the hot and cold water to be blended to a temperature that is sufficient to dissolve soils. A temperature within the range of 46°C (115°F) to 52°C (125°C) will be sufficient. If the water temperature is too high, people will not use them effectively, if at all.

    The pressure of the water contributes to the efficiency of hand-washing. Water pressure must be adequate for the intended purpose.

18. "Every receptacle, tray, tank, vat and utensil used for processing fish in a cannery and a fresh-fish, freezing or semi-preserving establishment shall be made of a non-corrodible material, other than wood, and shall have smooth surfaces free from cracks and crevices."

    Rationale: It is essential that equipment does not become a source of contamination of food products. Containers, including all boxes, receptacles, bins, tanks and trays used for fish processing must be of material that is smooth, durable and impervious and can be readily and repeatedly cleaned and disinfected. Receptacles used to hold fish, other than live fish, have provisions for drainage to prevent holding of wastewater. Cardboard or wood boxes can harbour micro-organisms and deteriorates rapidly in moist conditions, so it is not an acceptable material for use.

References

http://www.google.co.in/url?sa=t and source=web and cd=4 and ved=0CEUQFjAD and url=http per cent 3A per cent 2F per cent 2Fen.wikipedia.org per cent 2Fwiki per cent 2FBureau_of_Indian_Standards

http://www.google.co.in/url?sa=t and source=web and cd=1 and ved=0CBgQFjAA and url=http per cent 3A per cent 2F per cent 2Fwww.revistaaquatic.com per cent 2Faquatic per cent 2Fhtml per cent 2Fart303 per cent 2FAnexo

http://www.google.co.in/url?sa=t and source=web and cd=1 and ved=0CBYQFjAA and url=http per cent 3A per cent 2F per cent 2Fwww.codexalimentarius.net per cent 2Fstandard_list

http://www.google.co.in/url?sa=t and source=web and cd=2 and ved=0CB0QFjAB and url=http per cent 3A per cent 2F per cent 2Fwww.iso.org per cent 2Fiso per cent 2Fiso_catalogue per cent 2Fcatalogue_ics per cent 2Fcatalogue_ics_browse.

http://www.google.co.in/url?sa=t and source=web and cd=2 and ved=0CCgQFjAB and url=http per cent 3A per cent 2F per cent 2Fwww.bnet.com per cent 2Fblog per cent 2Ffood per cent 2Fgroups-clash-over-organic-standards-for-fish

– Chapter 26 –

Utilization of Fish Processing Waste

The three most common methods for utilization of aquatic waste (either from aquaculture or wild stock) are the manufacture of fish meal/oil, the production of silage or the use of waste in the manufacture of organic fertilizer. Several other options have been proposed, much of the fish waste is manufactured into value added products. The problem of aquatic waste disposal was approached in nearly a decade ago, at first with a view to waste disposal, then later with a view to manufacturing marketable products from waste.

Fish Meal and Oil

The traditional manufacture of fish meal usually involves the comminuting and cooking of waste in order to separate the oil from the rest of the material and to ensure the destruction of both pathogenic and spoilage organisms. Although there are a wide variety of processing conditions, in practice most fish meal cookers are designed to heat the minced fish to 95-100°C over a period of 18-20 minutes. Following this, the cooked material is pressed to separate solids (press cake) from liquids (press liquor) containing oil and water. The press liquor is further clarified by centrifugation to separate oil, water and solids, the water being subsequently evaporated and all solids are re-combined with the press cake which is then dried in an evaporator. The standard evaporator operates at 90-95°C whereas the evaporator for so-called "low temperature" (LT) meal is operated at 60-65°C.

The final product contains very little oil or water and is considered to be sterile or nearly so by virtue of the initial cooking process. This does not mean that problems related to non-sterility have not occurred in the manufacture of fishmeal. However, these problems are inevitably related to recontamination of the finished product by rodents or birds.

In general, aquaculture waste is not permitted for the manufacture of aquaculture feed and must be processed in facilities which are entirely separate from waste streams from the wild fishery. Also, special consideration must be given to offal which may reasonably be expected to contain chemical residues such as drugs and antibiotics. Offal which is destined for fish feed production must be heated to an internal temperature of at least 90°C to prevent the survival of fish pathogens which may be present.

"High risk" offal such as mortalities from fish farms, fish which show clinical signs of disease or animals which are slaughtered as a part of a disease control program, must be thermally processed to an internal temperature of at least 133°C and cannot be used for any type of meal.

Shrimp meal is usually manufactured from heads, guts and tail hulls and can be processed in a variety of ways. It may be manufactured by simple sun drying or may be cooked as in the traditional fish meal process. It is considered as an ingredient for aquaculture feed for two reasons. First, its amino acid profile is ideal for the culture of crustaceans, while the pigment (largely astaxanthin) is desirable in certain cultured fish. The pigment is however heat labile and the low temperature processes sometimes used for shrimp meal production cannot be considered adequate for the destruction of shrimp pathogens.

Fish Silage

Fish silage is produced by acidification of fish waste using organic acids such as formic acid which is added at a rate of about 3.5 per cent (w/w) or mineral acids such as sulfuric which is added at slightly lower levels. A third method sometimes used in tropical climates involves the addition of simple sugars such as molasses and a lactic acid bacterial culture which generates lactic acid through the natural breakdown of the sugar. The use of acid is necessary to inhibit spoilage bacteria which could produce off odors, flavours such as trimethylamine or ammonia and/or toxins such as histamine if left to ferment at neutral pH.

Fish and shrimp silage is highly nutritious and is traditionally fed as a protein supplement to swine, mink and poultry. It consists of autolyzed fish offal and is normally manufactured by the addition of fresh fish viscera which contain the necessary enzymes for autolytic breakdown. The liquified product has a pleasant "malty" odour and is often blended with dry feed ingredients to form a semi-moist diet.

Silage has also been used successfully as a low cost ingredient in aquaculture diets. In fact, shrimp silage has been used as a source of pigment as well as nutrition for farmed salmon(Fagbenro and Jauncey, 1993; Fagbenro *et al.*, 1994; and Fagbenro and Jauncey, 1995). Fermented fish silage produced by the addition of lactic acid bacteria and a carbohydrate source has been produced from offal from tilapia shrimp and salmon and subsequently used in aquaculture diets. One advantage of this process over the traditional organic acid processes is that there is a substantial saving in operating costs provided an inexpensive source of carbohydrate such as molasses. Another potential advantage of using silage rather than meal in aquaculture diets is the fact that most of the silage processes used to date (with a few notable exceptions) do not involve heat denaturation of the proteins. One exception is a Norwegian process in which silage is produced in the traditional manner and subsequently transported to a thermal processing facility where the silage is heated in a two-stage process to eliminate pathogen transfer.

Another exception is the mixing of silage with other dry feed ingredients and then processing by thermoplastic extrusion to produce feed pellets which are heated under pressure and then expand when exiting the extruder producing air voids and thus a lower density. This latter process also results in the evaporation of water which is a requirement for product stability since silage normally contains 65-80 per cent moisture before mixing with dry ingredients (Vanguard, 1991).

Compost and Other Products from Inedible Fish Waste

Hemophilic fermentation is one way of dealing with problem waste such as municipal sewage and fish mortalities. Processes for the production of fertilizers and other useful end products have been developed in various parts of the world. Hemophilic fermentation is a process which involves particle size reduction followed by bacterial fermentation at high temperature (usually 50-70°C) accompanied with aeration. The hemophilic process not only breaks down complex materials such as proteins, fats, carbohydrates, etc., but also generates heat which may or may not be utilized for other purposes. The production of heat during the process may result in the destruction of pathogenic microorganisms. Unfortunately, it is not always possible to obtain details about such processes since those which are in commercial production often contain proprietary information.

One such process was developed in Norway and has recently become commercialized. Trondheim, Norway, and involves the mixing of problem wastes such as animal manure, municipal sewage and aquaculture mortalities. A liquid compost is formed by aerobic fermentation at 60°C. The compost produced in the Norwegian process is currently used as an agricultural organic fertilizer. The Rubin Foundation claims that although the process is capable of destroying *Aeromonas salmonicida* and infectious salmon anemia, hemophilic fermentation was incapable of removing antibiotic residues sometimes found in aquaculture waste.

Another commercial composting process was developed by Thermo Tech Technologies in Langley, British Columbia, Canada. The process is patented and involves the aerobic hemophilic fermentation at approximately 70°C. The process has been used to compost municipal sewage sludges, fruits, vegetables, meats, dairy waste and fish products. The company claims that the process eliminates a variety of human bacterial and viral pathogens and is claimed to successfully destroy chlortetracycline, sulphamethazine and penicillin (Thermo Tech Technologies, 1998). It is therefore perhaps reasonable to anticipate that this process may be applicable to the destruction of fish pathogens. The finished product is dried, pelletized and used as an organic fertilizer.

- ☆ **Soup Powder from Trash Fish**: The soup powder prepared out of trash fish is a rich source of animal protein and other nutritive element.

- ☆ **Shark Fin and Fin Rays:** Dried shark fin is a valuable product of export from India.At the importing countries fins are processed for their fin rays which are utilized in soup preparation.
- ☆ **Shark skin leather:** Skin of fishes specially shark, seal,porpoise, dolphin is used for making leather novelties.
- ☆ **Extraction of sardine oil**: Sardine oil after separation of stearine has been found to be characteristic similar to synthetic oil.
- ☆ **Pearl Essence:** The lustrous appearance of the epidermal layer is due to GUANINE. The lustrous guanine can be extracted from fish scale.the suspension of the guanine crystal in a suitable solvent is called PEARL ESSENCE. It is great demand in Japan.
- ☆ **Fish Liver Oil:** From time immemorial fish liver oil were used for treatment of Vitamin A and D deficiency diseases.The most important fish liver oil is obtained from cod, haddock, and shark, halibut and tuna.
- ☆ **Fish Maws and Isinglass:** The word isinglass is derived from the Dutch and German words which have the meaning sturgeon's air bladder or swimming bladder. The bladder of deep water hake is most suitable for production.Isinglass dissolve more quickly in dilute alkali and acid. But insoluble in water. In hot water it produces opalescent gel.

  It is used as clarifying agent for beverages like wine, beer, vinegar.
- ☆ **Chitosan:** Obtained from exoskeletal material from the invertebrate. Chitosan is a linear polysaccharide composed of randomly distributed β-linked D-glucosamine and N-acetyl-D-glucosamine.

  Potential Uses – Absorb and bind fat, promote weight loss. Help to control blood pressure. Anti tumor and anti cancer property. Tissue and nerve regeneration.
- ☆ **Gelatin:** Protein have high amount of lysine and methionine. Can be extracted from skin and bone of fish.

Refernces

Arul James. Ensiled product from fish by microbial fermentation. Fish Tech.3;4:38

Biswas K.P. Advancement in Fish Fisheries Technology

Gopakumar K. Fish Processing Technology 475-482

http://www.fao.org/docrep/003/X9199E/X9199E04.htm

Nair, K.G. R. and Madhvan,P.1984. Fish Technology 21:109

Utilization of Fish Industry By-Products

Introduction

Parts of fish not used for human food such as intestines,head and gills as well as whole fish of less favoured spp. have been ground up,dehydrayed and converted to fish meal.these are known as fishery by-products

These products include

- ☆ Fish meal
- ☆ FPC
- ☆ Isinglass
- ☆ Fish glue
- ☆ Fish maws and Fish oil etc.

Fish Meal

- ☆ **Fish meal** is a commercial product made from both whole fish and the bones and offal from processed fish.
- ☆ It is a brown powder or cake obtained by rendering pressing the cooked whole fish or fish trimmings to remove most of the fish oil and water, and then ground. What remains is the fishmeal
- ☆ Fish meal is highly concenterated nutritious feed of high quality protein, mineral and vitamins.
- ☆ PROTEIN Conc.-50-70 per cent
- ☆ FAT CONC.-5-10 per cent

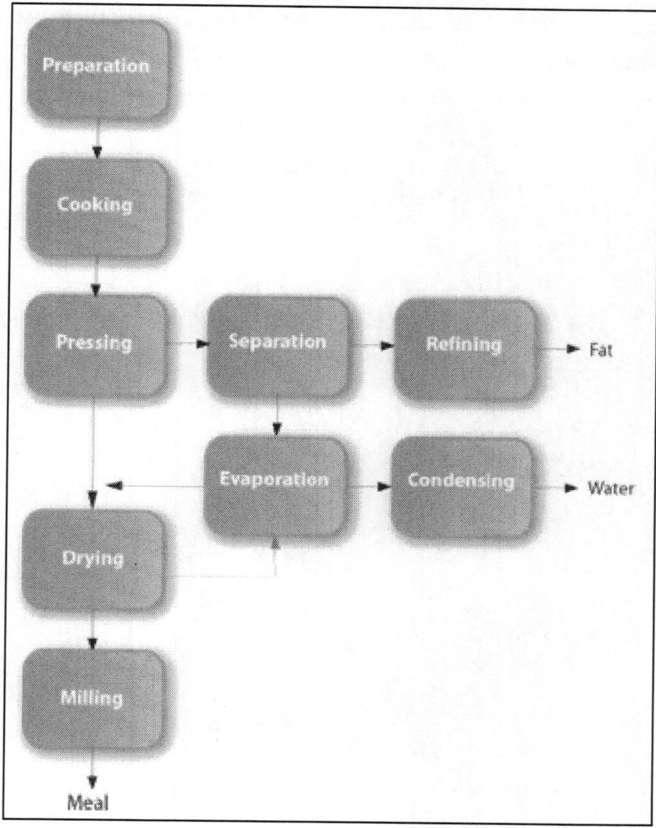

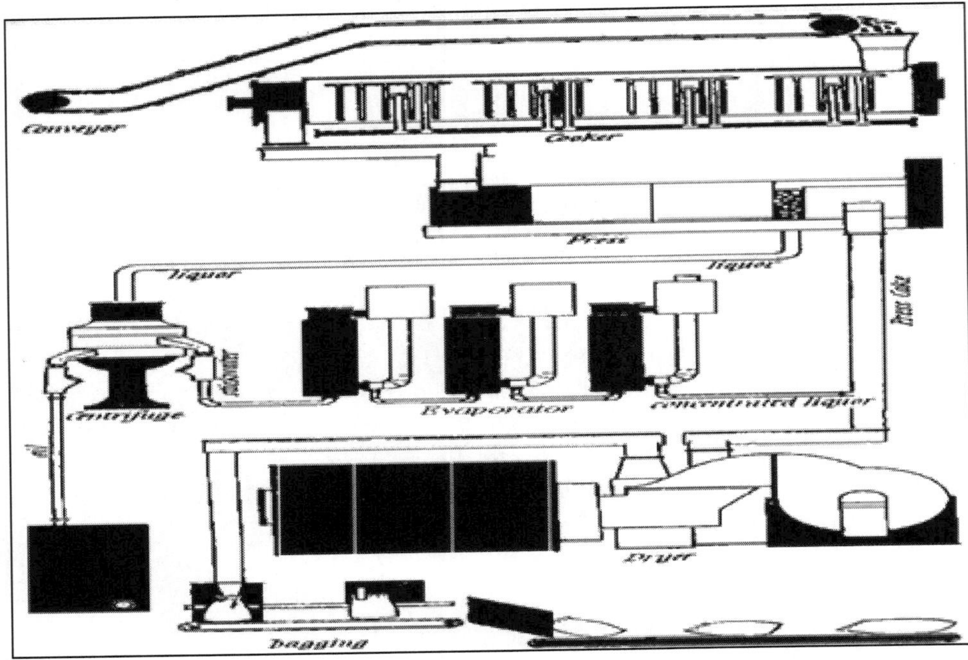

A Typical Process Diagram.

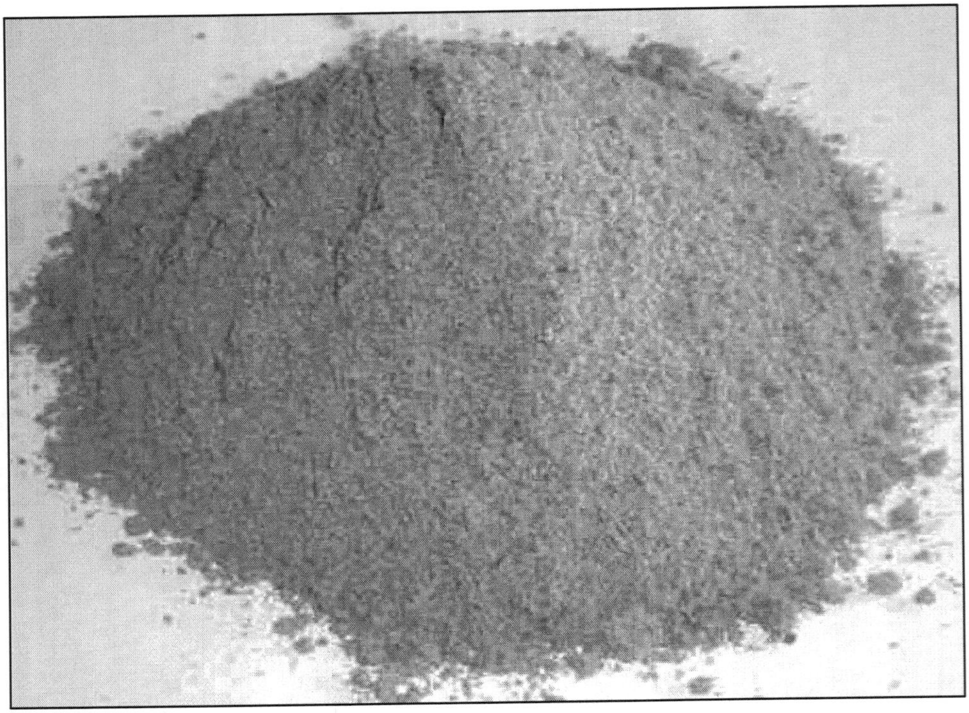

Fish meal has been widely used as a protein source for many years for fish. Two basic types of fish meal are produced;

- ☆ Produced from fishery waste (salmon, tuna, etc.) that are associated with the processing of various edible human fishery products and this fishmeal is rendered from fish offal, trimmings or cuttings, and other wastes principally from filleting and canning operations from the edible fisheries (*e.g.*, tuna, cod, haddock, hake, pollock).

When specific fish (Herring, Menhaden, Hakes, Jacks, Pollack, etc.) are harvested just for the purpose to produce fish meal. The fish can be dried directly drying or cooking prior to drying and oil extracted.

Most of these fishes are small, bony, with high content of oil, and considered of little edible use (*e.g.*, anchovies, herrings, capelin, menhaden)

Fish meal can be produced by:

- ☆ Dry rendering
- ☆ Wet rendering

How is Fish Meal Used?

- ☆ Fish meal in the UK was used mainly as a fertilizer until about 1910, but since then its high nutritional value has been far better utilized in animal feeding.
- ☆ The demand in the UK for fish as fish meal is far greater than the demand for fish for direct human consumption; therefore imports of fish meal to the UK are high.
- ☆ The pig and poultry industries producing large amounts of bacon and eggs, pork and chicken, at relatively low prices could not survive without large scale use of high protein animal foods like fish meal.
- ☆ Usually about 10 per cent of the diet of pigs and poultry consists of fish meal; 10 per cent is the upper limit for meal containing 10 per cent fat, because more than about 1 per cent of fish oil in the diet of the animal may taint the taste of its flesh.

Other uses of fish meal include:

- ☆ The feeding of mink,
- ☆ Farmed fish, dogs, cats and cattle.

Very small amounts of specially processed meals have been used in prepared foods for humans, and fish meal is also used in the preparation of certain antibiotics for the pharmaceutical industry

Fish Oil

Fish oil is oil derived from the tissues of oily fish.

Main source of fish body oil in our country is oil sardine

How are Fish Oils Used?

- ☆ Fish oils are produced whenever fatty fish are processed into meal.
- ☆ In Europe they are widely used in the manufacture of edible oils and fats, for example margarine.
- ☆ Other uses include the paint and varnish industry. In addition, there are several other specialized uses for small quantities of fish OILS.
- ☆ Fish oils, whether present as fat in the fish meal or as separated oil, are rich in omega3 fatty acids. When fed to food animals, these omega3 fatty acids deposit in the meat and depot fat.
- ☆ Fish oils usually have to be low in free fatty acids, less than 2 per cent, to obtain the best price; production of high quality fish oils depends on the use of fresh raw material, proper purification and good storage.
- ☆ **Cod liver oil** is a nutritional supplement derived from liver of cod fish.
- ☆ It has high levels of the omega-3 fatty acids, EPA and DHA, and very high levels of vitamin A and vitamin D

Therapeutic Uses

- ☆ Cod liver oil and fish oil are similar, but cod liver oil has much higher levels of vitamins A and D. Many adults do not meet the RDA for Vitamin D.
- ☆ Cod liver oil is effective in treatment of household burns because of its high vitamin content often leaving no burn-related blister.
- ☆ Cod liver oil may be an effective complementary measure for long-term treatment of multiple sclerosis.
- ☆ Use of cod liver oil during pregnancy is associated with lower risk of Type I diabetes in the offspring.This effect was found only in mothers taking cod liver oil, not in mothers taking multivitamin supplements.
- ☆ Cod liver oil taken by nursing mothers improves the breast milk by increasing the amount of fatty acids, which promotes brain development, and the amount of vitamin A, which helps prevent infections, but the level of vitamin D is unchanged.
- ☆ Cod liver oil is widely taken to ease the pain and joint stiffness associated with arthritis, but has also been clinically proven to have a positive effect on heart, bone, and brain as well as helping to nourish skin, hair, and nails.

Fish Protein Concentrates (FPC)

Fish protein concenterate is stable fish preparation intended for human consumption in which protein more concenterated than original fish

Why is FPC a Good Protein Source?

- ☆ First, of course, because it is concentrated: untreated and unprocessed foods do not generally contain more than about 20 percent protein, whereas FPC contains about 80 per cent.

☆ Secondly, the quality of the protein is high; by this is meant that the amino acids which make up the protein are present in just the right balance for human nutrition.

What are the Principal Types of FPC?

The Food and Agriculture Organization of the United Nations defines three types:

☆ Type A: a virtually odourless and tasteless powder having a maximum total fat content of 0 75 per cent.

☆ Type B: a powder having no specific limits as to odour or flavour, but definitely having a fishy flavour and a maximum fat content of 3 per cent.

☆ Type C: normal fish meal produced under satisfactorily hygienic conditions

How is FPC Used?

☆ Fish protein concentrate type A is an odourless, tasteless powder which is unattractive to eat by itself; there is therefore a real problem in finding ways to make most use of it.

☆ It has to be incorporated in other foods such as bread, biscuits, soups and stews at a level that does not affect their normal properties.

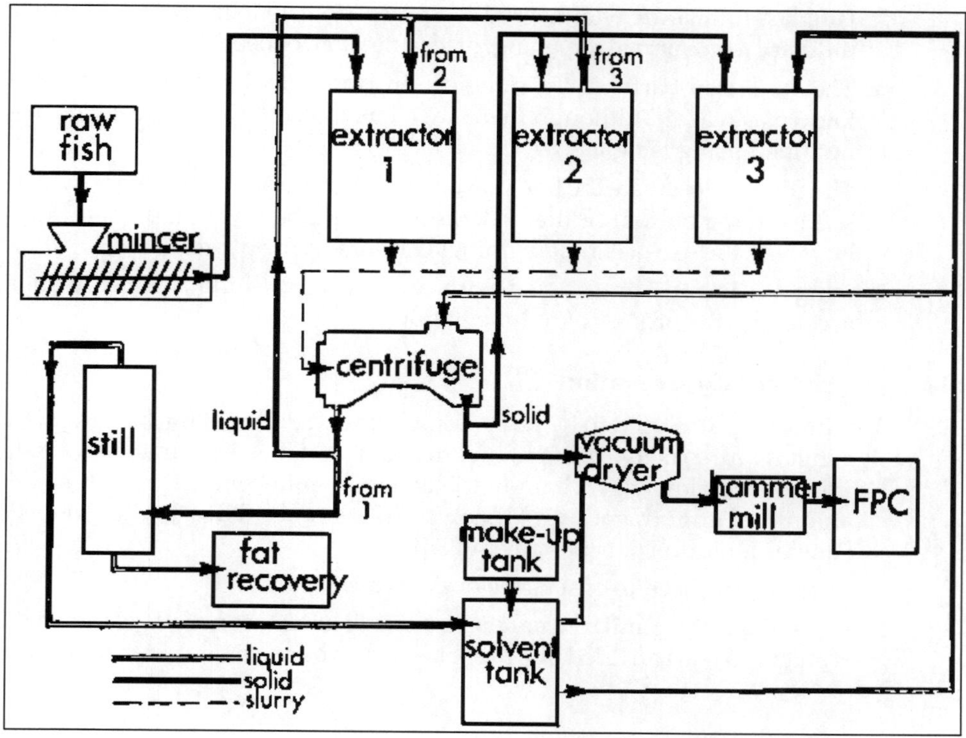

- ☆ Good results have been obtained with macaroni products, a milk shake drink, spaghetti sauce, infant foods, dietetic foods and breakfast cereals.
- ☆ There is less of a problem with other FPC products which have some flavour.
- ☆ A fishy flavour, even if a rancid one, is acceptable in food in some societies; thus the FPC can be eaten more or less as it is, or used as a flavouring in soups or stews.

Isinglass/Fish Maws

- ☆ **Isinglass** is a substance obtained from the swimbladders of fish (especially Beluga sturgeon).
- ☆ It is a form of collagen used mainly for the clarification of wine and beer.
- ☆ Isinglass is the purest form of animal gelatin
- ☆ To prepare isinglass, the bladder is taken from the fish and washed in cold water. Then the black outer skin is removed and the remaining part is washed again and spread on a board to dry. Next the inner skin is taken out by rubbing and beating.
- ☆ Next the bladder passes between rollers which reduce it to a thin, partly transparent ribbon which looks a little like watered silk.

Use in Foods and Drinks

- ☆ Isinglass finings are widely used as a processing aid in the British brewing industry to accelerate the fining, or clarification, of beer.
- ☆ They are used particularly in the production of cask-conditioned beers, known as real ale, although there are a few cask ales available which are not fined using isinglass.
- ☆ The finings flocculate the live yeast in the beer into a jelly-like mass, which settles to the bottom of the cask. Left to itself, beer will clear naturally; however, the use of isinglass finings accelerates the process.
- ☆ Isinglass is sometimes used with an auxiliary fining, which further accelerates the process of sedimentation.

Use in Parchment Conservation

- ☆ Isinglass is also used to help repair parchment. Pieces of the best Russian isinglass are soaked overnight to soften and swell the dried material. Next, it is cooked slowly in a bain-marie at 45°C while being stirred. A small amount of gum tragacanth, dissolved in water, is added to the strained isinglass solution to act as an emulsifier.
- ☆ It can also be used to coat tissue or goldbeater's skin.
- ☆ Here isinglass is similar to parchment size and other forms of gelatin but it is unique in that as a dried film the adhesive can be reactivated with moisture.

Fish Glue

- ☆ Fish glue is made by boiling the skin, bones and swim bladders of fish.
- ☆ Animal glue was the most common woodworking glue for thousands of years until the advent of synthetic glues such as polyvinyl acetate (PVA) and other resin glues in the 20th century.
- ☆ Today it is used primarily in specialty applications such as lutherie, pipe organ building, and antique restoration.
- ☆ Glass artists take advantage of hide glue's ability to bond with glass, applying hide glue to glass. As the glue hardens it shrinks, chipping the glass.
- ☆ It has several advantages and disadvantages compared to other glues. The glue is applied hot, typically with a brush or spatula; it is kept hot in a glue pot.

Pearl Essence

- ☆ It is a suspension of crystalline guanine in water
- ☆ Guanine combines with collagen and calcium phosphate yeilding silvery white shining
- ☆ Guanine is an iridescent material found in epidermal layer and scales of most pelagic spp. of fish like oil sardine, mackerel,herring etc.
- ☆ Pearl essence is used in manufacture of artificial pearls
- ☆ It is used as spray or dip for several items to impart an iridescent sheen reminescent of pearls.
- ☆ It is used on such diverse articles as shoe, pencils, fishing rod, spectacle frame, walking stick,vanity bag.

Fish Hydrolysate

- ☆ **Fish hydrolysate**, in its simplest form, is ground up fish carcasses. After the usable portions are removed for human consumption, the remaining fish body, (which means the guts, bones, cartilage, scales, meat, etc.), is put into water and ground up.
- ☆ Some fish hydrolysate is ground more finely than others so more bone material is able to remain suspended.

Enzymes may also be used to solubilize bones, scale and meat. If the larger chunks of bone and scales are screened out, calcium or protein, or mineral content may be lacking in the finished product form.

Uses of Fish Hydrolysate

- ☆ There is a lot of information on the many uses of fish hydrolsate - from its use as a fish-based fertilizer, to its use as an animal food, or even for human consumption.
- ☆ Antiproliferative activity of fish protein hydrolysate, which makes it eligible for listing as a nutriceutical.

Fish protein hydrolysates, particularly those developed from salmon, contain significant cancer growth inhibitors.

Products	*Source*	*Uses*
Shark fins	First dorsal fins,pair of pectoral fins of shark	Fish needles,fish nets etc.
Fish calcium	Backbone of tuna	Calcium supplement
Fish manure	Fish waste	Slow fertilizer b/c of organic constituents

References

Ismail,P.K.,Madhavan,P. and Pillai,V.K.1968.STUDIES on preparation of fish protein concenterates

www.fao.org/wairdocs/tan fao corporate document repository

Nair, K.G.R,2000.Project Report on Production of Isinglass

http://en.wikipedia.org/wiki/fish_products

http://jinhaiwan/product1.jpg

Nair, K.G.R. and Madhavan, P. 1984.Shark fin rays-Technology of Extraction.

www.foodmag.com.au/./isinglass.jpg

www.allproducts.com

– Chapter 26 –

Fishery Resources, Marine and Freshwater Fishes, Transportation, Processing, Preservation, Grading Standards

I. Fishery Resources of India

Introduction

The fishery sector in India is immensely contributing to the country's economy providing valuable foreign exchange and employment to millions of people. At the same time it also stimulates growth of a number of subsidiary industries and is a source of cheap and nutritious food besides being a foreign exchange earner. In world, India is third largest producer of fish and second largest producer of freshwater fish.

Fish Production Status In India

Fishing in India is a major industry in its coastal states, employing over 14 million people.

Fish production in India has increased more than tenfold since its independence in 1947. According to the Food and Agriculture Organization (FAO) of the United Nations, fish output in India doubled between 1990 and 2010.[1]

India has 8,118 kilometers of marine coastline, 3,827 fishing villages, and 1,914 traditional fish landing centers. India's freshwater resources consist of 195,210 kilometers of rivers and canals, 2.9 million hectares of minor and major reservoirs, 2.4 million hectares of ponds and lakes, and about 0.8 million hectares of flood plain wetlands and water bodies.[2] As of 2010, the marine and freshwater resources offered a combined sustainable catch fishing potential of over 4 million metric tonnes of fish. In addition, India's water and natural resources offer a tenfold growth potential in aquaculture (farm fishing) from 2010 harvest levels of 3.9 million metric tonnes of fish, if India were to adopt fishing knowledge, regulatory reforms, and sustainability policies adopted by China over the last two decades.

The marine fish harvested in India consist of about 65 commercially important species/groups. Pelagic and midwater species contributed about 52 per cent of the total marine fish in 2004.

India is a major supplier of fish in the world. In 2006 the country exported over 600,000 metric tonnes of fish, to some 90 countries, earning over $1.8 billion.[3] Shrimps are one of the major varieties exported. The giant tiger prawn (*Penaeus monodon*) is the dominant species chosen for aquaculture, followed by the Indian white prawn (*Fenneropenaeus indicus*). Shrimp production from coastal aquaculture during 2004 stood at approximately 120,000 tonnes. Farmed shrimp accounted for about 60 per cent of shrimp exported from the country.

Marine and freshwater catch fishing combined with aquaculture fish farming is a rapidly growing industry in India. In 2008 India was the sixth largest producer of marine and freshwater capture fisheries, and the second largest aquaculture farmed fish producer in the world.[4] Fish as food–both from fish farms and catch fisheries–offers India one of the easiest and fastest way to address malnutrition and food security.

Despite rapid growth in total fish production, a fish farmers' average annual production in India is only 2 metric tonnes per person, compared to 172 tonnes in Norway, 72 tonnes in Chile, and 6 tonnes per fisherman in China.[4] Higher productivity, knowledge transfer for sustainable fishing, continued growth in fish production with increase in fish exports have the potential for increasing the living standards of Indian fishermen.

As of 2010, fish harvest distribution was difficult within India because of poor rural road infrastructure, lack of cold storage and absence of organized retail in most parts of the country.

- ✰ Maximum fish production in India is as follows:-West Bengal (1359.10 tt) followed by Andhra Pradesh(856.93 tt) followed by Gujrat (747.33 tt) in 2006-2007 according to the Annual Report of Deptt. Of Animal Husbandry, Dairying and Fisheries.
- ✰ Minimum fish production in India is that of Dadra and Nagar Haveli abt. 0.05 tt in 2006-2007.

Other Highlights

- ✰ Total fish production during the year 2004-05 was 63.04 lakh tonnes comprising 27.78 lakh tonnes of marine fish and 35.26 lakh tonnes of inland fish.

- ☆ A network of 429 Fish Farmers Development Agencies (FFDA) has been set up covering all the potential districts in all the states and union territories for propagating freshwater aquaculture.
- ☆ 39 Brackish water Fish Farmers Development Agencies (BFDA) have been set up in all the coastal states and UT of Andaman and Nicobar Islands.
- ☆ Till 2004-05 about 6.74 lakh hactares of water area was brought under scientific fish farming through FFDA's.
- ☆ Govt. Of India has sanctioned 6 major fishing harbours, 58 minor fishing harbours and 189 fish landing centres.
- ☆ Fisheries sector, plays a very important role in the socio economic development of India.
- ☆ Fisheries sector provides employment to 7 million fisher men.
- ☆ India is endowed with vast and varied fishery resource, an outline of which is given below

Table 26.1: Fish Production of India (Lakh Tonnes)

Year	*Marine*	*Inland*	*Total*
2000-2001	28.11	28.45	56.56
2001-2002	28.30	31.20	59.56
2002-2003	29.90	32.10	62.00
2003-2004	29.41	34.58	63.99
2004-2005	27.80	35.20	63.04
2005-2006	28.16	37.55	65.71
2006-2007	30.24	38.45	68.69

Table 26.2: Growth in Export of Marine Products

Year	*Quantity("000 tonnes)*	*Value(Rs. In crore)*
2000-2001	502.60	6296.00
2001-2002	457.60	5815.00
2002-2003	520.70	6793.05
2003-2004	412.01	6086.83
2004-2005	482.22	6459.89
2005-2006	551.28	7018.68
2006-2007	563.39	7296.06

Fishery Resources

- ☆ 61 freshwater fish species (Saikia 2005)
- ☆ 54 indigenous; 5 exotics
- ☆ 8 protected species (Wildlife protection Act, 1972)

- ☆ 20 economically important
- ☆ 11 collect for ornamental trade

Highlights of Inland Fishery Resources

- ☆ Rivers and Canals.
- ☆ Estuaries.
- ☆ Food plains wetlands.
- ☆ Lagoons and Reservoirs.
- ☆ India has 14 major rivers, 44 medium rivers and innumerable small rivers and desert streams.

Different river systems of the country, having a combined length of 29000 km, provide one of the richest fish genetic resources in the world

Inland Fishery Resources of India

- ☆ Rivers and canals:0.20 million Kilometers
- ☆ Area under reservoirs:3.15 million Hectare
- ☆ Tanks and ponds: 2.25 million Hectare
- ☆ Beels, oxbow lakes and derelict water bodies:0.82 million Hectare
- ☆ Brackish water area:1.24 million Hectare
- ☆ Estimated annual potential:4.5 million tones

Highlights of Marine Fishery Resources

The harvestable potential of marine fishery resources in the EEZ has been revalidated by a group of experts constituted by the govt. Of India, ministry of agriculture at about 3.93 million tonnes (oct.2000) consisting of 2.02 million tonnes of Demersal, 1.67 million tonnes of Pelagic and 0.24 million tonnes of oceanic resources

Marine Fishery Resources of India

- ☆ Coastline: 8129 km
- ☆ Continental shelf: 0.50 million km^2
- ☆ Exclusive economic zone: 2.02 million km^2
- ☆ Estimated annual production potential: 3.90 million tones
- ☆ From area within 50-m depth:2.21 million tones
- ☆ From area beyond 50-m depth:1.69 million tones

Constraints of Fishery Development in India

Accurate data on assesment of fishery resources and their potential in terms of fish production, development of sustainable technologies for fin and shell fish culture, yield optimization, harvest and post harvest operations, landing and berthing facilities for fishing vessels and welfare of fishermen.

Conclusion

India's future need of fish has to come mainly from aqua farming. Moreover the hygienic and sanitation conditions in most of the harbours and fish landing centres are below the normal specifications. If these requirements are not met in the future, the marine products export may face trade restrictions, since most of the importing countries have stringent hygiene and sanitary conditions.

Refrences

Gopakumar K, Fish resources : Indian Scenario; Textbook of fish processing technology; 6-17.

Website:-www.dahd.nic.in

http://en.wikipedia.org/wiki/Fishing_in_India

II. Marine and Freshwater Fish

Freshwater Fish

Freshwater fish are fish that spend some or all of their lives in freshwater, such as rivers and lakes, with a salinity of less than 0.05 per cent. These environments differ from marine conditions in many ways, the most obvious being the difference in levels of salinity. To survive freshwater, the fish need a range of physiological adaptations.

41.24 per cent of all known species of fish are found in freshwater. This is primarily due to the rapid speciation that the scattered habitats make possible. When dealing with ponds and lakes, one might use the same basic models of speciation as when studying island biogeography.

Freshwater fish differ physiologically from salt water fish in several respects. Their gills must be able to diffuse dissolved gasses while keeping the salts in the body fluids inside. Their scales reduce water diffusion through the skin: freshwater fish that have lost too many scales will die. They also have well developed kidneys to reclaim salts from body fluids before excretion.

Many species of fish do reproduce in freshwater, but spend most of their adult lives in the sea. These are known as anadromous fish, and include, for instance, salmon, trout and three-spined stickleback. Some other kinds of fish are, on the contrary, born in salt water, but live most of or parts of their adult lives in freshwater; for instance the eels. These are known as catadromous fish.

Migrating Fish

Species migrating between marine and freshwaters need adaptations for both environments; when in salt water they need to keep the bodily salt concentration on a level lower than the surroundings, and vice versa. Many species solve this problem by associating different habitats with different stages of life. Both eels, anadromous salmoniform fish and the sea lamprey have different tolerances in salinity in different stages of their lives.

Freshwater Fishes of India

India is rich with inland freshwater fish, with about 940 species known from its rivers, lakes and estuaries. This constitutes about 38 per cent of the Indian Ichthyofauna and are of considerable economic and scientific value. Of these about 500 species are primary freshwater fish with around 65 per cent endemic, cloistered in the two hot spots of India, the Western Ghats and the North East. Many of these are unique to certain stretches of the various rivers especially the upper reaches and many more new species are being reported from these forested hills. However, threats to these faunaare aplenty, with urbanization, deforestation, habitat loss, pollution, over-harvesting, and culture of exotics. The only way for a fish enthusiast to save the fish and its habitats is creating awareness among the people. In this context, knowledge of the fish fauna of a region is the first step towards conservation.

Freshwater Fish of Australia

Freshwater fish of Australia are limited to approximately 280 species, even though the Australian continent is larger than the contiguous United States.

A large proportion of these species are endemic to Australia. Australia is unique in that the Percicthyidae (Temperate Perches) family and other families suspected in reality to lie within it (*e.g.* Gadopsidae, Nannopercidae) have risen to prominence in and dominate many of its freshwater systems, in contrast to the Northern Hemisphere where freshwater fish faunas are overwhelmingly dominated by the Cyprinidae (Carp) family. (no Cyprinid species is native to Australia). Due to the illegal introduction of Carp (*Cyprinus carpio*) the Cyprinidae family is now present in a destructive form in Australia. The Galaxiidae have also risen to unusual prominence in Australia, with the bulk of the world's Galaxias species found in Australia and its neighbouring land mass New Zealand.

The most important freshwater system in Australia is the Murray-Darling Basin which drains approximately 13 per cent of the continent and contains some of Australia's most significant freshwater fish species including the Murray Cod, Australia's largest freshwater fish.

Australian freshwater fish have not fared well since European settlement of Australia in 1788. The majority of Australian freshwater fishes are poorly understood and are under threat due to human activities such clearing of riparian vegetation and siltation associated with agricultural practices, snag removal, overfishing, river regulation through dams and weirs, introduced fish and diseases. Two native fish populations that may have been separate species or sub-species, the Richmond River Cod and the Brisbane River Cod, are extinct, and a number of other species are listed asendangered or critically endangered.

References

Borgstrøm, Reidar and Hansen, Lars Petter (red): *Fisk i ferskvann - et samspill mellom bestander, miljø og forvaltning*, Landbruksforlaget 2000.

Jonsson, Bror: «Fiskene» i *Norges dyr - Fiskene 1*, Cappelen 1992.

Freshwater Aquarium Fish Species

A vast number of species of fish have been successfully kept in the home freshwater aquarium. This list gives some examples of the most commonly kept species.

- ☆ Bichirs and redfish
- ☆ Catfish
- ☆ Armored suckermouth catfish (plecos)
- ☆ Airbreathing catfish
- ☆ Banjo catfish
- ☆ Talking catfish
- ☆ Squeakers and upside-down catfish
- ☆ Shark catfish
- ☆ Sea catfish
- ☆ Sheatfish
- ☆ Bagrid catfishes
- ☆ Long-whiskered catfish
- ☆ Tetras
- ☆ Pencil fishes
- ☆ Hatchetfish
- ☆ Headstanders
- ☆ Serrasalminae (pacus, piranhas, and silver dollars)
- ☆ Lake Malawi cichlids
- ☆ Lake Tanganyika cichlids
- ☆ Lake Victoria cichlids
- ☆ American cichlids
- ☆ Dwarf cichlids
- ☆ Barbs
- ☆ Cold-water cyprinids
- ☆ Danios and other danionins
- ☆ Rasboras
- ☆ Gobies
- ☆ Killifish
- ☆ Labyrinth fish
- ☆ Guppies and mollies
- ☆ Platies and swordtails
- ☆ Gambusia
- ☆ Loaches
- ☆ Pufferfish

- ☆ Rainbowfish
- ☆ Spiny eels
- ☆ Sunfish
- ☆ Gar

Marine Aquarium Fishes

Angel Fish (Large)

These big beauties are considered to be quite hardy, but because of their size may present a significant challenge to the potential keeper. They need huge aquariums, up to 180 gallons to house one for its entire lifespan.[1] Two angels might be kept in the same aquarium provided it is a large aquarium, they are properly acclimated as juveniles, and they have very different colouring and body shape.[2] However, because all Angelfish have essentially the same diet, mixing them is a feat that should be left to only advanced keepers. None are reef safe, and a potential owner should be aware that they need to have plenty of vegetable matter in their diet. They undergo major changes in colouration while maturing, and unless specified given descriptions are for adult specimens.[3][4][5]

Angel Fish (Dwarf)

Although Dwarf Angelfish are smaller and generally more manageable than their larger counterparts, they still have some specific care requirements. They are omnivores, but plenty of vegetable matter, preferably in the form of macroalgae, should be provided for their grazing pleasure.[20] Their suitability for reef tanks is hotly debated,[2] so add at your own risk. Specimens that have been successfully maintained inreef aquaria include the Flame and Coral Beauty angels. However, for obvious reasons they should not be put into tanks with expensive decorative macroalgae.[21][22]

Anthias

Although Anthias resemble damsels in shape and size, the two should never be confused. Where damsels are the goats of the Saltwater world, Anthias (also called "Fairy Basslets in) are finicky and many starve to death in captivity. In the wild, they eat zooplankton, and will not accept anything but in the aquarium. They also need to be fed nearly constantly, three times a day at least. The best way to ensure the health and longevity of an Anthias is to attach a refugium where you can grow copepods to "drip" into the display tank. Unlike many other saltwater aquarium inhabitants, they can be kept in groups.[35]

Bass and Groupers

In this exceedingly large group of fish, few are considered proper aquarium inhabitants, for various reasons including diet and size. Bassesvary greatly from species to species. Appropriate research should be done before purchasing a specimen. Many unsuspecting hobbyists bring home cute little specimens of popular aquarium fish such as the lyretail grouper, only to realize several months later that they do not have the resources to care for a meter-long that may cost hundreds of dollars a month to feed.[36][37][38][39][40]

Basslets and Assessors

Basslets and Assessors are small, long bodied fish strongly resembling Anthias. Their care requirements, however, are closer to those of damsels. They should be kept individually, and generally not with other fish of similar shape and colour. Feeding is easy: they will generally eat any meaty foods offered. Good water quality should be maintained at all times.[43]

Batfish

Batfish are gorgeous and striking fish that are not common in aquaria for one major reason: they get huge. A two or three hundred gallon tank is needed for one, minimum, and larger is better. They start out as tiny, manageable-looking cuties, which often fools aquarists into purchasing them for their small aquariums. However they quickly grow to gargantuan proportions, and require large amounts of food as well as space, so beware. They are not reef safe and should be fed plenty of large meaty foods. Batfish change greatly as they grow, however the potential aquarist is most likely to see them in their juvenile form, so that is the description of the colouration here. They all have generally the same body shape: disk-like with tall dorsal and anal fins, similar to a Freshwater Angelfish.

Blennies

Blennies are popular aquarium fish, and for good reason. They are peaceful, colorful, and many are downright helpful. For example, the aptly named Lawnmower Blenny will keep your green algae well trimmed and presentable. With the exception of Fang Blennies, Blennies are totally reef safe- in fact a reef environment is really best for them because they can be shy and the intricate rockwork of a reef provides ample hiding spaces. They are omnivores and should be fed a varied diet of frozen or live foods and plant matter. Blennies do not have teeth or functional jaw, so food must be small enough for them to swallow whole.

Blennies are often confused with Gobies, but there is an easy way to tell the difference. Gobies have two distinct dorsal fins, Blennies have a single dorsal fin that runs the length of their body. Also, Gobies' pelvic fins are fused to form a sucker, similar to Remoras.[45]

Boxfish and Blowfish

Members of the family Tetraodontidae, Boxfish, Blowfish or Pufferfish and their cousins Cowfishes and Porcupinefishes can be very personable and quirky pets, for the prepared.

They are not thought of as an ordinary aquarium tank mate, but are quickly gaining popularity. They do pose a hazard in the community tank however. They are capable of releasing a very powerful toxin which can kill other fish and in some cases, the boxfish itself. They generally only use it when threatened or dying, but can become disturbed easily with aggressive tank mates or overcrowded aquarium. Generally they are reef safe, though they will pick at invertebrates if not fed well enough.

Many people think puffed up Pufferfish, like in the picture, are cute, but an owner should never subject their pet to this as they are often unable to expel the air should they be out of the water. To prevent this, never remove a puffer from the water.[46]

Butterflyfish

Butterflyfish, when properly cared for, can make beautiful and distinctive additions to fish only marine aquariums. Often large and usually not suited for those with smaller aquariums, nor those of the faint of heart. Nevertheless, when fed a varied diet and kept in pristine conditions, Butterflyfish will usually thrive. That is, if you choose the right species. With Butterflyfish, usually a fish is going to survive, or it's not. Many species simply cannot be kept in captivity, and potential keepers must take care to only purchase those species that have a fighting chance. Also, be very picky about which specimen you choose- any sign of mishandling should be taken as a red flag.

The following species are relatively hardy and an experienced aquarist should have no trouble with them, so long as they are diligent.[47]

Cardinalfish

One of the few groups of shoaling fish commonly available to marine aquarists, Cardinalfish are nocturnal and tend to be quite shy. They require meaty foods and will often not take prepared foods such as flakes and tablets. For the best chance of success, keep a wide variety of frozen foods on hand. In the event of a hunger strike, they will almost always take adult brine shrimp. As far as other care requirements they are similar to damsels: not picky. So long as they are properly acclimated, they tolerate a wide range of parameters. A marine aqaurist should watch the ammonia/ nitrite levels of the environment, as cardinalfish are particularly sensitive to these chemicals.[48]

Chromis

Chromis are perhaps the ultimate reef fish. Generally peaceful, most species are easy to take care of and quite colorful. Like anthias, they will school, but in many cases this tendency disappears as they age. They are, nevertheless, at least ambivalent with their own species, as well as completely reef safe. Like Damsels and Anemonefish, their close cousins, Chromis are omnivores and will accept most foods offered. A flake staple is usually sufficient, but for best color and health supplement with frozen and live foods when possible.[50]

Clownfish

Clownfish, more technically known as **Anemonefish**, are the classic aquarium fish. Both hardy and attractive, they are perhaps best known for their symbiotic relationship with Sea Anemones, a relative of coral. In the wild, Anemonefish are always found with a host, leading many potential keepers to believe that an anemone is necessary to keep them. Anemonefish are easy to keep, but their cnidarian counterparts are inordinately finicky and need high light levels, and luckily Anemonefish will thrive without them. Aquarists often find that Anemonefish will host in other things, from corals and Feather Duster Worms to powerheads and other equipment. Anemonefish care is identical to that ofDamselfish, as they are actually very closely related.[51][52]

Damselfish

All Damselfish can be considered reef-safe, sometimes excluding larger, more aggressive Dascyllus varieties. Some Damselfish will host inanemones like clownfish. Most Damselfish are aggressive and difficult to catch once you put them in an aquarium.

Damselfish change gender as they grow larger and older. Small damselfish are ungendered. Eventually, they become males if no males prevent them from doing so. One or sometimes two males live with a female and guard over the eggs. Females are the largest fish and dominant over the males and juveniles. They will not allow other females into an area they have claimed as their territory without a fight. They may not allow new males or juveniles, either. Aggression increases with each change.[51][53][54]

Dragonets

Dragonets are often mis-categorized as gobies or blennies by fish sellers. They are bottom-dwelling fish that constantly hunt tiny invertebrates for food. Most starve to death in a marine aquarium unless you provide a refugium or place for the invertebrates to reproduce safely without any fish being able to reach them.[57][58]

Filefish

Less often kept than their relatives the Triggerfish and Puffers there are many filefish that make good aquarium residents, and a few that require specialized diets making it hard to sustain them in an aquarium.[63][64]

Frogfish

A type of Anglerfish, Frogfish are ambush predators with huge mouths. They are capable of eating fish up to twice their length so care should be taken in choosing tank mates.[65]

Hawk Fish

Attractive and relatively small, Hawkfish make excellent additions to fish only or FOWLR aquariums. With extreme caution taken, they could be kept in reef aquariums, but because of their propensity to eat small ornamental shrimps and other mobile invertebrates (usually leavingsessile invertebrates alone) they are not considered reef safe. Lacking a swim bladder, Hawkfish can often be found resting in crevices of rocks or among the branches of corals or gorgonians. Hawkfish are easy to care for and not picky at all about water quality. A varied diet, including spirulina and small meaty foods like Mysis is recommended.[69]

Jawfish

Jawfish are burrowers and require a sandy substrate of sufficient depth.[70]

Lionfish

"Lionfish" specifically refer to the genus *Pterois* within the family Scorpaenidae. They have venomous spines and should be treated with caution.[71] Other species within Scorpaenidae but outside *Pterois* may also have "lionfish" in their common names. Feeder goldfish are not the proper nutrition for a lion fish.

Pipefish

Pipefish are relatives of seahorses and require a similar level of care. They should only be bought by experienced aquarium owners. Captive bred specimens are sometimes available, and are significantly more likely to survive.[73]

Scorpionfish

Because they are relatively inactive fish, most species can be kept in smaller aquariums than other equally large fish, and 30 gallon tanks are not unusual. Because they are capable of eating fish that are surprisingly large, but will often be picked at by fish that eat invertebrates a species tank is often set up for them. Some fish will never accept anything but live food, typically these specimens are fed on gut packedguppies, mollies, or ghost shrimp. Similarly to the lionfish, care should be taken when handling these fish as they are also venomous.[78][79]

Seahorse

It takes a special aquarist to maintain these delicate beauties. A potential keeper must be dedicated and willing to throw artistic creativity to the winds- as what seahorses need is not always beautiful. They require taller tanks, live/frozen food, and many hitching posts, as well as very peaceful tank mates. In fact, beginners would be well-advised not to mix seahorses with any other species until they have more experience.

Seahorses found in stores are generally Captive Bred, but occasionally one might find a wild caught (WC) specimen. WC Seahorses should only be purchased by seahorse experts who are going to breed them, as they tend to be finicky and most are endangered in the wild.

One of the advantages of Seahorses is that many species stay small and can (in fact, some *should*) be kept in smaller tanks, making them ideal for aquarists who are pressed for space or money.[82][83]

Seahorses are among the few popular marine aquarium species that can be temperate. Species vary in their temperature requirement, so here an extra category has been added.

Sharks

Until recently only a few benthic species of shark, such as hornsharks, leopard sharks, catsharks, and zebra sharks, had survived in aquarium conditions for up to a year or more. This gave rise to the belief that sharks, as well as being difficult to capture and transport, were difficult to care for. A better knowledge of sharks has led to more species (including the large pelagic sharks) being able to be kept for far longer. At the same time, transportation techniques have improved and long distance movement of sharks is becoming easier.[1] One shark that never had been successfully held in captivity for long was the great white. But in September 2004 the Monterey Bay Aquarium successfully kept a young female great white shark for 198 days before releasing her back into the wild.

Tangs

Tangs generally feed on algae, though there are a few carnivorous species. Most tangs will not tolerate other fish the same color and/or shape as them. They have a spine on their tails that can cut open other fish and unprotected hands. All tangs should be given plenty of swimming room; try to have at least a 4' tank. Contrary to popular belief they will tolerate smaller (4' to 5') tanks just fine but tend to live better in larger tanks, over 5'.[89]

Triggerfish

While they are generally considered monsters that will chomp invertebrates, a few species can make great reef fish. Other more aggressive species such as the Undulated Trigger, and Clown Trigger will sometimes be so aggressive that it is necessary to keep as the sole inhabitant of the aquarium. All will require large tanks, with good filtration.[94][95][96]

Wrasse

A diverse group of fish with an equally wide range of characteristics. Some wrasse species are aggressive towards small fish andinvertebrates, others are reef safe. Some are quite hardy, some typically die within weeks.[98][99]

References

1. Michael, Scott (December 2003). "Beautiful Holocanthus Angels". *Aquarium Fish Magazine*. pp. 58–64.
2. Fenner, Robert (2001). *The Conscientious Marine Fishkeeper*. Neptune City, NJ: THF Publications.ISBN [[Special:BookSources/978-1-890087-20-9 | 978-1-890087-20-
3. "Aquarium Fish: Large Angels in the Home Aquarium, Part 1". Retrieved 2008-12-18.
4. "Aquarium Fish: Large Angels in the Home Aquarium, Part II". Retrieved 2008-12-18.
5. "Marine Angelfishes, Family Pomacanthidae". Retrieved 2008-12-18.
6. Froese, Rainer and Pauly, Daniel, eds. (2008)."*Genicanthus bellus*" in FishBase. July 2008 version.
7. Froese, Rainer and Pauly, Daniel, eds. (2008)."*Holocanthus bermudensis*" in FishBase. July 2008 version.
8. Froese, Rainer and Pauly, Daniel, eds. (2008)."*Pomacanthus zonipectus*" in FishBase. July 2008 version.

9. Froese, Rainer and Pauly, Daniel, eds. (2008)." *Pomacanthus imperator*" in FishBase. July 2008 version.
10. Froese, Rainer and Pauly, Daniel, eds. (2008)." *Pomacanthus paru*" in FishBase. July 2008 version.
11. Froese, Rainer and Pauly, Daniel, eds. (2008)." *Pomacanthus arcuatus*" in FishBase. July 2008 version.
12. Froese, Rainer and Pauly, Daniel, eds. (2008)." *Pomacanthus maculosus*" in FishBase. July 2008 version.
13. Froese, Rainer and Pauly, Daniel, eds. (2008)." *Pomacanthus semicirculatus*" in FishBase. July 2008 version.
14. Froese, Rainer and Pauly, Daniel, eds. (2008)." *Pomacanthus navarchus*" in FishBase. July 2008 version.
15. Froese, Rainer and Pauly, Daniel, eds. (2008)." *Holocanthus passer*" in FishBase. July 2008 version.
16. Froese, Rainer and Pauly, Daniel, eds. (2008)." *Holacanthus ciliaris*" in FishBase. July 2008 version.
17. Froese, Rainer and Pauly, Daniel, eds. (2008). " *Pygoplites diacanthus*" in FishBase. July 2008 version.
18. Froese, Rainer and Pauly, Daniel, eds. (2008)." *Genicanthus semifasciatus*" in FishBase. July 2008 version.
19. Froese, Rainer and Pauly, Daniel, eds. (2011)." *Apolemichthys xanthurus*" in FishBase. November 2011 version.
20. Hargreaves, Vincent (2006). *The Complete Book of the Marine Aquarium*. San Diego, CA: Thunder Bay Press.ISBN [[Special:BookSources/9871571457622 9871571457622
21. "What a Darling Little Angel: The Genus Centropyge". Retrieved 2008-12-18.
22. "The Pygmy Angelfishes". Retrieved 2008-12-18.
23. Froese, Rainer and Pauly, Daniel, eds. (2008)." *Centropyge multifasciata*" in FishBase. July 2008 version.
24. Froese, Rainer and Pauly, Daniel, eds. (2008)." *Centropyge bispinosus*" in FishBase. July 2008 version.
25. Froese, Rainer and Pauly, Daniel, eds. (2008)." *Centropyge argi*" in FishBase. July 2008 version.
26. Froese, Rainer and Pauly, Daniel, eds. (2008)." *Centropyge eibli*" in FishBase. July 2008 version.
27. Froese, Rainer and Pauly, Daniel, eds. (2008)." *Centropyge loricula*" in FishBase. July 2008 version.

28. Froese, Rainer and Pauly, Daniel, eds. (2008)." *Centropyge vroliki*" in FishBase. July 2008 version.
29. Froese, Rainer and Pauly, Daniel, eds. (2008)." *Centropyge heraldi*" in FishBase. July 2008 version.
30. Froese, Rainer and Pauly, Daniel, eds. (2008)." *Centropyge flavissima*" in FishBase. July 2008 version
31. Froese, Rainer and Pauly, Daniel, eds. (2008)." *Centropyge acanthops*" in FishBase. July 2008 version.
32. Froese, Rainer and Pauly, Daniel, eds. (2008)." *Centropyge flavicauda*" in FishBase. December 2008 version.
33. Froese, Rainer and Pauly, Daniel, eds. (2008)." *Centropyge potteri*" in FishBase. July 2008 version.
34. Froese, Rainer and Pauly, Daniel, eds. (2008)." *Centropyge ferrugata*" in FishBase. July 2008 version.
35. "Anthiinae - the Fancy Basses". Retrieved 2008-12-18.
36. "Aquarium Fish: The Hinds of the Genus Cephalopholis". Retrieved 2008-12-18.
37. "The Basses, Family Serranidae". Retrieved 2008-12-18.
38. "The Basses Called Hinds, Genus Cephalopholis". Retrieved 2008-12-18.
39. "The Soapfishes, Family Grammistidae, or Tribe Grammistini of the Serranidae, in part, or.". Retrieved 2008-12-18.
40. "Some Guys Like 'em Big:The Genus Plectropomus". Retrieved 2008-12-18.
41. "The Comet (Calloplesiops altivelis)". Retrieved 2008-12-18.
42. "The Roundhead Called the Marine Betta, Calloplesiops altivelis, Family Plesiopsidae". Retrieved 2008-12-18.
43. "Grammas". Retrieved 2008-12-18.
44. "Yellow Assessor, Assessor flavissimus". Retrieved 2008-12-19.
45. "Blennioids: Blennies and Blenny-Like Fishes". Retrieved 2008-12-18.
46. "All My Puffers, Tobies, Box, Porcupine, Cowfishes". Retrieved 2008-12-18.
47. "Butterflyfishes; Separating the Good Ones and Those You Don't Want". Retrieved 2008-12-18.
48. "Cardinals Not Named Pujols, Womack, or Edmonds:The Genus Cheilodipterus". Retrieved 2008-12-18.
49. Michael, Scott (2005). *Reef Aquarium Fishes, 500+ Essential-To-Know Species*. Neptune City, NJ: T.F.H Publications, Inc. ISBN 978-1-890087-89-0.
50. "Friendly Damsels? It Can't be Possible!...The Genus Chromis". Retrieved 2008-12-18.

51. "The Damsel and Anemonefishes, Family Pomacentridae". Retrieved 2008-12-18.
52. "Time to Quit Clownin' Around: The Subfamily Amphiprioninae". Retrieved 2008-12-18.
53. "Tiny (and one not so tiny) Terrors of the Sea: Damsels of the Genus Dascyllus". Retrieved 2008-12-18.
54. "Small-Man's Complex: The Genus Stegastes". Retrieved 2008-12-18.
55. "Firefishes, Dartfishes, Wormfishes, Family Microdesmidae, Subfamily Ptereleotrinae". Retrieved 2008-12-18.
56. "Worms Not Found in the Sandbed: The Genus Ptereleotris". Retrieved 2008-12-18.
57. "Mandarins, Psychedelic "Gobies", Dragonets, Scooter Blennies.YAH! Family Callionymidae". Retrieved 2008-12-18.
58. ".I'd like to buy a Mandarin!". Retrieved 2008-12-19.
59. "Mandarinfish, Synchiropus splendidus (syn. Pterosynchiropus splendidus)". Retrieved 2008-12-19.
60. "The Moray Eels, Family Muraenidae". Retrieved 2008-12-18.
61. "A Serpent For Your Reef Tank:A Look at Fish-Safe Eels". Retrieved 2008-12-18.
62. "Behold the Dragon!". Retrieved 2008-12-18.
63. "Filefishes, Family Monacanthidae". Retrieved 2008-12-18.
64. "Files Not Meant For Your Toolbox (or Reef Aquarium!):The Genus Pervagor". Retrieved 2008-12-18.
65. "The Bizarre Frogfishes, Anglerfishes, Order". Retrieved 2008-12-18.
66. "Mulling Over the Goatfishes, Family Mullidae". Retrieved 2008-12-18.
67. "Aquarium Fish: Gobies of the Genus Amblygobius". Retrieved 2008-12-18.
68. "The Fish Of Which Dreams (or Nightmares) Are Made: The Genus Valenciennea". Retrieved 2008-12-18.
69. "Hawkfishes, Family Cirrhitidae". Retrieved 2008-12-18.
70. "Let's Jaw About Jawfish". Retrieved 2008-12-18.
71. "The Scorpionfishes We Call Lions, Family Scorpaenidae, subfamily Pteroinae". Retrieved 2008-12-18.
72. "Twinspot Lionfish (Dendrochirus biocellatus)". Retrieved 2008-12-18.
73. "There's More to Pipes Than Just PVC:The Genus Doryrhamphus and Other Pipefish". Retrieved 2008-12-18.
74. "The Dottybacks". Retrieved 2008-12-18.
75. "The Fishes We Call Rabbits, Family Siganidae". Retrieved 2008-12-18.

76. "You Silly Rabbit: The Genus Siganus". Retrieved 2008-12-18.
77. "Blue-Lined Rabbitfish, Siganis doliatus". Retrieved 2008-12-18.
78. "The Rhinopias spp. The Ultimate Scorpionfishes". Retrieved 2008-12-18.
79. "Scorpionfish: Masters of Camouflage". Retrieved 2008-12-18.
80. "Aquarium Fish: Leaf Scorpionfish (Taenianotus triacanthus)". Retrieved 2008-12-18.
81. Michael, Scott (2005). *Reef Aquarium Fishes, 500+ Essential-To-Know Species*. Neptune City, NJ: T.F.H Publications, Inc. p. 54. ISBN 978-1-890087-89-0.
82. "Seahorse Care: A basic guide to starting your first herd". Retrieved 2008-12-18.
83. "Saddle Up, Cowboy! The Genus Hippocampus". Retrieved 2008-12-18.
84. "Squirrel- and Soldierfishes, Family Holocentridae". Retrieved 2008-12-18.
85. "But They Don't Look Like a Rat with a Fuzzy Tail:The Family Holocentridae". Retrieved 2008-12-18.
86. "KEEPING SHARKS IN THE HOME AQUARIUM". Retrieved 2008-12-18.
87. "Sharks For The Home Aquarium?". Retrieved 2008-12-18.
88. "The Epaulette Sharks (*Hemiscyllium* spp.) - The Perfect Aquarium Sharks". Retrieved 2008-12-18.
89. "Surgeons, Tangs and Doctorfishes, Family Acanthuridae". Retrieved 2008-12-18.
90. "Dussumieri Tang, Acanthurus dussumieri". Retrieved 2008-12-19.
91. "The Venerable Scopas Tang". Retrieved 2008-12-18.
92. "Redoing the Seafloor with Tile: The Subfamily Malacanthinae, Part I". Retrieved 2008-12-18.
93. "Redoing the Seafloor with Tile: The Subfamily Malacanthinae, Part II". Retrieved 2008-12-18.
94. "Aquarium Fish: Triggerfish". Retrieved 2008-12-18.
95. "Bruisers and Cruisers, the Triggerfishes, Family Balistidae". Retrieved 2008-12-18.
96. "Triggerfishes". Retrieved 2008-12-18.
97. "The Crosshatch Triggerfish (*Xanthichthys mento*)". Retrieved 2008-12-18.
98. "The Wrasses, Family Labridae". Retrieved 2008-12-18.
99. "Everybody Sing Together!:The Genus Coris". Retrieved 2008-12-18.
100. "The Cheeklined Maori Wrasse (*Cheilinus diagrammus*)". Retrieved 2008-12-18.
101. "Leopard wrasses (*Macropharyngodon* spp.)". Retrieved 2008-12-18.

III. Transportation of Fish

Introduction

There are two basic transport systems for live fish - the closed system and the open system. The closed system is a sealed container in which all the requirements for survival are self-contained. The simplest of these is a sealed plastic bag partly filled with water and oxygen. The open system consists of water-filled containers in which the requirements for survival are supplied continuously from outside sources. The simplest of these is a small tank with an aerator stone.

These systems will be discussed with respect to the problems of fish preparation for transport, types of vehicles and equipments, problems of water quality and its changes during transport, and chemical aids used during fish transport.

There is ample literature on fish transport and associated problems; however, the literary sources overlap and give partly differing interpretations of the recommended ways of transport. These are the reasons why this survey aims at comprising mainly those published results which have been fully verified in practice and which are, therefore, reliably instructive.

The basic factors and principles associated with any live fish transport systems, or influencing them, are evaluated before the actual ways of fish transport are commented on.

Factors and Principles Associated with Fish Transport

1. Quality of Fish

The quality of fish transported is a decisive criterion. The fish to be transported must be healthy and in good condition. Weakened individuals should be eliminated from the consignment, particularly when the temperature during shipment is high. When the fish are of poor quality, even a great reduction of fish density in the transport container fails to prevent fish losses. Weak fish are killed at a much higher rate than fish in good condition when the transport time is longer.

A need for adapting the fish to a lower water temperature may also arise before transport. Natural ice is used to cool the water; the ice of carbonic acid should be avoided. As a guide ratio, 25 kg of ice will cool 1 000 litres of water by 2°C. If the water contains fish during the cooling process, the temperature drop should not be faster than 5°C per hour. Direct contact of fish with ice should be prevented at the same time. The total temperature difference should not be greater than 12–15°C, with respect to the species and age of the fish

2. Oxygen

The most important single factor in transporting fish is providing an adequate level of dissolved oxygen. However, an abundance of oxygen within a tank does not necessarily indicate that the fish are in good condition. The ability of fish to use oxygen depends on their tolerance to stress, water temperature, pH, and concentrations of carbon dioxide and metabolic products such as ammonia.

The crucial factors underlying oxygen consumption by fish in relation with oxygen metabolism during transport are fish weight and water temperature. Heavier fish and those transported in warmer water need more oxygen. For instance, if the water temperature increases by 10°C (*e.g.*, from 10 to 20°C), oxygen consumption is about doubled. From the point of view of fish transport, for each 0.5°C rise in temperature, the fish load should be reduced by about 5.6 per cent; conversely, for each 0.5°C decrease in temperature, the load can be increased by about 5.6 per cent. Oxygen consumption also increases with fish excitement by handling. Excitement increases oxygen demand three to five times.

In water provided with an unlimited amount of oxygen, a fish at rest will consume a minimum amount of oxygen. In a fish transport system, the fish will require more than the minimum amount since they are not at rest. Furthermore, if they are excited at loading or disturbed during transport they may consume near to the maximum amount.

The amount of oxygen a fish consumes also depends on the amount of oxygen available. At high levels, the fish will consume at a steady rate. When water oxygen levels are low, fish consume lower amounts of oxygen than when oxygen levels are high, despite the degree of activity.

Fish transport systems often contain water with oxygen levels that do not provide enough oxygen required to satisfy the fish bodies. To offset this predicament, the fish will shift its metabolism to use the stored oxygen of the body. This condition is likened to that of a man who is at rest and suddenly performs strenuous activity before a proportionate amount of oxygen is taken in. For the man and the fish, an oxygen "debt" is created which must be repaid when favourable oxygen conditions are experienced.

The first hour after loading is a particularly critical time for fish in respect to their oxygen needs. They are excited and require a large amount of oxygen with a short time for adjustment. Significant differences in oxygen demand exist also within fish families. As asserted, for instance, when water temperature increases (4–14°C) during transport, the fry of*Coregonus lavaretus* consume 2.4 times more oxygen than the fry of *C. albula*. Fish size is also important. A large fish consumes less oxygen per unit weight than does a small one. Oxygen levels of water for most warm water fish should be above 5 $mg.1^{-1}$ for normal conditions. This level should prevent oxygen from becoming a major stress factor.

3. pH, Carbon Dioxide and Ammonia

Water quality is a function of the load of fish concentration and the length of time for which the fish are transported. The source of the water used during transport must have been tested before dispatching a mass consignment of fish. The water pH level is a control factor because the proportions of toxic ammonia and CO_2 contents are direct functions of pH.

With increasing transport time, CO_2 production through fish respiration shifts water pH towards acidity. Water pH levels about 7–8 are considered as optimum. Rapid changes in pH stress fish, but buffers can be used to stabilize the water pH during fish transport. The organic buffer trishydroxylmethylaminomethane is quite effective in fresh and salt water. It is highly soluble, stable and easily applied. This buffer has been used on 29 species of fish with no deleterious effects. Levels of 1.3–2.6 g/litre are recommended for routine transport of fish.

Elevated carbon dioxide concentrations are detrimental to fish and can be a limiting factor in fish transport. A product of fish and bacterial respiration, CO_2 acidifies transport water. Although this reduces the percentage of un-ionized ammonia in the water, it also reduces the oxygen-carrying capacity of fish blood. Fish may succumb if CO_2 levels are high, even though oxygen levels are seemingly adequate. Trout appear to tolerate carbon dioxide at levels less than 15 mg 1^{-1} in the presence of reasonable oxygen and temperature, but become distressed when carbon dioxide levels approach 25 mg 1^{-1}

Adequate ventilation is a necessity for transport units. Tight covers or lids on the units can result in a buildup of CO_2 which will stress the fish. Aeration of the water will reduce concentrations of dissolved CO_2, if there is adequate ventilation.

Another important factor is chlorine concentration in water, although - like carbon dioxide - chlorine is also removed from the water by aeration. The concentration of 0.5 mg/litre is considered as dangerous, though even lower chlorine levels, *e.g.*, 0.2 mg/litre disturb the fish respiration mechanism considerably (Shevchenko, 1978).

Ammonia (NH_3) builds up in transport water due to protein metabolism of the fish and bacterial action on the waste. Decreasing metabolic rate of the fish by lowering the water temperature, and thus lessening fish activity, reduces the production of NH_3. The production of NH_3 by bacterial action can be decreased by shipping fish only after food has been witheld long enough to void the stomach and intestine.

Temperature and time of last feeding are important factors regulating ammonia excretion. For example, trout held in water at 1°C excrete 66 per cent less ammonia than those held in 11°C water, and fish starved for 63 h before shipment produce half as much ammonia as recently fed fish. Fish larger than 10 cm should be starved at least 48 h; those 20 cm and larger should be starved 72 h The amount of un-ionized ammonia increases as water temperatures and pH increase.

4. Temperature

Water temperature is an important factor. When water temperature is low, the pH remains higher and fish metabolism decreases. The generally applicable zones of optimum temperatures for transported fish are 6–8°C for cold-water fishes and 10–12°C for warm-water fishes in summer, 3–5°C for cold-water fishes and 5–6°C for warm-water fishes in spring and autumn, and 1–2°C for all in winter.

5. Density and Activity of Transported Fish

Consideration should also be given to the factor of space. The ratio of the volume of the fish transported and the transport water should not exceed 1:3. Heavier individuals, *e.g.*, parent fish can be transported in a fish: water weight ratio of 1:2 to 1:3, but with smaller organisms this ratio decreases to 1:100 to 1:200. In the FRG recommendation (1979), the following ratios between fish weight and the volume of water in the transport tank (with good aeration of water at a temperature of 8–12°C during shorter transports lasting (1–2 h) are table carp 1:1, stock carp 1:1.5, table rainbow trout 1:3, stock trout 1:4.5, stock pike 1:2, herbivorous fishes 1:2.

The time of shipment experts its influence mainly on the larval stages of cyprinids; transport longer than 24 h always means some risk, although all conditions are otherwise good (Pecha, Berka and Kouril, 1983).

Salmonid stock densities in the transport container are always lower than the standard densities for cyprinids, owing to a higher oxygen consumption and a lower critical CO_2 concentration.

6. Biochemical Changes and Stress in Transported Fish

Shipment conditions also influence the composition of fish blood and the parameters of blood serum biochemistry. Increased temperature and a lower fish weight-to-water concentration ratio mean a higher number of erythrocytes and a greater haemoglobin concentration of fish blood. When fish were transported at higher densities, the levels of corticoids and glucose in the plasma increased and were retained when the transport was finished. Although mortality as a direct consequence of transport was low, the secondary effects of stress were responsible for delayed mortality, caused by the consequences of osmoregulatory disfunction and disease. It should also be noted that release of fish at the destination can be the most critical stage of the transport process. The fish are under some degree of stress in the transport unit and sudden exposure to water of different characteristies or low quality will further stress the fish, often beyond what they can stand. Poor-quality water may mean freshly pumped ground water with low oxygen or high carbon dioxide content. Different characteristics of water often mean a pH, temperature or gas saturation difference between the transport unit and the receiving water.

7. General Notes

Finally, several concluding notes, or technical and organizational considerations, can be quoted from the literature. The majority of authors recommend, irrespective of the guide numbers of stock density during transport, to consider the specific transport conditions in each case and to change the basic guide numbers if such a change appears necessary after a brief test. It is also recommended to use a fish density at which the time of transport can be prolonged at least 1.5 times to prevent the consequences of a possible delay during transport, *e.g.*, failure of a truck, failure to stick to the train or plane schedule, etc. When fish are transported for acclimation, or when endangered species are transported, the stock density should be lower: in such cases the economic aspects are not of primary importance and 100 per cent survival is required. Nevertheless, the economic side of transport can never be neglected; hence, when the transport costs are high and the value of fish of transported comparatively low, the stock density in the transport units can be increased though losses of fish may be expected to be higher.

Closed Systems of Fish Transport

The closed systems are represented by polyethylene bags and other sealed transport units. They are used mainly for the transport of the early fry, but also brood fish. The transport of fry in polyethylene bags with oxygen is particularly widespread in the world, being used as a very effective method. It substantially reduces the total volume and weight of transport water, enables public transport to be used for fish-transport purposes, makes it possible to prolong the transport time, and is economically advantageous.

1. Polyethylene Bags

The bags used for fish transport in water with oxygen atmosphere are produced in a number of modifications. They are manufactured from a thin (soft) or thicker (hard) transparent polyethylene foil and usually have the shape of sack or sleeve. The bags of the traditional shape (sacs) usually have the dimensions of 0.8–1.1 × 0.35–0.45 m. The upper end is usually fully open. The bottom either has a seam in the middle or consists of a rectangular piece of foil; the latter variant is better because it helps avoid losses of the fish squeezed in the corners. For safety reasons, the bags are sometimes duplicated: a thin (soft) bag is inserted in another thin bag, or a thin bag forms a lining in a thicker (harder) bag.

The other type of bags has the form of a sleeve. Its width usually is 0.4–0.5 m. The final length of the sleeve depends on where the sleeve is cut. One of the ends has to be completely closed, sealed: a suture is welded, or the folded end of the sleeve is fused in, after tightening with a rubber seal or a plastic adhesive tape, or binding with a rope. The welding is done with a special device, whereas for the fusing (sealing) the flame of a candle will suffice. Another possibility is to bind a knot on the end of the sleeve. It is important to make the knot as tight as possible. One sleeve equalling about 2.5 times the length of the future bag suffices, after binding a simple knot, to make a duplicated bag.

During transport the bags with fry are placed in outer cases protecting the bags against mechanical damage, mainly punching or tearing in contact with the ground. The case keeps the bags in the desired position, enables easier handling and/or provides thermal insulation of the bags.

These cases can be cardboard boxes, suitable plastic containers, wide polyethylene cans, polystyrene boxes. The kind of outer casing depends on the number of bags transported, length and method of transport, requirements for further handling (transloading), and on the differences between ambient temperature and the temperature of water inside the bag.

If water with transported fry is to be cooled, bags with ice should be placed under the fish-transport bags on the bottom of the polystyrene box. It is not recommended to put the ice inside the transport bag. The amount of ice depends on the size of the bag with water, transport time and difference of temperature. The volume of ice placed under the bag with transport water is usually 10–20 per cent of the transport water. This method of packing enables transport by public transport routes.

The water to be used for fry transport in a bag should comply with all requirements. It is best to use water of the same quality as that in which the fish were kept before transport, but there should be no organic pollutants and no dispersed mud of mineral origin. Sac fry, in particular, need transport water with air bubbles, *i.e.*, released air contained in water in oversaturated condition.

Before putting the fry in the bag, the procedure of catching, counting and distributing the fry in the bags should have been thoroughly prepared to finish the operation as quickly as possible.

The polyethylene sac, or sleeve with a closed bottom end, is first put in the outer transport case; if a double bag is to be used the inner bag is to have been inserted in the outer one. Then, water is poured in the bag, about 20 litres if the volume of the bag is 50 litres, and the fry are placed inside. Air is displaced from the space above water in the bag and a hose, connected to the pressure regulator of an oxygen cylinder, is introduced in the bag, the upper end of the bag being held tight around the hose by hand. Then, technical oxygen from the pressure cylinder is left to blow via the pressure regulator to the upper part of the bag. If the volume of water with fry is 20 litres, the volume of oxygen atmosphere should be 30 litres. The supply of oxygen is stopped when the bag is filled: the hose is quickly drawn out of the bag and the upper end of the bag is twisted to prevent oxygen from leaking and to produce some overpressure by reducing the volume. If the bag if to be transported in a horizontal position, the pressure should be 0.05 to 0.06 MPa but for vertical transport the pressure should be 0.02 to 0.04 MPs. In practice, this means that after filling the bag is tight: when pressed with thumb the foil quickly returns to its original position. During air transport the pressure in a vertically kept bag reaches -0.01 MPa, owing to the lower outside pressure. Finally the opening of the bag is closed. There are several ways of closing the bag; the simplest way is to tighten the end of the plastic foil with rubber, preferably duplicated. Rope or adhesive tape can also be used. The bag can also be closed with a metal screw cap.

After transport, or during control on a longer journey, the condition of the fry should be checked before release. The fry are examined for position, *i.e.*, swimming, lying on the bottom, staying in physiological position or turning to one side, for motility, readiness of reaction to light, touch, and/or number (proportion) of dead individuals.

The fish are released only when the temperature of the water in the bag reaches the same level as that of the receiving water. For sac fry the difference in water temperature should not be greater than 1°C, for older fry 2°C in both directions. To balance the temperatures it is best to put the closed bag on the surface of the receiving water. When the temperature difference is reduced to 2–3°C at the maximum, the bags are opened step by step and the receiving water is slowly added to the transport water. Releasing can start when about 50 per cent of the receiving water has been added to the bags.

If the bags are handled with maximum care, if they are closed in the most careful manner and transported in suitable outer cases, they can be used repeatedly. However, this is not a general recommendation because damage to the bags, however tiny it may seem, can never be avoided during fish release.

It is also possible to use bags - tanks, made of 4–12 layers of polyethylene foil ("sleeve" 80 cm in width), having a total volume of 300 litres. However, these types of bags are hard to handle and are used only for individual transports of large and broad fish.

Other Sealed Containers

Containers similar to polyethylene bags may be sealed. Generally made of cured plastics they can do the same job as bags and do not require as much care during handling, despite repeated use. However, their unit price is much higher.

Transport of Large Fish and Brood Fish in Bags:

Individual shipments of large brood fish can also be made in polyethylene bags. This possibility is suggested by several literary sources.

Naturally, when large fish of these species are transported for introduction or acclimatization, it is not recommended to apply the theoretical critical possibilities. The main requirement is to keep the fish healthy and physiologically intact throughout the transport, because brood fish are of a high potential value and their transport is to pay off in future. With respect to this, the safe transport densities of these fish, as recommended are 5 to 10 times lower than those of the fish of the same size transported to market.

The general principles, as recommended by a number of authors, *e.g.*, are that in every specific case the existing conditions and circumstances should always be considered and that the guide parameters should be adjusted on the basis of preliminary trials.

Open Systems of Fish Transport

The open systems have many technical variants, ranging from small transport fish-cans, containers for fish transport within the territory of a fish farm, up to special fish transport trucks and tank wagons.

1. General Technological Notes

In all cases of fish transport in open systems, it should be borne in mind that even a short-time transport of 10–30 m in open plastic or metal tanks should be done under the conditions of constant air or oxygen supply. This is very important to the welfare of fish even if dissolved oxygen content of water seems to be satisfactorily high in the tank. Transport longer than half an hour should be in completely filled and closed tanks to prevent splashing and injuries to young fish bumping into each other in the well of the tank.

The weight of fish that can be safely transported in a tank depends on the efficiency of the aeration system, duration of the transport, water temperature, fish size and fish species.

If environmental conditions are constant, the carrying capacity of a transport unit depends upon fish size. It has been suggested that the maximum permissible weight of trout in a given tank is directly proportional to their length. Thus, if a tank can safely hold 50 kg of 5 cm trout, it could hold 100 kg of 10 cm trout, and 150 kg of 15 cm trout.

Reported loading rates for fish vary widely among farms, and maximum carrying capacities of different types of transport units have not been determined.

Under ideal conditions, the maximum load of 20–28 cm rainbow trout is 3–3.1 kg/litre of water for 8 to 10 h. Similar loading rates are appropriate for brook, brown, and lake trout of the same size. If the trip exceeds 16 h, it is recommended that a complete water change be made during transport.

- 0.5 kg of 40 cm channel catfish can be transported per litre of water at 18°C;
- Loading rates can be increased by 25 per cent for each 5°C decrease in water temperature, and reduced proportionately for an increase in temperature;
- As fish length increases, the weight of fish per litre of water can be increased proportionally for an increase in temperature. For example, a tank holding 120 g of 10 cm catfish will safely hold 250 g of 20 cm or 500 g of 40 cm fish per litre of water;
- If the transport time exceeds 12 h, the loading rate should be decreased by 25 percent;
- If the transport time exceeds 16 h, loading rates should be decreased by 50 percent or a complete water change should be arranged;
- During the winter, transporting temperature of 7–10°C are preferred, whereas 15–21°C are preferable during summer months.

From the technical point of view, most tanks constructed in recent years are insulated, usually with styrofoam, fiberglass or urethane. Styrofoam and urethane are preferred materials because of their superior insulating qualities and the minimal effect that moisture has on them. A well-insulated tank minimizes the need for elaborate temperature-control systems and small amounts of ice can be used to control the limited heat rises.

Circulation is needed to maintain well-aerated water in all parts of the tank. Transport success is related to tank shape, water circulation pattern, aerator type and other design criteria. Warmwater transport tanks may be compartmented. Compartments facilitate fish stocking at several different sites on a single trip, permit separation of species, and act as baffles to prevent water surges. Tanks in current use have 1 000–2 700 litre capacities, averaging about 1 700 litres.

Although most tanks presently in use are rectangular, the trend in recent years has been towards elliptical tanks, such as those used to transport milk. This shape has several advantages: V-shaped, elliptical or partially round tanks promote better mixing and recirculation of water as the size of the tank increases. This shape also conforms to a truck chassis and holds the centre of gravity towards the area of greatest strength.

Water circulation systems are of various sizes and designs. Suction lines to the pumps lie on the bottom of the tank and are covered by perforated screens. Water is carried to the pumps and then forced through overhead spray heads mounted above the waterline. In most systems, oxygen is introduced in one of the suction lines just ahead of the pump. This usually is controlled by a medical gas-flow meter; because of the danger involved in handling and transporting bottled oxygen, care must be taken to follow all prescribed safety procedures.

Self-priming pumps powered by gasoline engines are used to circulate water in many transport units. Pumps may be close-coupled or flexibly coupled. Although the former type is more compact, it tends to transfer heat to the water. Depending upon ambient air temperature, close-coupled pumps may increase the temperature of 1 500 litres of water by about 4°C an hour, whereas flexible coupling will reduce heat transfer to approximately 1.7°C per hour (Piper *et al.*, 1982).

A method of circulating water with 12-volt mechanical aerators uses carbon rods and micropore tubing for dispensing oxygen. Aerators alone may not be sufficient to provide the oxygen needed to transport large loads of fish, but a supplemental oxygenation system can increase the carrying capacity of the transport tank. Some advantages of aerator systems over gasoline-driven water pump systems are (Piper *et al.*, 1982):

- ✰ Temperature increases from aerators are less than 0.5°C per hour, compared with 1.3°C with pumps;
- ✰ Aerators and the oxygen injection system can operate independently. There are advantages to carrying small sizes of certain species of fish on oxygen alone. Oxygen also can be used as a temporary backup system if aerators fail;
- ✰ Usually, aerators have fewer maintenance problems;
- ✰ Costs of recirculating equipment and aerators strongly favor aerators;
- ✰ Use of aerators eliminates the space required between the tank and truck cab for pumps and plumbing.

The most efficient tanks have the highest water circulation rates, but circulation rates must be balanced with water capacity. Pumping or aerating systems should be able to circulate at least 40 percent of the tank water per minute when 20–22 cm salmonids are transported, though lesser rates are appropriate for smaller fish.

Railway Fish Transport

The wagon is designed for the transport of 8–12 tons of fish, usually market cyprinids. The amount of fish transported depends on temperature because the wagons usually have no cooling system. In the variant, the dimensions of the tank are 3 × 3 × 1.4 m. Oxygen cylinders are kept as a reserve to replace, in case of failure, the air compressor used during the journey. When the transport time is longer, water is completely replaced in the tank in the marshalling yards. The mud deposited on the bottom is drained from the tanks during the trip.

Chemical Methods for Water and Fish Treatment during Transport

The chemical methods of treating the transport medium, aimed at increasing the capacity volume of the transport units and preventing physiological and health damage to the fish. They include the use of anaesthetics, water-hardening and oxygen-producing chemicals, bacteriostatics, buffering and antifoam chemicals.

Use of Fish Tranquilizers

During transport, sedation of the fish is desirable, since oxygen consumption and CO_2 and NH_3 production are all decreased. However, deep sedation is undesirable because the fish may fall to the bottom, pile up and smother. If pumps are used, the fish may be pulled into the screen, the air may move the deeply sedated fish about and cause a loss of scales. It is best to sedate the fish in the holding facility for 30 min before loading and then to continue exposure to a lower concentration of sedative during transport. The use of anaesthetics should not be relied on for increased load carrying capacity. Other methods are safer and dependable. The use of anaesthetics on food fish that will be consumed soon after exposure is not legal. Consideration should always be given to the legal status of a chemical and possible consequences to the consumer.

Anaesthesia usually applies only to transported brood fish. In practice, the fish are first tranquilized with the normal dose and put into the transport tank, where original concentration is diluted by 50 percent by adding the same amount of freshwater. The brood fish will remain tranquillized well in that diluted solution.

It is not recommended to use anaesthetics on small fish transported on small distances, since in such conditions the space factor has a greater influence on the health of the fish than the accumulation of metabolic products.

It is recommend to anaesthetize the fish for transport only in cases of temperatures above 15°C.

Among the broad spectrum of anaesthetics, tricaine methanesulfonate (MS-222) and quinaldine appear to be used most frequently.

Application of Sodium Chloride and Calcium Chloride

Handling stress and delayed mortality of fish can be decreased by the addition of sodium cloride (NaCl) and calcium chloride ($CaCl_2$) to the transport water. The sodium ion tends to "harden" the fish and reduce slime formation, and the calcium ion suppresses osmoregulatory and metabolic disfunction. Calcium chloride may not be needed in hard water already containing high concentrations of calcium.

Chemicals as Oxygen Sources

There are contradictory views concerning the use of chemicals as oxygen sources during fish transport. The use of one drop (1 ml = 20 drops) of hydrogen peroxide (6 percent concentration), applied to 1 litre of water, increased the oxygen content by 1.5 $mg.1^{-1}$ when the temperature was 24°C. CO_2 content and water pH were not influenced by the addition of hydrogen peroxide.

Bacteriostatic Chemicals

Antibacterials are also used to check the development of bacteria in transport units. Among the wide spectrum of bacteriostatic drugs, the following are used most frequently: nitrofurazone (furacin) at 10 $mg.1^{-1}$, acriflavin at 1 to 2 $mg.1^{-1}$, oxytetracycline (terramycin) at 20 $mg.1^{-1}$ Combiotic at 15 $mg.1^{-1}$ and neomycin sulphate at 20 $mg.1^{-1}$.

Antibacterials may strengthen the resistance of fish, but they are probably of little value as bacterial checks in transport tanks.

Buffers

Among other chemical additives, buffers such as "tris-buffer" (tris-hydroxylmethyl-amino methane) are helpful in controlling pH at a favourable value of 7 to 8. The accumulation of carbon dioxide in bag transport allows for a decrease in pH, because carbon dioxide is an acid. Since 2.2 to 4.4 $g.1^{-1}$ or 1.1 to 2.2 $g.1^{-1}$ of tris-buffer are required to control pH in bags with only moderate loads, the use of tris-buffer in tank transport usually is impractical because of cost.

Ammonia Control

To control ammonia concentration in the transport bags when the transport is expected to be long, it is recommended to use clinoptilolite, a zeolite mineral. Amend *et al.* (1982) tested with success the dose of 14 g of clinoptilolite per litre, Bower and Turner (1982) tested the doses of 10–40 $g.1^{-1}$; the concentration of non-ionized ammonia nitrogen never exceeded 0.017 $mg.1^{-1}$ in bags containing even the lowest dose of clinoptilolite, whereas concentrations as high as 0.074 $mg.1^{-1}$ were recorded in the control bags left without clinoptilolite.

Antifoam Chemicals

The formation of foam and scum, especially when drugs are used in transporting fish or on water which is heavily laden with organic material (secretions and excretions, such as mucus and excrements) often becomes quite bothersome. The foam interferes with oxygen exposure at the water surface and also makes it difficult to observe the fish being carried. Water with NaCl foams less than water without NaCl, but NaCl may interfere slightly with the effectiveness of anti-foam chemicals. In some cases, a 10 per cent solution of Dow Corning Antifoam AF Emulsion is used at the rate of 0.05 $ml.1^{-1}$ of water (Leitritz and Lewis, 1976; Dupree and Huner, 1984). The advantages of using anti-foam chemicals are not so great, but their use does keep the water more clear so that the fish can be observed better.

References

Amend, D.F., *et al.*, 1982 Transportation of fish in closed system; methods to control ammonia, carbon dioxide, pH and bacterial growth. Trans.Am.Fish.Soc., III (5): 603–11.

Anon., 1979 Gutachten über tierschutzgerechte Hälterung und tierschutzgerechten Transport von Fischen - überarbeitete Fassung vom 15. Dezember 1978. *In* Fisch und Umwelt. Stuttgart, Gustav Fischer Verlag, pp. 1–24.

Anon., 1980 Capacity boost for truck. Fish Farm. Int., 7(1):48.

Anon., 1980a Semi-trailer carries live fish fry. World Fish., 29(11):17.

Anon., 1982 Live elvers survive 2 000-mile road trip from UK to Hungary. Fish Farm.Int., 9(1):14.

Anon., 1984 Transporter moves live fish. Fish Farm.Int., 11(12):19.

Astapovich, J., 1974 Khimicheskii method obogashcheniya vody kislororodo (Chemical method of water enrichment with oxygen). Rybov.Rybolov., 5:15.

Barekyan, A. Sh., *et al.*, 1975 Gidravlicheskie issledovaniya rubovoznogo avtokonteinera s ezhektornym blokom pitaniya. (Hydraulic studies of a fish-transport truck tank with an ejector feed system). Rybn.Khoz., 8:37–40.

Bodgan, E., 1972 PrzewoŸenie narybki letniego sielawy, siei i pelugi. (Transport of the yearlings of great maraena, vendace, peled). Publ.Inst.Rybaetwa Sródladowego, Olsztyn, (55):16 p.

Bower, C.E. and D.T. Turner, 1982 Ammonia revomal by clinoptilolite in the transport of ornamental freshwater fishes. Progr.Fish.Cult. 44(1):19–23.

Carmichael, G.J., 1984 Long-distance truck transport of intesively reared largemouth bass. Progr.Fish. Cult., 46(2):111–5.

Demchenko, I., 1970 Kakim transportrom luchshe? (Which transport system is better?) Rybov.Rybolov., 13(3):11 p.

Dupree, H.K. and J.V. Huner, 1984 The status of warmwater fish farming and progress in fish farming research. Washington, D.C., U.S. Fish and Wildlife Service, pp. 165–76.

Dyagilev, S., 1974 O rezhime ekspluatatsil zhivorybnoi mashiny (On the regime of the use of a live-fish transport truck). Rybov.Rubyolov., 1974(6):8–9.

Emerson, K., *et al.*, 1975 Aqueous ammonia equilibrium calculations: effect of pH and temperature. J.Fish.Res.Board Can., 32(12):2379–83.

Fereira, J.T., J.J. Schoonbee and G.L. Smit, 1984 The use of benzocaine-hydrochloride as an aid in the transport of fish. Aquaculture, 42(2):169–74.

Garádi, P. and I. Tarnai, 1983 Százhalombatti anyahalak szállítása Iránba. (Transportation of brood carp and brood herbivorous fishes from Szazhalombatta/Hungary/to Iran). Halászat, 29(3):82–4.

Gilev, G. and G. Krivodanova, 1984 Konteiner dlya transportirovki lichinok i molodi ryb (Container for the transport of fish larvae and fry). Rybov.Rybolov. (11):8.

Hamman, R.L., 1981 Transporting endangered fish species in plastic bags. Progr.Fish-Cult., 43(4):212–3.

Hartman, P., 1976 Pokus s pouzitím persíranu amonního k okyslicování vody pri preprave ruby (A trial with the use of ammonium persulphate for water oxygenation during fish transport). St.rybárství, o.p., C. Budejovice, (MS).

Hatting, J., *et al.*, 1975 The transport of freshwater fish. J.Fish.Biol., 7(4):447–9.

Heiner, H., 1982 Sauerstoff sichert neue wirtschaftliche Produktionsformen. Lebendfischtransport mit Flüssigsauerstoff. Osterr.Fisch., 35(10):207–9.

Heiner, H., 1983 Begasung sichert neue wirtschaftliche Formen der Zucht. Lebendfischtransport durch Flüssigsauerstoff leichtgemacht. Allg.Fischwirtochaltztg. (13/14):532–34.

Horváth, L., G. Tamás and I. Tölg, 1984 Special methods in pond fish husbandry. Seattle, Halver Corporation, 146 p.

Huilgol, N.V. and S.G. Patil, 1975 Hydrogen peroxide as a source of oxygen supply in the transport of fish fry. Progr.Fish-Cult., 37(2):117.

Ioshev, L., 1980 Transportirane na zhiva riba u nas - problemi i normi (Live fish transport in our fish culture - problems and standards). Izv.Inst.Sladkovodno Ribovod., Plovdiv, 14:35–42.

Johnson, S.K., 1979 Transport of live fish. Aquacult.Mag., 5(6):20–4.

Kavalec, J., 1973 Neobvyklý transport ryb (An extraordinary fish transport). Rybárství, 28(3):54–5.

Kozlov, A.A., *et al.*, 1977 Spravochnik po akklimatizatsii vodnykh organizmov (Bulletin on the acclimation of aquatic organisms). Moskva, Izd.Pishchevaya Promyshlennost, 174 p.

Kruzhalina, E.I., I. Averina and G. Vol'nova, 1970 Ispytanie zhivorubnykh emkostei. (Investigation on live-fish capacities.) Rybov.Rybolov., 13(5):13 p.

Kruzhalina, E.I., O.A. Leis and T.I. Ovchinnikova, 1984 Razrabotka metodov transportirovaniya vodnykh organizmov (On the methods of the transport of aquatic organisms.) Rybn.Khoz. (4):75–6.

Leis, O., 1978 Metod rascheta (Capacity calculation method) Rybov.Rybolov. (5):14–5.

Leis, O., E. Kruzhalina and T. Ovchinnikova, 1980 Prognozirovanie i podderzhanie temperaturnogo rezhima v transportnykh emkostyakh (Determining and maintaining the temperature inside transport tanks.) Rybov.Rybolov. (3):8–9.

Leis, O.A., E.I. Kruzhalina and S.E. Dyagilev, 1975 Opredelenie plotnostei posadki vodnykh organizmov v aeriruemye transportnye emkosti (Determination of fish densities in aerated transport tanks). *In* Akklimatizatsiya ryb i bezpozvonochnykh v vodoemakh SSSR, 1975, vol. 103 pp. 274–9.

Leitritz, E. and R.C. Lewis, 1976 Trout and salmon culture (Hatchery methods). Fish Bull.Calif.Dep. Fish Game, (164):128–37.

Lusk, S. and J. Krcál, 1974 Preprava plôdika lososovitých rýb s kyslíkom (Transporting the fry of salmonids with oxygen.) Polov.Rybár. (2):32.

Máchová, J., 1984 Peroxodisírany jako okyslicovadla v rybárství (Peroxodisulphates as oxidizers in fishery). Vodnany, VURH, 3 p. (mimeo).

Mackevich, I. and I. Shiyanov, 1984 Sovershenstvovanie zhivorybnoi mashiny (Improving the fish-transport truck.) Rybov.Rybolov. (11):9.

Mishra, B.K., D. Kumar and R. Mishra, 1983 Observations on the use of carbonic acid anaesthesia in fish fry transport. Aquaculture, (3/4):405–8.

Okoniewski, Z., 1975 Hodowla ryb ciepolubnych w USA. 8. Transport ryb (Warm-water fish culture in the USA. 8. Fish transport). Gospod.Rybn. (10):19–22.

Orlov, Yu, I, *et al.*, 1973 Normy posadok promyslovykh ryb v transportnye emkosti zakrytogo tipa (Standard densities of farmed fish in closed-type transport tanks) Rybn.Khoz. (6):17–9.

Orlov, Yu. I., E.I. Kruzhalina and I.A. Averina, 1975 Raschet norm posadok vodnykh organizmov v transportnye emkosti zakrytogo tipa (Calculation of the density standards of aquatic organisms in closed-type transport tanks) *in* Akklimatizatsiya ryb i bezpozvonochnykh v vodoemakh SSSR, 1975, vol. 103 pp. 268–70.

Orlov, Yu. I., *et al.*, 1974 Transportirovka zhivoi ryby v germeticheskikh emkostyakh. Spravochnoe posobie (Live fish transport in hermetically sealed containers. Information manual) Moskva, Izd. Pishchevaya Promyshlennost', 97 p.

Orlov, Yu., 1971 Kakoe kolichestvo vodnykn organizmov sleduet pomeshchat v transportnye emkosti (What amounts of aquatic organisms should be kept in transport tanks) Rybov.Rybolov., 14(2): 12–3.

Orlov, Yu., 1973 Mozhno-li uvelichit' davlenie v paketakh (Is it possible to increase pressure in transport bags?). Rybov.Rybolov., 16(1):19.

Orlov, Yu., 1975 Raschetnyi sposob normirovaniya (Calculations for determining fish density standards). Rybov.Rybolov., 1975, (4):8–9.

Pavlov, Yu., 1973 Zhivorybnaya mashina iranskogo proizvodstva (Fish transport truck of Iranian produce) Rybov.Rybovlov., 16(1): 11.

Pecha, O., R. Berka and J. Kouril, 1983 Preprava pludku v polyetylénovych vacích (Fry transport in polyethylene bags) Ser.Metod.VURH Vodnany, (10):16 p.

Piper, R.G., *et al.*, 1982 Fish hatchery management. Washington, D.C., U.S. Department of the Interior, Fish and Wildl. Service, pp. 348–71.

Popov, E.P., 1975 Transportirovka lichnok ryb i kormovykh bespozvonochnykh v zhestkoi polietilenovii tare s kislorodom (Transport of fish larvae and feed invertebrates in a hard polyethylene container with oxygen). *In* Biologicheskoe obosnovanie vosproizvodstva sigovykh i ich znacheniya v povyshenii ryboproduktivnosti vodoemov, vol. 104, pp.180–4.

Powell, N.A., 1970 Striped bass in air shipment. Progr. Fish-Cult., 32 (1):18.

Proske, Ch., 1982 Uberlandfahrt im kühlen Wasser. Der Transport von Fishen bringt im Sommer eine Menge Probleme. Landwirtsch.Wochenbl., 172(15):11–2.

Rzanicanin, B. and I. Balcer, 1973 Transport sarana uz dodatak trankilajzera MS-222 (Carp transport with the addition of the MS-222 tranquilizer). Ribarst.Jugosl., 28(3): 49–51.

Rzanicanin, B. and I. Balcer, 1974 Istrazivanja o moguænosti transporta sarana uz dodatak trankilajzera MS-222 (Studies on the possibilities of carp transport with the use of the MS-222 tranquilizer). Ribarst.Jugosl., 29(5): 93-97.

Shevchenko, V., 1982 Normativy i kachestvo perevozimoi ryby (Standards and the quality of transported fish). Rybolov. (7):9–10.

Shevchenko, V.V., 1978 Khranenie i transportirovanie zhivoi ryby (Storage and transport of live fish). Moskva, Izd. Ekonomika., 71 p.

Smorodinskaya, M. and I. Khasman, 1973 Problema perevozki zhivoi ryby (Problem of the transport of live fish). Rybov.Rybolov. (4):10–1.

Snow, J.R., D. Brewer and C.F. Wright, 1978 Plastic bags for shipping sac fry of largemouth bass. Progr.Fish-Cult., 40(1): 13–4.

Strebkova, T.P., 1971 Ispol'zovanie narkoticheskoi smesi pri transportirovke zhivoi ryby (The use of a narcotic mixture in the transport of live fish). Rybn.Khoz. (12):19–20.

Studnicka, M., *et al.*, 1982 Zastosowanie œrodka antystresowego w transporcie pstraga (The use of an anti-stress preparation in the transport of trout). Gospod.Rybn., 34(3):10–1.

Uryn, B., 1971 Sposoby obliczania norm transportowych przy przewoŸeniu wylegu siei i sielawy (Methods of determining transport standards in the shipment of great maraena and vendace fry).Gospod.Rybn., 23(11):4–7.

Varga, I., 1984 Magyar anyahalak egyiptomi halkeltetö telepen (Transportation of brood carp and brood herbivorous fishes from Hungary to Egypt). Halaszat, 30(3):88–9.

Vollmann-Schipper, F., n.d. Transport lebender Fische. Hamburg and Berlin, Paul Parey, 104. p.

Woynarowich, E. and L. Horváth, 1980 The artificial propagation of warm-water finfishes - a manual for extension. FAO Fish.Tech.Pap. (201): 138–47. Issued also in French and Spanish.

IV. Processing of Fish

Catching and Preparing Fresh Fish

As fish spoils very quickly, measures must already be taken on board the fishing boat to limit spoilage. First of all, the fish must immediately be kept out of the salt water so that the fish does not get contaminated by bacteria in the salt water. Apart from preventing contamination, one should also prevent outgrowth of bacteria which are already present. The best way is to remove

the intestines and gills of the fish on board the fishing boat. After that the fish must be washed with clean water to rinse off any blood or other remains. It is recommended to transport the fish on ice to shore. However, cleaning and transporting the fish on ice is often difficult and expensive to realize. All that can be done then is to transport the fish as quickly and carefully as possible to the shore. To prevent the bacteria in the intestines, liver, gills and on the skin of the fish from increasing, the fish must be kept in a clean boat and in the shade.

Cleaning Fish

To clean fish, first of all one needs good and clean tools. Personal hygiene is also important. It is important that the fish is not cleaned on the ground but on a clean table or bench. The table should be at working height and can be made of wood, metal or concrete. The surface of the table must be smooth and easy to clean. It is also handy to clean the fish on a cutting board so that the table is not damaged. Knives are the most important tools for cleaning fish. Short knives are used for small kinds of fish, long flexible knives to fillet larger kinds of fish and a thick, strong knife to cut open large fish. The knives must be sharp. To salt, dry and smoke fish, it is important that the surface area of the fish be increased. Then the salt and smoke particles can penetrate easily into the fish and moisture can work its way out. The method used to clean fish depends primarily on the size and kind of fish. (1) With very small kinds of fish, such as chovies, sardines and others smaller than 10 cm, usually only the intestines are removed. Whether or not this is done depends on local customs and the purpose for which the fish is to be used. For some fermentation processes the intestines are not removed. (2) Fish larger than 15 cm are, apart from being cleaned, also cut crosswise so that the surface area of the fish is increased and the flesh becomes less thick. Preservation methods work faster with a larger surface area of the flesh. (3) In addition to cleaning and splitting fish that are larger than 25 cm, one also makes extra cuts in the flesh. Sometimes the fish are cut into chunks or completely filleted. The way in which the fish are cleaned depends not only on the size of the fish but also on the wishes of the consumer. Some consumers, for example, want the fish with its head intact while others especially want it cut off. The last thing to be discussed is a brief description of how to gut, split and fillet fish.

Gutting and Scaling

1. Place the fish on a clean board and hold it by its head. Scrape the scales off starting at the tail and working towards the head. Try not to damage the skin of the fish while doing so.
2. Wash the fish in clean (drinking) water and remove all loose scales.
3. Lay the fish on its side on a clean board and cut into the fish along its gills with a sharp knife. Do the same on the other side but do not cut the head off.
4. Cut the gills free by cutting the ends free from the head and body with the point of the knife.
5. Slit the abdominal wall open from the anal opening towards the head of the fish. Cut deep enough but try not to damage the intestines of the fish.
6. When the fish has been opened up, the gills and intestines can be removed by placing one's fingers under the gills and pulling everything out.
7. Scrape any remaining blood out with the knife.
8. Clean the abdominal wall with clean (drinking) water.

Splitting

Small and Medium-Sized Fish

1. Place the fish on a clean board with its back facing you and its head to the right if you are right-handed. Slit the fish open down the middle from the head to the tail, along the middle fish bone, but do not cut into the underbelly.
2. Open the fish and remove the intestines and gills. Wash the fish thoroughly with clean (drinking) water.

Large fish

Extra cuts are made in the flesh of large fish to increase the surface area and to decrease the thickness of the fish.

1. Place the fish on a clean board, with the abdominal side facing you and the head to the right if you are right-handed. Make a cut in the fish from the gill arch to the tail so that a strip of fish-flesh is left.
2. Turn the fish over and open it up. The strip of flesh must remain attached at the back.
3. Place the fish with its head to the right and the abdominal side facing you. Split the head open and cut towards the tail so that a second strip of flesh is formed. In doing so, the abdomen is also cut open.
4. Open the fish and remove its intestines and gills. Then wash with clean (drinking) water.

Filleting

Small Fish

One can use a fish which has not been cleaned for this.

1. Place the fish on a clean board with its back facing you. Place the head on the left if you are right-handed. Cut along the contours of the gill arches until you hit the backbone.
2. With one slice, cut the fillet loose from the backbone from the head to the tail. In doing so, the abdomen is cut open.
3. When the fillet is loose, you can see the intestines and other organs.
4. Turn the fish over so its abdominal side faces you.
5. Repeat steps 1, 2 and 3.
6. If necessary, cut the fins from the fillets. Then wash the fillets with clean (drinking) water.

Large Fish

1. Place the fish on a clean board with the stomach facing up. For right-handed people the head must be on the right. Cut along the contours of the gill arches.
2. Remove the head and intestines.

3. Place the fish on its side. For the first fillet, start at the head end and cut the fish in the direction of the tail to halfway along the backbone. Cut as close to the backbone as possible.
4. Also cut the other side of the fillet loose.
5. Turn the fish so that its tail is to the right.
6. Remove the other fillet from the backbone. If necessary, remove the fins from the fish. Wash the fillets with clean (drinking) water. With all preservation methods it is important to use fish of the same size within one batch so that a uniform final product is made.

V. Grading Standards of Fish

Introduction

Commercial fish farming involves many steps between producers and end users of aquaculture products. One important step in this process is the sorting or grading of live fish. Grading allows the producer to maximize profits when prices vary with fish size. Large fish mixed with nailer ones can affect the appearance of a shipment of fish. Smaller fish may appear less attractive, and the shipment may be considered of poor quality. Fish should be graded for economic reasons either to increase the value of the crop, to increase fish yields or both. In some markets and production systems, however, there are no advantages to grading fish. Many methods and types of equipment can be used successfully to grade fish. Sorting can be accomplished in ponds, holding vats, tanks and raceways. As with any live fish handling practice, there are safe ways and proper methods that will influence the success in sorting and maintaining live fish in good condition. When grading is required, proper equipment and techniques reduce scale loss, stress and mortalities. Grading involves holding. It is essential that fish be in good health and condition prior to grading, and that the water and environment in the holding facility are of good quality to reduce stress and associated problems. Whenever possible, grading should be done in ponds to reduce the number of fish to be transported to holding facilities before returning them to ponds as unusable.

Advantages of Grading

Many fish are sold by size or grade. Grading increases the crop's market value by supplying the sizes or grades of product desired by customers. For example, smaller minnows are worth more per pound than larger fish. Feeder fish of the same species may be worth twice the price of larger fish used for bait. Catfish are sold by the inch and categorized as small to large fingerlings just like redfish, striped bass and their hybrids. State laws may prohibit marketing certain fish species, especially game fish, that are longer than a specified length. When fish of a similar size and age are stocked in a pond, differential growth among individuals produces fish of various sizes at the end of the grow-out cycle. This is more pronounced in ponds where fish are graded only at the time of harvesting. Some markets do not accept pond-run, ungraded fish of mixed sizes. Some species are cannibalistic and periodic size grading is important to obtain good survival and yields and to eliminate runts. Largemouth bass and striped bass and their hybrids are examples of cannibalistic fish. These and other species may require frequent grading when maintained at high densities in tanks or troughs. Grading is also required during the various stages from fry to food-sized fish in outdoor pond culture. Frequency of grading depends on the growth rate of fish and their uniformity in size. The first 2 months are usually the most critical to minimize losses from cannibalism. Grading also allows more accurate sample counting to estimate fish numbers from a weight-number relationship. This is important to baitfish retailers who sell fish of a uniform desired size by the number. Fish of mixed sizes make this counting method more difficult because of a wider size variation. The process of grading provides an opportunity to remove unwanted fish species, undesirable organisms, and nuisance aquatic plants that could become established in, or contaminate stocked waters. Species separation is required in polyculture systems where more than one species of fish are grown together in a pond. Each species may require sorting because of different market outlets or processing requirements.

Often it is desirable to separate males from females, or to determine the numbers of each sex for breeding purposes. Sexes of fathead minnows can be effectively separated using a 15/64- to 16/64-inch bar spacing. Other species like channel catfish and tilapia exhibit growth differences between sexes. This fact can be important, depending on how fish are used after grading. Sometimes a special variety of fish species with unique breeding or market characteristics is desired, or fish with deformities or poor breeding traits may need to be culled. Accurate length, weight or size information may also be required for research purposes. Food fish growers may want to grade fish to avoid harvesting fish too small for marketing or processing. Processors may want to have fish graded because of differences in the value or demand of fish by size. Grading requires additional labor, time and equipment but in many markets it is essential and may improve profits.

Grading and Sorting Equipment

A variety of commercial graders is available. Many producers construct grading devices specially designed for use in their facilities. Based on the market situation, know the size or sizes of fish that require sorting before purchasing or constructing a grader. Grader panels or grills can be purchased and inserted into homemade frames to save money. PVC pipe is a popular material used in making graders. Plastic netting is also available in various meshes and can be used for grading small fish when the material is strong and well supported. Fish are injured less if the grading material is smooth and non-abrasive, without any sharp edges or roughness. Mechanical bar graders often have 3/16-inch parallel aluminum or bronze rods that are separated by measured distances in a frame. The spacing between the bars determines the size of fish retained or allowed to pass through. These graders may be vertical panel graders like those often used in holding vats and raceways, or grader panels may be mounted on rollers or wheels for easy movement across the tank bottom. The manually pulled panel graders should have handles for easier use. To compensate for any slight difference in the widths of holding vats, some type of flexible sheeting, like rubber stripping, can be placed around the frame to provide a snug fit. To sort fish into a variety of sizes, multiple panel bar graders of various spacings work well. Grading boxes are used to sort large numbers of minnows or fingerling fish. These boxes vary in size from small units for use in tanks to larger ones designed to handle more fish in ponds. The boxes usually float. Both pond and tank grader boxes can be constructed with frames that accommodate standard sized grader panels with various bar spacings. Some commercial boxes have simple adjustable or interchangeable bar graders.

Polyethylene fish baskets have a square mesh of 5/16 inches and can grade out small fish.

A series of grading baskets with various bar spacings can be used to sort mixed sizes of fish. The grading boxes can be enclosed on the sides and bottom with galvanized hardware cloth, but plastic coated wire cloth is preferred because of greater durability and less injury to fish. The series can be built as nest boxes and should have long handles that permit easy use and support by the walls of the holding vat Sorting or grading tables work well when hardy species require accurate processing for research or breeding purposes. Tables can be portable or permanent. The tables are of various dimensions but all have smooth surfaces and slots in at least the corners and sometimes sides. Slots should be large enough to allow passage of fish sizes anticipated. Fish can be collected in containers filled with fresh, oxygenated water. A chute from the slots properly directs fish to containers. If fish are sorted by length, reference length easurements can be inscribed into the table surface, or rulers can be located on the sides. Every time fish are crowded with a harvesting seine, some rough grading occurs. Net graders of various types can be used to sort fish. Fish of a minimum desired size can be harvested by selecting a harvesting seine of the proper mesh size. Nylon nets should be treated with a net coating material. Polyethylene nets require no special treatment. Seines can be ordered or made with end panels of a desired mesh for grading. This means fewer seines for storage and use. Live cars or socks can be used to further grade fish after they are seined. These grading or holding nets, usually 10 to 20 feet wide, 10 to 60 feet long and4to41/2 feet deep, are commonly used by catfish producers to sort and hold both fingerlings and food-sized fish. They usually have an 18-inch wide skirt inside the net with floats to prevent fish from jumping out of the enclosure. These devices are equipped with a 3-foot by 5-foot tunnel and metal frame attached to the harvesting seine by a drawstring. Fish pumps equipped with grader boxes can be used both to load or transfer and grade fish simultaneously. Fish pumps are used in the salmonid industry where fish are commonly grown in concrete raceways. They are also used in some other countries. Until now, fish pumps have not been widely used with warmwater fish. Specially designed dewatering towers are required to separate water from fish.

Recommended Bar and Mesh Spacing

Bar spacings or mesh sizes should conform with the desired sizes of fish to grade. Commercial grader basket spacings range from 12/64 to 74/64 inches. Net or seine square mesh sizes normally range from ¼ to 3 inches. Whether or not a fish is retained by a grading device depends on its body shape and dimensions. Another factor is the number of days off feed before grading. The condition factor of fish will also determine lengths of fish retained; thin or fatter than normal fish will affect lengths graded. The following tables are recommended dimensions or guidelines to grade various fish species to different desired sizes. There is always a range between the largest and smallest fish in a length group; the fish sizes reported are approximate values. The length-weight relationship of catfish and other species varies depending on the condition of individual fish. Differences are greater with smaller fish because a l-inch length increment can result in a big difference in weight between different populations or lots of fish.

Repeated trials are required to determine bar spacings or mesh sizes required to grade other species to desirable sizes.

Grading and Sorting Techniques

There are various methods for using different types of grading devices. The technique should be compatible with the species of fish and grading situation, and should consider the behavior and water quality requirements of the fish. For example, baitfish grade well through the sides of a grader box, while catfish grade more efficiently through the bottom. Golden shiners are very excitable and more difficult to handle when water temperatures are above 60° to 65° F. Fish are especially delicate to handle for sorting purposes during July through September when pond temperatures are highest. Striped bass and its hybrids should preferaly be handled and graded at water temperatures less than 60° to 70° F. The risk of mortality is greater if fish are graded in soft water with low chlorides at higher water temperatures. Fish should be allowed at least 2 hours to recover after seining or transport before they are graded. Fish stomachs should be empty and any unwanted debris that hampers sorting should be removed either before or during grading. Fish are crowded during grading and oxygen can be depleted quickly in a localized area. It is essential to maintain dissolved oxygen levels at least 5 ppm to 6 ppm in the grading or holding area at all times. If large fish are held overnight, the top of the vat should be covered to prevent loss of fish from jumping. To minimize stress, all sorting should be conducted in a shaded area to prevent brightness from direct sunlight or warming effects from radiation. Factors that influence the grading process are the degree of fish crowding, fish condition (normal, thin or plump), water temperature, level of fish activity and grading time. Fish require crowding for efficient grading, and most are more active and grade faster at higher temperatures. During colder winter temperatures catfish, especially, require more time for pond grading to prevent many small, off-sized fish being harvested. Use of larger than normal mesh sizes also helps grading when temperatures are cold. Some fish can be attracted through a grader by a flowing water current. This is most applicable when a pond is drained into an outside harvest basin.

Select graders by visually estimating the sizes of fish. Use a test sample of fish in the selected grader or graders, and examine fish for uniformity in size. An additional grader is needed if there is an excessive or unacceptable size difference among fish graded to one size. If no fish or very few fish remain in a grader then that grader should not be used. Occasional large fish can be sorted manually.

For grading in vats or tanks, floating grader boxes or baskets work well. Fish are dipped into the graders and are retained or pass into other graders or the tank. A simple method to grade fingerlings uses a series of two, three or four grading boxes that nest inside each other. There should be enough space between boxes to accumulate 10 to 30 pounds of fish of a similar size. The inner box may have l-inch mesh with other boxes having l/2-inch, l/3-inch and l/4-inch meshes. The nested boxes are put in the tank, and ungraded fish are dipped or poured into the inner box. Fish pass through the different meshes until they can no longer pass. The smallest sized fish may be collected outside the outer box. When enough fish of a given size accumulate, the boxes are separated and fish can be processed by counting, weighing or passing to another tank or compartment. Splashing inside the grader box speeds grading time. Minnows grade faster when thumping sounds are made on the water surface by snapping the fingers. The loading rate of fish in a grader box should not exceed 5 pounds per cubic foot of water. When using a sorting table, a thin sheet of water should be kept on the surface for easy movement of fish. A short block of wood or other material can be placed in front of the slot opening to avoid accidental entry of unwanted fish if the table is heavily loaded. Fish should be worked up quickly. Sorting during cooler months of the year greatly reduces handling stress. Catfish withstand this type of handling and are less active during colder temperatures. Other more delicate species can suffer severe losses after processing on a sorting table. Whether or not the fish require restocking or will be killed should be considered before this method is used. In ponds, large floating grader boxes or a net device can be used. Larger fish are easiest to remove when a grading or cutting seine of the appropriate mesh is pulled inside a harvesting seine of smaller mesh. Much labor and time are required to sort fish manually. In other cases, a harvesting seine may have end panels of various meshes and the seine ends can be used like grading seines once the fish are crowded. One problem with any net grader is the possibility of gilling fish or trapping fish in the mesh net. Bass and their hybrids snag easily in nets by their fins and operculum, or gill flap, if a seine with an improperly sized mesh is used to grade widely mixed sizes. water well. The live car can also be used to hold two lots of sorted fish by putting the center of the sock over the harvesting boat to form two separate compartments. This works well to select and sort males and females. Fish loading rates in live cars should not exceed 5,000 pounds per 10-foot length; lower fish loads are recommended at temperatures above 60° F. Handling of fish in tanks is reduced by using vertical panel graders that are built to fit the holding tank. To use this type of grader simply move it from one end of the tank to another. This forces the fish to either pass through the bar space or be trapped. at the other end of the tank. Disturb the water in the confined area to move as many fish as possible through the grader. Sorting more than one size is accomplished by repeating the process with panels of desired bar spacings. The vertical panel graders require less handling of fish and cause less stress compared to forcing fish through hardware cloth grading boxes. Different lots of fish in tanks can be separated by transferring them to another tank or by using blocking screens to form several compartments in the same tank. Blocking screens can be placed in recessed grooves in the tank wall or wedged tightly between the side walls and bottom. Suspended nets inside wooden frames (hapas) can also be used to segregate fish. Be patient when grading and check to be sure that your efforts produce the desired results. Remember that fish are crowded and excited and maintaining good water quality is essential. Live cars or socks work well for inpond crowding and grading of catfish. Provide adequate aeration during grading or holding, especially during summer. It is important to secure the net enclosure firmly into the pond bottom. Support it with harvesting stakes to prevent rolling up the sock and killing fish from currents created by an aerator or water well. The live car can also be used to hold two lots of sorted fish by putting the center of the sock over the harvesting boat to form two separate compartments. This works well to select and sort males and females. Fish loading rates in live cars should not exceed 5,000 pounds per 10-foot length; lower fish loads are recommended at temperatures above 60° F.

Handling of fish in tanks is reduced by using vertical panel graders that are built to fit the holding tank. To use this type of grader simply move it from one end of the tank to another. This forces the fish to either pass through the bar space or be trapped. at the other end of the tank.

Disturb the water in the confined area to move as many fish as possible through the grader. Sorting more than one size is accomplished by repeating the process with panels of desired bar spacings. The vertical panel graders require less handling of fish and cause less stress compared to forcing fish through hardware cloth grading boxes. Different lots of fish in tanks can be separated by transferring them to another tank or by using blocking screens to form several compartments in the same tank. Blocking screens can be placed in recessed grooves in the tank wall or wedged tightly between the side walls and bottom. Suspended nets inside wooden frames (hapas) can also be used to segregate fish. Be patient when grading and check to be sure that your efforts produce the desired results. Remember that fish are crowded and excited and maintaining good water quality is essential.

– *Chapter 27* –

Post-processing Value Added Meat for Export-Integration, Poultry and Fish Processing and Marketing

Introduction

Sustained livestock production to provide livelihood and ensure food and nutrition security to a large population is dependent upon efficient utilization of livestock product. Processing meat to value added products contribute to sustained demand for meat and efficient marketing of meat to earn reasonable return. At present about 2 per cent of total meat is processed into product while it is above 60 per cent in developed countries (N. Kondaiah 2004). There are about 170 processed units in India, mostly small scale units, licensed under MFPO 1973. (http://nopr.niscair.res.).

Value Addition

It is to economically add value to a product and form characteristics more preferred in the market place.

Scope of Value Added Meat Product in India

India ranks top in animal and cattle population. The present production of meat is estimated at 6.3 million tons in 2010 (FAO, 2012), which is 2.21 per cent of the world's meat production (4th rank). But in meat production we are still lag behind the developed countries and the meat and meat processing industry is still to come up (www.fnbnews.com). A large proportion of meat animals are spent (aged) whose meat is tough and less palatable but more suitable for processing to products both on economic and quality consideration. It is necessary to produce quality value added meat products to check the large scale imports to detriment of domestic sector and to promote export.

Purpose of Value Addition

- ☆ To produce value added products and provide variety of meat products.
- ☆ To increase demand and meet life style requirements.
- ☆ To utilize different carcasses efficiently.
- ☆ To combine and compliment different meats with advantage.
- ☆ To incorporate non meat ingredients for quality and economy.
- ☆ To preserve, transport and distribute meat and meat products to larger population.
- ☆ To facilitate export and compete with imports from different countries.
- ☆ So many times there is excess supply of meat that can be stored after processing to be released into market at appropriate time (especially in poultry).
- ☆ Different important value added meat products are meat balls, patties, nuggets, pakoda, Kabab, sausages, hotdog etc.

Export Status of India Regarding Meat

In terms of export from India, processed meat recorded 54 per cent growth during financial year 2011-12 over the same period of last year.

Andhra Pradesh, *West Bengal, Maharashtra, Kerala, Delhi, U. P., Rajasthan, Goa are the key areas of Processed meat production in India.*

Major Export Destinations (2011-12) are Myanmar, Vietnam Social Republic, United Arab Emirates, Australia and Seychelles. (http://www.apeda.gov.in)

Regulations for Safe Meat Export

Processing of meat is licensed under the Meat Food Products Order, 1973.

Export (Quality Control and Inspection) Act 1963, Raw Meat (Chilled and Frozen).

Export of Processed Meat, 1992.

Registration and licensing of abattoirs and meat processing plants is done by the Agricultural and Processed Food Export Development Authority (APEDA), Ministry of Commerce and Industry, Export Inspection Council and Food Safety and Standards Authority of India (FSSAI).

Inspection of the meat processing plants is carried out by a committee of experts according to Meat and Meat Products Order (1973) of FSSAI, Government of India.

Inspection focus is on hygiene and sanitary conditions maintained by the plant, ante-mortem and post-mortem inspections, infrastructure facilities etc.

Steps have been initiated to grade the plants on the basis of adoption of international quality systems such as HACCP.

The Government of India has notified 3 agencies namely

I. State Directorates of Animal Husbandry,

II. Directorate of Marketing and Inspection:- it helps in enforcing hygienic standards and to exercise quality control. It has Veterinary Biological Control Laboratories (VBCLs) to support field inspection and analysis of meat food products samples.

III. Environmental Impact Assessment (EIA).

Steps that should be taken for the development of meat industry are:

a. Industry has demanded some immediate measures like financial assistance for up gradation of export oriented abattoirs/processing plants.
b. Inclusion of buffalo meat under APEDA's Transport Assistance Scheme for new markets in Africa/CIS where freight cost from India for reefer containers is much higher than from competing countries.
c. Exemption from Service Tax on transportation of meat products processed for exports.(this is presently applicable only for fruits, vegetables, eggs and milk for domestic consumption).
d. Apply World Class Sanitary and Phytosanitary Measures in the abattoirs.
e. Strict Surveillance of Diseases Confirming to WTO must be done.
f. Strict monitoring of Infective Agents/Drug Residues/Antibiotics is crucial.

Note: Indian government made Mandatory HACCP, ISO 9001 certification requirement.

What are the Opportunities for Export in India?

- ☆ India is strategically located.
- ☆ Animals fed on natural feed so less cost of production.
- ☆ Animals are free from BSE, CBPP and Rinderpest.
- ☆ Indian meat is 93 per cent chemically lean.
- ☆ Indian meat is free from radiation.
- ☆ Indian meat blends well with other meats.
- ☆ Genuinely Halal meat is available so good for processing and acceptable.
- ☆ Guidelines of Codex Alimentarius practiced so safer.

Some Important Rules for International Trade

The undersigned official veterinarian must certify that:

There has not been any outbreak of FMD or contagious infectious disease in the previous 90 days at the area of production and around which within a radius of 25 km.

The buffalo or livestock from which product/s were produced:

Were subjected to FMD vaccination programme.

Born, raised and slaughtered only in republic of India.

They have not been sacrificed as a consequence of contagious-infectious or parasitic disease eradication programme, not precede from areas subject to quarantine control measures to imply risk for its commercialization.

Before export of meat :- The meat/offal confirmed to following bacteriological specification:

1. Total bacteriological count within limit of 1-10 million per gram.
2. E coli count within limit of 100 per gram.
3 The buffalo meat/offal free from Salmonella.

Poultry Processing

It refers to the processes associated with poultry and poultry products between the time birds are caught, and the time the final product is delivered to the customer.

It includes:

Transport/procurement of bird, Withdrawal of feed supply, Ante mortem examination. Slaughter – stunning and bleeding, Scalding, Defeathering/picking, Pinning, Singing, Washing, Removal of feet and evisceration, Post mortem examination, Washing and cleaning, Processing giblets, Chilling, Storage.

Transport/Procurement

Coops, cages, crates or specially built vans are used. Avoid overcrowding of birds. It should be done in cooler hours of day, either morning or evening time.

Withdrawal of Feed

It should be done 24 hr before the slaughter.

Ante Mortem Examination

Inspection of birds for abnormal conditions as follows:

1. Reject grade – unfit for slaughter
   a) For example:- limber neck, fowl cholera, black head, infectious coryza, neural lymphomatosis, IB, CRD, Ranikhet disease, ornithosis etc
   b) Evidence of localized conditions: - severe injuries, discoloration of comb and wattle, bloody diarrhoea, bruishes etc.
   c) Birds with morbid conditions: - due to heat stroke or traumatic injury, greenish, yellowish- brownish/bloody diarrhoea, gasping and extreme emaciation.

2. Removal of birds and treatment: if respond then remove.

   Slaughter: It include stunning and bleeding.

   Stunning: Electrical stunning – water bath stunner is most commonly used. Other methods are: grid stunner, CO_2 stunner.

   Bleeding: There are different methods of bleeding. Modified kosher method is most commonly used. it leads to 35-50 per cent bleeding in 1-2 min.

   Scalding: it is defined as submerging killed birds in hot water.

   It is of 4 types:

   I. Soft scalding :- 50-51.5 ° C for 2.5 min. hand pinning required (no complete defeathering)

   II. Semi scalding: - 53-55 ° C for 1-2 min. for broiler and heavy fowl.

   III. Sub scalding:-56-60 ° C for 30 – 75 sec. easy defeathering and uniform skin color.

   IV. Hot/hard scalding: - 82 – 86 ° C for 30-60 sec. for water fowl, turkey, spent hen, causes discoloration of skin.

   Defeathering/picking: feathers removal done mechanically, 2 type:- dry picking -used for domestic purpose; Wet picking - for commercial purpose, done either by hand or mechanically.

   Pinning: It is removal of pin feather.

   Singeing: done for removal of hair like appendages called filoplumes.

   Washing: by spraying water before evisceration to reduce microbial load.

   Removal of feet and evisceration: Remove the feet at tarsometatarsal joint., Remove oil glands and head.Open abdominal cavity, remove viscera, gall bladder, crop and wind pipe carefully without breaking intestine. Take out lungs, ovary, oviduct or testis.

   Washing and cleaning: from both outside and inside with cold and clean water.

Postmortem Examination

Rejected and declare unfit in following cases:- CRD, coccidiosis, erythroblastosis, erysipelas, aspergillosis, infectious coryza, infectious laryngotracheitis, pullorum, fowl typhoid, Ranikhet disease, listeriosis, T.B. etc.

- ☆ **Processing Giblets**: include gizzard without contents, heart without pericardium and liver without gallbladder. Separately cleaned, wrapped and stuffed inside the eviscerated carcass.
- ☆ **Chilling and packing**: It is done at 2.2 – 4° C.
- ☆ **Different value added chicken products are:** Chicken casserole, Chicken curry, Chicken salad, Chicken salami, Chicken sambhar, Chicken samosa, Chicken sandwich, Chicken chow mein, Chicken sausage, Chicken soup, Chicken tikka, Chicken biryani, Chicken nuggets, Chicken roll, Chicken risotto.

Marketing of Poultry and Poultry Products in India

The domestic poultry market size is estimated at more than Rs. 47,000 crore. Indian poultry sector has been growing at around 8-10 per cent annually over the last decade and at more than 15 per cent in last three years. The processed chicken market is expected to grow at a much stronger pace of more than 25 per cent. Domestic poultry industry has few large scale integrated players like Venkateshwara Hatcheries (VH) group, Suguna Poultry Product Limited, Godrej Agrovet Limited, Charoen Pokphand (India) Private Limited, Arambagh Hatcheries Limited, etc (*www.icra.in*)

Outlook

The annual per capita poultry meat consumption in India though increasing from 0.7 kg in 2001 to 2.5 kg in 2010 remains one of the lowest globally with vast gap even between NIN (National Institute of Nutrition) recommended levels of 11 kg of poultry meat per person. Population is increasingly converting to a non-vegetarian diet. Poultry meat is preferred over other meat products as it is considered more hygienic and is available year around throughout the country at relatively lesser prices than fish/mutton. This offers a tremendous opportunity for further integration and growth in industry.

Fish Processing and Marketing

Introduction

Fishing is one of the oldest occupations of man. About 18000 fish species are found in India.

It is playing an important role in the economy of the country. As it helps in augmenting food supply, generating employment, raising nutritional level and earning foreign exchange by export.

Fish is a highly perishable item (high moisture and nutrient) and reportedly, bulk of the catch is sun-dried after salt curing which is certainly an unhygienic process. Kerala, Goa, Maharashtra, Gujarat, Orissa, Tamil Nadu, West Bengal and Karnataka are the leading states in fisheries.

It refers to the processes associated with fish and fish products between the time fish are caught or harvested, and the time the final product is delivered to the customer.

Processing is done to preserve the fish.

All methods are designed to arrest the autolysis and bacterial action.

Handling of Fish

It is done to preserve the quality of fish by bringing down the temperature near 0° C as quickly as possible.

Transportation

Keep the temperature down by using ice or kept in refrigerator.

Some good practices that should be followed before or during processing are:

- ☆ Avoid warming of fish.
- ☆ Avoid mishandling (prevent skin and flesh damage).
- ☆ Fishes caught at different time should be kept separately. Also separate small and large fishes.
- ☆ Keep the container clean used for transportation.
- ☆ Adopt good hygienic practices.

Storage

Different methods are:

1. **Chilled Storage**: different methods are- iced storage (1:1 ratio of fish and ice), chilled seawater storage (better than ice alone), chilled freshwater storage and refrigerated seawater.
2. **Freezing method**: (temp -18 to -40° C, most commonly -35° C),
   a) *Air freezing*: *e.g.* - sharp freezing, tunnel freezing, plate freezing, etc
   b) *Liquid immersion freezing*: cryogenic freezing liquid N_2 (-196° C) or subliming CO_2 (-80° C or sometime CCl_2F_2 is also used.

Note: In frozen thawed cooked fish quality is maintained by using – antioxidant(BHA, BHT, ascorbic acid etc), dip in 6-15 per cent NaCl solution for 20 sec before freezing, eliminating O_2

Canning

Destruction of micro organism by using heat.

Use of appropriate container inhibits the re-entry of microorganisms and further spoilage.

Salient features of canning:

- ☆ Consumer safety
- ☆ Ready to consume products
- ☆ Concentrated product as only edible part is packed.
- ☆ No special storage facility needed.
- ☆ Very long shelf life
- ☆ Processing methods simple.

Procedure

Selection and preparation of raw materials: variety of fin fishes(tuna, sardine, seer fish etc) and shellfishes (shrimp, crab, oyster,clam etc) are suitable.

Preparation: descaling, beheading, gutting, removal of fins,tail and cutting in smaller pieces.

In some shellfishes, purification (by starving18-24 hr) is done.

Blanching/Pre-Cooking

It is done in two methods:

1. **Cold blanching**: - here dressed fish is immersed in a salt solution. Dipping time and concentration vary depending on the species and size of the fish.

   It helps in removal of blood, dirt, gives firmness to texture and imparts a salty taste to product.

   It also reduces bacterial population.

2. **Hot blanching**: - done for shellfishes including shrimps and crabs.

   Here we use boiling brine.

   It gives characteristics red color, curls and shrinks in size permitting adequate filling into cans.

Note

Blanching/precooking in steam removes 15-30 per cent of body water

Most commonly used container is OTS cans (open top sanitary can which is made up of 98 per cent steel and 2 per cent tin coating on either side. Internally coated with a sulphur resistant lacquer. It prevents black discoloration of fish.)

Exhausting: Removal of air from contents and headspace of the can before it is seamed.

It minimizes strain on the seam through expansion of air.

Remove oxygen (decreases chances of corrosion), Ensures proper vacuum, Decreases oxidation of fat so deterioration chances less.

3 methods:

1. **Heat exhausting**: heating time is adjusted to obtain a core temperature 85° C, circulating steam is used. It is most widely used.
2. **Mechanical exhausting**: filled cans are sealed in a vacuum seaming machine, air is drawn out and sealed. Steam injection:- a jet of steam is used for vacuum creation.
3. **Can coding**: Can must have some information like:

   Details of product, date and year of production, producer's name etc. Code should be in English and numerals. Code marking should not damage lacquer or tin coating.

Seaming (sealing can):- it is done:

To provide air tight seal. And To prevent micro-organisms entry.

Heat Processing

It is the most important part of canning. Heating at a high temperature (110 ° C or above) to sufficient length of time to destroy or inactivate all micro organisms(specially *Clostridium botulinum*). After heating cool immediately (to 37 ° C), to decrease the temperature and pressure.

Curing of Fish

Traditional, oldest and cheapest method of processing. Include salting, drying, smoking and pickling.

Drying

It decreases moisture level and water activity so decreases the microbial activities.

2 methods

1. Sun drying: - traditional method using natural weather. No control over operation.
2. Artificial drying: - expensive method. A blast of hot air is passed over material.

There are different types of dryer:- cabinet dryer, tunnel dryer, multi deck tunnel, fluidized bed dryer, contact dryer (vacuum, rotary and drum dryer)

Salting, Curing

One of the oldest method of preservation of fish.

Usually done as such or in combination with drying or as a pretreatment to smoking. Osmotic transfer of water out of fish and salt in the fish. Different methods of salting:- dry salting, wet salting, pickle salting etc.

Smoking

Curing is done by smoke.

Salted and partially dried fish is used for salting. Source of smoke is wood, saw dust or coconut husk. Smoking of fish is either cold (28–32°C), hot (70–80°C), liquid and electrostatic.

It gives particular flavour, decrease moisture content of fish, have bactericidal property.

Fish protein and other substances get concentrated and product becomes harder. No much change in nutritive value (however some protein denaturation, lipid oxidation, decrease digestibility occur). Preservatives used in cured fish: - benzoic and sorbic acid (most common), nitrites, BHA, BHT etc.

Fish Marketing in India

Fishery and aquaculture are two very important facets of the Indian economy.

India is the second largest in aquaculture production in the world. The fish production during 2010-11 is estimated to be 8.29 million tonnes. The domestic fish marketing system in India is neither efficient nor modern and is mainly carried out by private traders with a large number of intermediaries between producer and consumer. Andhra Pradesh accounts for about 25-30 per cent of India's total seafood exports. Major Fish Manufacturers and Exporters of India are:-

Sea Star Marine Service, Aksa Sea Foods, M S Exim Corporation, Ved Agro Agency, Poonam Ice and Cold Storage, Oceayanic Groups, Mekatronics Products

Pvt. Ltd., Hiran Fish Aquarium, Aksha Fish Meal and Oil, Samudram, Richu Exports and Imports etc. Most of India's fish exports have gone to Japan closely followed by United Arab Emirates, U.S.A. and the Southeast Asian countries like Thailand, Singapore, China and Malaysia. India's main import is fishmeal. Another product imported from Bangladesh is the Hilsa.

Problems in Fish Marketing

It include high perishability, bulkiness of material, high heterogeneity in size and weight among species, high cost of storage and transportation, no guarantee of quality and quantity of commodity, low demand elasticity and high price spread and a large number of intermediaries.

Conclusion

There is an urgent need to frame a right strategy for the development of meat and poultry production in the country. This will certainly bring prosperity to millions of our rural citizens and create employment in rural India. As after white revolution, green revolution, there is full scope of Pink Revolution in country's meat and poultry processing sector.

References

Kondaiah, N. 2004. Value added meat products and Development of processed meat sector. Izzatnagar I.V.R.I., 34: 281-283.

http://nopr.niscair.res.in/bitstream/123456789/9435/1/NPR per cent 203(4) per cent 20281-283.pdf

http://mofpi.nic.in/ContentPage.aspx?CategoryId=173

http://www.assocham.org/events/recent/event 523/Dr SK_Ranjhan.pdf

http://en.wikipedia.org/wiki/Smoked fish

http://www.indg.in/agriculture/fisheries/value-added-products-from-fish

http://dahd.nic.in/dahd/WriteReadData/Annual per cent 20Report per cent 20English per cent 202011-12.pdf

Poultry production and management by Jagdish Prasad

Handbook of Fisheries and Aquaculture, ICAR.

http://www.icra.in/Files/ticker/Poulltry-Note-June-2011.pdf

www.fnbnews.com)

– *Chapter 28* –

Storage and Packaging of Poultry and Fish Products

I. Food Packaging materials

1. Paper: Paper and paper based containers, fiber board or cardboard cellulosic material grass, soft wood. Laminates, lebeling wrappers etc.
2. Glass containers: Limited use
3. Metal containers: Limited use
4. Plastics
5. Rubber

Clasification

1. Rigid containers: Difficult to deform, Product take the shape of container-glass, fiber board, metal container.
2. Semi rigid containers: Definite shape, not influenced by shape of content, but can be dented *e.g.* Molded pulp container, egg containers, Aluminium foil of higher gauge.
3. Flexible: Acquire shape and contour of product *e.g.* Plastic films, paper, Al. foil in thinner gauge.

Rigid Containers

Glass

Versatile, multiple application, In poultry – limited use, storage of albumen flakes/egg powder replaced by laminated pouches. glass jars- poultry meat spreads, Chicken essence solid contents 10-11 per cent.

Composition of Glass

Silica (SiO_2)73 per cent, lime (CaO)11 per cent, soda ash (Na_2O) 14 per cent, Alumina (Al_2O_3) 1 per cent. MgO, FeO, Potash, decolouring agent may be used to impart specific property. Green, blue, amber colour to prevent light penetration. For more transparency- Selenium, Cobalt used.

a) Amber colour: iron oxide, C and S in the melt.
b) Green colour: iron, manganese and chromium oxide in traces.
c) Blue colour: cobalt oxide is used.
d) Pyrex/Borosil : Silica, Barium oxide.

Advantages

(i) Transparency (ii) Non flexible (iii) Chemically inert (iv) Non-leachable (only in highly alkaline hot solution may cause leaching of glass container) (v) excellent barrier- water vapor, gas (vi) versatile –different size, shape (vii) recycled.

Disadvantages

(i) weight- add to cost of transport (ii) fragile (iii) not suitable to high pressure packaging, canning etc., low mechanical strength.(iv) thickness-thinner glass container resist thermal treatment (retort packaging) differential expansion an heating- crack at junction.

Forms of Glass Container

(i) bottle (Narrow necked) (ii) jar (wide mouthed) - pickles (iii) tumbler neck less, top open (iv) Carboy: shipping containers 10gal (cap) (v) Vials and ampoules: pharmaceutical, chicken essence.

Metal Containers

Materials

(a) Mild steel plates (low carbon)
(b) Tin plates: mild steel plate coated with tin layer.
(c) Terne plate: mild steel coated with tin/lead alloy layer outside and inside.
(d) Galvanised steel: zinc coated steel
(e) Stainless steel: Nickel, chromium steel.
(f) Aluminum: more common metals, tubes, cans, box etc.
(g) TFS: Tin free steel
(h) Tin plate container

Tin Plate Can

Low carbon tin plate 0.15-0.5mm thickens coated with thin layer of tin on both sides, corrosive resistant.

Seam

Joining of two pieces. seam is the most weak area- rupture, break or dent during process.

Seamless can: molded cans.

Soldering: Use alloy to join the ends.

Welding: electrically (heat+ pressure), pure tin difficult to coating, so tin + impurities

Types of metal cans: Tin plates.

(1) Hole and cap: HAC narrow hole on the top, difficult to fill the food material. Hole is sealed by a cap by soldering.

(2) OTS: (open top sanitary) cans = 25 per cent of total cans, top is open completely. Cap is separate, easy filling and removal.

Thickness of tin plate: considerably reduced by double cold reduction process (DCR) this very tensile strength (forces against stretching) is increased - this process also lowers the thickness of tin plates without affecting any stiffness or strength.

High Tin filled can/(HTF) can: Made from tin plate, coating of tin is 2.8gm/cm^2 on either side *i.e.* contains higher content of tin per unit area 5.6gm/m^2 by hot dipping or molten bath. Now it is electrolytic or electroplating process - very thin coating or differential coating is possible.

Low Tin coated steel can/(LTS) can: 1.1g/m^2 area of tin plate - Thickness of coating tin, uses: canning of chicken soup, meat balls in gravy, beef curry, meat curry.

Tin Coating

(i) Hot dipping or conventional method. Passing steel plate in molten tin bath, no control of thickness, even up to 11-28g/m^2, only reduce duration of contact, give thick and non-uniform coating, but finish is bright.

(ii) Electroplating or electrolytic coating: is done now-a-days, thickness reduced to desired level, differential coating (outside + inside) can be done. Coating down to 2.8g/m^2 on each side or 5.6g/m^2 both sides.

(iii) Flow brightening: Thin plating in electroplating, dull appearance. Removed by flow brightening, hot dipping in hot oil/electro heating.

Corrosion in tin plate: Electrochemical reaction involving transfer of electron.

(i) O - food contain entrapped O, act as catalyst

(ii) Moisture- more O, Sn -ve, Fe +ve.

(iii) Electrolyte

leaching out of tin layer, react with food, acidic food- corrosion more.

Changes due to Corrosion

(i) Discolouration

(ii) Flavour
(iii) Toxicity

Degree of corrosion: following are the factors.

(i) Acidity of food -more acidic more corrosion
(ii) Presence of Sodium nitrite/nitrate.
(iii) Amount of head space- more head space, more corrosion
(iv) Residual O - trapped in food.
(v) Processing time and temp.
(vi) Storage condition.

Corrosion of Tin Plate

Tin plate is a mild steel plate coated on each side with a thin layer of tin. Dissolution of tin by the food products or atmospheric condition is known as corrosion. Since tin exciting is thin and is not 100 per cent complete, particularly after fabrication of can due to rigor or stress produced during conversion of tin plate into container. Attach on steel wall due to dissolution of tin layer may lead to pin holding of the container.

Corrosion leads to discoloration (due to production of iron oxide), off flavour development and toxicity. Hence lacquer coating is done to protect the inner wall of the container from corrosion brought about by food stuff.

Mechanism

Corrosion is an electro-chemical reaction evolving transfer of electrons. when two dissimilar metals are immerged in water or some other electrolyte (conducting solution) and then connected, a current flows and there is a galvanic cell or electric cell. If water (since water is poor conductor of electricity) is absolutely pure only very little current will flow. The two metals in such a cell are called electrodes'. One is a anode (+ ve). The flow of current is due to flow of electrons from anode to cathode (*i.e.* from + ve to –ve).

The loss of electrons from a metal anode leaves the metal below the liquid surface as a positive ion which is soluble and slowly dissolving in the electrolyte. In case of tin plate container the two metals tin and steel in contact with as electrolyte. If the tin is anode and steel is cathode then tin is dissolved in the electrolyte foodstuff and steel remains unaffected. Hence tin is sacrificial anode because by its dissolution it protects steel.

However the electrochemical behaviour of tin is influenced by other factors *i.e.* oxygen in the head space or foodstuff. If oxygen is less then acts as a anode and steel as cathode a desirable condition because tin is dissolved and remain unattached. But if oxygen concentration is higher then tin acts as cathode and steel plates causing perforation of the container.

Polarization

The passage of electric current through a electrolyte leads to production of hydrogen (H) gas at cathode (-ve) pole, most of hydrogen escapes, but gas bubbles deposit at the cathode and cause the current to flow in the opposite direction. This reduces the overall flow of current and the phenomenon is called polarization.

In case of corrosion any factor which reduces the current flow *i.e.* increases polarization reduces the corrosion rate. Conversely any factor which reduces polarization will accelerate corrosion. Thus gives explanation of the effect of dissolved oxygen in food products as the corrosion of steel in contact with tin. High O content in food react with H deposited at cathode, thus making unavailable of H_2 at cathode and reduces the polarization process and thereby allowing electric current to be restored and promotes corrosion.

O and H are two factors necessary for corrosion of item. The corrosion product is iron oxide. Any factor which interferes with the normal function of electrolyte (here tin and steel) or the electrolyte may slow down or even stop corrosion process. Conversely any factor promotes their function will accelerate corrosion.

Stress Corrosion

Due to stress brought about by cold drawing or too severe drawing in fabrication of containers, electro chemicals reaction between stressed anodic area (+ve) and unstressed cathode area (–ve).

Passivity

A passive state of metal electrode which ceases to dissolve depend upon electrolyte *e.g.* metals like iron the passivity is formed by alkalinity but tungsten metal become passive in acidic environment.

Lacquer

An organic protective layer given on tin coating to prevent discoloration, staining of canned food, (syn: lining, enamel, organic protective coating).

Inhibitors, Corrosion of Tin Plate

(i) Inhibitors are added in electrolyte during coating *e.g.* cystine, gelatin, agar agar, edible gums, Carboxy methyl cellulose. These substances interfere with the functions of the electrolyte or electrodes thus inhibit corrosion.

(ii) Nitrate introduced corrosion: Thiourea, carbon disulfide, diphenyle thiourea - minimize liberation of H.

(iii) Can Lacquers: to protect food can against corrosion should be nontoxic, economic heat stable, no odour to product, uniform coating. Two types,

  (a) Acid resistant lacquers : For semi acid for pH 4.5 or more *e.g.*

  (i) Oleoresins Congo gum, rosin,(ii) plant oils *viz.* Tung oil, castor oil(dehydrated).

  (b) Sulphide Resistant Lacquers : (i) vinyl resins (ii) Phenolic resins (iii) epoxide resins.

ZnO is invariably a constituent of acid resistant lacquers. ZnO 10 per cent is added to it to make it sulfur resistant lacquers. Because ZnO+FeS form zinc sulphide so sulfur is not available. So blackening color is minimized.

Tin Free Steel (TFS) Cans

Base plate mild steel, there is a coating of chromium oxide. Coating is done by electrolytic process, little costly, high resistance to corrosion induced by acid, alkali, salt, sulfur, better printing.

Aluminum Cans

Light wt. container, non toxic, better thermal treatment, pure aluminium sheet is difficult to mold. Si, Cu, Fe, Mn, Mg added in trace amounts to pure Al. to enhance physico- chemical properties, not good for acid food, may be used for meat, fish, dairy products.

Composite Cans

Made of more than one metal, body may TFS, top and bottom Al etc. *e.g.* packs of tinopal, toothplaste.

Semi Rigid Containers

Al. in higher gauges, 0.1to 0.2 mm generally, not commonly used for meat used as component of laminates.

Physico-Chemical Properties of Metal Containers

1. Thickness of tin coating expressed as
   E (Electrolytic) 11.2/10.5(inside/outside)
   H (Hot dipping) 2.4/2.4(inside/outside)
2. Particle size of tin coating: coarse or smooth, fine etc.
3. Dimension: of metal containers
   Cylindrical can = diam x height 705x512 inch
   Rectangular can = LxWxH = old practice $7\ {}^{5}/_{16}$ X $5\ {}^{12}/_{16}$

Now a days expressed in mm *i.e.* 400 x 250x 400mm

Corrosion testing: chemical testing is done.

1. Chemical extraction method: normal storage condition, metallic ions leaching under simulating condition, estimated in atomic absorption spectrophotometer

2. Electrochemical testing: done by measuring of magnitude and intensity of electric flow. if current flow more, there is more corrosion.

Limit of metal constituents in canned meat products.

Arsenic 1ppm, Lead 2.5 ppm, Copper 20 ppm, Zinc 50 ppm, Tin 250 ppm

Other Tests for Ductility

1. Ductility: tests for resistance of tin plate to stress during bending.
2. Jenkins test: A sample is placed in a machine and subjected to bending at 90° in one direction and then other direction until it breaks, number of bends before break is counted.
3. Erichson test: A piece of tin plate is clamped and pressure is applied using pneumatic pump until it splits. At this point the pressure is measured.

Fiber board containers: Paper, cellulose 30 per cent, hemicelluloses 10-20 per cent, cellulosics/paper/card board/fiber board made from fibrous grass, wood, recycling of paper. Mostly used as secondary packages for transport, less use in poultry.

I. Rigid Containers

1. Solid fiber board container: made for fibers, Kraft paper by gluing with sodium silicate as adhesive, thickness to 0.8 to 2.8mm, wet resistance depend upon type of wood pulp, no. of plies, adhesives used for joining the plies mainly used for boxes in transportation.
2. Corrugative fiber board container: made from Kraft paper board corrugated single wall, double or triple flutes. Used for egg transportation, secondary packaging.

Type of flutes: A, B,C, and E. nos. of corrugation/meter length.

A: (Broad) 105-125 - 4.5-4.7 mm

B: (Narrow) 150-185-2.1-2.9mm

C: (Medium) 120-145-3.5-3.7mm

E: (Micro) 290-320-1.1-1.5mm

Factors for selection of fiber board container:

(1) Wt of content (2) Dimension of content (3) Mechanical strength - bursting strength, tensile strength, tear resistance (4) type of opening - easy open, self locking device (5) moisture resistance (bitumen is used for this) by product of refinery of crude oil. (6) Easy printing.

Wooden Creates

Transport of birds, now replaced by plastic creates- wt, easy cleans.

Plastic Packaging Material

Plastic containers were introduced around 1950 for packaging of food products. First commercial film was introduced in 1924 as cellophane.

Plastics (Polymers)

Most plastics or polymers used for food packaging are thermoplastic *i.e.* they can be softened by heating and hardened by cooling repeatedly provided that no chemical decomposition occurs. Thermo sets cannot be softened and hardened repeatedly. They undergo an irreversible change on heating and do not softened. They get charred at higher temp. Since their molecular structure is a complex three dimensional bonded network. Main uses of the thermosets are bottle caps and in most cases contact with food does not occur due to use of liners as a barrier.

In food packaging applications thermoplastics are preferred since basic polymer has to undergo several heating and cooling cycles during its conversion into containers or films. Most thermoplastics are chemically regarded as derivatives of ethylene ($CH_2=CH_2$). They are also often referred to as venyl plastic, since they contain the vinyl groupings($CH_2=CHR$) or polyolefins since all monomers contain an olefin linkage before polymerization.

Monomer: single unit of a substance.

Polymer: repeating monomer units resulting high mol. wt. units.

Homopolymer – Polymer of only one substance.

Copolymer : Blend of two or more types of polymer.

Condensation polymerization: Chemical reaction in which the two more molecules combine with the separation of water.

Film: Sheet having thickness not more than 0.25mm.

Ethylenic (or polyolefins) Thermoplastic

1. Polyethylene

Minimum 85 per cent polymer of ethylene and 15 per cent copolymer. PE can be defined as polymer of ethylene gas obtained as a byproduct from petrochemical industries. It is done by addition polymerization using catalysts, largest vol. film used in flexible packaging industries, manufactured by addition polymerization process.

LDPE

LDPE is produced by polymerization of ethylene gas at high pressure (1000-3000 atm.) and at high temp. (150-200°C). this process result in a macromolecule with high degree. of branching *i.e.* a mixture of single long chain and chains with branches linked at right angles to the main chain. But when low pressure process is used-then formation of long parallel linear chains occurs. Density 0.9084 to 0.9384 at 27°C. The molecular formula of the polymer is $(CH_2)n$.

The carbon atoms are linked by strong covalent bonds at a distance of 1.54A° (15.4nm) at an angle (α) = 109°

For food grade thermoplastic, especially PE the units of additives as follows: Catalysts for polymerization (0.2 per cent) of finished product

1. Catalysts for polymerization(not more than 0.2 per cent of finished products
2. Lubricants(not more than 0.3 per cent of finished product)
3. Emulsifying agent (not more than 0.03 per cent of finished product)

4. Antistatic or antifoaming agent(not more than 1.5 per cent)
5. U-V absorbers (not more than 0.5 per cent)
6. Antifungal agent (not more than 1.0 per cent)
7. Pigments/clays/filler
8. Anti blocking agent: the agent to control sticking (adhesion) between touching layers of plastic during storage, application of heat, pressure etc.

The neighbouring chains are stabilized by a much weaker van der waal forces, which account for much of the plasticity of LDPE of the same thickness as that of HDPE, more flexible.

Branched chain polymer of LDPE- The branch chain prevents close packing of the polymer chain and hence the finished polymer is a low density. The branching of chains also lowers crystallinity.

Types: two types- LDPE and linear LDPE (LLDPE)

LDPE Properties

Elasticity tend to recover their original size and shape when deformed

1. Tough, transparent and flexible
2. Excellent resistance to most chemicals below 60°C, but above this temp the polymer becomes soluble in hydrocarbon solvents.
3. Good barrier to water vapor but less for gases *e.g.* O_2
4. Lower softening (melting pt.) hence not suitable for packaging of food products which are to be heat sterilized.
5. Because of flexibility and heat sealability properties, it is easily converted into film for packaging of fresh frozen foods.
6. Suitable for coating into other materials such as paper and Al foil.
7. Moderate tensile strength.

HDPE

Density 0.9384 to 0.9634 at 27°C, is produced as low pressure and temp *i.e.* 50 to 75°C, 10 atm or 60-100°C, 40 atm.

Types: two types-HDPE and high molecular HDPE (HMHDPE)

Properties of HDPE

1. Stiffer, harder, less transparent.
2. High melting or softening pt. (increased solubility to heat hence seam sterilized)
3. Better resistant to oils and greases.
4. lower permeable to water vapor and gases than LDPE

Polypropylene (PP)

It is the polymer of propylene and the structural formula is as follows. One of hydrogen atoms of ethylene has been replaced by CH_3 group. (Polypropylene monomer)

1. **Atactic Form:** irregular arrangement of CH_3 group *i.e.* the methyl groups (CH_3) are randomly distributed on either side of the main chain *i.e.* exists as irregular macromolecule of polypropylene.
2. **Isotactic form**: regular arrangement of CH_3 gr., produced by using stereo specific catalysts and low pressure which results in the regular arrangement of the methyl group onto the same side of the polymer chain, has high crystalline due to regular arrangement of CH_3 group but not as high as HDPE, as a result this polymer (pp) is harder and has high softening point than HDPE but low shock resistance especially at low temp.

Properties of Isotactic Form

1. PP is more rigid, stronger and lighter than PE
2. The film has low WVTR,good grease resistance
3. It has high temp. resistance and good gloss, hence good printability

Types

1. Unprinted PP film: Generally not used in food packaging it has low temp. stability and poor gas barrier.
2. Oriented film: Monoaxially- stretching the film in one direction.

Biaxially- stretching in two directions. PP film is generally used in oriented form by stretching the film monoaxially or biaxial (film is stretched in two direction at right angles under suitable temp. condition, the resulting film has (i) good tensile properties to water vapor and gases (ii) high tensile strength (iii) high abrasion resistance (iv) good gloss and clarity (transparency)(v) very high melting point.

Uses

1. As biaxial oriented film (BOPP) in flexible packaging.
2. As one of the plies in lamination.
3. As rigid container- jar, bottles, trays

Food Packaging Application

1. Container for food storage.
2. Drinking straw
3. Wrapping of foods and biscuits

(3) Polyvinyl Chloride (PVC)

It is the polymer of vinyl chloride. Polymerization is done in the presence of catalysts. By addition of plasticizers, flexible film is obtained. Structural formula - one of the hydrogen atoms in the ethylene molecule is substituted by halogen (chlorine).

Properties of PVC

1. The film is hard, stiff, clear and glossy surface.
2. Excellent moisture barrier.
3. Low gas permeability.
4. Good grease resistance.

Uses

1. Rigid containers such as jars, bottle, trays (for carbonated drink, mineral water, edible oil)
2. Flexible film in biaxially oriented form for shrinks packaging of meat and chunk.
3. Film used as copolymer *i.e.* component of laminate.

(4) Polyvinylidine Chloride (PVDC)

Saran film or cryo-vac film is the polymer of vinylidine chloride. The structural formula of vinylidines chloride (VDC) *i.e.* two atoms of hydrogen in the ethylene molecule have been substituted by chlorine atoms. It is generally used as a copolymer with PVC (13 to 20 per cent)

Properties

1. The film is clean, good mechanical strength.
2. Low WVTR and gas permeability.
3. Good grease resistant
4. Insoluble in many organic solvents.

Uses

1. Used as film (saran film) for packaging of meat.
2. As a component of laminate (copolymer)

Food packaging application: meat, sausage, cheese, dried fruit wrapper.

(5) Polystyrene (PS)

It is the polymer of styrene. Styrene consists of an ethylene molecule in which one of the hydrogen atoms has been substituted by a phenyl radical.

PS: Because of the bulky nature of phenyl radical, polymerisation of styrene, results in amorphous macromolecular chain. The phenyl radical during polymerization prevent close packing of polystyrene (PS) molecule.

Properties

1. Is transparent
2. Good barrier to gases
3. Poor barrier to water vapor

4. Soluble in alcohol, ketones, esters and aromatic and chlorinated hydrocarbons.

Disadvantages

It is brittle and hence often copolymerized with butadiene and/or acrylonitrile.

Uses

1. As molded tubs, cups dairy products (ice cream, cheese, cream)
2. As a copolymer
3. PS slabs (laminates) for insulation in card board boxes.

The polystyrene film is brittle and hence is biaxial oriented to reduce the brittleness.

(6) Polytetrafluoro Ethylene (PTFE)

It is polymer of tetrafluoro ethylene, in this case the ethylene molecule has been fully substituted with fluorine atoms. The PTFE is highly crystalline and has very high mol.wt.

Properties

1. Extremely inert to chemical.
2. Very low coefficient of friction producing non stick surface and can withstand wide range of temperature.

Uses

As a coating on frying pans and other cookery wares.

Non Ethylenic Thermoplastics

(1) Polyamides (Nylons)

These are polymer prepared by Condensation Polymerization process of a diacid and diamine.

The reaction is presented below.

$$\underset{\text{Diamine}}{HN(CH)NH} + \underset{\text{Diacid}}{COOH(CH)COOH} = \underset{\text{Polyamides}}{[\text{-}NH(CH)NHCO(CH)CO\text{-}]_n}.$$

The first compound produced was nylon 6,6 made from adipic acid and hexamethylene diamine. Some polymers in these series are obtained by self condensation of one molecule only *e.g.* nylon6 prepared from omega- amino caproic acid.

Properties

1. Very strong, tough (excellent strength)
2. High melting point
3. Low friction and hence high abrasion resistance.
4. Low gas permeability and water vapour permeability.

Uses

1. Boil-in-bag type application for convenience foods.
2. As a component of laminates.

Polycarbonates

These are linear polyesters of carbonic acid.

Properties

1. Tough, stiff, hard and transparent
2. Withstand wide range of temp. (up to 300pC)
3. Soluble in chlorinated hydrocarbon solvents.
4. Not a good barrier to water vapor/gas.
5. Resistant to weak acids and alkalis.

Uses

1. As a flexible film, not generally used cost is prohibitive.
2. As a rigid, semi-rigid containers *i.e.* thin walled bottle, baby feeding bottle, oil, fruit juice.
3. Heat sealable film.

(2) Polyester

It is the condensation product of polyalcohol (or **mylar**) with a diacid or its anhydride.

Metalized polyester: is done by coating the plastic film with small quantity of metal (aluminum) by vaporization. The resulting film is transparent and abrasion resistant.

Properties of Polyester

1. Excellent tensile strength, tear resistance
2. Not heat sealable
3. Wide temp. Resistance.

Uses: in laminates *e.g.* retortable laminates.

(3) Polyvinyl Acetate

Polymer of vinyl acetate

Uses

1. As a coating on paper
2. As a copolymer (for sausage casings)

(4) Polyvinyl Alcohol

Prepared by hydrolysis of polyvinyl acetate.

Properties: soluble in water but insoluble in organic solvent, hence used for packaging oils and fats.

(5) Rubber

Polymer of isoprene (CH) monomer

Natural Rubber

Made from coagulation of latex obtained from rubber tree, contains 95 per cent hydrocarbons with some proteins, lipids and inorganic salts.*e.g.* rubber hydrochloride (pliofilm)

Synthetic Rubber

Made from byproducts of petroleum industry. Ethylene, propylene, butadiene, styrene and acrylonitrile are used as monomers.

Properties: flexible elastic, tough, waterproof and impermeable to air.

Rubber Hydrochloride (Pliofilm)

Made from natural rubbers by treatment with HCl.

Properties

(i) stretchable (ii) non-toxic (iii) resistant to grease and oil (iv) unaffected by weak acids and alkalis (v) Heat sealable.

Uses

1. As wrapper bags for meat, cheese.
2. As a liner of thermoplastic bags.
3. Sealing rings for cans, glass bottle.
4. Stopper for bottles/flasks
5. Conveyor belts
6. Rubber aprons and gloves.

Types of Synthetic Rubber

1. Styrene and butadiene rubber (SBR): has more abrasion resistance, elasticity, slightly inferior to natural rubber, process superior heat ageing characteristics.
2. Butyl Rubber: resistant to vegetable oil/grease/solvents.
3. Nitrile Rubber: is a copolymer of butadiene and acrylonitrile, excellent resistance to solvents/oils.
4. Silicon Rubber: excellent résistance to oil/grease excellent temp. resistance(-75 to 260°C)

(6) Cellulose/Cellophane

Cellophane "cello" means cellulose. The cellulose is treated with NaOH soln. and carbon disulphide to produce xanthate which is dispersed in NaOH to produce viscose: The viscose is extruded through a slot into acid salt bath to produce regenerated cellulose film which contains 70 per cent cellulose and 30 per cent additives.

Types: (1) Plain and transparent cellophane (PT) : The regenerated cellophane is washed, desulphured, bleached, softened, dried and wound as plain and transparent film.

Properties

(1) Non moisture proof (2) Not sealable.

Use

As wrapper for food

MST Cellophane: (moisture proof heat sealable and transparent). The cellophane film is coated on one or both sides to make it moisture proof and heat sealable. By application of various coating several grades of cellophane are available. MST/MSAT cellophane 300,400 or 600 plain/or coated grade 300 means 300g/10m^2 of film.

(a) Nitrocellulose coated cellophane: (NC coated) good water vapor barrier, flexible, heat scalable, not good barrier to oxygen.

(b) Saran coated cellophane: coated with PVDC.

(i) Flexible (ii) Heat sealable (iii) Good barrier to water vapor (iv) Good barrier to oxygen.

Uses: coated (saran) cellophanes are used for

(i) Meat wrapping film (ii) As a component of laminates (iii) Baked goods (cakes, breads, biscuits) vegetables confectionary.

Copolymers

Homopolymer : Repeating units of single monomer.

Copolymer: Two or more repeating units of monomers produced either by addition polymerization or condensation polymerization. The properties of a copolymer often differs markedly from either of the homopolymers and depends on :

1. Composition of the monomers used.
2. Arrangement of the monomers along the chain.

Examples of Copolymers

(1) Ethylene-vinyl Acetate (EVA)

It is made from the copolymerization of LDPE and vinyl acetates. Vinyl acetate may be up to 20 per cent in the copolymer.

Properties of EVA

1. More flexible than LDPE, more stretchable
2. Not good barrier to water vapour and gas.
3. Film is cleaner than LDPE
4. Impact strength is excellent
5. Unstable at high temperature but very stable and versatile at low temp.
6. Can be heat sealable.

Disadvantage

EVA has tendency to block due to polar nature of side chain in copolymer *i.e.* high coefficient of friction. Hence antiblocking agents are added to control adhesion (sticking) of both touching layers of plastic during storage or use.

Uses

1. As a coating to bags or industrial sacks
2. Shrink film packaging.
3. Suitable for low temperature storage of food products.

(2) Vinyl Chloride Copolymers

Vinyl chloride is copolymerized with

1. Vinyl acetate (VA)- VC/VA for increased flexibility.
2. Vinylidene chloride (VDC)- VC/VDC for flexible packaging and for better protection of food from water vapor/gas.
3. Polypropylene (PP) – VC/PP (up to 10 per cent) for making bottles.
4. Acrylonitrile (AN)

(3) Polystyrene Copolymer

1. SAN (Styrene and Acrylonitrile) – rigid containers (bottle, jars)
2. ABS (Acrylonitrile butadiene styrene): Three monomers are used, manufacturing of tubs, tray, boxes and as a liner of refrigerator.

These two copolymers possess impact resistance than polystyrene alone.

These monomers are member of ethylenic thermoplastic

(4) Polypropylenic/Ethylenic Copolymer

PP is a good barrier to water vapor/gases, has low impact resistance at low temp. Hence a copolymer made of PP/PE offers increased impact resistance to low temperature.

Other Films (Plastic)

(a) TPX = Chemically closely related to ethylene manufactured from polymerization of 4- methyl pentene-1 transparent, low density (0.83) compared to any plastic material. High melting pt. (474pF) hence used for hot filling and cooked food application. Disadvantage: Highly permeable to gases/water vapor.

(b) Acrylic film: (XT): excellent clarity, oil/grease resistant, gas permeability very low. Good impact but poor resistance to aromatic and chlorinated hydrocarbon.

Uses: Rigid container

(c) Polyurethane (PU): Tough, strength, abrasive resistance excellent oil/grease resistance uses motor oil packaging and boil- in- bag and flexible packaging of meat.

Laminates or Composite Films

Layers of individual material bonded together by adhesives, coated and co-extruded. No single polymer possesses all the desired properties, which may be required for efficient packaging of particular food stuff. In other words monolayer flexible packaging materials offer limited desired properties which may be achieved to a greater extent, by the use of coated or laminated packaging material. Consisting of two or more laminates depending upon the specific packaging needs of a product.

Types

1. All plastic laminate.
2. Laminate based on paper/Al.foil/thermoplastic.

Numerous possible combinations of individual layers of material for production of laminates are possible which depends on the specific requirements of the food to be packaged.

Examples

2-ply Laminates

1. Glassine 38 GSM/LDPE 150G
2. Grease proof paper 38 GSM/LDPE 150G
3. Litho paper 100 GSM/LDPE 100 G
4. Kraft paper 100 GSM/LDPE 100 G
5. Cellophane/LDPE
6. PVDC/PVC copolymer (or saran or cryovac)

3-Ply Laminates

1. Paper/Al foil/LDPE- Non retortable pouch
2. Polyester/Al foil/LDPE-Non retortable pouch

Retortable

can withstand processing temp. 135°C.

1. Poly amide (Nylon)/Al.foil/PP.

2. Polypropylene/PE copolymer
3. Polyester/Al. foil/oriented nylon/PP.
4. PP/Al.foil/PP

Non Retortable

1. Cellophane/PE
2. Nylon/PE
3. Paper/Al foil/PE (tetra brick)- milk, fruit juice, soft drink.
4. Polyester/Al foil/LDPE.

Meat, Cooked Meat, Brined Meat

Pouches of made of

1. PE/PVDC/PA
2. PE/metalized polyester
3. PE/Al.foil/Polyester.

In India the following packaging materials are being manufactured:

LDPE, Linear LDPE,HDPE, High molecular HDPE,PP,PE,PS and PVC.

Rigid bottles/jars/containers: Are made from HDPE,PP,PE and high impact PS.

PET bottles/jars/containers: Polyethylene terephthalate containers are made by blow molding or by co-extrusion process. These are food grade kitchen containers for stock of solids, semi-solid and liquids. PET containers are transparent, light weight, $^{1}/_{15}{}^{th}$ of glass jar wt. of same dimension, unbreakable.

Coloured PET bottles/jars: of diff- shape, sizes. Amber/green/blue/clear transparent.

Mfg: (i) M/S Pearl polymers Ltd. PET containers in India- BIS, FDA approved.

Heat seal strength of film/laminated pouch is influenced by :

1. Type and thickness of sealing medium
2. Composition of laminates/films
3. Sealing temp. and duration of sealing (time)
4. Pressure applied
5. Cooling timer
6. Area to be sealed.

Sealing

1. Hot jars sealing (temperature and Pr.)
2. Impulse heat sealing
3. Cold sealing by use of adhesives.

Retortable/Autocleavable Pouches

Usually heat sterilizable *i.e.* canning in pouches.

1. Polyester/Al foil/PP
2. Polyamide (nylon)/Al foil/PP
3. PP/Al foil/PP.

Boil-in-bag/cook in bags: For convenience packaging.

1. The bags should withstand the cooking,frying, baking, roasting or oven simmering temp.
2. Should reduce losses due to excessive dehydration during cooking.
3. Should require selectively shorter time to bring the food to desired temp. during cooking.
4. The package or bags should be strong to protect the food from the time of packaging, storage, handling and retailing.

Ideal Materials

1. Polyester (Mylar) film
2. Polyamides (Nylon) film

Physico-chemical properties flexible packaging material:

A knowledge of these packaging material is necessary for

1. Selection of appropriate packaging material for packaging of particular food products.
2. To select appropriate types of material to be converted into laminate.
3. To make economic use of packaging material thus reducing wastage due to wrong selection.

1. Thickness

Influence the rigidity, transparency, strength and salability of the film, thickness of thermoplastic films is measured by a suitable micrometer fitted with a dial gauge reading correct to 0.01 mm and expressed in gauge.

100 Gauge = 1/1000 inch or 0.001 inch

= 0.0025cm = 0.025 mm

Paper is not uniform in structure. Its properties varies from one sheet to other and from place to place in the same sheet. Hence it is expressed as GSM *i.e.* g/m^2.

2. Heat Seal Strength

Expressed as gm/cm width

3. Barrier Properties

(i) Water Vapour transmission Rate (WVTR):

A Knowledge of WVTR of plastic/paper/laminate is essential to select a material which is a good barrier to water vapor permeability.

- ☆ High moisture food- fresh meat (desiccation)
- ☆ Low moisture food- dehydrated meat pick up of moisture (<10 per cent)
- ☆ Intermediate moisture food(20-40 per cent) moisture requiring barrier to as well as to prevent condensation of water vapor. Aluminum dishes are filled with suitable desiccant *i.e.* anhydrous calcium chloride in the form of small lumps, sealed with the test material of known surface area (50cm^2 or 25 cm^2) with the help of wax and stored in a conditioned atmosphere (humidity cabinet maintained at 27pC to 65 per cent R.H. for a definite period of time or 38pC and 90 per cent R.H. The WVTR is computed from the ratio of increase in weight of the dish assembly. The cumulative wt. increase (in mg) is recorded at suitable intervals when the constant rate of increase attained, the expt. is discontinued

$$\mathrm{WVTR} = \frac{240x}{A \times y}$$

where, x= is weight increase in mg over a period of hr. for an exposure Area of A cm^2. WVTR expressed as= g/m^2/24hr. at 27p C, 65 per cent R.H.

OTR (Oxygen Transmission Rate)

Oxygen permeability by Beckman gas analyzer (*i.e.* CO_2, O_2, N_2)

OTR is expressed as cc/m^2/24hr at 27pC, 65 per cent R.H. at atmosphere pressure.

Table 28.1: Physical Properties of Plastic Films

Physical Properties	*Polyamide (Nylon)*	*Polycarbonate*	*LDPE*	*HDPE*	*PP*	*PVC*	*PVDC*	*PTFE*	*PS*
Mol.wt.	–	10u	1-3x10t	10u	10u	10t	–	10v	10t-10v
Crystallinity (per cent)	–	–	55-70	80-95	65-70	<5	–	93-98	–
Density (g/cm)	1.04	1.20	0.915-0.935	0.945-0.965	0.90	1.4	1.6-1.7	2.1-2.2	1.04-1.05
Softening pt. (°C)	175	135-165	86	120-130	150	70-80	100-150	–	78-103
Melting Pt. (°C)	185	220-230	112	137	168	220	–	342	240

PTFE: Coating of nonstick kitchenware.

PS: Egg cartoons, porous in nature.

Nylon: Lack of heat sealing but high mechanical strength, main use laminates, polycarbonate: not used in meat and meat products.

(4) Mechanical Properties

Elongation (at break) or stretch (per cent)

Bursting strength (kg/cm^2)

Tear resistance (g)

(i) Tensile Strength and Elongation (kg/15mm width)

Tensile strength is the measure of the resistance of test piece to rupture when tensile force (load) is applied. Higher tensile strength is desired to (1) to hold heavy packaged articles (2) For semi semi-automatic or automatic pouch forming machine (3) In operations such as laminating, coating and printing. It is expressed as kg force/15mm width of test material. For majority of thermoplastic film the TS range form 3 to 6kg/15mm width.

LDPE or HDPE in higher gauge (400 to 500) has more tensile strength (up to 15kg) among plastic films, both PS and PVC have poor tensile strength. Lamination of paper/foil/PE or polyester/foil/PE have high TS. Elongation property of flexible packaging material gives a measure of toughness or resistance to rupture. In food packages which are likely to experience drops during retail distribution require material of higher elongation. In general paper has low elongation value (2-5 per cent) whereas plastic such as LDPE or HDPE has 300-400 per cent elongation. The material to be tested is cut into strips in machine and cross (transverse) direction Length 200-250mm, width 10-50mm.The specimen are conditioned at the testing temperature and R.H. They shall be free from creases or wrinkles.

Both the ends of test strips is tightly clamped and tensile forces (load) or pulling force is applied to stretch the test piece and force (load) or tensile load is recorded from the load scale at the instant of break or rupture. The speed of machine is so adjusted that the fracture or rupture occurs in not less than 30 or more than 45 seconds. The readings are taken in each direction and average is reported.

Similar elongation (stretch) is recorded on stretch or elongation indicator at the instant of break and expressed as per cent elongation (per cent increase length over initial value)

Both tensile strength and per cent elongation are measured on the same machine. Tensile strength is generally more in machine direction (M.P) than transverse direction where as per cent elongation is generally more in T.D. than M.D.

Table 28.2: Physico-chemical Properties of Some Thermoplastics/Paper/Laminates

Thermoplastics and Paper and their Laminates	WVTR (g/m²/ 24 hr at 38°C and 90% RH	Tensile Strength Kg/15mm		Per cent Elonation		Bursting Strength (kg/cm²)	Tear Resistance (g)	
		MD	TD	MD	TD		MD	TD
LDPE(100G)	10.7	3.7	2.0	300	175	0.98	27	32
LDPE(200G)	5.7	2.9	2.2	>250	>250	1.4	120	120
LDPE(300G)	4.1	1.8	0.90	>250	>250	2.2	>120	>120
HDPE(100G)	3.8	7.0	4.2	305	110	0.70	34	47
HDPE(200G)	1.8	5.2	4.7	270	240	1.54	38	95

Contd...

Table 28.2–*Contd...*

Thermoplastics and Paper and their Laminates	*WVTR (g/m²/ 24 hr at 38°C and 90% RH*	*Tensile Strength Kg/15mm*		*Per cent Elonation*		*Bursting Strength (kg/cm²)*	*Tear Resistance (g)*	
		MD	*TD*	*MD*	*TD*		*MD*	*TD*
HDPE(300G)	1.4	3.6	3.2	>250	190	1.97	52	52
PVC(120G)	2.7	2.7	2.6	5	3	2.7	4.4	6.4
Polystrene (PS) (150G)	66	2.9	2.4	0.3	0.3	1.34	7.8	10.2
Polyester(PS) (100G)	13.1	8.3	6.7	58	81	4.64	20	30
PP(140G)	6.7	3.6	2.6	602	937	–	–	–
Kraft Paper (124GSM)	4260	9.6	5.8	3.0	5.0	2.39	87	165
Kraft/LDPE (124GSM/100G)	19.2	10.3	6.8	5.0	5.5	2.88	143	138
Glassine (40GSM)	1920	4.1	1.9	2.0	6.6	1.27	12	19
Glassine/LDPE (40GSM/150G	10.6	5.1	2.8	3.0	5.0	2.39	87	105
MSTcellophane (100)	27	6.7	2.9	16.5	58.5	–	–	–
PET/Al.foil/PE (12μ/0.009/150G)	Nil	11.6	11.1	56	60	–	–	–

Table 28.3: OTR (cc/24hr/m² at 27°C and atmospheric pressure)

	OTR	*Resistance to*	
		Acids	*Alkalies*
LDPE(185G)	8181	Excellent	Excellent
LDPE(365G)	3380	Excellent	Excellent
HDLP(330G)	2228	Good	Good
PP(140G)	6682	Good	Good
PET/Al.foil/PE(Nylon)	Nil	–	–
Cryovac/Saran/PVC/PVDC)	0.1-0.2 cc/100 sq.inch/24hr at 72°F		
Nylon(polyamides)	1.0 cc/	"	"

Table 28.4: Grease Resistance of Film/Laminates

Cellophane/LDPE (150G)	*A (Exudation time>30min)*
HDPE(300G)	A
PVC (120G)	A
Polystyrene(100G)	B (between 2min and 30 min)

Contd...

Table 28.4–*Contd...*

Cellophane/LDPE (150G)	*A (Exudation time>30min)*
HDPE (100G)	B
Kraft/LDPE	B
LDPE (100G)	C(Exulation times between 30sec. and 2 min)
Glassine	C

MD: Machine direction TD: Transverse direction.

PE has higher tear resistance

Laminates : " " (about 100g)

PVC and PS have poor tear resistance (4.4 to 7.8g)

Tear Tester (Elmendorf Type)

The machine is provided with two clamps - one fixed and other carried on a pendulum. On releasing of pendulum the centre tongue is subjected to load of pendulum which is recorded through a spring loaded friction pointed on the pendulum.

The test piece is cut with a template and the outer tongue of the test piece is held by fixed clamps and the centre tongue of test piece is held in the moving clamps. The pendulum is released and the load (g) necessary to continue tear is recorded.

(a) Grease Resistance

This property of packaging material is important since seepage of oils or fats from the product into the outer surface of package may result in (1) removal or smudging of the printed surface and (2) decrease in the protective function due to swelling of the packaging material.

Paper

Among paper glassine has better grease resistance (60 sec.)

1. Than grease proof (20sec) and Kraft paper
2. Cellophane, PVC and HDPE, Polystyrene. Polyester have good grease resistance
3. LDPE has poor grease resistance
4. Laminate of paper/PE or cellophane/PE had moderate grease resistance.

Grease resistance is expressed as transudation times in seconds:

Below 30 seconds- D

Between 30 seconds and 2 min- C

Between 2 min and 30 min- B

More than 30 min – A

Package Design and Packaging Equipments

Two Things

Functional role protection and Aesthetic feel

Convert raw material to package – shape, size, color, graphic pattern.

1. Selection of packaging material
2. Testing for its compatibility with the proof
3. Attractive labeling
4. Attractive shape and size for consumer satisfaction
5. Convenience to use, efficient disposal.

Steps to be taken while Designate

1. Idea generation, new package for a new product, modified package or existing package.
2. Initial market appraisal – assistance of market potential.
3. Idea screening
4. Design concept- develop questionnaire, intervening consumer.
5. Development of the package- packaging engineer play important role.

   Contour, shape, size, color, mechanical strength property, shelf life, stakability, unit pack/bulk package, cost – economics etc.
6. Actual performance testing
7. Business analysis – sale, cost, profit
8. Prototype development: small scale mfg.
9. Final market testing.

Packaging Machineries (Equipment)

Four types

1. Machinery manufacturing raw material for package.
2. Converting machineries raw material into container.
3. Machine for testing package performance-WVTR, mechanical strength, oxygen, permeability, transparent stress, impact resistance, drop test, tearing resistance.
4. Packaging machineries to package finished food into the container.

Sealer: (i)Impulse sealer- LDPE, HDPE, PP. (ii) hot jaw sealer for laminates mostly (iii) heat and pressure sealer - copolymer.

Sealing agents- PE, cold sealing - use of additives.

Packaging machine- Semiantimate, automatic.

Form fills and seal machine: *e.g.* pouch packaging of milk, packaging of egg powder.

Filler machine: Predetermined quantity of food is packaged.

Vacuum Packaging Machine

1. Metal tube type- most commonly for dressed chicken, metal tube suck the air, then automatic sealing, operator hold the pack.
2. Chamber type - automatic sealing
3. Jaw type – more sophisticated, adjust vacumization, keep minimum head space of bars, four control knobs- vacuum control knob, heating knob, cooling knob, gas knob

   OR Flusher: flushing out air.

   Chamber type: control switch vacuum switch, flushing switch etc. now more commonly used highest speed 1000/hr. cap. Trade name, multivac, swissvac, Autovac etc.,

II. Packaging Safety

Evaluation of packaging material for safe use in contact with food stuff. Plastic containers (rigid, semi-rigid, and flexible) are more or less chemically inert, so plastic widely used in food packaging. However improper manufacture and inanimate use of plastic material may endanger the safety of food material for human consumption. Therefore, there is growing concern over the migration of the trace amount of chemical constituents (monomer, additives) originally employed their manufacture.

All plastic including basic polymers contain a number of other substances during their manufacture and processing polymers are of very high mol.wt. Inert, of limited solubility in aqueous and fatty systems. Therefore polymers an unlikely transferred into the food to any significant effect. Even if fragments of polymer are accidentally swallowed they would not react body fluids of digestive system.

Concern over safe use of plastics as food packaging material arises principally from the possible toxicity of low mol. wt. constituents (*i.e.* monomer and additives). These constituent may get leached into the food stuffs during storage, such constituent arise from two sources:

1. Polymerization residues: ending monomer, oligomer mol.wt. upto 200, catalysts mainly metallic salts, organic peroxides, solvents, emulsifiers, wetting agents, raw material impurities, plant contaminants, inhibitors, and decomposition and side reaction products.
2. Processing aids such as antioxidants, anti-blocking agents, antistatic agents, heat and light stabilizers, plasticizers, lubricants, pigments, fillers, mould release agents and fungicides. These constituents are added to help production processes or to enhance the properties and stability of the final product.

Since compounds of first group are present inadvertently, there not a lot that can be done to remove them. However with optimum manufacturing practices the adjuvant used in polymerization (category1) can be kept to a minimum level. The greatest danger to human health is from the additives of the 2nd category.

Type of Additives Used in Manufacture of Plastics

1. **Antiblock agents:** Added to prevent blocking (adhesion of the surface of the film *i.e.* touching layers of films.) which develop under Pressure during storage or use. Silica most commonly used, because poor solubility in most polymers. It helps to increase the surface concentration. It makes the surface of the films rough hence prevent them. sticking together during processing fatty acidamides- are used to reduce mobile frictional forces.
2. **Antistatic agents:** Since all plastics are good electrical insulators (hence used in large scale for this purpose) they retain electrostatic charges produced by friction from contract with processing machinery. Accumulation of static electricity can cause problems such as pick up to dusts, adhesion between layers, sparking, electrical stock, sometimes fire hazards. Hence antistatic agents glycol derivatives or quarternary ammonium compounds are used which increase the electrical conductivity.
3. **Antioxidants:** Added to prevent the degradation of polymer from atmospheric oxygen. During moulding operation at high temp. or when used in contact with hot foods. Derivatives of phenols and organic sulphides are most frequently used. Some of these components are called heat stabilizers.
4. **Lubricants:** used to reduce frictional forces (low to medium mol. wt. hydro carbons).
5. **Plasticisors** used to make the plastic more flexible and less brittle, of high mol.wt. esters *e.g.* phthalates.
6. **U.V. stabilizers:** protect the product from deterioration by sunlight or supermarket lighting.
7. **Catalysts:** used to enhance polymerization process *e.g.*NaCl, KCl, $NaNO_3$, KNO_3.
8. **Antifungal agents:** to prevent fungal contamination *e.g.* Ascorbyl palmitate.
9. **Pigments fillers, dyes:** shall be permitted substances.

As the migration of toxic chemical constituents/additives of the packaging materials into the food, make the food unsafe for human consumption, therefore, qualitative and quantitative estimation of migrants into the food under actual use condition are carried out to assess the safety of such plastics for food contact application. Hence the test involves:

Fixing the Limits for Migrants

Migration refers to transfer of substances from the package (usually a packaging material) into the food staff. The substances which are transferred to food as a result of contact or interaction between food and packaging material are referred as migrants. Migration is a two-way process, since constituents of food can also penetrate into the plastic.

Two Types of Migration

1. Specific migration: refers to migration of a single mobile compound only which is identifiable and of toxicological interest or a labeled compound used in experiments to elucidate the extent or mechanism of migration of a particular migrant.
2. Global migration or total migration: is the sum of all mobile packaging components transferred into the food whether they are of toxicological interest or not and will include some of the substance which are physiologically harmless, they may have effect on organoleptic characteristics of food.

Advantages

The global migration test obviates the need to identify each and every individual migrant. It also serves as a screening test which saves time and expensive analytical resources, where no particular hazard is expected.

Disadvantages

Does give any indication of/about a particular migrant.

Mechanism of Transfer of Migrants

1. Diffusion

Regarded as main controlling mechanism. There are natural tendency for materials to diffuse from area of high cone to low, come until at equilibrium, when no concentration gradient exist. Not only the components of plastic diffuse into the foodstuff, but it may be possible for the constituents of food to penetrate the plastic. The latter may depend on the random motion of the plastic polymer chains into whom liquid food can penetrate when food (or extractant) penetrates into the plastic (polymer) a boundary layer is formed (boundary phase) swollen-polymer and diffusion coefficient in this phase will not be the same at that of the unswollen area.

The rate of diffusion is dependent on:

1. Type of polymer and thickness
2. Temp. and time of contact between food and plastic
3. Nature of food.

(b) Adsorption

It is a type of adhesion which occurs at the surface of a solid or a liquid in contact with another medium, resulting in the increased concentration of molecules in the immediate vicinity of the surface. Constituents of plastic (monomer and additives) may get adsorbed on the surface of food.

Types of Migration Process

Interaction may occur among three components – *i.e.* plastic, food and environments. In packaged food, the plastic a container is interposed between food and environment. In case of food packaged in a container/package impervious to gases and water vapour (*i.e.* gaseous state of water), interaction occurs between food and container. But since not all plastics are not impervious to gaseous transfer, hence tainting may occur or in reverse direction, food may loose aroma. Migration is concerned with the interaction of plastic and foodstuff in which environment takes no part.

Types of Class of Migration

1. Non migration: dry or hard food packaged in inert containers (salt, sugar, dry hard fruits, vegetable). In this case only the monolayer of component present on the inner surface of plastic container can be dissolved and hence transferred into the foodstuff.
2. Independent migration: *i.e.* migration not contributed by food. *e.g.* diffusion of gases component *i.e.* Vinyl chloride monomer (VCM) from the plastic into the food. VCM is a gas at ambient temperature and is a known carcinogen by inhalation rates. When VC M is present as residue monomer in the PVC resin, it is likely to be diffused from the resin to food.
3. Dependent migration: *i.e.* migration is dependent on food. In these situation food penetrates into the plastic leading to swelling of the plastic which increases as penetrates proceeds. The swollen layer is not homogeneous system and diffusion rate increases with time or duration of contact.

Toxicological Aspects

Toxicology is the study of the interaction between chemicals and biological (living) system.

1. Acute effect: Short term effect of poisonous compounds.
2. Sub acute: Intermediate between acute and chronic effect.
3. Chronic effect: Long term effects resulting from the ingestion, inhalation, contact of a low level of toxic compounds over a long period of time.
4. Cumulative effect: Most of the toxicological studies on plastic compounds used as packaging material have been done on laboratory animals *i.e.* rat, mice etc. In toxicological study, dose- response relationship is of fundamental importance. LD50 (lethal dose) by which 50 per cent of the population of test animals are killed) is usually expressed in units of mg of compound/kg of animal under test. Since the response of the test animal to the stimulus (tonic constituent) depends on
   - (i) Species of the animal.
   - (ii) Route of administration of stimulus
   - (iii) Sex, age and nutritional states of the animal.

Hence experimental condition is defined in toxicological evaluation of plastic container. The results obtained from the toxicology study of animals serve as a guide to the safety of a compound to human and in defining an acceptable daily intake (ADI) for a given food additive in the human diet.

Carcinogenic Risk of some Monomer to Human

Hazard is related to the presence of residual monomer and not to the polymer. All monomers are suspected to be toxic, however toxicological study on VCM and AN have been carried out in detail.

(a) Vinyl chloride monomer (VCM) : toxic effects in man

1. Lesions of bones in the terminal joints of fingers and toes (*i.e.* aero osteolysis)
2. Tumours (carcinogenic)
3. Damage to liver and spleen (*i.e.* angiosarcoma of the liver, brain, lung and haematolymphopoitic systems.

(b) VDC (vinylidene chloride monomer): less known about its toxicology in man and animals.

1. VDC affects the activity of rat liver enzyme and decrease the glutathione reserve.
2. Prolonged exposure of rat and rabbit to VDC results in tumour development.

(c) Acrylonitrile monomer (AN)

1. Causes mutation *i.e.* has mutagenic effect.
2. Carcinogens (tumour)

(d) Styrene

1. Potent mutagen (causes chromosomal aberrations).
2. Neurological changes in humans.

Determination of Monomers

1. Colorimetric/sphectrophotomatric method.
2. Gas chromatography
3. Mass spectrometry
4. Infrared spectrometry
5. Radioactive labeled compounds are used in migration experiment.

First the monomers are extracted from the sample (Polymer/foodstuff). Polymers are dissolved or dispersed in order to release any free monomer prior to analysis. Food stuffs are even more complex in chemical composition than the polymers. Hence, migration experiments are often carried out with the use of stimulants in the place of real food.

Head Space Gas Chromatography (HSGC)

It is carried out to estimate monomers. In HSGC, the vapor space above the sample (liquid/solid) enclosed in a gas tight container (vial) is taken for analysis rather than an injection of sample dissolved in a liquid as is done in case of conventional.

Procedure

The vial containing test sample is held at preset temp. until equilibrium of volatile exponents of the sample between the gaseous and liquid phase has been established.Then a portion of gaseous phase is transferred to the GLC column with a gas tight syringe and chromatography is performed. Similarly Internal standard of monomer under test is also chromatographed. Quantitative measurement made by computation of peak area (or height) ratio of test sample and the standard.

Simulants

Used since the most of the foodstuffs are complex chemical composition. Hence the choice of particular simulant for a food product depends on the nature of food. Some foods are aqueous; some are fatty where most of the foodstuffs are admixture of both aqueous and fatty system.

1. Distilled water: for aqueous food.
2. 3 per cent (w/v) acetic acid- for acidic foods, vinegar, pickles.
3. Olive oil for fatty foods.
4. 15 per cent (v/v) ethanol-for spirits.

Test Conditions

Are selected keeping in view the practical condition of contact time and temp. in actual use of the packaged food.*i.e.* conditions at which the test material remain in contact with the stimulant.

Procedure

In principle the extractability of a compound from a plastic can be determined by placing the plastic of known surface area in contact with food under defined condition of temp and time. Then an appropriate analytical technique is used to determine the amount of compound present in food and is usually expressed in PPM (*i.e.* mg/kg or mg/liter) or mg/dm^2)

In practice, the test becomes difficult due to:

1. The compound present in plastic under test may be unknown and may have been degraded during processing.
2. Many compounds are difficult to determine in a complex system like food, particularly when only small amounts are present in the extract.
3. Compounds other than the one of interest may be extracted and may subsequently interface the analytical determination.
4. Appropriate test conditions are not easy to define since wide variations may exist between the actual condition of contact encountered in practice during storage in warehouse, supermarket, household storage etc. Though it is desirable that food to be tested should be used for extractability testing (migration), but in practice it is seldom possible, hence food simulants are used.

Food Simulants

Food consists of a complex mixture of water, fats, proteins, carbohydrates as well as minor constituents such as vitamins, minerals and additives such as preservatives, color, antioxidants, flavouring agents etc. Simulants used to simulate the migration of a substance from a plastic into food. This creates a problem in selecting a food stimulant which can accurately reflect the extraction characteristics of such a mixture. Thus in order to simplify the situation foods are often classified into groups such as:

(a) Dry solid foods: Dehydrated meat soup powder, egg powder.
(b) Acidic food: Pickles
(c) Fatty food

Thus food simulants are classified into:

(a) Distilled water for aqueous food.
(b) Dilute solution of acidic (*i.e.* acetic acid 3 per cent soln.)
(c) Ethanol/water mixture (fatty-**cum**-aqueous system in food)
(d) Fatty food simulants (*e.g.* n-Turpentine, diethyl ether, ethanol, olive oil, lard, sunflower or coconut oil etc. synthetic triglycerides

Influence of Time-Temperature on Migration

Accelerated tests at elevated temp are carried out.

Table 28.5: Test Conditions to Simulate Migration under Real Time and Temperature

Real Time/Temp.	*Simulating Condition*
Storage for 9 months at -18°C	48 hr at 45°C
Storage for 6 months at -25 °C	10 days at 45°C
Bottling/filling at 70°C	1 hr at 70°C
Pasteurization in the packet	½ hr at 100°C
Sterilization in the packet	½ hr at 120°C

In practice it is not flexible to practice the simulating condition as test of actual use condition, hence accelerated test at higher temp is generally carried out. It has been suggested that a simulating test for10 days at 45 °C is roughly equivalent to 6 months of storage at- 25°C.

Global Migration or Total Migration Measurement

(a) Gravimetric Test

A sample of packaging material of known surface area is placed in contact with a food stimulant (ethanol/water bath) under specified conditions of temp and time. At the and of the test, the simulant (*e.g.* chloroform ethanol etc.) is evaporated off and the residue is dried and weighed. The result is then expressed as mg of residue/dm^2 surface area of the material.

Disadvantage

(1) Volatile materials (VCM) will be lost during evaporation stage. (2) This method cannot be used for fat simulant like olive, coconut and sunflower oil as they can be evaporated.

(b) Fat Test

In case of fat simulant such as olive oil, coconut oil, sunflower oil etc. the evaporation technique can not be used. In this test, samples of plastic of known area are weighed before and after contact with the fatty simulant test piece of known surface area are conditioned at 20°C and 50 per cent R.H. Prior to emerging it in the fatty stimulant. Global migration (GM) is calculated as follows:

$$GM\,(mg) = \frac{w_1 - w_2}{S}$$

where,

w_1 = wt. of sample before contact with the stimulant.

w_2 = wt. of sample after contact with the stimulant.

S = surface area of the test piece (sample)

In practice w_2 usually greater the w_1 despite migration of compounds from the plastic into the oil, since more quantity of oil is absorbed by the plastic than the quantity of compound leached out of the plastic. Hence the change in wt. as calculated above has to be corrected and an allowance is made for weight of oil absorbed by the plastic.

$$\text{Now, } GM = \frac{(w_1 - w_2) + F}{S}$$

where, w_1, w_2 and S represent same as indicated earlier.

F = wt. of oil absorbed by the plastic which is determined by GLC using triglyceride as standard. Several method, they different in choice of simulant, method of oil absorbed determination.

1. Since a test sample may gain or loose moisture with the change in R.H. of atmosphere hence test sample are conditioned at 20°C, 50 per cent R.H.
2. Method in GLC.

Specific Migration (S.M.)

It is the study of the migration of a single chemical compound from the plastic into a foodstuff or food simulant.

Method

(1) Conventional chemical method for detn.of specific migrant in aqueous, alcoholic and fatty simulants used for examination of migrant compounds GC, GLC, MS, Atomic absorption spectrophotometer.

Radio Tracer Method

(a) It is widely used in most cases, compounds or additives are labeled with either carbon (^{14}C) or tritium (^{3}tt). The next step is to determine the specific gravity of the compound and then introduce a known wt. of the compound in the plastic under test and is taken to ensure that the labeled compound is distributed evenly throughout the thickness of the test material.

(b) Then the specimens are tested in a special cell filled with a known food simulant in a controlled test condition. Plastic and food simulant kept in contact at controlled temp./time

(c) After the contact period the radioactivity of the extractant is measured which is directly proportional to the mass of labeled compound transferred.

Composition and Toxicological Aspects of Glass

Table 28.6: Composition of Typical Commercial Glass

Type	SiO_2	Al_2O_3	Na_2O	K_2O	*Mgo*	*CaO*	*BaO*	*PBO*	B_2O_3	Fe_2O_3	SO_3	*F*
Colourless	73.3	1.93	14.07	0.46	3.76	5.82	0.34	–	0.04	0.37	0.23	0.06
Amber	72.5	1.45	13.71	0.61	3.77	7.34	0.29	–	–	0.08	–	0.26
Pyrex	81.0	2.2	3.6	0.2	–	–	–	–	0.13	–	–	–

Chemically glass is highly resistant to attack of water, aqueous solution, organic compounds. Water and acids have very little effect on silica, although they may attach other constituents of glass. Alkaline solution are generally much more corrosive to glass, especially when hot.

Test for Migration of Constituents of Glass

Glass containers are autoclaved with test liquid under defined conditions. Evidence of attack is determined by measurement of loss of wt. or by chemical analysis of the test liquid extract for compounds present. Toxic compounds leached out from glass are mainly lead, or cadmium, zinc, fluorine.

Table 28.7: WHO Recommended intake of Metal in Total Diet

Metal	*Food*	*Intake (μg/Person/Week)*
Lead	Canned meat, fish, vegetable	3000
Cadmium	"	400-500
Mercury	"	300
Zinc	"	35000-150.000
Chromium	"	140-3500
Cabalt	"	14-3500
Manganese	"	14000-21000
Arsenic	"	0.35mg/kg

Paper and Paper Products

Limits of impurities such as arsenic,Cu,Fe,Pb,glycerine and other substance specified.

Metal Cans

Limits indicated to safeguard the consumers' health.

III. Packaging of Meat and Meat Products

Introduction

Packaging of meat and meat products is the important aspect of meat preservation. This is because poor wrapping and packaging techniques or wrong selection of packaging material leads to deterioration changes of meat and meat products. Packaging system depends on processing, preservation, storage, distribution, marketing etc. Also the packaging method depends on inherent quality of fresh or processed meat product, storage condition and desired shelf-life.

1. Fresh Meat

Highly perishable, characteristic colour, flavour, texture that is required to be protected.

- ☆ **Colour:** most important for marketability, eye appeal. Natural colour – Mb, Hb – purplish red. Short exposure to O_2 – oxymyoglobin – bright red: desirable, Mb – O_2Mb reversible reaction, in absence of oxygen for long time, prolonged exposure to O_2, then Mb-MMb, brown colour, poor quality.
- ☆ **Surface dehydration** of fresh meat affects texture, may cause discolouration – conc of pigments increases on surface because dissolved pigments migrate to surface.
- ☆ Light affect colour of meat UV light oxidation Mb, desiccation oxidation of UFA.
- ☆ Natural flavour affected, hydrolytic rancidity (enzymatic) and Oxidative rancidity promoted by light and exposure to O_2.
- ☆ Microbial growth – dev. off-flavour and pick-up of forgeign odour, functions of package of fresh meat should:
  - i) Control dehydration
  - ii) Maintain desirable bright red colour
  - iii) Prevent pick up of foreign odour and further microbial contamination.

Packing material should therefore be moderate barrier to oxygen but a good barrier to water vapour.

Packaging Material: I. Fresh Meat

1. Wrapping

NC coated cellophane (nitrocellulose is coated in one side of film. The uncoated side remain in contact with meat.

2. Film Packaging

i) LDPE 200G film or 250 gauze, ii)Highly plasticized PVC film (100G) to increase O_2 permeation and reduce dehydration, make it stretchable, so skin tight package. iii)Pliofilm (Rubber hydrochloride), iv) EVA (ethylene vinyl acetate film) v) Biaxially oriented polystyrene film (BOPS).

Storage

Fresh meat stored at 0-2°C to prevent microbial spoilage. R.H. 85 to 90 per cent maintained to prevent desiccation, at condition kept for 5 to 7 days.

3. Tray Packaging

packaging retail cuts of fresh meat, cut up portion of chicken, earlier days trays from moulded pulp, are rigid, absorb drip from meat, but loss of strength due to excessive moisture absorption and adhesion to meat. eg. (1) Moulded pulp trays (2) paper board trays. Now (1) moulded expanded polystyrene foam trays. (2) clear polystyrene trays (transparent). The retail meat cuts are placed in the trays, overwrapped with transparent film. The blotter is kept underneath the trays to absorb excessive meat juice. Kept 10 days at 0°C, 85 to 90 per cent RH,desirable colour maintained only for 10 days. Recently clean polystyrene trays – imporved visibility – overwrapped with plastic film of moderate OTR 5000 ml/m^2 24 hrs at 24°C. The packaging films are (i) PE (ii) PP (iii) PVC (iv) PVDC.

Shrink Film Packaging

Large irregular cuts of fresh meat, uneven cuts of carcass, quarters, dressed whole chicken. Cryovac used for storage under frozen condition, shrink film offer neat appearance, Contour package convenient to handle dressed whole chicken or meat is vacuum packed and dipped in water bath at 90-95°C or passed through hot air tunnel to effect shrinking of film. (i) cryovac (copolymer of PVC/PVDC)(ii) shrinkable PE (iii) Oriented PP (BOPP) (iv) PVC, PVDC (v) PVDC coated polyester (Mylar)

4. Vacuum Packaging

Longer shelf-life 2 to 3 weeks, purple-red colour of meat – not popular in retail shops. Bigger cuts/Primal cuts vacuum packed – sold in institutional packs to hatels, hostel, hospital, catering establishment.

(a) Conventional vacuum packaging – use of non-heat shrinkable film.

(b) Vacuum shrink packaging – use of heat shrink film laminate should be a good barrier to water vapour and gases, good mechanical strength.

- Aerobic bacteria inhibited.
- *e.g. Pseudomonas, Achromobacter* – spoilage bacteria
- Facultative anacrobes not inhibited.

Packaging Material

1. Polyester/PE laminate

2. Polyamide (nylon)/PE
3. PVC/PVDC copolymer (cryovac)
4. PVC film (5) polyamide film.

Shelf-life: 2 to 3 weeks at 0-2°C and 85-90 per cent RH.

Disadvantage: colour not optimum, bone- in meat not suitable.

Gas Packaging (Modified Atmosphere Packaging) MAP

Extend shelf life of fresh meat, atmosphere inside the package modified; use of CO_2, N_2, O_2.

Beef and Mutton: fairly high O_2 content to maintain bright red colour.

Pork: due to high fat content (UFA) – less O_2, some N_2 for glow.

Chicken: as compared to beef and pork, needs little O_2 and reduced amount of CO_2 which can flavour the meat.

(a) 75 per cent O_2 + 15 per cent CO_2 + 10 per cent N_2 red meat 15 days at 40°C.

(b) 80 per cent O_2 + 20 per cent CO2 fresh meat 15d at 4°C – this combined not ideal in obtaining attractive meat colour and restrict bacterial growth in providing reasonable shelf-life.

Advantage: attractive colour

Disadvantage: (i) shorter life than vacuum packaging; (ii) require more space during storage; (iii) not suitable for frozen storage of meat.

2. Frozen Meat

A. Raw Frozen

Convenience products prone to dehydration, loss of texture, freezer burn, oxidation. Package – minimize moisture loss good barrier to O_2, light, accommodate contraction and expansion during freezing and thawing operation impermeable odour/flavour, raw meat – prepackaged blast frozen (-40°C) for 4 to 12 hr depending upon size and shape, content meat – repackaged in corrugated fiber board boxes (are waxed internally or on bothe sides) and stored at -18°C for 9-12 months.

Packaging Materials

1. LDPE (200 to 300G) – low cost, clarity, low temperature toughness resist freezing and thawing contraction and expansion.
2. Polyester/PE laminate
3. Polyamide/PE (4) Cryovac (PVC/PVDC copolymer)

B. Pre-cooked Frozen

Chicken patties, nuggets, chicken curry – prone to oxdn., desiccation hamburger, fried meat Chunk, meat in gravy. Packaging material must protect moisture loss, exposure to air, resist thawing/heating operation).

Packaging Material

1. Tandoori, barbecue, meat gravy. (1) HDPE (200-300g) – short term package, (2) PVC, (3) Saran or Cryorac (PVC/PVDC copolymer)
2. Boil-in-bag (should have double line seal): meat in gravy is first preformed into frozen block before putting into bag. The product can be thawed and heated either. (a) Polyester/PP (b) Polyamide/PP.
3. Aluminum mould: in boiling water. Meat products like hamburger, hot dog, patties require double purpose packaging to hold the product together in addition to provide general protection – it is achieved by stretch or shrink wrap but such film are not suitable for microwave heating.

Hence, alternately glassine bag (glassine is the densest and most compact form of paper formed of small cellulose fibers whichis hydrated until the mass become gelatinous with the application of heat and pressure then converted into smooth and transparent) is used. The glassine bag is folded loosely around the roll of hamburger, hot dog etc but no seal is applied at the ends. The bagged rolls in a dozen or so are then packed into a shallow plastic coated wire basket to hold them together during freezing. The rolls may be thawed and heated in glassine bags in a microwave oven after unfolding the end of the bag.

Fried Chicken/Fried Chips

Shall be immediately frozen without wrapping because of their fragile nature. Once hard they may be vacuum packed in laminated paper bags or pouches for long term strorage under frozen condition.

Cooked Meat

1. Canning: Most cooked meats are canned and have a canning storage life of 1-2 yrs. Tinplates, TFS and Aluminium cans are used. The cans are lacquered internally with epoxy phenolic meat lacquers.
2. Unit package retortable (120°C)
   a) Use of Aluminium trays lined with PP
   b) Use of plastic trays – polyamide/PP higher gauges
   c) Use of laminated pouches – polyomide/Al foil/PP or polyester/Al. foil/PP.

Cured Meat

impart desirable pink colour, typical cured flavour, enhance shelf life. Ham, bacon, luncheon meat, sausage, frankfurters etc have a shelf-life of 2 to 3 weeks at 2-4°C and 80-85 per cent R.H. depending upon the degree of curing (level of nitrite etc.) nitrosomyoglobin – during curing desired pink colour but unstable colour. High storage temp and light also responsible for nitroso Mb – MMb; when cured meat is smoked nitrosoMb – nitrosochromogen by heat a stablilized colour pigment.

Packaging Requirements

1. Prevent dehydration
2. Prevent fading of desirable pink colour
3. Retention of characteristic cure meat flavour.
4. A good O_2, WV, light barrier.

For short term storage of cured meat- Whole cured chicken, Cut up cured chicken

(A) Plastic Films and Foil Laminate

a. LDPE/HDPE, PVC, PVDC
b. Paper/Al. foil/PE laminates
c. Heat shrink film – PVC/PVDC copolymer (cryovac a saran)

Vacuum packaged, then heat shrinked in hot water 90-95°C or passing through a hot air tunnel.

(B) Chub Packs

done for ground cured meat. Chub packs are tubes stuffed with cured minced meat and the ends of the packs are twist-tied or clipped. The film used for club packs is generally PE or cellopham/PE.

3. For Longer Storage

(a) Vacuum/Gas Packaging

Sliced bacon, sliced luncheon meat, chicken, turkey breast meat, cured chicken etc. can be vacuum/gas packed.

Ideal material for vacuum or gas packaging:

Cellophane/PVDC/PE, Polyester/PVDC/PE, Polyamide/PVDC/PE, Metalised polyamide/PE, Metalised polyester/PE.

Shelf-life: (a) vacuum packed slice bacon 2-3 months at 0-4°C and 6 month at -18°C.

(b) Control Atmosphere Packaging

Gas mixture of 85 to 90 per cent N_2+ 10-15 per cent CO_2 can be flushed either through displacement of air and conducting the filling and sealing operation in a gaseous atmosphere.

4. Dehydrated Meat Products

Ideal for military ration, expedition, space travel etc.

(a) Hot air drying of pre cooked ground meat results in a poor quality product generally not practiced (poor reconstitution, protein denaturation).

(b) Freeze drying: widely accepted method of meat dehydration.

Water removed by sublimation process: solid state to gaseous phase under control condition of temperature 40°C and vacuum (1.5 mm Hg). Freeze dried meat rehydrated or reconstituted in water at 90-95°C

Causes of Deterioration

1. High susceptility to oxidative rancidity.
2. Porous mass, needs protection against mechanical damage.
3. Water absorbed from atmosphere, textural changes rancidity and non-enzymatic browning.
4. Needs to be compressed to reduce density and eliminate air trapped in the porous texture.
5. Protein denaturation, poor solubility

Packaging Material

Should be impermeabl to WV, O_2, protect against light, foreign odour/flavours.

Laminates (Impermeable to Moisture and Gases)

1. Paper/Al.foil/PE as outer wrap and inner cellophane wrap ideal for compressed bar of dehydrated minced meat.
2. Vacuum sealing in metal cans, packaging in metal cans under nitrogen
   (a) Polyester/Al. foil/PE
   (b) Cellophane/Al. foil/PE
   (c) Polyamide/Al. foil/PE

Shelf-life: 1-1 ½ years at ambient temperature when vacuum/gas flushed.

5. Thermoprocessed Meat Products

1. Meat balls
2. Corned beef/pork/chicken
3. Meat curry/kema/chicken biryani
4. Chicken gravy/meat soup
5. Boneless chicken

Metal cans: OTS, TFS and Al. cans used.

(a) Canning: traditionally hermetically sealed and processed in metal cans. Commercially sterile canned meat are shelf-stable for many years at ambient temperature generally 1-2 years storage life.

(b) Packaging in flexible pouches or retortable pouches, retortable at 120°C.
   1. Pslyester/Al. foil/LDPE
   2. Polyamide/Al. foil/LDPE
   3. Polyster/Al. foil/PP
   4. Polamide/Al. foil/PP

   More ideal the the first two.

References

Bharti,A. and Sahoo, J. (1999). Modified atmosphere packaging of meat and meat products – aspects of packaging materials, packaging environments, and storage temperature.Indian Food Industry, 18 (5): 299-310.

Sahoo, J. and Anjaneyulu, A.S.R. (1995). Modified atmosphere packaging of muscle foods : Technology, shelf life and safety aspects.Indian Food Industry, 14 (3): 28-36

IV. Packaging of Poultry and Poultry Products

The principal role of fresh meat package is:

- ☆ To prevent moisture loss
- ☆ To offer the product to the consumers in most desirable colour-red bloom
- ☆ To prevent further bacterial contamination of meat
- ☆ To arrest pick up of foreign flavour and odour by meat
- ☆ To control oxygen transfer

Poultry meat is high in protein, low in calories and easy to chew and digest, but poultry fat is unsaturated and is very prone to the development of oxidative rancidity. Shelf-life of poultry varies according to type of processing, nature of processing environment, initial flora and post-slaughter treatment. Packaging of poultry meat is undertaken immediately after the dressing operations are over. Unpacked refrigerated storage may result in surface dehydration, freezer burn, characterised by surface discolouration, tough texture and diminished juiciness as well as flavour loss. Poultry is usually packed as whole dressed poultry, cut up poultry and poultry organs. Dressed poultry have a shelf-life of 5-7 days at refrigerated storage conditions of 0-5°C.

Packaging Materials

Over-wraps

Packaging of whole dressed chicken halves or cut-up parts are done in plastic films like polyethylene, polypropylene, PVDC, rubber hydrochloride or nylon. These are films of 150 to 200 gauge in thickness. Polyethylene is the most widely used packaging material in our country because of low cost and easy availability. These thermoplastic film sheets can be fabricated into bags. Each dressed eviscerated bird is inserted into a bag. Giblet of individual bird is wrapped in waxed paper or parchment paper and placed into the body cavity before bagging. The problem of body fluid accumulation is avoided by putting an absorbent pad or blotter on the pack of each bird to soak up the liquid. The bag is then heat sealed or twist-tied or clipped shut.

Tray with Over-wraps

Small whole dressed chicken, broilers, roasting chickens are placed in a polystyrene foam tray and over-wrapped with transparent plastic film. A blotter underneath absorbs the excessive meat juice accumulated. Chicken thus wrapped has a shelf-life of 7 days at 4°C in refrigerator.

Shrink Film Over-wraps

Many thermoplastic films such as polyethylene, polypropylene, poly vinylidene can be biaxially oriented to stay stretched at ambient temperature. Dressed chicken is overwrapped with such films and passed through hot air tunnel or dipped in water tub maintained at 90°C for a few seconds to effect shrinkage of the film.

Vacuum Packaging

The ideal materials for vacuum packaging of poultry are laminates of polyester/ polyethylene (PE), polyamide/polyethylene, PVDC co-polymer film, nylon/EVA.

Modified Atmosphere Packaging

In this technique, the atmosphere surrounding the product in the pack is modified by flushing carbon dioxide, nitrogen and oxygen alone or in combination. Mixture of 60 per cent nitrogen and 40 per cent carbon dioxide or 50 per cent nitrogen and 50 per cent carbon dioxide is ideal for modified atmosphere packaging of chicken meat.

Table 28.8: Typical Gas Mixtures used for some of the Meat Products

Product	*Temperature in °C*	*O_2 Per cent*	*CO_2 Per cent*	*N_2 Per cent*
Fresh meat	1-2	70	20	10
Cured meat	1-2	0	30	70
Pork	0-2	80	20	0
Poultry	0-2	0	20-40	80-60

Table 28.9: Changes in Meat, Fish and Poultry as Brought about by Modified Atmosphere

Changes	*Results*
Enzymatic ageing process	Unaffected
Microbial spoilage	Increased CO_2 reduces growth of aerobic spoilage organisms by penetrating membranes and lowering intracellular pH
Fat oxidation	Reduced O_2 reduces oxidation of fats, although oxidation can still occur at low O_2 tension
Oxidation of myoglobin	Increased CO_2 promotes metmyoglobin formation and colour darkening

VI. Modern Trends in Meat and Poultry Packaging

Introduction

Modern food preservation and packaging technologies make foods available thousands of kilometers away from the places of their origin and weeks, months and even years beyond the day of their production. Packaging is the key link in the supply chain that delivers wholesome, safe, nutritious, convenient and quality foods to the consumer. Packaging functions at several levels. At the most basic level – occasionally it is the most sophisticated one – is the primary package, which is in direct contact with the product. It provides the initial and usually the major protective barrier. It is frequently the primary package, which the consumer sees and purchases at retail outlets and uses. Other levels of packaging that include secondary package, *e.g.*, a corrugated fibre-board box that carries a number of primary packages, and a tertiary package such as stretch-wrapped pallet of corrugated boxes, perform mainly the distribution function. A total packaging system consisting of these different levels performs the four major functions of containment, protection, providing convenience and communication. Increasing demands on shelf-life extension, product safety, consumer convenience, retail operations, cost-effectiveness and environmental issues are shaping the present and future food packaging technologies.

1. Active and Intelligent Packaging

Recent research efforts are focused on development of active and intelligent packaging. Active packaging changes the condition of the packed food to extend shelf life or to improve safety or sensory properties, while maintaining the quality of the packaged food. Food condition here includes various aspects that may play a role in determining the shelf life of packaged foods, such as physiological processes (*e.g.*, respiration of fresh fruits and vegetables), chemical processes (*e.g.*, lipid oxidation), physical processes (*e.g.*, staling of bread, dehydration), microbiological aspects (*e.g.*, spoilage by microorganisms) and infestation (*e.g.*, by insects). Intelligent packaging systems monitor the condition of packaged foods to give information about the quality of the packaged food during transport and storage. They can be external (attached outside the package, time-temperature indicators) or internal (oxygen, carbon dioxide, microbial growth indicators).

2. Aseptic Packaging

It has revolutionized the way fluid foods are delivered – cartooned fruit juices, milk and other dairy beverages, soya drinks, tomato puree, soups, puddings, RTD tea, wine and now low-acid and particulate foods. Recent aseptic packaging innovations include injection molded reclosable plastic closures, PET bottles for still beverages and HDPE bottles for refrigerated still beverages, flexible aseptic pouch, octagonal and wedge shaped cartons in both paperboard/aluminium/plastic and transparent silica-coated PET lamination, thermoform/fill/seal systems for barrier plastic cups with heat-seal flexible closures and snap-on plastic overcaps and vertical form/fill/seal aseptic stick pack machine for tubular packages.

Modern Trends in Meat and Poultry Packaging

With the development of new meat products entering the market, high quality alternative packaging materials are also emerging. The consumer is becoming more discerning in his or her choice of food products and there is a trend, which shows a shift from traditional food items and eating habits. Some of the recent trends in the meat packaging industry are covered here.

1. Retortable Flexible Pouch

A retort pouch can be defined as a flexible package into which a food product is placed, sealed and then sterilized at temperatures between 110 °C to 140 °C. The finished product is commercially sterile, shelf-stable and does not require refrigeration. A retortable pouch Dressed Chicken Packed in Plastic Pouches is made of polyester, polyamide or oriented polypropylene provides support and physical strength to the composite. The middle layer of aluminum foil acts as a barrier against water vapour, gases and light. The inner layer of polyethtlene, polypropylene or PVDC provides heat sealability and food contact. The different laminates used for a retort pouch are polyester/aluminum foil/modified high-density polyethylene or polyester/aluminium foil/polypropylene-ethylene co-polymer.

2. Roast-in-bags

It is an oven stable vacuum skin package that can be used to cook meat at a temperature up to 204 °C. it is fabricated from polyethylene terephthalate (PET) film due to its unusual properties such as it does not become brittle with age, has long shelf-life, has resistance to most chemicals and moisture and is dimensionally stable.

3. Microwave Packages

Convenience food fall into two categories, frozen and retortable. The current trend in frozen food is dual oven-ability *i.e.* products that can be heated in a microwave oven and conventional oven. Shelf-stable retortable food are better suited to microwave heating. Owing to the growing importance of microwave ovens, other materials are overtaking the conventional aluminium trays. While selecting thermoplastics for dual ovenable packages, the critical properties to be considered are dimensional stability up to 200°C to 250°C, good impact strength at freezer temperatures and microwavability. Heat resistant plastic trays made from materials like polyester, polypropylene, nylon and polycarbonate can be used in combination or as monolayers. They are easy to handle, sturdy, attractive, cost competent and can be compartmentalized for multicomponent food items. They are self-serving and reusable.

4. Cryovac Packages

Pre-cooked meat packages with shrink film are an innovation with equipment made and supplied by Cryovac. In this system, there is a double chamber machine. In the longer chamber the meat is placed in the film bag and the mouth of the bag is drawn into small chamber. In the longer chamber a low level of vacuum is just drawn to balloon the bag in order to eliminate formation of air pockets. A high level of vacuum is then drawn into the smaller chamber where the mouth of the bag is placed. When both the chambers are at maximum vacuum an automatic clipper closes the bag. The packaged meat is then sent to the shrink tunnel. Cryovac package forms a skin tight package. This together with the use of a film with low oxygen permeability stabilizes the products and increase the shelf-life.

5. Thermoprocessed Meat Products

Meat products like meat balls, corned beef, corned pork, meat gravies, meat soups, liver sausages, chicken curry, boneless chicken etc. are hermetically sealed and processed in metal cans to preserve the desirable flavour, texture and appearance. Commercially sterile canned meats are shelf stable for a number of years at room temperatutre but standards in many western countries recognize the storage life of canned meat products only for two years. Thinplate cans have been the leader in this field. These are coated on the inner side with a sulphur-resistant lacquer. Aluminium cans have also made a substantial headway but they are not used as extensively as tinplate cans in meat canning industry. Shallow-drawn aluminium cans with internal lacquer have been successfully used for certain meat products. Meat Food Products Order-1973 prescribes the maximum limit (ppm by weight)for the poisonous metals in canned meat products. These are 2.5, 20, 250 and 50 ppm by weight for lead, copper, arsenic, tin and zinc respectively.

The present trend in packaging thermoprocessed meat products is the use of flexible retort pouches. These pouches are self-stable for a period of one year. generally composite film/foil/film laminates are used for this purpose. The outer plastic film made up of polyester, polyamide or oriented polypropylene provides support and physical strength the composite. Aluminium foil in the middle layer contributes excellent barrier peroperties and inner layer consisting of polyethylene, polypropylene or PVC provides heat sealability. Meat products like pork, luncheon meat, chopped pork, corned beef etc. are vacuum packed in a polyester film/aluminium foil/ polyolefin film laminate pouches, autoclaved and put in a printed board carton. The packaged meat products are processed in a retorts using pressured steam cook to achieve commercial sterilization. The products have ample shelf-life in addition to good consumer appeal due to transparency, gloss and agreeable feel.

Some Emerging Technologies

Processors are not satisfied even with the present main function of protection and major role in marketing of food products. They have as well started assigning specified functions to packaging which require its active involvement in the extension of shelf-life such as packaging has been named as **active or smart packaging**. In dehydrated and hurdle treated shelf stable foods, humidity build up in the package due to carbohydrate and fat metabolism can be checked by **moisture scavengers** such as diatomaceous pad in the packaging system. It restricts the growth of yeast and molds. In oxygen sensitive foods, head space oxygen can be climinated by incorporating **oxygen scavengers**. Similarly, carbon dioxide build up in a pack can be checked by **carbon dioxide scavengers.** On the contrary, carbon dioxide can be regularly generated in the package by placing a carbon dioxide filled sachet to control oxygen concentration. Ethylene scavangers may be placed in the packages of fruits and vegetables to retard maturity and enhance their shelf stability.

Biodegradable Packaging

Plastic packaging materials and polymers of synthetic origin have posed the problem of after-use disposal throughout the world. This is adding to the misery of environmental pollution. In Indian cities, the problem of blockage of sewer lines has acquired a stupendous proportion and many municipal corporation have banned their use to overcome this problem. Hence, efforts are being made to come up with environment friendly biodegradable packaging. The natural biopolymers are films of vegetable origin. Polysaccharide films may be derived from starch and its derivatives, cellulose and its derivatives, gelatin, gum, glutenetc. These have good mechanical and optical properties but their limitations are susceptibility to moisture and low water vapour barrier properties. On the contrary, biopolymer films made up of lipids and waxes or their derivatives are a good barrier to water vapour but are fragile opaque and prone to rancidity. Such a situation has forced the technologists to look for viable alternatives. Hence, the concept of mixing synthetic polymers and biopolymers has been invented. Starch is the base of most of these mixtures. A potential example of these type of composite packaging materials is gelatinized starch/ hydrolysates copolymer/polyethylene. Another alternative is the use of starch hydrolystates alongwith polyesters which are prone to microbial degradation. Yet another example is thermoplastic corn starch incorporating the use of plasticizers such as glycerol sorbitol etc.

We are familiar with the sugar and chocolate coatings on candies for a long time. With the development of all vegetable biopolymers the area of edible films and coatings has acquired a new dimension. Now edible packaging is an emerging field and improved starch and pectin films have been proposed for coating red meats also. These films and coatings help in maintaining the desired colour without affecting other sensory attributes. People wish to buy consume perishable livestock products in as much fresh condition as possible. They look forward to the labeling with shelf life dating on the food products itself as an assurance of quality, nutrition and safety. Quality indicators are now being proposed to be inbuilt in packaging material or fastened on to packages. The indicators can respond to storage temperature fluctuations with a colour change and give an idea about the probable loss of shelf life. Further intensive research work is required in this area to come up with reliable time-temperature on packaged livestock products.

Cost Effective Packaging

The most recent development for the paperboard carton is the retortable carton that is likely to compete with the retort pouch and tray. Its main advantage compared to retort pouch is the fast filling speeds of 400 per min, which is comparable to conventional metal can lines. In a country like India, where nearly a third of the population lives below the poverty line, one cannot afford to have high levels of food wastages resulting from inadequate use of packaging. The view that packaging is an unnecessary cost arose due to ignorance of the crucial role that a package plays in protecting and delivering the product. India, in fact, is a pioneer in evolving cost-effective packaging systems that cannot be found in markets of developed countries. Flexible pouches for milk and edible oil are two shining examples. Recent market successes of packaged atta, cartoned fruit juices and ready-to-eat foods in retort pouches point to the consumer trends and increasing appreciation of value addition through packaging.

VII. Marketing of Poultry Products

Market

Interaction between potential buyers and sellers- commercial based for their services.

Free Competition

Neither buyer market nor seller market in sorround market.

Marketing

A comprehensive term include all the processes involving transport of commodities from producers to the consumers, totality of activity, assurance of needs of consumer.

Marketing survey, Marketing intelligence, Marketing research - Gather required information about potentiality of buyers

Product Developement - Creating proper environment(both Micro innermost and Macro outermost)

By marketing personnells – salesmen, commission agents, manager. Internal planning – pricing product

Selling - retailers - transformation of commodities into cash, giving to consumers.

Terms: Basis of area	*Basis of commodities*
Local market	Raw produce
Urban market	Processed produce
Rural market	Capital market
National market	Vegetable market
International market	Fish market Broiler market

Perfect Market

Buyers and sellers aware of price.

Imperfect Market

No free competition – different prices for same commodity

Organized Market

Dealing eggs and meat market rules and resolution, business activation by marketing bodies *e.g.* poultry farmers cooperative market, Traders association, chambers of commerce, vyapar mandal.

Regulated Market

By Govt. regulation, public authorities NECC- National Egg Coordination Committee.

Consumer Market

Where buyers buy to consumer commodity not for sale.

Wholesale Market

Primary and Secondary market.

- ☆ Primary: village hats, seller market.
- ☆ Secondary: Mandies, cities areas, rules regulations.

Terminal Market

These markets in which produce is either disposed off directly to the bulk consumers or processors or assembled for shipment to foreign or distributing other consuming areas *e.g.* Delhi is terminal for eggs. Situated in large cities, Sea ports. Communications, warehousing excellent.

Need

A pen, what deprived of Want: Blue pen. Want + purchasing == demand

Demand

1. Negative: Target consumer dislike a commodity.
2. No demand: Product not liked at all
3. Latent demand: Hidden demand consumers want to purchase, but products not available.
4. Falling demand: dg or reduction of demand, due to sudden increase in price, or income or trade barriers (govt. rules)
5. Irregular demand: impt for eggs. Seasonalvariations, misconceptions
6. Full demand: in peak
7. Elastic demand: changes or varies greatly due to slight increase in price.
8. Inelastic demand: demand hardly changes *e.g.* milk for babies
9. Price: elastic of demand ratio = $\frac{\text{\% change in demand}}{\text{\% change in price}}$

Expressed in negative sign, because of increase relation of

Marketing Channel

Distribution channels

Perishable shortest channels required.

Produce – retailer-consumer: two channels

Produce – commission agent- retailer- consumers: three channels

Produce – consumer – zero channel.

Producer –commission agent- wholesaler- retailer – consumers: four channels

Marketing channels: cost of margin increase.

Factory

Issue information about demand forecasting, supply and demand (marketing information).

Marketing Intelligence

Collection of day to day marketing information gathers from newspaper, commercial activity in wider geographical areas, trade public consumers, distribution, salesman. Competitors, product quality, price- vol. of sale- govt./private marketing consultants.

Egg Marketing Board

Information to producers to increase/decrease product, domestic/foreign market- current observes forecasting of market- assessment.

Future Demand

Of future demand of a commodity impt for poultry.

Poultry Reporter

Factors (1) customers need (2) religious culture etc.

Advertisement

Boosting of sale, promotion of idea.

Communication Leaflets, pictorial display superiority over other product.

Sales promotion : giving incentives

Prices Spread syn: Marketing margin:

- ☆ Is the producer's share in the consumer's price or difference in the price paid by the consumer and received by the producer, difference is taken away by commission agents, packers, graders wholesalers, retailers etc. In our country price spread is much wider- because of no organized markets in poultry or egg. Middlemen get big chunk, so neither farmers/producer get resalable price, consumer exploited by middlemen.

Factors, Marketing Margin

Degree of processing and marketing services *e.g.* of egg-grading, cleaning, transport mode, brokers negotiate position of articles- no physical possession, commission agents take commission.

Perishability

Marketing margin is high.

Seasonality of Production

GNP: Gross national product – is the yard stick of measurement of the overall expenditure of a nation's economic activities.

NI

Net income

Label

Carrying information about the product.

Questionnaire

Marketing survey intelligence research feed back to organization of information important of marketing system.

Micro Environment

Organization immediate involvement influences mark *e.g.* supply demand mark channels competition.

Macro Environment

Demographic factors, sex, family size, economy, food habit, religion

MFPO

Marketing of eggs and poultry products.

Egg Marketing

1961-66 Third five yr. plan. initiated organizing market. Integrated poultry Dev. Federation- state level Poultry marketing federations10-12 Nos., marketing dominated by middle men- wholesalers, brokers, commission agents, assemblers.

NAFED

Marketing eggs in Delhi, terminal market. Farmers cooperative soc.

NECC

Nation Egg Coordination Committee 1982 organization of farmers, operated by farmers, run by farmers HQ: Pune, major role wholesale price fixed, even 2/3 rd eggs in the hand of middle men. State, district, village cooperative society - no poultry Govt. scheme yet, no governing system followed, eggs cartoons introduced, egg washing in cities.

Suggestion

1. Setting up of well organizing State District region by National Egg and Poult. Dev Board. Safe guard producers, consumers 3 tier system. Nation-State- District apex body.
2. Strengthening of Poultry Coop Societies
3. Setting up eggs processing unit- for egg products.
4. Cold storage for lean period and release in peak period.
5. Packaging, handling, quality control and transport system.
6. Gracing be encouraged
7. Marketing intelligence report- Monthly arrivals eggs, source of arrival, mode of transport holding area, type of middle men in distribution channel, cold storage, warehouses facility, variation in regional demand, price spread, competition, competitive forecasting for supply and demand, export potential

8. Sales promotion: consumer education removes misconceptions.

   Set up more retail outlets: egg cart system (MP) now lunched by NABARD+ NECC, finance nationalised banks, products:egg omelets, scrambles

   Poultry meat: about 25 per cent of total meat product.

   (i) Cooperative Marketing: of farm by farms benefit shared by farmers.

   (ii) Private Traders.

   (iii) State Poultry Market corp.

Difference between Selling/Marketing

Selling	*Marketing*
(i) Concerned with needs of the seller to convert his product into cash	(i) Concerned with needs of the buyer *i.e.* satisfy the needs of buyers or consumers.
(ii) Starts with existing product, calls for heavy-selling, promoting to achieve profitable sells.	(ii) The assessment of target consumers wants and needs, interference with all activities that lead to consumer satisfaction. Producers achieve profit through creating and maintaining consumers satisfaction

Needs

State of felt deprivation in a person.

Wants

(Selective choice) shaped by a person's culture and individuality, governed by curiousity, desire of a person (*e.g.* prefer brown shell eggs).

Demands

Unlimited wants but limited resources, wants become demands when backed by purchasing power (factors purchasing power, seasonal variation)

Product

Which satisfy want or need.

Exchange

Act of obtaining a desired product from some one by offering something in return. producers sell good in exchange of money.

Transactions

Unit of measurement of exchange. a transaction consists of a trade value between two parties.

Marketing Management Process

1. Analysis of market opportunity (a) demographic market (b) geographic market
2. Selection of target markets (a) demand measurement and forecasting.

3. Development the marketing (a) product (b) price (c) place (d) promotion
4. Managing the marketing efforts.

Marketing Information System (MIS)

1. Internal reports system
2. Marketing intelligence system
   (a) From newspaper, periodicals, trade publications
   (b) Talking to consumers, suppliers, distributors, salesman sales representatives.
   (c) Salesman/sales representative
   (d) Company motivates distributors, retailers.
   (e) Gathering of information about the competitor's product
   (f) Purchase of information from outside intelligence suppliers (private agencies).
   (g) Establishment of an intelligence section by the company.

Marketing Research System (MRS)

Marketing research system is the systematic design, collection, analysis and reporting of data and findings relevant to a specific marketing situation relates to the determination of :

(a) Market characteristics,(b) Market potential,(c) Market Share analysis, (d) Sales Analysis (e) Business trends, (f) Competitive product studies, (g) Short/long range forecasting, (h) New product acceptance and potential, (h) Pricing pattern, (i) Export and international study.

Steps Involved in Marketing Research Activities

1. Identification of problem and research objectives
2. Development of information sources -secondary data and primary data.

Primary Data

(a) Research approaches- (1) observational research (2) survey research (3) experimental research.

(b) Research instrument: (1) questionnaire (2) mechanical instrument - (i) Galvanometer (ii) tachistoscope

(c) Sampling plan: (i) Sampling unit (ii) sample size (iii) sampling procedure (simple random sample) stratified sample Nonprobability sample (convenience sample judgment sample, quota sample).

Contact Methods

(i) Telephone interviewing (ii) mail questionnaire (iii) personal interview (iv) group interview.

Collection of information/data, Analysis of information/data, Presentation of finding

Marketing Environment

(a) Micro environment - firm's immediate environment.

(b) Macro environment - larger societal forces that affect firm's micro environments.

Micro

Marketing intermediary's middleman agent/merchant, physical distribution firms (warehouse, transport) marketing service

Financial intermediate agencies (research firms, banks, credit company, advertise agency, media insurance, market consultancy firm etc.

Macro

Demographic, population growth, geographic, economic, natural, technological, political, cultural, legislation PFA, MEPO, EDA education, religion, family, age, sex, form.

Consumer Market

All the individual buyers and households.

Industrial Market

Producer or business market all the individuals and organization who acquire goods and services that enter into the production of the products or services that are sold, rented or supplied to the consumers.

Inelastic Demand

Nor affected by he price changes

Flucturing Demand

Tends to be more volatile

Measurement of Current Market Demands

(a) Total market demand (b) Area market demand (c) actual sales (d) market shares of he product.

Forecasting future demand: It is the art of anticipating the demand of a product under a given set of conditions.

Techniques Followed

a. survey buyers intention
b. sales force opinions
c. expert opinion
d. time services analysis
e. statistical demand analysis

Brand

A name, term, symbol, design or combination

Brand Name

That part of the brand which can be uttered *i.e.* Avon, Atlas

Brand Mark

Symbol or design but not uttered can be recognized.

Trade Mark

A brand which is given legal protection it may be not be copied.

Copy Right

Exclusive legal rights to reproduce publish or sell the matter.

Life Cycle of a Product

1. Introduction stage
2. Growth stage
3. Maturity stage
4. Decline stage

Elastic Demand

Changes greatly as a result of small change in prices

Inelastic Demand

Hardly change with small change price

$$\text{Price elasticity of demand} = \frac{\text{\% change inequality demands}}{\text{\% change in price}}$$

Pricing Demands

(1) Cost of production (2) marketing cost (3) profit desired (4) competitions price (5) demands of the product.

Marketing Channels (Distribution Channels)

Function

(1) research information (2) sales promotion (3) contact (4) matching (5) physical distributions.

Types of Marketing Channels

Direct- zero level channels or direct marketing channel

Indirect- One level channel – produce retail consumer

Two level channel – produce wholesale- retailer- consumer

Three level channel – producer assembler- wholesales- packer- retail- consumer

Retailing

Selling directly to final consumer

Wholesaling

Selling to those who buy for reselling

Consumer Cooperatives

It is a retail firm consumer themselves decide policies elect from themselves

Producer's Cooperative

Owned by farm members.

Brokers

Brings buyers and sellers together assist in negation they do not take physical possession of goods

Commission Agents

Take physical possession of products and negotiate sale

Assemblers

Gather farm products, make larger lots for transport to food processors, bakers, govt.

Trade Restricticons

Tariff

A tax levied by the foreign govt. against the imported products.

Quota

It is the limit on the amount of goods which is the importing country will accept.

Embargo

Ultimate form of quota in which import of a particular item is completely banned.

Exchange Control

Regulation of control over available foreign exchange and its exchange rates over other currencies

Non Tariff Barrier

Its discriminations against certain products quality

Group 77

In order to liberalize and foster trade between nations the general agreement in traffic and trade (GATT) an international organization has been established. It prescribed an international agreement on the level of tariffs throughout the world.

EEC

European Economic Community- major Western Europe countries, 11 in number, striving to reduce tariffs with in the community, reduce prices and expand investment and employment within the community.

LAFTA

Latin American Free Trade Association

CACM

Central American Common Market

CMEA

Council for Mutual Economic Assistance of Eastern European Countries

– Chapter 29 –

Preservation Methods of Poultry Meat and Fish Products

Preparation of Meat before Preservation

Only a brief description of how to butcher livestock is given here. The storage life of consumer meat and meat products depends on the quality of the fresh meat. Meat must therefore be as clean as possible after being butchered so that microbial decay is avoided. The chemical reactions which occur are also important. After being killed, the animal is hung upside down so that the blood can drain from the carcass. After bleeding dry, the head can be removed. Subsequently the hooves and the hide are removed from most kinds of animals. After a thorough inspection for visible abnormalities, the carcass can be divided into four parts and each part can be hung up. Pigs, after being killed, hung up and bled, are heated so that the hide with the hairs can be scraped off. The butchering of sheep and goats is comparable to that of pigs. It is best after butchering to store the parts of the carcass in cooling cells. However, as cooling facilities are often absent, the meat must be consumed or processed as quickly as possible (within several hours).

Cutting Meat into Pieces for Drying

After hanging up the carcass quarters, the meat is trimmed. This means the membranes within which the meat is enclosed are cut away. Bad parts in the meat such as damaged areas, discolourations, insect or parasite affected parts must also be cut away. After this the bones are cut out of the carcass, during which the flesh should be damaged as little as possible. Then pieces of meat of good quality must be selected for preservation. For the drying of meat, for example, one can best use lean meat of an animal which has been slaughtered when it is middle-aged. The larger pieces of meat are cut into smaller ones following the anatomical lines. The larger muscles are left in one piece but one piece of meat may contain a number of smaller muscles. Subsequently the pieces of meat are cut into strips. There are two ways to cut the pieces into strips:

1. Place the meat on a board and cut it into strips.
2. Hang the meat up and cut strips off it.

In both cases the meat must be cut in the direction of the muscular tissue.

The length of the strip can vary from 20 to 70 cm. Short strips of meat take more time to be hung up, but longer strips can break under their own weight when drying. The thickness of the meat is important in determining the necessary drying time of the meat. In one batch it is important that all the meat strips are equally thick so that after drying you are not left with too dry or not dry enough pieces of meat.

Examples of different thicknesses which are used are:

- ✰ Strips of 1 × 1 cm
- ✰ Flat strips of 0.5 × (3, 4 or 5 cm)

The exact shape of the strips depends on the preservation method to be used. It is very important that a clean working surface and knife are used so that the starting material for preservation is good. Personal hygiene is also very important. Further preparatory work such as salting is described under the appropriate preservation method in the following.

Preservation Methods

1. Salting

General Information

By salting food, storage life is prolonged. Salt absorbs much of the water in the food and makes it difficult for micro-organisms to survive. For salting, it is important that the fish or meat has been prepared in such a way that the salt added can quickly draw into the flesh and the moisture can leave the fish or meat. Large pieces of flesh must be cut into thin slices to allow this. Fish are divided in half or even in quarters depending on their size. Fish smaller than 10 cm (anchovies, sardines) usually only have their intestines removed. Fish of ± 15 cm are split open so that the surface area of the fish is increased, salt can penetrate better, and the flesh of the fish therefore becomes thinner. Large cuts can be made in fish 25 cm or longer, or these can be split a number of times. To learn how to salt fish, for example the amount of salt needed and the effect of those quantities on the firmness and the taste of the fish, it is recommended at first to use small amounts of different kinds of fish that are easily available. It is easier to start with non-fatty kinds of fish. Lean fish is recognizable by its white or very pale flesh. More fatty fish usually have a darker colour. The quality of the starting material to be used must be good. Old, rotten fish or fish of poor quality is not improved by salting it and is certainly not storable for longer. Salt intended for salting fish should be as clean as possible. The salt may not contain any dust, sand, etc. Salt can contain bacteria which can survive despite a very high salt concentration. These bacteria can therefore also cause salted fish or meat to spoil. Strongly contaminated salt can be recognized by a slightly pink colour. It can be heated on a metal plate over a fire to kill the bacteria. Salt can be very fine or have large chunks; a mixture of fine and coarse salt is best.

During the salting of fish and meat in the tropics, attention must be paid to the following:

1. Use the cleanest salt available.
2. Use enough salt. Note that salting products is not the same as using a lot of salt. Large amounts of salt give fish and meat a very salty taste. At the same time many of the nutrients are lost if too much salt is used.
3. The water which is to be used must not be contaminated; it must be clean and clear (drinking water quality).
4. The most effective way of preserving fish and meat is to combine salting with smoking or drying.

Salting Fish

Three ways of salting fish are described here: dry and wet salting (in technical jargon: kench salting and pickle curing) and brining. The first two methods result in fish with a relatively high salt content, the third method is usually used if one wants fish with a relatively low salt content.

For kench salting and pickle curing, 30-40 kg of salt is used per 100 kg of **cleaned** fish. Using more salt does not improve the process and only leads to unnecessarily high costs: salt is expensive.

Dry Salting Fish: Kench Salting

Coarse salt is more suitable for dry (kench) salting. Fine salt will draw water too quickly from the outside of the fish, making the outside hard. As a result the water inside the fish cannot escape and the salt cannot penetrate deep into the fish. Therefore the fish spoils despite being salted. This is known as.salt burn. Coarse salt does not have this effect. Kench salting is very suitable for mainly lean kinds of fish.

You will need:

- ☆ Split fish or fish fillets (see Chapter 3). If the flesh is thick, make cuts in it so the salt can penetrate well.
- ☆ Salt. Use 30-35 kg of salt for 100 kg of cleaned fish. Use more salt where deep cuts have been made or where the flesh is thicker.
- ☆ Baskets or other perforated containers from which moisture can drain.

Method of Working

1. Split fish or fish fillets.
2. Rub the fish well with salt, especially in the deep cuts.
3. Put a thick layer of salt in the bottom of the basket or container.
4. Place one layer of fish with the skin facing up on the salt. The fish are not allowed to overlap.

5. Follow with one layer of salt, one layer of fish, etc. until the basket is full.
6. Cover the basket with a layer of plastic but do not put any weights on it.

By adding salt to fish, moisture is drawn out of the fish. This moisture, with the salt dissolved in it, is called brine. Place the basket on some stones so the brine can drain. Take care with this method that the fish is piled in such a way that the brine can drain easily and will not collect in spots. If it does, it causes an uneven preservation. After a day the fish must be stacked anew so

that the fish which was originally on the bottom now lies on top of the pile. The salt is thus distributed more evenly (replenish it if necessary) and you will not get the effect that the fish on the bottom of the pile has a different amount of salt than the fish on top. After being salted, the fish must look clear and see-through. The fish must feel firm and have a whitish salt layer all over it. A fishy smell and the smell of brine must dominate. Strongly salted fish, if it is properly covered, can be stored for a long time. A disadvantage of this method is that the brine drains away, leaving the fish standing dry. Fatty kinds of fish can then turn rancid as they are exposed to air. Scavengers can easily get to the fish and bacteria and moulds cause decay there where insufficient salt has been used.

Wet Salting Fish: Pickle Curing

Wet salting is a good way to preserve fatty fish such as herring, sardines, anchovies and mackerel. With this method the fish is better protected against vermin and a more uniform salt distribution is achieved.

You will need:

- ☆ A clean watertight barrel with a lid of a smaller diameter than the barrel itself. It must not be made of iron, zinc or aluminium because of corrosion. Plastic, wood, clay or stainless steel is acceptable.
- ☆ Large stones washed clean to be used as weights.
- ☆ Salt. Use one kg of salt for three kg of fish, which is equal to 30-35 kg of salt for 100 kg of fish.
- ☆ A bucket or large pan in which to make brine.
- ☆ Fish. With small fish (<10 cm): leave the fish whole.
- ☆ With large fish (>10 cm): remove the intestines.

Method of Working

1. Put a thick layer of salt on the bottom of the barrel.
2. Put one layer of fish on the salt with the skin facing up.
3. Cover the fish with a layer of salt and make sure that no parts are left uncovered. Use more salt at deep cuts or thicker flesh.
4. Alternate one layer of salt, one layer of fish, etc. Make sure the fish do not overlap. Finish with a layer of fish with the skin facing up.
5. Cover the final layer of fish with a thick layer of salt.

6. Cover the barrel with the lid and distribute the weights evenly on top of it.

   As explained above, by adding salt to fish, moisture is drawn out of the fish. This moisture, with the salt dissolved in it, is called brine. Because more and more water is drawn out of the fish, the brine in this wet method becomes diluted. The brine must be topped up with salt to keep it saturated. This can be done by hanging a jute bag filled with fine salt in the brine.

7. Keep the brine saturated. This can be done by hanging a jute bag filled with fine salt in the brine. Using unsaturated brine will lead to spoilage.
8. If, after several hours, the level of the created brine does not reach the lid, a saturated salt solution must be added.
9.. The salt solution is made of at least 360 grams of salt dissolved in each litre of water. Heat the solution in a pan and let it boil for 10 minutes. Let the brine cool down until it is warm to the touch. Then add the brine to the barrel with fish until it reaches the lid.
10. Keep the barrel in as cool a place as possible

After being salted, the fish must look clear and see-through. The fish must feel firm and have a whitish salt layer all over them. A fishy smell and the smell of brine must dominate.

Check the container regularly. If foam appears on top of the brine (a result of fermentation), replace the old brine with a fresh brine solution

Brining

With this method, fish is soaked in a solution of water and salt (brine). The use of a light salt solution ensures a decrease in bacterial growth on the surface of the fish during the smoking or drying process. It also protects the fish against insects and other vermin; however the protection provided is not complete.

You will need:

- ☆ A clean watertight barrel with a lid of a smaller diameter than the barrel itself. It must not be made of iron, zinc or aluminium. Plastic, wood, clay or stainless steel is acceptable.
- ☆ Salt. To make brine, very fine salt is best. Use one kg of salt for three kg of fish.
- ☆ A bucket or large pan in which to make brine.
- ☆ Cleaned, washed large stones to be used as weights.
- ☆ Chicken wire or a bamboo rack.
- ☆ **Small fish**: leave the fish whole but remove the intestines.
- ☆ **Large fish**: clean large fish and divide them in two. If the fish is larger than 30 cm, cut it into pieces. Make cuts in large, fatty fish.

Method of Working

1. Wash the fish with clear, clean water (preferably of drinking water quality).

2. Soak the fish for 30 minutes to 1 hour (1.5 hours for large fish) in not too strong brine. Make this brine by dissolving 300 grams of salt in every four litres of water. By submerging the fish in this brine, the blood and slime are removed.
3. Next, wash small fish with clear, clean water.
4. Do not wash large fish but let them drain briefly on a bamboo rack, keeping the fish from overlapping.
5. Next, place the fish in a saturated brine solution: 3.0-3.5 kg of salt in 10 litres of water.
6. Mix the brine well before the fish are put in it; all of the salt must be dissolved. If the fish sink, add more salt.
7. Cover the container with a clean board or mat and put clean washed stones on top of that until the fish are covered by the brine.
8. Leave the fish for 5-6 hours in this brine. Leave larger fish longer in the brine than smaller fish.
9. Take the fish out of the brine.
10. Put the fish on the chicken wire or bamboo rack to drain, taking care not to let the fish overlap.
11. Cover the fish with a clean white cloth or mosquito netting. Do not let the netting touch the fish. The fish is now ready to be dried or smoked.

Salting Meat

The methods of salting meat are very comparable to those for fish. To get good results, one should start with fresh meat.

Dry Salting Meat

This method of salting is used for meat which is to be dried after being salted.

You will need:

- ☆ Fresh, raw meat in long strips that weigh 1.5-2 kg and are about 1cm thick.
- ☆ Salt. Use 30-35 kg of salt for 100 kg of meat.
- ☆ Clean wood or plastic sheets, perforated.
- ☆ Heavy stones.

Method of Working

1. Always take care to work in a hygienic way; for example wash your hands well at every step of the process to prevent cross contamination.
2. After cutting the meat, wash it in clean, running water and let the strips drain briefly in the shade.
3. Place the meat for 1 hour in a saturated salt solution (brine). This brine is made by dissolving at least 360 grams of salt in every litre of water. Dissolve the salt completely before placing the meat in the brine.

4. Next, hang the meat up above the brine to let it drip dry.
5. Rub the meat thoroughly with salt; use a total of 30-35 kg of salt for 100 kg of meat.
6. Put a 1-2 cm thick layer of salt on a (perforated) wooden or plastic board, or if possible, a concrete or stone slab with diagonal grooves.
7. Put the meat on top of this layer of salt. Put another 1-2 cm layer of salt on top of the layer of meat. Alternate one layer of meat, one layer of salt, etc., until the pile is about 1-1.5 meters high.
8. Cover the pile with a wood or plastic board on which there are several heavy, clean stones to weigh it down. The liquid which comes out of the meat must be able to drain away.
9. The next day, rotate the layers by putting the top layers on the bottom and the bottom layers of meat on top. Again, use salt. If after two days the liquid starts to come out of the pile, and no more liquid drips out of the meat, the process can be stopped. If this is not the case, keep on rotating the layers of meat until no more moisture comes out of the meat. Only then can the drying process start.

Wet Salting Meat

One can also wet salt meat by placing it in brine (pickling). In that case it is not necessary to dry the meat. This salting process gives the best results when the process and the storage of the final product take place at as low a temperature as possible.

Pickling

You will need:

- ☆ Fresh, raw meat in strips that are 2-3 cm thick and weigh 0.5-1 kg.
- ☆ Salt: use 10 kg of salt for 100 kg of meat.
- ☆ A clean watertight barrel, with a lid of a smaller diameter than the barrel itself. It must not be made of iron, zinc or aluminium because of corrosion. Plastic, wood, clay or stainless steel is acceptable.
- ☆ Large stones.
- ☆ A large pan in which to make brine.

Method of Working

1. Cut raw meat in strips.
2. Spread a layer of salt on the bottom of the barrel and put a layer of meat on top of it. Alternate one layer of salt, one layer of meat until the barrel is full.
3. Place the lid on top of the meat and push it down using the stones. Let the meat stand for two weeks, during which time brine is formed from the salt and the moisture leaving the meat.
4. Take the meat out of the brine and rinse it with cold (drinking) water.
5. Make a brine solution of at least 360 grams of salt per litre of water.

6. Boil the brine for several minutes.
7. Let it cool until it is warm to the touch.

Put the rinsed meat in a clean, empty barrel. Fill the barrel with the boiled, saturated brine. In this way the meat is preserved for later consumption.

Alternative Method of Pickle Brining

Below an alternative pickling method is described which can be used as an initial preparation for drying meat.

For what you need (materials) see: pickling.

Method of Working

1. Follow the method described above; let the meat cure for two weeks during which time a brine is formed from the salt and the moisture leaving the meat.
2. Soak the meat in boiled water for 2-3 hours to remove any excess salt. Refresh the water 2-3 times with clean, freshwater.
3. The meat is now ready to be sun-dried.

Brine Salting

With this method, meat is soaked in a solution of water and salt (brine). **Brining is not used as such as a preservation technique but as preparation for the smoking or drying of meat**. The use of a light brine solution slows bacterial growth at the surface of the meat during the smoking or drying process. It also protects the meat against insects and other vermin; however, it does not provide complete protection.

You will need:

- ☆ Fresh, raw meat in long strips of about 1 cm thick.
- ☆ Salt. Use a 15 per cent salt solution (150 grams of salt per litre of water).
- ☆ Very fine salt is best for making brine.
- ☆ A strainer.

Method of Working

1. Submerge the strips of meat in the brine as soon as the salt has dissolved in the water. Leave the meat in the brine for 5-10 minutes.
2. Let the meat drain in a strainer. Catch the brine for re-use. The meat can now be dried and/or smoked.

Preparing Salted Fish and Meat for Consumption

Before salted fish can be used it must first be soaked in clean, cold water for 48 hours. When the weather is very warm the fish must not be left any longer. The water must be replaced several times by clean, freshwater. Fish can also be broken up into pieces before being soaked. If the fish is very salty it can also be slowly heated in water (until just before boiling) for about 1 hour. However, the preservedfish, salted, dried and/or smoked, must eventually always be heated to 100 °C (212 F) before being eaten.

Meat

Heavily salted meat must be soaked for at least a day prior to use in cold (drinking) water. The water must be replaced regularly by freshwater. One can also let the meat boil gently for several hours over a low fire. If the meat is very salty, soak it in (drinking) water and also boil it for about an hour. How long one should soak the meat, or let it boil gently, depends on the final taste desired.

2. Drying

General Information on Natural Drying

Spoilage of fish and meat is slowed when water is drawn from the fish or meat. This can be achieved by salting as described in Chapter 4 but also by naturally drying fish or meat. The best results are achieved by combining salting with drying. Salting the fish or meat is not essential but has great advantages and is therefore strongly recommended before drying. The salting ensures, among other things, that during drying the micro-organisms at the surface are inhibited and insects and other vermin are kept away. Thus the spoilage of material is slowed. After drying, salt gives a more stable product with a longer storage life. The use of salt before drying and the manner of salting depend on the availability of salt and local customs. Generally very small fish are dried unsalted. Large fish will spoil before the drying process is completed and therefore salting is necessary. It is important that fish and meat be prepared in such a way that salt can be quickly drawn into the flesh and moisture can quickly leave. To achieve this, try to keep the flesh of the products thin and the surface area of the product as large as possible. Be sure to work as hygienically as possible. Make sure that a batch of meat or fish to be dried is made up of pieces of roughly the same size. This ensures that the whole batch dries evenly and that after drying part of the product is not too dry or actually not dry enough. Very fatty fish or meat is difficult to convert into a good salted and/or dried product. The problem is that the fat forms a barrier to salt penetration and/or loss of moisture.

Preparation

Salting is part of the preparation for drying, and depends among other things on the availability of salt and on local customs. After salting, the excess water formed must be removed from the fish or meat. With meat, it can be done by passing the larger pieces of meat through a wringer (two wooden rolls 1.5-2.0 cm apart). In doing so, the surface area is also increased which reduces the time needed for drying. A somewhat simpler method for removing moisture is to press meat and (mainly whole) fish. Put the fish on a clean, level surface and, using sheets of *e.g.* wood with weights on them, press the fish or meat as flat as possible. Subsequently the fish and meat is hung up before drying to speed up the drying process.

Hanging Fish and Meat up to Dry

Fish can be hung up in several ways on horizontal sticks to dry. It is advisable to hang fish on hooks or with string tied around the tails Meat to be dried is hung on hooks or on strings. The pieces of meat are then evenly spaced on sticks hanging horizontally in such a way that the pieces of meat do not touch. With this method of drying, air is free to circulate all around the meat and the product will dry quickest and most uniformly. If there is no free air circulation, some parts will remain moist. Spoilage by bacteria or insect damage (they are carriers of bacteria) can especially start at such places. Whole fish, fish fillets or meat can also be dried on drying racks made of chicken wire or bamboo poles. The disadvantage of this method is that, due to the contact between the meat or fish and the poles or wire, there is a chance the product will remain moist in places and thus cannot dry completely.

The Drying Process

Drying must take place carefully and uniformly. The best results are achieved in dry weather with a lot of wind. Take care that the meat or fish does not get so hot the fat starts to melt or that a crust is formed on the surface. The inside of the fish or meat would then stay moist which would make it spoil quickly. Therefore do not put the meat or fish to be dried directly in the sun at the start of the drying process. In the early morning or the late afternoon sun, the product to be dried will stay relatively cool, but in the middle of the day it must be protected against overheating by temporarily putting it in the shade. Experience will teach you what the best method is. If drying racks are used, the pieces of fish or meat must be turned every two hours so they dry uniformly. The product to be dried must be protected as much as possible against vermin and insects. Insects are carriers of various bacteria which can cause the product to spoil.

Bluebottle or carrion flies lay their eggs on the still damp product and their larvae eat the flesh. Beetles of the species Dermestes lay their eggs especially in the already dried product. Try to prevent such insects from nestling in or near the material to be dried. To do so, remove all animal waste from the immediate vicinity. This is a highly suitable breeding place for these kinds of insects. Using a good salting technique helps to keep the insects at a distance during drying. Also use mosquito netting to keep insects, and especially the bluebottle/carrion flies, away. Do not let the netting touch the material to be dried. Put the drying rack at least one metre above the ground so that other vermin do not get a chance to get to the product. Put the legs of the rack in a pan of water to which a little oil has been added. The meat or fish must be protected against dusty wind, rain and dew. The products can be covered with banana or palm leaves or plastic. They can of course also be put under an awning or in a shed. However, put the products to be dried out in the sun again as soon as possible to let them dry further.

Dried Fish: Storage and Use

How long fish must dry depends on the type of fish, its size and the weather. The final moisture content must be less than 25 per cent to prevent microbial spoilage. Weighing the fish before and after the drying process can tell you whether the fish is dry enough. If during the drying process the weight of the fish does not decrease further, it is sufficiently dry. In general, naturally dried fish needs about 3-10 days to dry. After drying, the dried fish is difficult to bend. Some of the dried fish products are very crumbly and breakable and must be handled with care after being dried.

In dry climates it is possible to store dried fish in sealable, sturdy boxes or wooden crates in which ventilation holes have been made. The holes must be covered with mosquito netting to keep out insects and vermin. In humid conditions dried fish can take up moisture from the air and must be packed airtight. An additional advantage of airtight packaging is a delay in the onset of rancidity in fatty fish. Strong plastic bags can be used which are then closed properly. These provide protection against insects and moisture. However, the bags should not be placed in the direct sun or in warm places. The product can then start sweating; there is, after all, some moisture left. This moisture can cause mould to grow on the fish. When such moisture is seen, the fish should be re-dried in the sun for several hours and re-packed. Store the packed, dried fish in a cool, dry, well-ventilated and dark place. Before unsalted or salted dried fish can be eaten, it must first be soaked in clean, cold water for 48 hours. In very warm weather, the fish should not be left standing longer than that. The water must be replaced several times by clean, freshwater. Fish can also be broken into smaller pieces before being soaked. If the fish is very salty, it can be slowly heated in water (until just before boiling) for about 1 hour. However, preserved fish, whether salted, dried and/or smoked, must eventually always be heated to 100°C (212°F) before being eaten.

Meat

Experience will help you determine when meat is dry enough. Often this is after 5 days, depending on the weather. Well-dried meat has a uniform appearance after being broken. The colour is the same throughout the product and is often dark red. The consistency is hard and when it is pushed with a finger, it does not give. The smell and taste of dried meat is different to that of fresh meat. Light oxidation of the meat fats gives a typical dried meat taste. Meat which has any signs of spoilage should not be stored any longer nor eaten. After drying, the meat can be packed and stored. In dry climates it is possible to store dried meat in sealable, sturdy boxes or wooden crates in which ventilation holes have been made. These holes must be covered with mosquito netting to keep out insects and vermin. One can also store-dried meat in closed (jute) bags hung from the ceiling to keep out any vermin. In humid conditions dried meat can take up moisture from the air and must be packed airtight. Strong plastic bags can be used which are then closed properly. Keep the packed meat in a cool, dry, well-ventilated and dark place. In such conditions, well dried meat can be kept for months. Before using salted or unsalted dried meat, it must first be soaked in boiling water or be boiled gently. How long the meat is soaked or heated depends on the desired taste and consistency.

Solar Drying

Natural drying of fish and meat sometimes has disadvantages. Long periods of sunshine are required, the drying speed is slow and in areas with a relatively high humidity it is often difficult to dry the fish and meat adequately. An alternative for conventional sun drying is solar drying.

Improved Sun Drying for Fish

A solar tent dryer can be used for solar drying. This is the simplest and cheapest way of solar drying. Solar dryers work by retaining the heat of the sun's rays. A higher drying temperature and thus greater drying speed can then be achieved. The moisture content of the final product is lower than that achieved with conventional sun drying. All this means that the chance of spoilage occurring during the drying process and storage is smaller. The higher temperatures in a tent dryer slow down bacterial growth on and in the product and kill insects and their larvae if they are present in the product. Product loss due to insect damage is thus less than with sun drying. A tent dryer is almost completely sealed so the product is protected against rain, dust, vermin, etc. Inlet and outlet openings can be covered with taped-on pieces of mosquito netting if necessary. All these factors ensure that the final product is of higher quality. It is relatively easy to make a tent dryer and it requires little material. The dryer consists of a tent-shaped frame of bamboo or wooden poles covered with a piece of strong plastic. For the sun side of the tent and the two sides, transparent plastic is used. For the shadow side and the ground, black plastic is used. The black plastic absorbs and retains the heat from the sun. Along the whole length in the middle of the tent a drying rack is placed on which the products are spread. Put the drying rack about 30 cm above the ground. By opening one side panel the drying rack can be put inside the tent. Close this side again well by putting sand or stones on the base of the plastic.The transparent plastic on the front side is wrapped around a stick at the bottom. In this way the plastic can be rolled up or let down to allow air into the tent and to regulate the temperature a bit. The air entering is heated in the tent and absorbs moisture when it flows past the fish on the rack. The humid air can leave the tent through both air outlets in the top of the tent. disadvantage of tent dryers is that they are light in weight which makes them susceptible to damage in windy weather. The tent dryer also requires the use of a lot of plastic, which can be costly. Experience will help you determine when the fish is dry enough and can be packed. The drying time depends on the kind and the size of the fish.

3. Smoking

General Information

Raw fish and meat can also be preserved by smoking. The preserving effect of the smoke is a result of drying (withdrawal of moisture) of the product during the smoking. The smoke particles, absorbed by the flesh, also have a preserving effect which, however, is less than the drying effect. The smoke particles, after being absorbed by the product, inhibit bacterial growth on the surface of the product. The smoke particles also have a positive effect on the taste and colour of the product. The heat of the fire dries the fish or meat during the smoking process and if the temperature gets high enough, the flesh is cooked. This means that bacterial spoilage and spoilage due to enzyme activity is prevented. Drying and cooking of the flesh when being smoked play an important role in the preservation. If a product is well dried during smoking then it can be stored for a long time. There are three ways of smoking:

1. **Cold smoke method**: the temperature during the smoking is at most 30 °C (86°F) which means the product does not get cooked.
2. **Hot smoke method**: during this process the product does get cooked but not dried (temperature varies between 65 and ±100 °C [149-212°F])
3. **Smoke drying**: during this process, the product is first hot smoked, so that it gets cooked, and then, with continued smoking the product is dried (temperatures vary between 45-85 °C [113-185 °F]). Cold smoking gives a product which is not cooked. It is therefore susceptible to spoilage and must be kept cool. The storage life of a cold smoked product is not greater than that of fresh fish or meat. Furthermore, it is difficult to control the process in high ambient temperatures; the temperature may not rise above 30 °C (86 °F). The process demands strict hygiene and the danger of spoilage occurring during the smoking process itself is present. Because of these disadvantages, this process will not be described further in this chapter.

Hot smoking, during which the fish or meat is heated without being dried, extends the storage life of raw products by at most two days. Hot smoking will also therefore not be described further. Most traditional smoked products in the tropics belong to the third category. They are hot smoked and subsequently dried under continued smoking (smoke drying). The process takes about 12-18 hours or even days, depending on the product. Sometimes the product is salted and/or pre-dried (see Chapters 4 and 5) before being smoke dried. The smoke drying method will be described further below. Because smoking is virtually the same for meat and fish, no further distinction will be made between the two.

Preparation

Fish can be smoked whole, cleaned, split or filleted, depending on local preferences and the desired final product. Meat must be cut into strips 5 cm wide and 1 cm thick before being smoked. An important fact is that the greater the surface area of the meat or fish, the greater the amount of smoke particles which can be absorbed during smoking and the better the product can dry. It is advisable to kench salt or brine the product in a saturated salt solution before smoking. This extends the storage qualities of the final product. Remove excess salt after salting by rinsing the raw material in clean (drinking) water, since salt can form a hard, impenetrable crust during smoking. It is also advisable to dry the raw product for an hour in the sun before smoking it. This prevents the outer layer of the fish or meat from sealing shut (case hardening) during smoking. That would mean the outer layer (which in the case of fish is their skin) would no longer allow moisture to pass through and therefore the inside of the fish would not be able to dry properly. Insufficiently dried fish or meat cannot be stored long. Furthermore, pre-drying fish gives it a nice shiny surface layer. Whether or not a product is salted and/or dried before smoking depends on local customs and preferences. The fish are threaded on stakes or tied to them using string or hooks. Meat is attached to sticks using string or hooks. Products which are hung up may not touch each other during smoking. The smoke would then not be able to reach everywhere and the product would not dry uniformly.

Wood

The best smoke production is obtained from a smouldering fire of wood shavings and hard wood blocks. One can best begin the smoking process by burning damp wood. After that, smoke with dry wood. Some kinds of wood (such as oleander) are not suitable for smoking as they contain poisonous substances. All wood from deciduous trees and pines is reported to be safe. A disadvantage of smoking is that a lot of wood is needed. If wood is scarce, one can also use papyrus, palm kernels, peeled maize-cobs and coconut husks as fuel.

Smoking Ovens

The smoking process has the best results in a dry environment. It is therefore often better to work in a smoke house rather than in the open air. A few types of smoking ovens which can be made at a reasonable price are described below.

Simple Ovens

The simplest oven is open grating on which the meat or fish is placed with a smouldering fire underneath. The capacity is small, however, and there is much loss of smoke. An improvement is an oven made of layers of dried mud or clay or oil drums, with a grating on top. The grating is best made from wood; steel can scorch the fish. A number of these small ovens can be put in a hut.

Oil-drum Smoking Ovens

Another possible model is a few oil drums placed on top of each other. The rims must fit well. A damp sack is placed over the rim of the top drum. This system uses the smoke more efficiently. The order of the drums, or of the meat in the drums, must be changed regularly as the lowest drum gets most of the heat and the smoke. Oil drums and mud ovens can only be used to make smoked products. One disadvantage of these kinds of oven is that the temperature is difficult to control and in the end the products are not equally or uniformly smoked. The ovens are sensitive to the influence of rain and wind. An advantage is, of course, the low cost of materials to make these ovens.

The Chorkor Oven

This large, rectangular smoking oven is especially suited for smoking smaller fish. It consists of a rectangular fire box onto which a number of shallow wooden framed wire mesh trays are stacked. Fish are placed on the trays and firewood is burnt in the fire box. The fire box can be constructed in different ways:

- ✰ Clay and mud shaped by hand
- ✰ Packed mud faced with cement
- ✰ Clay mud blocks and mortar
- ✰ Cement blocks with mortar.

The use of cement is more expensive, but the oven will last longer. The stoke holes should be arched for structural strength. The oven should be low, for ease of stacking up to 15 trays, but the flames of the fire should be at least 50 cm removed from the lowest tray, hence a 10-20 cm fire pit is required for each stoke hole. The smoker is designed so that wooden trays will rest along the midlines of the oven walls. The top tray may be covered by a sheet of plywood or corrugated iron. During the smoking process trays can be exchanged. This way the fish are smoked more uniformly. Tray capacity: 15 kg fish.

Smoke House

The last suggestion is to build a smokehouse. This house should have a floor space of about 2 by 2 metres. Place an oil drum on an earthen or stone floor. Fireproof the place where the drum stands with stone walls. Remove the bottom from the drum and build a grate for the fire a little above the bottom. Make a door in the drum to regulate the oxygen flow and cut smoke holes in the top. Build shelves above the drum on which to put the meat. Leave enough room to let the smoke permeate the house. Instead of shelves, the walls can have supports to rest removable beams on. The meat and fish can be hung from these beams. The walls and the roof must be closed so that the smoke cannot escape. Build a ventilation valve or flap into the roof. This can be used to control the smoke circulation. When one builds a completely closed smokehouse, the fire can be made directly on the floor. Hang the meat on ropes or hooks above the oven.

Smoke-Drying Process

Start the smoking process with a smouldering fire using some damp wood so that a lot of smoke (at ± 45 °C/113°F) is produced. This damp smoke forms a layer of moisture on the surface of the product which allows smoke particles to be absorbed quicker. Next, slowly raise the temperature (to ± 85 °C/185°F) by allowing more oxygen to enter. With fish do not allow the temperature to rise too quickly as the skin may split and case hardening can occur. Case hardening can also occur during the smoking of meat. The product is then cooked for a short time (2-4 hours) at ± 85 °C (185°F). It must be remembered that at such temperatures fat will leak from the product and be lost. You will therefore be left with a final product which has a lower fat content. If the smoking is continued after 2-4 hours at a lower temperature (±50 °C/ 122°F) for several hours, the product will slowly dry further. Lower the temperature of the smoke by reducing the oxygen flow to the fire. Smoke the products at this temperature until they are sufficiently dried. A cheaper alternative is to do all or part of the drying using solar energy.

The smoked and dried final product should be clearly brown, nice and dry and have a hard structure. If the final product is well dried, it can be kept for several months. Experience will help you determine when the fish or meat has been properly smoked and dried. The total smoking time also depends on the oven used and the kind of fish or meat. Smoke-dried fish or meat can be stored in the same way as dried fish or meat. The final product can be eaten dry or cooked well in clean (drinking) water.

Smoking of Meat

Introduction

Smoking of meat was known to man as an aid in preservation for a long time, although the chemical basis was a mystery. Now it has become well known that smoke contain a large number of wood degradation products such as aldehyde, ketones, organic acids, phenols etc. Which exerts bacteriostatic effect besides imparting characteristic smoky flavour. Preservation of smoked meat is also due to surface dehydration, lowering of surface pH and antioxidant property of smoke Constituents. Curing and smoking are interrelated and often practiced together, *i.e.* cured meat is commonly smoked and vice versa.

Purpose of Smoking

The primary purposes of smoking are:

1. Development of aroma and flavour.
2. Preservation.
3. Creation of new products
4. Development of color
5. Formation of a Protective skin on emulsion type sausages.
6. Protection from Oxidation.

Smoking of meat and creation of new flavours have developed entirely different group of meat products. The brown color developed on the surface of many processed meat products is also enhanced by smoking. The browning or Maillard reaction is responsible for development of the characteristic brown color on the surface of smoked products.

Source of Smoke

A variety of fuels have been used for smoking of meat, varying from animal dung, to corn cob, through a variety of soft and hard woods. Since there is considerable variation in the composition of various fuels, the components of smoke vary widely. There are two types of smoke being used.

1. Wood Smoke
2. Liquid Smoke

Wood Smoke

Wood is composes of Cellulose, hemicelluloses, and lignin. Upon heating cellulose breaks down to form 1, 6 – anhydroglucose, apparently by first forming glucose and than by dehydration to 1, 6 – anhydroglucose, further heating decomposes 1, 6 anhydroglucose in such products as acetic acid, phenols, water and acetone.

Hemicelluloses are composed of pantosans and upon thermal decomposition produce furans, furfurals and acids. The pentosans yield a larger quantity of acids than either cellulose or lignin. Phenolic compounds are the major products of thermal degradation of lignin. Lignin also yields methanol, acetone, a variety of simple organic acids, a number of phenols. There is also some evidence that both lignin and cellulose produce polycyclic hydrocarbons at high temperatures, particularly in absence of oxygen.

Earlier smoldering cord wood was used as fuel for producing smoke, however it was soon replaced by green or partially cured woods that give better control of temperature and a denser or heavier smoke. Today most commercial smoking operations have abandoned cord wood and gone to saw dust. Which is easier to utilize and gives a greater volume of smoke.

Hard woods have generally been reported to be best for smoking and soft woods such as pine have been largely avoided. Hickory has come to be the standard of excellence for smoking meat, but it is almost impossible to obtain good hickory saw dust in its pure form. Therefore, sawdust is most often a mixture of hard woods.

Liquid Smoke

Now a days, liquid smoke is being used by many processors and has several advantages over natural wood smoke. First, it does not require the installation of a smoke generator. Secondly, the process is more repeatable, as composition of liquid smoke is more constant. Thirdly, liquid smoke can be prepared so the particle phase is removed and thereby possible problems by carcinogens can be alleviated.

Liquid smoke is generally prepared from hard woods, although soft wood can also be used if precautions are taken to remove the tarry substances. The tarry droplets and polycyclic hydrocarbons are removed by filtration.

The final product is composed of vapor phase that contains mainly phenols, organic acids, alcohols, and carbonyl compounds. Analysis of several liquid smoke preparations has shown that they do not contain polycyclic hydrocarbons, especially benz(a)pyrene.

Composition of Smoke

More than 200 different compounds have been isolated from wood smoke. The chemical compounds most commonly found in smoke include phenols, organic acids, alcohols, carbonyls, hydrocarbons and some gaseous components such as carbon dioxide, carbon monoxide, oxygen, nitrogen and nitrous oxide.

Phenols

About 20 different phenols have been isolated from wood smoke and identified. Among them are guaiacol, 4-methyl guaiacol, phenol, 4-ethylguaialcol, o-cresol, m-cresol, p-cresol etc. Phenols appear to play a there fold role in smoking of meat and other foods :

1. They act as antioxidants.
2. They contribute smoky note to the flavour of smoked products.
3. They have a bacteriostatic effect that contributes to preservation.

Alcohols

A wide variety of alcohols are found in wood smoke. The most common and simplest of these is methanol or wood alcohol because it the one of the main product obtained on destructive distillation of wood. The role of alcohol in wood smoke appears to be that of a carrier for the other volatile components. The alcohols are probably one of the least important classes of components in smoke, although they may exert a bacteriostatic effect.

Organic Acids

Formic, acetic, propionic, butyric and isobutyric acids contribute to vapor phase of smoke, whereas valeric, isovaleric, caproic, heptylic, caprylic, nonylic and capric acids are located in the particle phase. Organic acids have little or no direct inference on the aroma or flavour of smoked products. They have a minor preservative action, which results as acidity on the surface of smoked meat. The acids do play an important role in skin formation in some kinds of sausages. They also contribute to the red color of smoked products.

Carbonyls

A large number of carbonyl compounds contribute to smoke. Similar to organic acids, they occur in steam distillable fraction and also in the particle phase of smoke. Well over 20 compounds have been identified : 2 pentanone, crotanaldehyde, ethanol, isovaleralehyde, acrolein, isobutyraldehyde, diacetyl, 3-methyl-2-butanone, pinacolene, etc. These carbonyl compounds contribute to smoke flavour and aroma, or more probably, the level of corbonyls in smoke is much higher and thus imparts the characteristic aroma and flavour to smoked products.

Hydrocarbons

A number of polycyclic hydrocarbons have been isolated from smoked foods. Out of which at least two of the compounds benz(a)pyrene and dibenz(a,h)anthracene, are recognized as being carcinogens.

Fortunately, the polycyclic hydrocarbons do not appear to impart important preservative or organoleptic properties to smoked meat. Several liquid smoke preparations have been subjected to analysis and have been found to be free of benz(a)pyrene and dibenz(a,h)anthracene. Thus smoke fractions can be prepared that are free of the undesirable hydrocarbons found in whole smoke. Fibrous casing prevent penetration of the hydrocarbons during smoking of meat.

In a study conducts by Karl *et al.* (1996) on the polycyclic aromatic hydrocarbons in smoked meat products from different kilns, they found that the average benzo(a)pyrene (BaP) concentration of 35 samples from commercial smoking kilns with external smoke generation was 0.1 mg/kg (wet weight) and the sum of carcinogenic compounds *i.e.* benz(a)anthrence, chrysene, benzo(b)fluoranthene, benzo(k)fluoranthene, benzo(a)pyrene, dibenze(a,h)anthraane, and indeno(1,2,3,c,d,) pyrene did not exceed 4.5 mg/kg (wet weight). The average concentration of the sum of the carcinogenic compounds was 9.0 mg/kg.

Gases

The gaseous component in smoke that is probably of the greatest significance is nitrous oxide, which has been linked to formation of nitrosamine and nitrite in smoked foods. Nitrosamines can form either directly by interaction of nitrous oxide with the secondary amines in the food or indirectly by formation of nitrites, which may then react with sec. amines to form nitrosamines. The pH of meat being in acid range may not favor the direct reaction of nitrous oxide with secondary amines to form N-nitrosamines, since this reaction occurs best under alkaline conditions. The cure accelerators (erythorbate and ascorbate) are known to prevent formation of N-nitrosamines during curing.

Deposition of Smoke on Meat

The amount and rate of smoke deposition is influenced by following things.

1. Smoke density.
2. Smoke house air velocity.
3. Smoke house relative humidity.
4. The surface of the product being smoked.

The relation of smoke density is obvious, since the denser the smoke, the greater the smoke uptake.The air velocity in the house also facilitates uptake, since more rapid movement brings more smoke into contact with meat surface.Relative humidity can influence not only the rate of deposition but also the nature of the deposity. Higher humidity favors smoke deposition but limits color development.The moisture or lack of moisture on Product surface also influences smoke uptake, a moist surface favors uptake and a dry surface retards it.

Smoking Methods

Earlier smoking practiced was a very simple process, but it became more complex but also more repeatable as it was industrialized. Basically, there are three types of smoke houses, namely:

1. Natural – Air Circulation
2. Air conditioned or forced air
3. Continuous.

These are, in addition, many modifications of the three types.

1. Natural Air Circulation

This is designed so that natural ventilation will occur. Regulation of the volume of air controlled by the opening or closing of a series of dampers, thus providing natural circulation. The fire pit may be designed to use either logs, sawdust, or a combination of the two.

Modification of the Natural Air Circulation

It consists of an end less chain, to which the meat is attached. The endless chain keeps the meat in continuous motion. This system is particularly useful where curing is carried out on one level and smoking on another, since it eliminates the need for an elevator. However the higher labour requirement associated with this type of smoking has placed them at a marked disadvantage.

2. Air Conditioned or Forced Ventilation Smoke House

In this method the air circulation is controlled by a fan, so the air can be recalculated, exhausted, or a portion of the air exhausted and part recalculated. Thus this type of smoke house gives uniform air movement to good control of temperature.

3. Continuous Smoke House

The continuous smoke house comprises part of the continuous processing system and was developed specifically for frankfurter production. It has advantage of occupying less space than conventional smoke house of similar capacity and also has a much lower labour requirements per unit of finished product. The continuous smoking system also permits better control of shrinkage. It allows more specific control of processing time, temperature and relative humidity. However the large capital investment and high output limit its usefulness.

Application of Liquid Smoke

There are a number of ways of adding liquid smoke to food products.

- ☆ Adding it directly to meat emulsion.
- ☆ Dipping the product directly into smoke solution.
- ☆ Spraying the smoke solution over the product.
- ☆ Atomizing the liquid smoke into a dense fog and injecting it into the smoke house.
- ☆ Vaporizing the liquid by putting it on a hot surface and
- ☆ Adding by way of smoked treated casings.

The liquid smoke preparations are usually diluted before applying to meats. Commercially prepared liquid smoke solutions are diluted with water, or frequently with vinegar or citric acid. A typical liquid smoke solution prepared and used by meat processors consists of 20-30 parts liquid smoke, 5 parts citric acid or vinegar and 65-75 parts water. Citric or acetic acids are used to enhance skin formation on skinless frankfurters and other small sausages products. Although skin formation can be achieved by spraying with liquids smoke alone, a higher concentration of smoke is required. This acid added to the smoke solution reduces the cost of smoking.

Quality of Smoked Poultry Meat

1. Physio-chemical Quality

(a) Formation of Furfurals

When a meat is smoked formation of furfurals takes place due to enzymatic browning reaction and the maillard reaction. Black or brown colored furfurals or hydroxymethyl furfurals are formed. This gives smoked product a characteristic appearance also.

(b) Retards Rancidity of Fats

Smoking has definite influence upon the development of rancidity by virtue of its antioxidant activity. This extends the shelf life of smoked meat products and helps to account for their desirability. Phenols present in the smoke act as antioxidants.

(c) Helps in Skin Formation on Sausages

Smoke helps in formation of skin on the skinless sausages and frankfurters. Organic acids are present in the smoke which helps in the coagulation of the surface protein which forms a outside covering on skinless frankfurters and sausages.

(d) Occurrence of Carcinogenic Hydrocarbons

A number of polycyclic hydrocarbons which are carcinogenic in nature house been isolated from smoked products. Among them benz(α)pyrene and dibenzanthracene are commonly found in smoked foods. The average concentration of the sum of carcinogenic compounds was 9.0 mg/kg (Karl 1996).

(e) Occurrence of N-Nitrosamines

Various studies have shown that smoking increases the amount of nitrosamines content in the meat. These nitrosamine are also carcinogenic in nature. An investigation done by Rywotychi (1999) in different meats revealed a clear relationship between the smoking process and subsequent increase in nitrosamine content of meat.

2. Microbiological Quality

The most important property of smoke is its effect upon the bacterial population. Smoking of meat has been shown to greatly reduce the number of surface bacteria and to extend its storage life. This is due to bactericidal and bacteriostatic properties of smoke. These properties are attributable to certain components in the smoke, such as phenols and acids. Unquestionably, removal of moisture from the surface of meat during smoking also retards the bacterial growth.

3. Sensory Quality

(a) Development of Flavour

A typical smoky flavour is generated by the smoking of meat which is very much liked by consumer. Phenols are present in the smoke which gives a smoky note to the product. The role of alcohol is to carry components of flavour, thus alcohol also serves in generation of flavour and aroma.

(b) Development of Color

Smoke helps in development of color to the meat being smoked. Especially brown or black color development takes place on the skin of the meat. Browning reaction or the maillard reaction is responsible for development of the characteristic brown color on the surface of smoked product. Some of the carbonyls present in the smoke also contribute to color of meat.

4. Curing of Meat

Introduction

Meat curing was used originally almost entirely as a means of preserving meat during times of plenty to carry over to times of scarcity. Ancient man was well aware of preservative action of salt, which was probably discovered by accident. Farley dry cured meat products were extremely variable in quality, often too salty and lacking in uniformity of cure. As the art progressed, additional substances were added to meat for curing purpose. As a result, the term meat curing eventually came to be understood as the addition of salt, nitrates, sugar, or in some instances, other ingredients like phosphates, sodium ascorbate, erthorbate, potassium sorbate etc. for the purpose of processing and flavouring meat.

With the advent of wide spread refrigeration, the need for preserving meat by curing done has greatly diminished and factors such as flavour, color and yield have become of much greater relative importance than the amount of preservation provided.

Various Ingredients Utilized in Meat Curing

The basic ingredients used in curing are salt, sugar or some other sweetener, and nitrite and/or nitrate. In addition, phosphates are commonly added to pickle cures in commercial operation. A number of other compounds are some times used in curing mixtures, such as various spices, baking soda, sodium erythorbate, hydrolyzed vegetable proteins and Monosodium glutamate (MSG).

1. Salt

From the ancient times salt is being used as the basic ingredient necessary for curing. Salt acts by dehydration and altering of the osmotic pressure so that it inhibits bacterial growth and subsequent spoilage. However if we use salt alone for curing, it gives a harsh, dry, salty product that is not very palatable. In addition, salt alone results in a dark, undesirable colored lean that is unattractive and objectionable to consumers. As a consequence of undesirable effects of salt on flavour and appearance, it is generally used in combination with both sugar and nitrate and/or nitrite. Only food grade salt should be used in curing since impure salt can cause flavour and color problems. An acceptable level of salt in ham has been reported to be about 3 per cent and about 2 per cent for bacon. Addition of sodium chloride to the meat in the form of brine causes a reduction in the nitrosamine content (Rywotychi – Ryszard 1999).

Low Salt Cured Meats (Replacement of NaCl with KCl)

The aim of lowering the salt (NaCl) level in meat is to reduce the sodium intake for those individuals sensitive to dietary sodium (Kolari 1980) Partial replacement of NaCl with KCl, upto 50 per cent replacement was generally successful without the major -ve effects of KCl on flavour. Increasing the KCl proportion was accompanied by increased bitterness and off flavour. Research indicates that 25-40 per cent replacement appears to be the range at which the flavour impact is not noticeable.

2. Sugar, Corn Syrup and Honey

Sugar is added to cure primary for flavour. Sugar softness the product by countering the harsh hardening effects of salt by preventing some of the moisture removal and by direct moderating action on flavour. Sugar also interacts with amino groups of proteins and when cooked, forms browning products, that enhance the flavour of cured meat. Most processors use only 20-30lb per gallon of brine, Studies shows that consumer prefer about 2 per cent sugar incured hams. This would require about 160 lb sugar per 100 gallon brine.

Corn Syrup and Solids

Corn syrup is not as sweet and is less soluble than sugar. However, both corn syrup solids and corn syrup are used widely for curing meat because they cost considerably less. The amount of corn syrup solids is limited to 50 lb per 100 gallon brine under federal inspection regulations.

Honey

Honey can also be used in curing meat. It imparts a sweet taste and is used primarily in honey glazed or honey cured hams and singular poultry products. Although it costs more than the other sweetness, some consumers prefer its flavour and will pay a premium for honey cured products.

3. Nitrite and/or Nitrate

The nitrite or nitrate is used in curing of meat for following functions.

1. Stabilize the color of the lean tissue.
2. To contribute to the characteristic flavour of cured meat.
3. To inhibit growth of a number of food poisoning and spoilage micro organisms.
4. To retard development of rancidity.

It has been clearly demonstrated that nitrite is effective in preventing the growth of *Clostridium botulinum*. Nitrate serves principally as a source of nitrite. Although nitrate was originally approved for color fixation in cured meat, it has largely been replaced by nitrite.

Role of Nitrite and/or Nitrate in Meat Color

Nitrite and/or nitrate are used in curing meat to counteract the undesirable effects of salt upon color. Not only is the color of fresh meat is protected from degeneration, but also the pigments react with nitric oxide to produce the stable pigment characteristic of Cured Meat. Nitrite requires one step less in stabilization of color as shown in series of reactions below:

1. $\text{Nitrate} \xrightarrow[\text{Organisms}]{\text{Nitrate Reducing}} \text{Nitrite}$

2. $\text{Nitrate} \xrightarrow[\text{Absence of light and air}]{\text{Favourable Conditions}} \underset{\text{Nitric oxide}}{NO} + \underset{\text{Water}}{H_2O}$

3. NO (Nitric Oxide) + MB (Myoglobin) —Favourable Conditions→ NO (Nitric Oxide) MMB (Met Myoglobin)

4. NOMMb —Favourable Conditions→ NOMb

5. NOMb + Heat + Smoke → NO - Hemochromogen Nitrosohemochromogen Stable Pink pigment

Since nitrite reacts quicker and less is required for color stabilization, it is being used widely in place of nitrate. Many processors prefer to use a combination of nitrite and nitrate, which gives a source of additional nitric oxide. They believe the slower release of nitric oxide from nitrate gives them an additional safety factor over nitrite alone. Trends have been toward decreased use of nitrate by the industry.

Nitrosamines

The reaction of nitrous acid (which is formed by break down of nitrite) with secondary amines to produce nitrosamines is a well known reaction in organic chemistry.

$$(CH_3)_2NH + HONO \longrightarrow (CH_3)_2N\text{-}NO + H_2O$$

Dimethyl amines nitrous acid Dimethyl nitrosamine

Research has shown that nitrosamines are carcinogenic compounds and has raised the question of the occurrence in cured meat.

Levels of Nitrite and/or Nitrate

Federal meat regulation permits the use of the following quantities of nitrate :- 7 lb to 100 gal pickle, 3½ oz to 100 lb meat (dry cure), and 2¾ oz to 100 lb chopped meat. The same regulations permit use of nitrite at the following levels. 2 lb to 100 gal pickle at 10 per cent pump level, 1oz to 100 lb meat (dry cure), and ¼ oz to 100 lb chopped meat. The regulation further state that the use of nitrite, or nitrate, or a combination of both, shall not in more than 200 ppm nitrate in finished products.

4. Phosphates

Phosphates are added to the cure to increase the water binding capacity and thereby the yield of finished product. The action of Phosphates in improving the water retention appears to be two fold.

1. Raising the pH

2. Unfolding the muscle proteins, there by making more sites available for water binding.

Only alkaline Phosphates are effective for improving water binding since acid Phosphates may lower the pH and cause greater shrinkage. Phosphates also chelate trace metal ions especially Ca and Fe and retard development of rancidity in meat products. The binding of Ca ions aids in restoring the meat to prerigor state by breaking the bonds between actin of myosin. Chelation of iron, on the other hand, aids in prevention of oxidation, since iron is pro-oxidant.

Phosphate is used in various forms like Trisodium Phosphate (TSP), Sodium hexameta Phosphate, Sodium acid pyrophosphate (SPP), Monosodium Phosphate (MSP), Mono Potassium Phosphate (MKP) etc. Legal limit for added residual phosphates are set at 0.5 per cent in the finished product.

In a study conducted by Kim and Marshall (1999) shows that TSP has greater antimicrobial activity than MKP, SSP or MSP. Dipping chicken legs in 5-10 per cent TSP could extend shelf extend shelf life upto 8 days during refrigerated storage without adversely affecting sensory quality.

5. Sodium Ascorbate and Erythorbate

The salts of ascorbic acid and erythorbic acid are commonly used to hasten development and to stabilize the color of cured meat. This group serves four main functions.

1) Ascorbates take part in the reduction of metmyoglobin to myoglobin, there by accelerating the rate of curing.
2) Ascorbate reacts chemically with nitrite to increase the yield of nitric oxide from nitrous acid.
3) Excess ascorbate act as anti oxidant, there by stabilizing both color and flavour.
4) Under certain conditions ascorbate have been shown to reduce nitrosamine formation. (Rywotycki *et al.*, 1995).

The antioxidant property of ascorbate or erythorbate not only prevents development of rancidity but also prevent fading of color of sliced meat. When ascorbate is depleted, the heme pigments are degraded and apparently catalyze lipid oxidation.

Federal regulations permit addition of 0.75 oz ascorbic acid or erthorbic acid (0.875 oz sodium ascorbate or erthorbate) per 100 lb sausages emulsion, or addition of 75 oz Ascorbic acid (87.5 oz of Sodium Salt) per 100 lb gal pickle for primal cuts. Pickle containing both sodium nitrite and sodium ascorbate is stable for at least 24 hrs. when maintained at 50° f and pH 6.0 or higher.

6. Potassium Sorbate

Sorbic acid and its Potassium salts, Potassium sorbate are widely used as antimicrobial agents and thus as preservatives. These compounds are particularly effective in inhibiting mold growth in meat products. It is also soluble in water which makes its use easy and effective. This is readily metabolized and relatively non-toxic.

A study by Binstok *et al.* (1998) has shown that reaction between potassium sorbate and sodium nitrite results in formation of mutagenic products (ethyl nitrolic acid and 1, 4-dinitro-2-methyl pyrrole). Results highlighted the need for minimizing the combined use of nitrites and sorbates in food products.

7. Mono Sodium Glutamate

MSG has been widely used in a number of products to enhance the flavour. It has not, however, been widely used in the meat industry as there is limited advantage in its use in good meat products, although mixed meat dishes may benefit from its meat flavour enhancing properties.

8. Hydrolyzed Vegetable Protein

Addition of HVP to sausages and other meat products has been utilized by some processors. It is used to improve flavour and effectively increase the protein content. Its use in meat products has, however, gained little acceptance by the processing industry. Some smaller processors have also used HVP in cured hams.

9. Sodium and Potassium Lactate

They are used to prevent spoilage and to extend storage life. Generally sodium lactate is preferred over potassium lactate because the later product has a bitter taste. However, the potassium salt can be substituted in producing low sodium products as described earlier.

10. Ginger Extract

Ginger extract can be used to enhance tenderness, flavour, and juiciness of the meat. In corporation of ginger extract in the curing solution also improved the shelf life of smoked chicken. The study conducted by Naveena (2000) showed that ginger extract at a level of 2.5 per cent in the standard curing solution effectively improves the sensory and keeping quality of smoked spent hen meat.

11. Ethyl Maltol

Ethyl maltol, previously used in fruit juices, jams and jellies biscuits and dairy products, is now used in meat products to improve the flavour and color of products. When it is applied in combination with Fe Salts, it prevented degradation of myoglobin by chelating the Fe atom in myoglobin. Liu (1998) worked out the optimum dose as 0.02-0.2 per cent and should be added to meat product at salting stage. It was used successfully to replace nitrates or nitrites. Meat products containing ethyl maltol maintained their original pink color.

Curing Methods

Although these are a number of curing method, they are all modifications or combination of two fundamental procedures.

1. Dry curing
2. Pickle curing

In dry curing the curing ingredients, - usually salt, sugar, and nitrite and/or nitrate are added to meat without additional water. In this method the curing ingredients draw enough moisture from the meat to form a brine, which serves to transport the ingredients into the meat by diffusion. In pickle curing, the ingredients are dissolved in water, which forms a brine that acts in the same general manner as that formed by the natural meat juices and the curing ingredients.

In actual practice, there are the several modifications of the dry and pickle curing procedures, which are a result of combining the two methods. These modifications are as following :

(1) dry salt curing (2) Conventional dry curing (3) Conventional pickle curing (4) artery pumping (5) Stitch plumping (6) thermal/hot cures and (7) Curing of speciality products.

Dry Salt Cure

In this method salt is used alone or in combination with nitrite and/or nitrate. The cure is primarily used in excess and mainly for fatty cuts, such as fat backs, clear plates, jowls, or heavy bellies.

Advantage of Dry Salt Curing

1. It is safe, *i.e.* there is little if any spoilage.
2. It is easy.

Disadvantage

The end product is too salty and the color is lost.

Color degradation may be prevented by adding nitrite and/or nitrate to the cure. However, there is only a restricted and relatively low priced market for dry salt cured products.

Conventional Dry Curing

This curing involves salt, nitrite and/or nitrate, and sugar is sometime utilized by the industry. However this dry curing is not the predominant method now, but is used mainly for speciality products, such as dry cured bacon, and country – cured-hams. Time required for dry curing is usually 2 - 2½ days per lb for hams and shoulders. Bacon cured by this method usually requires about 10 – 14 days.

The mixture of curing ingredients in dry curing varies some what, put a common recipe is 6.0 lb salt, 2.5 lb sugar, and 2.5 oz of nitrate or 0.25 oz nitrate per 100 lb meat, or 10 g of curing mix per lb meat.

Disadvantage of Dry Curing Method

1. High cost due to poor space utilization and the amount of labour required.
2. High inventory due to slowness of curing.
3. Harsh salty flavour of the final product.

Advantages of Conventional Dry Curing

1. A relatively high priced speciality product is produced.
2. Cuts are less perishable because of dryness and firmness.

Pickle Cure

The pickle curing procedure uses the same ingredients as dry curing except the cure is dissolved in water to form a brine or pickle. The cuts are submerged in the pickle until the cure has completely penetrated the meat. All cuts can be cured by the conventional pickle curing procedure.

The strength of brine is expressed in terms of degree brine, which is essentially a measure of density. A salometer or salinimeter is used to determine strength of the brine, and its strength is adjusted to the desired level. The water used should have a high degree of purity. The usual pickles are 60°- 70° brine, 70° brine being most common. Those containing sugar in the brine are sometime referred to as sweet pickle cures.

Disadvantages

1. Poor Utilization of space
2. Slow turnover of meat inventories.

Advantages

1. Pickle cure gives a product with a milder flavour than dry curing.
2. It requires less labour than dry curing.

Artrey Pumping

Artery Pumping is said to have been developed by a New Zealand undertaker who decided that principles utilized in embalming the dead could be applied in curing of meat. Thus the method makes use of pumping a pickle or brine into the cuts through the arterial system. This procedure is almost entirely limited to curing hams only because disassemble carcasses do not maintain the intact arterial system. The needle is usually inserted in front of the branch in the femoral artery so that the pickle goes into entire ham.

The curing ingredients are essentially the same as for dry curing, except the brine is dissolved in water to make a pickle. It is common practice to also use phosphates to aid in water retention and increase yields. The pump pickle is usually a 65-80° brine, 65° being the most common. Sugar is at a level of 20-30 lb/100 gal brine. Nitrite is used at a level of 150 ppm.

Advantages

1. The speed is curing is fast.
2. The attendant reduction of inventories.
3. High yield which is usually further improved by use of alkaline phosphates.

Disadvantages

1. It is largely limited to curing of hams and picnics.
2. Special care is required in cutting to maintain the artery intact.
3. Hams cured by this procedure are perishable and require refrigeration.

Single Needle Stitch Pumping

Stitch pumping utilizes a needle having several openings, so it can be adapted to a variety of cuts. It is not dependent upon the arterial system. Usually, the operator makes 3-5 stitches per cut of meat, delivering about 3 oz brine for injection. Stitch pumping gives a somewhat wetter product than artery pumping and requires special care to produces a good quality product. This is because the brine often accumulates at the injection site, so a longer time is required for cure diffusion by stitch pumping.

Multiple Needle Stitch Pumping

The regularity in shape and freedom from bone makes bellies ideally suited for curing by injection pumping, Hams, both bone-in and boneless are also cured. The results have been greatly reduced labour costs and a reduction in time required for production. Pickle injection has also increased yields, all of which have contributed to lower production costs. The quality of the final product is not as high as for dry cured bacon, since the flavour is less desirable cooking shrinkage is greater. Since the pickle enters through a large number of needles spaced relatively close together, the distribution of pickle is excellent. This results in rapid curing.

Thermal or Hot Cures

Hot pickle cures can best be applied by artery pumping or stitch pumping. There are advantages in raising the temperature of the products either before or immediately after injection. This can best be achieved by placing them in the heated pickle. Best results with the hot-pickle method have been achieved using a 70° pickle at a temperature of 135 to 140°F. Hams should not be held in the hot pickle for periods longer than 1 hr., while 30 min is adequate, following the heating period, the hams can go directly into the smoke house. Holding overnight before smoking gives the best results. Hot dry cure is not well adapted to large cuts but can be used to produce dry-cured bacon.

Advantages

1. Rapid curing with reduction of inventory.
2. Greater amounts of smoke flavour, as smoke also penetrates the performance.
3. Increased yields over dry-curing, although lower than injection – cured bellies.
4. Absence of pickle pockets, and
5. improved flavour

Disadvantages

1. Problems in heating and applying the cure and the reduced yields as compared to injection curing.
2. Also hot dry curing is adapted only to relatively thin cuts.

Double Mixer Process for Raw Cured Meat Products

A new process, the double mixer process, in which the meat pieces are mixed with a specified quantity of nitrite curing salt under specified conditions has been developed by Lyimen (2000). This process gives high quality product with a uniform consistent salt content. This process is quicker than dry salting and gives better firmness, etc, than brine injection. Environment pollution with salt in minimized, as only the amount of nitric curing salt which will be taken up by the meat product is used.

Cured-Product Quality

1. Physico-chemical Quality

(a) Formation of Pink Color

The role of nitrite has been described before in the formation of nitric oxide hemoglobin which in turn forms nitrosohemochromogen which is pink in color. Only 1 ppm of sodium nitrate is required for inducing pinking in chicken breast.

(b) Availability of Essential Amino acids

The proteolytic changes occur during dry curing which increases the nutritional quality (Toldra 1993). Sodium dodecyl sulphate polyacrylamide gel electrophoresis revealed the breakdown of several muscle proteins in dry-cured muscles. Peptide analysis by reverse phase chromatography separation or free solution capillary electrophoresis confirmed the intense proteolysis. Dry cured ham also showed large amounts of free essential amino acids : valine, methionine, isoleucine, leucine, phenylalanine, tryptophan and in particular, lysine.

(c) N- Nitrosamine Problem and Nitrate free Curing System

As explained earlier nitrate on reaction with secondary amines forms nitrosamines which is a carcinogenic chemical. Now a days emphasis is on using such a curing ingredients which do not have nitrate in it. Such a Nitrate free Curing mixture was formulated by Shaidi *et al.* (1993). These mixtures were effective in reproducing the color, oxidative stability and flavour, as well as antimicrobial effects of nitrite without the problems of N-nitrosamine problems.

(d) Increasing the Water Binding Capacity

Phosphate added to the cure increases the water binding capacity of the meat. It works by raising the pH and unfolding the muscle proteins thus making more site available for water-binding.

2. Microbiological Quality

(a) Growth of Staphylococcus

The effect on the growth of *Staphylococcus aureus* by curing was studied by Szczawinski (1994). He concluded that sodium nitrate exerted little inhibitory effect on *S. aureus*, however, it caused lag time extension, increase of exponential growth rate, decrease of generation time and maximum population density of staphylococcus in samples of cured meat.

(b) Black Spot in Cured Meat Products

A rust like color on the surface of cured meat products was studied to determine the reason for its presence by Arnau (1993). The defect was found to be caused by microbiological agent, a G-ve bacterium being responsible. The presence of these rust-like areas, which turn black with in a few hours, can be prevented during the manufacture of meat products by adding potassium bisulfide and sodium nitrite, as well as sugar other than dextrose, maltose or dextrin.

(c) Effect of Curing on Bacteriocin Production by Lactobacillus

In a study conducted by Leroy (1999) showed that sodium chloride and sodium nitrite interfere with the growth of *Lactobacillus sakei* CTC 494. Sodium chloride dramatically influenced bacterocin production by decreasing both biomass production and specific bacteriocin production. Sodium nitrite however, had no effect on specific bacteriocin production and decreased bacterocin production only because of its effect on cell growth.

(d) Effect of Dry Cured Ham Process on Growth of Pathogens

The dry curing process for ham to control *Salmonella* spp., *E.coli*, *Listeria monocytogences*, and *Staphylocollus aureus* was evaluated by Reynols (2001). The study showed that salt conc. (8 per cent) pH (5.5), storage temperature (20°C), ham aw (0.92) limited staphylococcal proliferation and also effected growth of other bacterial population.

3. Sensory Qualities

There is an increase in the sensory qualities of meat by curing like there in an increase in flavour, taste and palatability of meat. Preference by people increase after curing of meat. Texture also becomes tenderer.

(a) Development of Color

The curing ingredients like Nitrites, sodium erthorbic acid, ascorbic acid helps in development and stability of color of cured meat.

(b) Stabilizing Flavour and Aroma

Monosodium glutamate gives the meat a characteristic flavour and helps in development of new products. Other ingredients like hydrolyzed vegetable proteins, sugar and salt also contribute significantly to the flavour and aroma of cured meat. Browning reaction occur on cooking and burnt flavour arises which is preferred by consumers.

References

1. Arnau J., Garriga M. (1993). Black Spot in cured Meat Products; *Fleischwirtschaft* 73(12); 1412-1413, c.f. CAB Abstracts 1993-1994.
2. Binstok G., Campos C., Varela O., Gerschenson LN (1998). Sorbate-Nitrite reactions in meat products. *Food Research International*; 31(8); 581-585 c.f. CAB Abstracts 1998-1999.
3. Karl H., Leinemann M. (1996); Determination of Polycyclic Aeromatic Hydrocarbon in smoked fishery products from different smoking kilns; *Zeitschrift – Furlebensmittel Unteruchung* 202(6) 458-464 c.f. CAB Abstracts 1996-1997.
4. Kim CR., Marshal DL. (1999); Microbiological, Color and sensory changes of refrigerated chicken legs treated with selected phosphates. *Food Research International*; 32(3); 209-215 c.f. FTA 35(5) 2000.
5. Kramlich WE., Pearson A.M., Tauber F.W. (1973). Processed Meats AVI Pub. Connecticut. Ch. Smoking and Curing.
6. Leroy Frederic, Devuyst Luc(1999). The presence of salt and Curing agent reduces bacteriocin production by *Lactobacillus sakei* CTC 494, a potential starter for sausage fermentation; *Applied and Environmental Microbiology*, 65(12); 5350-5356.
7. Liu, W.W. (1998). Property and Application of Ethyl maltol to meat products; *Meat hygiene* (9); 19-21 c.f. FSTA (1999).
8. Lyimen S. (2000). Raw Cured Meat Products, Guaranteed Salting to the desired extent; *Fleischwirtschaft* 80(1); 33-34 c.f. FSTA 2000.
9. Naveena B.M.; Mendiratta S.K., Anjaneyulu ASR; (2000). Use of ginger extract for production of cured and smoked products from spent hen meat; *Indian Journal of Poultry Science* 35(3); 291-296.
10. Price J.F.(a. Pearson A.M. (Ed.), Duston T.R. (Ed.) (1997). Production and Processing of healthy meat poultry and fish products. Blackie Academic Pub. London. Ch-Low fat/Salt cured meat products 251-256.
11. Reynold A.E., Harrison M.A., Rose Marrow R and Lyon C.E. (2001). Validation of dry cured ham process for control of pathogens; *Journal of Food Science* 66(9); 1373-1379.
12. Rywotcki-Ryszard (1999). The effect of various combination of functional additives on nitrosoamine contents in beef ham as a result of curing, pasteurization and smoking. *Medycyna-Weterynaryjna*; 55(8) 550-555 c.f. CAB Abstracts 1999-2000.
13. Rywotcki R. (2001). Nitrosoamine concentration in beef ham, influence of smoking and diversified combination of functional additives; *Fleischwirtschaft* 81(8); 104-108, c.f. CAB Abstracts 2001-2002.
14. Shahidi f.; Pegg R.B.; Waldron K.W. (ed.) (1993). Nitrate free meat curing system and the N-nitrosoamine problem; *Food and Cancer prevention: Chemical and Biological aspects*, Pub- Royal Society of Chemistry (RSC); Cambridge. 82-86 c.f. CAB Abstracts 1993-1994.

15. Szczawinski J., Szczawinska M. Szule M.(1994). Growth of *Staphylococcus aureus* in cured, irradiated meat as affected by Sodium nitrate and radiation dose; *Annals of Warsaw Agricultural University SGGW-AR, Veternary medicine*, (18); 91-95 c.f. CAB Abstracts 1996-1998.

16. Toldra F. (1993). Availability of essential aminoacids in dry cured ham; *International Journal of Food Science and Nutrition*, 44(3);215-219.

5. Fermenting Fish

General information

Fish is an important source of protein in the daily diet. However, fish also has the disadvantage that it spoils quickly. If fish is not boiled, salted, dried, smoked or preserved in some other way, it will quickly spoil. In South-East Asia, fermentation is the most important way of preserving fish. Fermented fish pastes and sauces have a much more important place in the daily diet than salted or dried fish. Fish sauces and pastes provide a welcome variation in the monotonous South-East Asian diet which often consists mainly of rice. Although fermented fish products are a good source of protein, they can be consumed only in limited quantities because of the high salt content of these products. Fermentation of fish is especially used in situations where drying of fish is not possible because the climate is too wet and where cooling and sterilization of the product is too expensive.

Fermentation

During the fermentation of fish, protein is broken down in the presence of a high salt concentration. The fish protein is mainly broken down by enzymes which come from the fish itself. These enzymes are mainly present in the gut. In the traditional fermentation methods in which the intestines are removed from the fish, fermentation will often be slower as there are fewer enzymes present in the flesh.

Role of micro-organisms

Micro-organisms probably play no role in the breaking down of protein during fermentation. However, micro-organisms which can tolerate salt (because of the high concentrations of salt which are used during fermentation of fish) do seem to contribute to the specific taste and smell of the fermented product. In some traditional fermentation techniques, such as in the production of sushi, a fermentable source of carbohydrates such as boiled rice is added to the fermented fish product. This combination stimulates the growth of lactic acid bacteria. The rice is a source of sugars for the lactic acid bacteria. Due to the formation of lactic acid, which is desirable in these products, the pH of the fish mixture is lowered making the product safer and easier to keep.

Salt

Salt is used to draw liquid out of the fish and to control the fermentation. Thus the high salt content (20-30 per cent) ensures that spoilage due to bacteria is prevented and that the number of bacteria present drops as quickly as possible during fermentation. From a nutritional point of view, however, it would be best to use as little salt as possible. The high salt concentration also slows down the fermentation speed.

Traditional Fermentation Methods

The fermentation methods described in this chapter are traditional methods. That is to say that the fermentation is allowed to take place by chance and is guided by experience. No control is exerted over the fermentation. If enough salt is added, some 30 per cent by weight of fish, and there is no influx of air during the fermentation process (anaerobic environment), the fermentation will proceed by itself. The fermentation methods are more or less standard for a given region. Local adaptations or changes in the procedure can, of course, be found. Experience will help determine whether or not the fermentation has gone well. If the product is different than normal, for example if it has a different colour or smell, the product should not be eaten.

Traditional products are divided into two groups:

1. products which, in the presence of salt, are fermented by the enzymes present in the fish flesh and intestines;
2. Products which are fermented in the presence of boiled or roasted rice.

Usually in South-East Asia boiled rice is added to the fish-salt mixture.

There are three kinds of fermented fish products:

1. The fish flesh is converted into a liquid fish sauce;
2. The fish is converted into a paste;
3. The fish, whole or in pieces, retains as much as possible of its own structure.

Fermented fish products are eaten mainly in South-East Asia. Protein consumption is relatively low in those countries and the most important sources of protein are fish and fish products. Fermented fish products are an important protein supplement. They contain a number of essential amino acids which can form an important addition to the daily diet. For example, fish sauce contains a lot of the amino acid lysine. This amino acid is found only in small quantities in rice.

The quality of the resulting product depends on the fat content of the fish, the enzyme activity in the fish flesh, contaminations in the salt used and the temperature. Contaminated salt can be recognized by its slightly pink colour and can be purified by heating the salt on a metal sheet over a fire. If the same fermentation process takes place at a higher temperature, a completely different product results.

Fish Used

Often the surplus or the side catch of the main catch are fermented. These fish would otherwise be lost to spoilage. Mainly small kinds of fish are used.

Product Group

Species

Saltwater fish Anchovies, herring, deep-bodied herring, fimbriated herring, mackerel, round scad, slipmouth

Freshwater fish Carp, catfish, climbing perch, gourami, mudfish

Shellfish and crustaceans

Shrimp, mussels, oysters, octopus

Fermented Fish Sauce with 20-25 per cent Salt

Fish are washed and left intact. The fish are then packed with large quantities of salt in earthenware or wooden containers. Usually 1 kg of salt is used for 3 to 4 kg of fish. The containers are filled to the rim so that no air is present and sealed so as to create an anaerobic environment. The fish protein is broken down as a result of the activity of the enzymes present in the fish. After several months a clear, amber coloured liquid will have been formed which is separated from the residue by squeezing it out. Sometimes a fish sauce can also be made during

the preparation of fish paste. Fermentation of fish sauce takes longer than that of fish paste because all of the flesh must be broken down to create a clear liquid. A number of methods are given below for making the most common **fish sauces**.

South-East Asia

Nuoc-mam

The basic principle of nuoc-mam preparation is the breaking down of fish protein by enzymes in the presence of large amounts of salt. The fish, usually anchovies or mackerel, which are not cleaned, are kneaded by hand and mixed with salt (1 kg of salt to 3 kg of fish). The mixture is put in an earthenware pot. The pot is filled to the brim so that no air is present. The pot is then closed carefully and put in the ground. After several months the pot is dug up and opened. The liquid thus made is nuoc-mam. On a larger scale the fresh, not cleaned fish are mixed with salt and put in bamboo vats fitted with a tap. 4 to 5 kg of salt are used for 6 kg of fish. The fish are put in the vats in alternating layers with the salt, the final layer being salt. After 3 days a cloudy and bloody liquid,.nuoc-boi., can be tapped. After tamping the fish-salt mixture down, the nuoc-boi is again added to the vat so that the fish is 10 cm underwater. The vat is covered and stones are put on top of it so that the mass is put under pressure. After months of fermentation, several months for small fish and 12 to 18 months for large fish, the nuocmam can be tapped. Figure 18 illustrates a vat for the preparation of nuoc-mam. After the first nuoc-mam has been taken, lower-quality products can be made by extracting more from the residue using boiling water.

Sometimes caramel, roasted rice or molasses are added to fish to get a dark colour and a certain taste. This improves the keeping qualities of the qualitatively inferior nuoc-mam. At a fermentation temperature higher than 45°C (113°F), the nuoc-mam loses its characteristic taste.

It is therefore best to keep the vats somewhere cool.

Nampla

This product from Thailand is made in the same way as nuoc-mam. The ratio of salt:fish is 1 kg of salt to 4 kg of fish. The fermentation time is 6 to 12 months. The sauce is ripened for another 1 to 3 months in the sun.

Patis

In the Philippines a sauce comparable to nuoc-mam is made. The procedure for making patis is more or less the same as that for nuoc-mam. After the first patis yield, which has a characteristic taste, a saturated brine solution is used to obtain the second yield of patis of an inferior quality. Patis is usually made of small fish. Small shrimp or alamang, goby fry, herring fry and anchovies give the best results. Enough salt must be added to saturate the moisture which oozes from the fish. One kg of salt to 3.5-4 kg of fish gives a final product with 20 to 25 per cent salt content. Patis is also a by-product of the preparation of the fish paste bagoong.

Japan

Shottsuru

A Japanese variation of the nuoc-nam of South-East Asia is soy-sauce, made from soya beans. However, another sauce, shottsuru, is also made in Japan from sandfish. Sardines, anchovies and molluscs can also be used as starting material. The fluid is filtered and boiled and can be kept for years. Soya bean sediment or koji, which is fermented with wheat, can be added to shottsuru.

Fish Pastes and Whole Fish

A considerable part of the protein consumption in a number of Asian countries comes from the consumption of fish pastes, which are of greater importance from a nutritional point of view than fish sauces.

There are two kinds of fish pastes in South-East Asia:

1. Fish-salt mixtures
2. Products which are fermented in the presence of cooked or roasted rice on which yeasts and moulds are present.

The general method of preparation of fish pastes is the same as that described for fish sauces. Only the fermentation time is shorter, as not all of the fish flesh needs to be broken down. Fish paste must be mixed regularly to keep the salt evenly distributed.

South-East Asia

Bagoong

Bagoong, a fish paste from the Philippines, is made by fermenting well-cleaned whole or minced fish, shrimp, fish or shrimp eggs in the presence of salt (1 kg of salt to 3 kg of fish). The salt-fish mixture is put into earthenware pots and covered with cheesecloth for 5 days. The covered pots are then put in the sun for 7 days. After that, the product is fermented for a further 3 to 12 months. As a by-product, the fish sauce patis can be harvested by separating the liquid above from the paste. The paste is sometimes coloured by adding.angkak., rice which has been treated with the red yeast-like organism Monascus purpureus. Bagoong can be stored for several years.

Balao-balao

Balao-balao, which comes from the Philippines, is a fermented rice shrimp product. Balao-balao is made by mixing boiled rice, whole raw shrimp and salt (20 per cent of the weight of the shrimp). The product is stored in jars and is fermented for 7 to 10 days. The mixture becomes less sour the longer the fermentation takes place. The shells of the shrimp become red and soft and the mixture, including the rice, becomes liquid. In the general preparation it is fried with garlic and onion after fermentation. It is eaten as a sauce or as a complete meal in itself.

Belachan

Belachan is a paste made of small shrimp to which a relatively small amount of salt has been added (4 to 5 kg per 100 kg of shrimp). The mixture is dried on mats on the ground in the sun. After 4 to 8 hours of drying, during which 50 per cent of the moisture is lost, any contaminants in the shrimp are removed. The shrimp are then chopped up and squeezed into wooden vats so that no more air is present. The paste which results is fermented for 7 days. After 7 days the substance is taken out of the barrel and is dried for 3 to 5 hours in the sun. The paste is again ground up after which it is put back in the wooden vats. The paste should now be fermented for one month.

Ngapi

Small anchovies are washed with salt water and dried in the sun for 2 days. One kg of salt is added to 6 kg of dried fish in bamboo baskets. The mixture is pounded until it is fine and is then packed into wooden crates, after which fermentation takes place for a period of 7 days.

Next, the mixture is again ground up and the same amount of salt is added. The mixture is dried in the sun for 3 to 5 hours. Further fermentation takes place for 1 month in wooden crates.

Prahoc

In Kampuchea, prahoc is prepared as follows: after the fish (cyprinids) are beheaded they are kneaded by hand so that the scales and intestines come loose. The fish are then washed in drinking water, during which care is taken to remove all scales. The fish are placed in a basket and covered with banana leaves and stones for 24 hours in order to drain. The fish are salted and, after leaving them for half an hour, they are dried on mats for 1 day in the sun. The fish are then pounded into a paste. The paste is put into open jars and placed in the sun. At night, the jars are closed so that insects cannot get at the fish. Fermentation now takes place. The liquid which appears on top is removed. The paste can be eaten when no more liquid comes out.

Trassi

Trassi is a fish paste made in Indonesia. Trassi udang is made of shrimp and trassi ikan of fish. The fresh shrimp or fish are mixed with 15 per cent salt. The mixture is spread out on mats and is dried for 1 to 3 days in the sun. The moisture content of the fish or shrimp drops from 80 to 50 per cent. The substance is kneaded and pounded until it is a paste. The paste is dried in thin layers in the sun. It is then packed in cylinders made of bamboo or nipa leaves after which it is allowed to ripen as long as is needed to get a typical trassi smell. Three kg of shrimp give 2 to 2.5 kg of trassi. Rice and potato peelings are sometimes added. Trassi must never be eaten raw but must always be heated in some way, such as boiling or frying, before consumption. Trassi is used as a seasoning. As a supplement to fish sauces and fish pastes, **entire fish are also fermented** in South-East Asia.

Colombo Cure

The intestines and gills are removed from mackerel or non-fatty sardines after which the fish are washed in drinking water. The fish are 62 Preservation of fish and meat mixed with salt (1 kg of salt to 3 kg of fish) and put into jars. Dried fruit pulp or tamarind (a tropical fruit) is added to the salt and fish to lower the pH (8 kg of tamarind to 100 kg of fish). The fish are kept covered with brine with the help of weighted mats and are fermented for 2 to 4 months. They are transferred to wooden barrels and care is taken to keep them covered with brine. The fermented fish can be kept for one year.

Pedah-siam

This product is made of salted mackerel. During the preparation, the intestines are removed through the mouth. The fish are then salted, 3 kg of fish to 1 kg of salt, and stored for 24 hours. Ripening takes place under anaerobic conditions. The brine formed is removed regularly. A red colour appears after ripening.

Japan

Sushi

Sushi is a group of preserved fish products which are formed through the addition of boiled rice to fermented fish and salt. The low pH which results from the growth of lactic acid bacteria contributes to the preserving effect. The general preparation is as follows. The intestines of the fish are removed and the fish is mixed with 20 to 30 per cent salt. After being stored for 1 to 2 months the fish are de-salted and the liquid is removed. Boiled rice and.koji. (fermented wheat) are placed on the bottom of a basket and the de-salted fish are alternated in layers with boiled rice or koji. The amount of boiled rice added is equal to 40 or 50 per cent of the weight of the fish, the amount of koji is half the amount of boiled rice (rice: fish:koji = 2:4:1). The fermentation continues for another 10 days.

South America

Anchoa

Anchoa is a product found in a few South American countries, including Peru, Chili and Argentina. Whole anchovies are mixed with 35 per cent Fermenting fish 63 salt and placed in barrels. The fermentation, a result of enzyme activity, takes place for a period of 3 to 4 months.

Africa

Momone

Momone is product from Ghana. In its general preparation, the intestines and gills of the fish are removed and the fish are washed in water. They are then rubbed with salt and packed in layers in barrels, alternating with layers of salt. The salt:fish ratio is 1:9. Fermentation takes place for 7 days. After that the fish are dried for 1 to 3 days on mats in the sun.

6. Canning

General Information

First, some general information about canning of fish and meat will be given. This covers the advantages and disadvantages of the process, packaging materials and materials needed. After this general introduction, the following will be described: preparation of fish and meat, processing techniques and storage of the product. A lot of canning equipment is manufactured in the U.S. Therefore pressures and temperatures will be given both in metric and American measuring units (*e.g.* pounds/inch^2 and degrees Fahrenheit).

Principle and Limitations

The canning process involves placing foods in cans or jars and heating them to a temperature that destroys micro-organisms that could be a health hazard or cause the food to spoil. Canning also inactivates enzymes that could cause the food to spoil. As the cans or jars are sealed hermetically, re-contamination from outside is prevented. In general, canned products can be stored for a long time without refrigeration. Chemical quality loss (in taste, colour and amount of certain essential nutrients) will slowly continue though. Not all products can be heated in the same way. The amount of time and the temperature needed depends on:

- ☆ The number and kinds of micro-organisms and the form (active cells or spores) in which they are present
- ☆ Water content of the product
- ☆ Acidity of the product
- ☆ Presence of salt and/or other inhibitors of bacterial growth
- ☆ Fat content of the product
- ☆ Shape and size of the tin can or glass jar
- ☆ Storage temperature

In fish and meat the number of micro-organisms initially present may be large, the internal water content is high and the pH is close to neutral. It is therefore difficult to kill all micro-organisms present and to get a safe product. The only safe way to sterilize low acid products such as fish and meat is by prolonged heating in a pressure canner or sterilizer in which temperatures higher than 100 °C (212°F) can be reached. The main reason pressure canning is necessary is the hazard of the *Clostridium botulinum* bacterium. Though the bacterial cells are killed at boiling temperatures, they can form spores that can withstand these temperatures. The spores grow well in low acid foods, in the absence of air, such as in canned low acid foods (vegetables and meats). When the spores germinate and grow to high numbers, they produce the deadly botulinum toxins (poisons). The spores can be destroyed by canning the food at a temperature of 115-121°C (240-250°F) for the correct length of time. This temperature can only be reached in a pressure canner.

As the canning of fish and meat requires a lot of energy, clean water and a large investment in equipment, usually it can only be done at a small-scale industrial level. It is less suited for household-level preservation.

Advantages and Disadvantages of the Canning Process

Advantages of Canning

- ✰ The product can be stored longer and more safely.
- ✰ A good-quality product is ensured with fish and meat; it is better than that of foods preserved by other methods like drying in the sun. The best quality is achieved by using fresh, healthy products and by exactly following the heating specifications for that product.

Disadvantages of Canning

- ✰ The high price of the preserved foods due to the following:
    - Glass or tinned steel packaging materials must be used, and may be expensive and difficult to obtain. Glass can be reused.
    - The processing equipment is, when compared with sun drying or smoking, very expensive. The costs for canning in glass jars are less.
    - The process requires a lot of fuel.
- ✰ The process requires more clean water than other methods do.
- ✰ The extended heating at high temperatures causes both a decrease in taste and vitamin losses. The nutritional value of the food, compared to the fresh product, is therefore somewhat lower. Nutrients dissolving in the brine are lost if these juices are not consumed.

Packaging materials

General

Cans made of tinned steel plate are especially used to store fish and meat products. Sometimes it is better to use glass; acid products, for example, corrode cans and are therefore better packed in glass. The shape and volume of the vessels must be chosen according to the quantity to be processed. Big bulky products such as pieces of meat must be sterilized in small or flat tin cans or jars which allow the heat to penetrate quickly to the centre of the product. Small products and products in brine, etc., can be packed in all shapes and types of tin cans or jars. The contents of an opened tin can or jar must be consumed as quickly as possible (in any case within 24 hours), which implies that the amount of food put in one can or jar should be adjusted to the amount of food consumed during one meal or in one day. Of course, it is true that the larger the tin cans or jars, the cheaper the packaging material will be per kilo of processed product. But in general, larger tin cans or jars with meat must be heated longer, which means that the quality is usually somewhat lower than that of meat in smaller tin cans or jars.

Tin Cans

Tin cans are steel cans which are covered with a thin layer of tin. They are used especially for sterilizing and are very suitable for sterilizing larger amounts. Unfortunately they can only be used once. There are many different types of tin cans available with varying capacities and shapes (cylindrical = long and thin, flat = wide and shallow). Tin cans can also vary according to the presence or absence of a layer of varnish on the inside. For fish and meat unvarnished tin cans are often suitable. Every tin can has a lid which can be hermetically sealed with a tin can seamer. Various types of seamers are available, ranging from simple hand operated tools to new, automatic machines. The seam must be made correctly so as to prevent leakage. This can be checked by closing the tin can with a little amount of water and immersing it in boiling water. If, after a few minutes, steam escapes, the seaming machine must be readjusted and a newly seamed can must be checked again. New tin cans delivered from the factory are fairly clean and do not require extra washing. However, do check that they were not contaminated during storage. Do not use damaged or corroded cans. Store them upside down to keep dirt out. If they are not clean, wash them in hot soda water (1.5 wt per cent sodium carbonate), rinse with hot water and let them drip dry on a clean cloth. The lids must also be clean.

Glass Jars

Glass jars can be used for sterilizing under pressure and for bottling. Glass is used less frequently for fish and meat as large pieces of fish or meat are difficult to get out and the product does not look as nice. However, glass is a good option for small and acidic products. Furthermore, at the (large) household level sterilizing products in glass jars in a pressure canner may be an economically feasible option. Glass has the advantages that it can be reused after the product has been consumed and it does not affect the product. The fragility of glass, its weight, poor heat conduction and the fact that light can get to the product are some disadvantages. Jars and lids must be cleaned before use with soap (soda) and hot water. Keep clean jars in hot water until they are needed. Jars come in different sizes. Manufacturers have their own rings, lids and sometimes clamps which fit on jars. The best results are achieved when all parts are obtained from the same manufacturer.

Processing Equipment

The items needed for the whole process are:

- ☆ Tubs for washing and rinsing fish, meat, tin cans, jars, etc.
- ☆ Cutting equipment: tables, knives
- ☆ Kettles for heating, boiling, pre-boiling, processing
- ☆ Shallow open pans for sterilizing at 100 °C (212°F) for acid products like fish in tomato sauce

- ☆ A sterilizer (autoclave) or pressure canner for sterilizing at temperatures higher than 100 °C (212°F) for.low acid. products. These include almost all meat and fish products.

Note: There are various types of pressure canners.Not all pressure cookers are suitable as canners. In a good canner a pressure of at least 1 atmosphere (101.3 kPa or 14.7 pounds per square inch) above atmospheric level should be attainable.

- ☆ A thermometer to check the temperature
- ☆ Cans or glass jars with lids
- ☆ (Hand-operated) seaming machine for seaming tin cans

Preparation

Clean and tidy work pays off in lower levels of micro-organisms and a greater chance the process will be successful. A few remarks are made below about preparations specific to the canning of fish and meat.

Fish

For the canning of fish, it is also important that the fish to be canned is brought ashore as quickly as possible. The mechanization of fishing boats, transporting on ice and cooling facilities are useful for that. Especially fatty kinds of fish spoil quickly, due to oxidative rancidity.

Good personal hygiene among fishermen and processors and hygienic conditions in harbours and factories are also necessary for the proper processing of the fish. Not all kinds of fish are suitable for canning. When boiling fish with white flesh, the flesh will rapidly fall apart leaving hard bones. Thus these kinds of fish are unsuitable for canning. Fish with a high fat content (usually fish which swim in schools such as herring, mackerel, tuna and sardines) have much firmer flesh and softer bones. When cooking such fish, the bones get soft before the flesh starts to fall apart. The fish thus retain their original shape and are very suitable for canning. Another advantage of canning fatty kinds of fish is that the oxygen entrapped in the can will be consumed during sterilization and this will prevent fat oxidation and rancidness, which is not achieved with simpler preservation methods such as drying, etc. Start with fresh, healthy fish. Wash them and gut them in such a way that the intestines do not touch the flesh while being removed. Remove the head and tail, and the bones of large fish, then wash the fish thoroughly in cold water. The fish can be tinned raw, but preferably fried or cooked. Fish is often also salted, pickled, smoked, etc. after being cleaned and before canning. The protein thus denatures which makes the flesh stay firm and not shrink after canning. Use as little herbs and spices as possible. These are often a source of contamination with bacterial spores. Put small fish straight up in flat oval cans (herring). Big fish have to be cut into smaller pieces to get them into small tin cans.

Meat

Bottling meat at 100°C (212°F) is not advisable but sterilizing it at 115-121°C (240-250°F) is possible. Use only clean, fresh pieces of meat. Remove the bones, cut the meat into smaller pieces (a few cm thick) and season as desired. Brown the meat by roasting or frying; big pieces should be partially cooked before frying. For small pieces in sauce, stock or brine, various sizes of tins and jars can be used. For bigger pieces, use flat tin cans. In general, almost all meat products are suitable for canning. Only products which are eaten raw such as raw dry-cured ham or dry sausage are not suitable.

Processing Techniques

A simple description of the process of canning fish or meat is given below:

- ☆ Prepare fish or meat (Chapter 3)
- ☆ Precook (or roast/smoke) meat and fish; this reduces volume and makes the flesh firmer.
- ☆ Fill tin can with fish or meat and filling liquid.
- ☆ Remove excess air from can, but keep the required headspace.
- ☆ Seal can shut with seamer.
- ☆ Apply heat treatment (115-121°C/240-250°F for most fish and meat products or 100 °C/212 °F for sour products)
- ☆ Cool can, wash it and affix label.

Filling and Closing Containers

After initial preparation, the products, which are still warm or heated to the filling temperature, are put into tin cans or glass jars as quickly as possible. These are then filled with hot water, hot broth, hot salt solution or hot oil to about half a centimetre under the rim. This is called the headspace; it is needed to give the food inside the jar room to expand during heating and to create a vacuum in the jar after cooling. Take care that no air pockets are sealed in with the product. Glass jars can be closed at this point. The lid should fit well, but (for example in the case of a screw cap) it should not be twisted tightly closed, because some air should be allowed to escape while the jar is being heated. Immediately after the heating process the lid should be closed tightly. This way a vacuum will develop in the jar as the product cools and the food inside has no more chance of coming in contact with outside air and becoming contaminated. Tin cans can be sealed after adding the liquid, as long as the middle of the product has reached the sealing temperature. Always measure the temperature in the middle of the tin can. The sealing temperature must not be lower than 60-80 °C (140-176 °F), depending on the product and the size of the can. If it is lower, the cans must be quickly reheated in a shallow water bath until the temperature in the middle of the tin can is equal to or higher than the indicated temperature. This procedure ensures that the can will not deform at the sterilizing temperature and that a proper vacuum is created after cooling. The time between filling, sealing and sterilizing must be as short as possible. Never use damaged cans or jars.

Sterilizing Using an Autoclave or Pressure Canner

In low acid products spores of pathogenic (disease causing) microorganisms, which are not killed at 100 °C/212 °F can grow and multiply. To kill those spores sterilization for 60 minutes or longer at 121 °C (250 °F) may be necessary. At 115 °C (240 °F) spores will be killed too, but it takes longer (Table 3). Sterilizing below 115 °C (240 °F) is generally not safe. To sterilize at temperatures higher than 100 °C (212 °F), a pressure canner or autoclave is needed. These high temperatures can be reached only through increased pressure. At sea level water boils at 121 °C (250 °F) when the pressure inside an autoclave is one atmosphere (equivalent to 101.3 kilopascal) above atmospheric pressure. At 0.7 atmospheres above atmospheric pressure, water boils at 115 °C (239 °F). In higher areas, greater pressure is needed to attain the required temperature. As a rule of thumb, 0.1 atmospheres (1.5 pound/square inch) of extra pressure is needed per 1000 metres above sea level. Many household canners are fitted with counterweights of 5, 10 and 15 pounds as pressure regulators. Above 300m (1000 ft) the 15-pound weight should be used.

The general method of working is as follows:

- ✰ Cover the bottom of the pressure canner with water.
- ✰ Place the basket with the jars in the pressure canner. The holes in the basket must not all be blocked, as steam must be able to pass through. Remember to unscrew the jar lids a little bit.
- ✰ Seal the pressure canner and open the ventilation system. Apply heat. The autoclave may be heated by gas or by electricity and in an industrial setting frequently saturated steam is directly injected in the retort.
- ✰ After steam has escaped for 10 minutes, close the ventilation system (the air has by then been evacuated) and let the pressure build up.
- ✰ When the required temperature is reached, the cooking time starts. Cooking times depend on the product, can shape and size, temperature and pressure. Keep the temperature and pressure as constant as possible during cooking by regulating the heat source.
- ✰ Tin cans: After the process, let the steam escape slowly. This can be done faster with small tin cans than with bigger ones, but nonetheless should be done slowly and carefully as the cans can deform or even burst. When the pressure is again normal, the lid of the canner can be opened. Remove the tin cans and immerse them in cold water, replacing the water now and then to keep it cold. When the tin cans have cooled down enough (*i.e.* when they feel hand-warm), they still contain sufficient heat to dry by themselves if stored in the open air.
- ✰ Glass jars: Wait until the pressure canner cools down and the pressure inside has gone down before opening the lid. Remove the jars and tighten the lids immediately. A disadvantage of glass jars is that they cannot be cooled quickly. The safest way to cool them is to leave them in open air until they are hand-warm and then to put them in cold water.
- ✰ A second technique for sterilization with an autoclave uses more energy and water but gives a slightly better product. The autoclave is completely filled with water and the tin cans and jars are put in it. The process proceeds as above. The cooling can be quickened by slowly removing the hot water and adding cold water to the autoclave after sterilization. During cooling, the pressure in the autoclave must be reduced gradually.

Sterilizing Sour Products in a Boiling Water Bath

Sour fish products, such as fish in tomato sauce, are barely heated (*e.g.* 5 minutes at 100°C/212°F) as most micro-organisms will not survive in an acidic environment anyway. A boiling water bath is used to preserve sour products. To prevent glass jars from breaking, start with hot but not yet boiling water. Tin cans can go straight into boiling water. Cans or jars should be completely under water. Start timing the process from the moment the water boils again, making sure that the water remains at a rolling boil during the entire sterilization period. An open water bath boils at 100 °C (212 °F) at altitudes of up to 300 metres above sea level. At greater altitudes, water boils at a lower temperature and the products must be sterilized longer to achieve the same effect, After heating, the cans can be cooled in cold water, which should be changed occasionally to speed up the cooling. Glass jars should be put into cold water only when they are lukewarm. The cooling can be speeded up by gradually adding cold water to the hot water in the sterilizer. When doing so, one should use chlorinated water (water containing 0.01 wt per cent chloride of lime = bleaching powder, available worldwide) so that the cans with possible micro leaks are not contaminated.

Storage

Store the canned foods in a cool place. Label them so that you know the contents. The storage temperature should preferably stay below 20 °C (68 °F); the cooler the better, as chemical quality degradation still continues after canning. With conventional canning techniques not all bacterial spores may be killed. Fortunately, these heat resistant survivors do not grow at temperatures below 35 °C. If you want to store the product for a long time (up to 2 years) in tropical conditions with higher temperatures (of 35 °C or more), than a much more intensive heat treatment at 121 °C (250 °F) is necessary so that all micro-organism spores are inactivated. This is expensive in terms of fuel and will lower the quality of the canned product. Do not pile the preserved foods too close to each other; air should be able to circulate. The storeroom should also be dry and kept at a constant temperature. Only ventilate with dry air; avoid ventilation in warm, humid weather, as condensation could rust the tin cans. Always consume the oldest preserved foods first. Check each product for spoilage. Pasteurized meat products (heat treatment at 80 °C/176 °F) can be kept in cooling cells (2-4 °C/ 35.5-39 °F) for up to 6 months.

7. Chilling and Freezing

General Information

The storage life of fish or meat, or of a fish or meat product, depends on the acidity and water content of the product. External influences such as oxygen (from the air), micro-organisms, storage temperature, light and water secretion are all also important determining factors.

Fresh fish and meat spoil very quickly in the high ambient temperatures of the tropics. If you want to keep fish or meat more than one day, you will have to preserve it. Another preservation method is to cool or freeze the products.

There are two possibilities for storing fresh fish or meat at low temperatures:

1. Cooling at -1°C+4°C/30-39 °F, which inhibits the growth of micro-organisms
2. Freezing at -18°C-30°C/-0.5 -22 °F, which completely stops bacteria from growing.

Because of the low temperatures, all (bio)chemical, physical and micro-biological processes are slowed down so decaying does not occur.

To increase the storage life of the product, it is important to lower the temperature very quickly so as to preserve its quality. If the freezing goes too slowly, large ice crystals are formed which affect the structure of the product.

To cool meat, one needs a large cooling cell. Cooling of fish is often done by keeping it on ice. This requires ice-making machines. Very expensive and advanced freezing equipment is needed for the freezing of fresh fish or meat. Furthermore, these preservation methods require a lot of energy and a large investment in the necessary materials. The supply of fish or meat must be large to cover these costs and there must also be a good market for cooled or frozen fish or meat. Therefore cooling and freezing can only be done at an industrial level. As we are mainly focusing on preservation methods which are feasible at household level, these methods will be described only very briefly. For further information, please read other relevant literature.

Cooling and Freezing Fish

Whole fish, with the intestines and gills removed, and fish fillets are often cooled (at 0°C/32°F) by putting ice on them. Alternating layers of fish and ice are put in a box. Be sure to use at least as much ice as fish. One should always end with a layer of ice. When the ice has melted, new ice must be added to keep the fish at 0 °C (32 °F). Especially with fatty fish it is important to cool quickly so that oxidation of the fat is slowed down. Fish can also be stored in cooling cells. The temperature there is just above freezing point, so ice lying on the fish melts and the fish stay fresh. This way fish will not freeze. The boxes in which the product are kept must not be kept on the ground, against a wall or against each other, but in clusters on pallets and slightly away from walls so that air can circulate freely. If one wishes to store fish for more than 2 or 3 weeks, it must be frozen. For the freezing of fish in freezing cells, a temperature of -30°C/-22°F is recommended. If good quality fish is frozen at -30 °C/ -22°F quickly after being caught, then it can be stored for a very long time. The storage life which one achieves depends on the quality of the fish and the storage conditions (*e.g.* how constant the temperature is).

Storage Life of Fish at different Temperatures

Product	*Temperature (°C/F)*	*Storage Life*
Cooling:		
Cod fillets	0/32	11 days
	3/37	5 days
	10/50	25 hours

Contd...

Contd...

Product	Temperature (°C/°F)	Storage Life
Bred trout (cleaned and vacuum packed)	0/32	18 days
	5/41	10 days
South American hake (cleaned)	0/32	11 days
	5/41	5 days
Freezing:		
Cod	0.30/0.22	8 months-4 years
Herring	0.30/0.22	6 months-1 year

Refrigeration and Freezing of Poultry

Introduction

Early man used different techniques for preservation of his food, which included sun drying, salting, smoking fermentation etc. He also found the cold of winter climates could be used for preserving foods. It is impossible to point out the date, that artificial freezing of foods originated. Early records, however, indicate that in 1865 fish were frozen in the US by placing in pans surrounded by ice and salt. In about 1880, ammonia refrigerated machines began to be used for freezing fish. Commercial freezing of meat probably began in New Zealand for keeping mutton in good condition during transport ot England. In 1891, New Zealand exported over two million frozen mutton carcasses. The future growth of frozen foods will be influenced by a number of economic and technological factors which are population, growth in personal income, relative cost of frozen versus other forms of foods; changes in food tastes and preferences, technological advances in freezing etc.

Freezing is a unit operation in which the temperature to a food is reduced below the freezing point and a portion of water undergoes a change in state to form ice crystals. The immobilization of water to ice and the resulting concentration of dissolved solutes in unfrozen water lowers the water activity of the food. Preservation is achieved by low temperatures and reduced water activity.

Mechanism of Refrigeration

During freezing, sensible heat is first removed to lower temperature of a food to the freezing point. This is known as heat load and is important in determining the correct size of freezing equipment. Latent heat of crystallization is then removed and ice crystals are formed. If the temperature is monitored at the thermal center of a food as heat is removed, a characteristic curve is obtained. It include 6 steps.

1 – 2: The food is cooled to below its freezing point Q_f which with the exception of pure water, always 0°C. At point S the water remains liquid, although the temperature is below the freezing point. This phenomenon is known as super cooling and may be as much as 10°C below the freezing point.

2 – 3: The temperature rises rapidly to the freezing point as ice crystals begin to form and latent heat of crystallization is released.

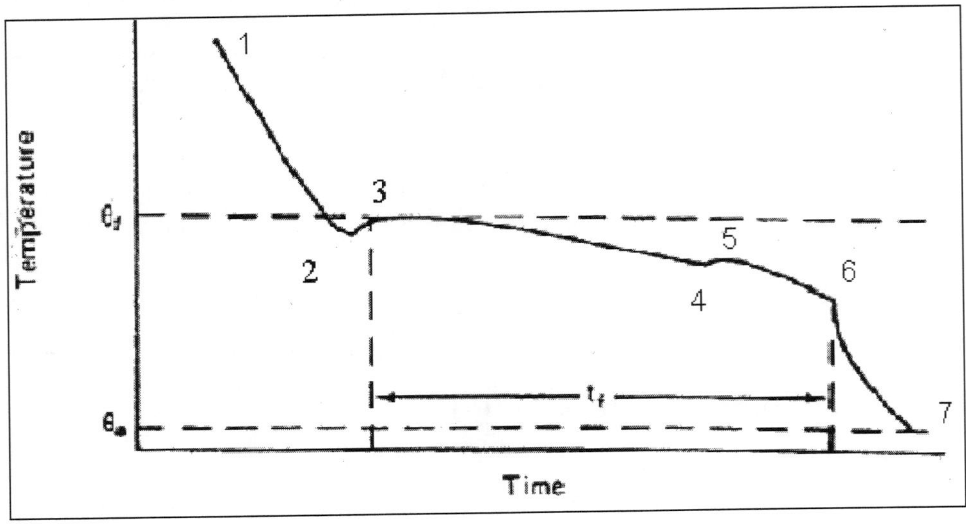

3 – 4: Heat is removed from the food at the same rate as before. Latent heat is removed and ice forms, but the temperature remains almost constant. The freezing point is depressed by the increase in solute concentration in the unfrozen liquor and the temperature, therefore, falls slightly. It is during this stage that the major part of the ice is formed.

4 – 5: One of the solutes become supersaturated and crystallize out. The latent heat of crystallization is released/and the temperature rises to eutectic point for that solute.

5 – 6: Crystallization of water and solutes continues. The total time T_f taken (freezing plateau) is determined by the rate at which heat is removed.]

6 – 7: The temperature of the ice-water mixture falls to the temperature of the freezer. A portion of water remains unfrozen at the temperatures used in commercial freezing; the amount depends on the type and composition of food.

Thermodynamics

To understand the operation of a refrigeration system, it is necessary to understand the principles of thermodynamics. Thermodynamics is the study of energy, its transformations, and its relation to states of matter. The unit of measurement representing the amount of heat is the calorie. A calorie is the amount of heat required to raise the temperature of 1 g of water 1°C.

Refrigeration involves removal of heat from an object or area. Heat always flows from a warm to a cold body and follows the first and second law of thermodynamics. Different forms of energy are interconvertible, and a definite numerical ratio exists for each conversion. Heat is a form of energy that transfers from one system to another by temperature difference. A refrigeration system transfers heat from a low temperature region to a high temperature region.

The characteristic thermodynamic properties such as internal energy and enthalpy are not directly measurable. However, at states of equilibrium these properties are functions of measurable parameters like pressure, temperature, and volume.

Several thermodynamic relationships important to understanding a refrigeration system are described as follows:

1. The constant-temperature (isothermal) process. In this process temperature remains constant and pressure (P) is inversely related to volume(V).
2. The constant-pressure (isobaric) process. In this process pressure remains constant and temperature is related to volume.
3. The adiabatic process. In such a process no heat transfer takes place between the system and its surroundings.

Refrigerated Poultry/Chilled Poultry

The most common method of prolonging shelf life of meat is refrigeration meaning storage at temperatures between -2°C and 5°C (28-41°F). Refrigeration is the single most important means of preservation fresh poultry meat.

Dressed poultry of fish chilling by immersion in ice or ice-water till the internal temperature of meat reaches 4°C. Beef, pork, lamb and veal carcasses chilling in forced air movement coolers (<0°C).

Effect of Fast Chilling

To determine the effects of carcass chilling rate on some major qualitative and quantitative indices, 2 series of experiments were carried out in which 88 cattle sides were chilled rapidly or slowly (22 sides in each variant). Rapid chilling involved initial cooling to – 5 or – 8 to - 10°C at cold air speeds of 1-2 m/s, RH of 90-100 per cent and chilling times of 115 or 212 min, followed by holding in a cold chamber at 0-4°C, air speed 0.2 m/s and RH approx. 95 per cent. Analyses included determination of limit of cold shortening, changes in meat and carcass temp., tenderness scores, shear and penetrometer values, sarcomere length and surface aerobic bacterial counts. Results showed that rapid chilling led to a significant decline in meat tenderness as a result of cold shortening. This effect was observed when the SE index (the rate at which the meat temp. declined, in °C/h, at $\Delta t = 17$°C, *i.e.* from 35 to 18°C at specific measuring points) was > 7.70 in the centre of the round, or > 3.10 in the centre of the shoulder. Wt. loss aerobic bacterial counts were lower with rapid chilling than with slow chilling (Miesnego, 1997).

Methods of Freezing

Air Freezing

Freezing with still air results in a slow frozen product because the air is not moved away from the poultry as it becomes warmed after removing heat from the product. Despite this limitation, still air freezing is used in home freezers and small freezer operations with satisfactory results providing appearance is of no concern.

Frozen carcasses are usually held in holding freezers after they have been quick frozen. Such freezers generally have a temperature of around (-29°C). Which may rise to around 0°F. When loaded with an incoming product. Generally, the air is not circulated in holding freezers.

Blast Freezing

Freezing with a continuous blast of cold air is the most prevalent method used in freezing poultry. With this system air is moved around the products at 1300-1500 r.p.m. **Advantages** of the blast freezer compared to liquid freezing:

1. Air blast systems are more flexible because they can freeze other products in addition to poultry.
2. Different methods and types of materials handling equipment can be used;
3. The freezer can be overloaded because the air temperature rises and freezing occurs at slightly higher temperature and higher plant capacity;
4. The plant capacity is higher with air blast freezers.

Van den Berg and Lentz in a study of factors affecting the freezing rates and appearance of eviscerated air blast frozen poultry reported that the color of eviscerated vacuum packed poultry depended upon the freezing rate. The lightness of color increased rapidly when air velocity was increased from 0 to 700 f.p.m. or when the temperature with a velocity of 500 f.p.m. was lowered from 10°F. to 20°F. Beyond these ranges of temperature and velocity improvement in color was relatively small. Boxing and close stacking of boxed poultry for freezing resulted in non-uniform appearances and long freezing times.

Immersion Freezing

Liquid freezing entails immersing the product after packaging in circulating super-cooled solutions of calcium chloride, glycols, or other appropriate solutions until a crust is formed and then completing the freezing in a conventional freezer.

Advantages for Liquid Freezing

1. The finished product has a good color.
2. It operates at higher suction pressure.

Disadvantages

1. A lack of flexibility.
2. Greater floor requirements.
3. The need for finish freezing after the surface is frozen;
4. Larger cartons because the bird is "sprawled out" during freezing;
5. Contamination if the bag is broken;
6. Dripping brine from the package;
7. Loss and contamination of the brine.

Liquid immersion freezing using methanol at - 20°F. takes an immersion period of 20 min. for 4– to 6-lb. chickens and 40 min. for 15-lb. turkeys to obtain optimum appearance. The initial temperature of the carcass influences the freezing rate and appearance of the carcass after freezing but Cryovac packaging has no affect. The appearance in storage changes in two weeks when the carcasses are frozen at 20°F., in six weeks when frozen at 0°F and the color holds indefinitely when frozen at - 20°F.

Cryogenic Freezing

At present time, the cost of freezing by this method is higher than by other methods. However, the products are of higher quality. Some products which can not be frozen by other methods can be frozen by the use of liquefied gases.

With liquefied gas freezing, the product is frozen completely rather than just the surface. Cryogenic liquids are liquefied gases of extremely low boiling point such as liquid can with boiling point at -196°C and -79°C. Liquid N is most commonly used. Each Kg of gas at -196°C absorbs 186 kg in rising in temperature rise from -18°C.

Advantages of Cryogenic Freezing

1. It undergoes slow boiling at -196°C, which provides a great driving force for heat transfer.
2. Liquid nitrogen, like other immersion fluids, intimately contacts all portions of irregularly shaped foods, thus minimizing resistance to heat transfer.
3. Since the cold temperature results from evaporation of liquid nitrogen, there is no need for a primary refrigerant to cool this medium.
4. Liquid nitrogen is nontoxic and inert to food constituents. Moreover, by displacing air from the food it can minimize oxidative changes during freezing and through packaged storage.
5. The speed of liquid-nitrogen freezing produces frozen foods with a quality unattainable by non cryogenic freezing methods. Although many products do not require such fast freezing for good quality, some products such as mushrooms cannot be frozen by other methods without excessive tissue damage.

Disadvantage of liquid Nitrogen freezing generally cited is its high cost.

Plate Freezing

Plate freezing is adapted only to packaged poultry. Plates which contain a refrigerant flowing through them come into contact with the package so that there is a direct transfer of heat from the package to the plate. Generally plate contact is made with both the top and bottom of the package.

Freezing Equipments

Today freezing equipment can be divided into two main groups: integrated in the processing line and operating in batches. According to the heat-transfer method, there are basically three main types of equipment:

- ✰ Air-blast freezers, which use air for heat transfer. Because air is the most common freezing media, this method of heat transfer has probably the largest range of designs.
- ✰ Contact freezers, Heat transfers occurs through conduction. A refrigerated surface is placed in direct contact with the product or package to carry away the heat. Alternatively, the product is immersed in a cold liquid-brine.
- ✰ Cryogenic freezers. These freezers. These freezers use liquefiable gases, nitrogen or carbon diozide to produce vapors that precool and freeze the products.

Air-Blast Freezers

Air is most common freezing medium, and for that reason a number of designs can be found. Even if a storage room should never be considered as a piece of freezing equipment, it is sometimes used for this purpose. However, freezing in a storage room involves so many disadvantages that it should be used only in exceptional cases. The freezing is so slow that the quality of almost all products will be affected adversely.

Sharp Freezer

Basically, a sharp freezer or blast room is a cold storage room that has been especially constructed and equipped to operate at low temperatures for freezing. Even if this room is equipped with extra refrigeration capacity as well as fans for air circulation, there is normally no controlled airflow over the products, and for that reason freezing is normally slow. This type of equipment is however, still used sometimes for bulk products such as beef quarters but not for processed food products.

Immersion Freezers

The immersion freezers consist of a tank with a cooled freezing medium, such as salt, sugar, or alcohol solution in water. The product is immersed in this brine or sprayed while being conveyed through the tank.

This type of equipment has been quite commonly used for surface freezing of turkeys and other poultry on markets where a light color is demanded. It is necessary to protect the product from contact with the brine by using high-quality packaging materials with absolutely tight seal. Brine residues on the packages are washed off with water at the freezer exit.

A Sodium chloride brine was earlier sometimes used in direct contact with the product in the fishing industry.

Cryogenic Freezers

Cryogenic freezers differ from all other types of freezers in one fundamental respect: they are not connected to a refrigeration plant. The heat-transfer medium is nitrogen or carbon dioxide liquefied. This type can be found as straight-belt, multitier, and spiral belt as well as immersion designs. The size and mobility of cryogenic freezers allow for flexibility in design and redesigning a processing plant.

Key attributes of the equipment are high heat-transfer rates, low investment costs, and rapid installation and startup. In a typical belt liquid nitrogen at 196°C is sprayed into the freezer in which the atmosphere is circulated by small fans. The freezant or liquid nitrogen partially evaporates immediately leaving the spray nozzles and on contact with the products. The cold gas is circulated -196°C by fans toward the infeed and precooling the products entering the freezer and thereafter extracted by an exhaust fan.

The freezant thus passes in countercurrent to the movement of products which is an advantage in terms of quality for some special products. The quick freezing may also result in cracking of the product surface. The freezant consumption is in the range of 1.2-2.0 kg per kilogram of product. Typical products are meat cuts, fish poultry fillets, seafood, fruit berries, pies, and pastries

Physico-chemical Properties of Meat

Hydrolytic and Oxidative Changes in Lipids

The changes in free fatty acid (FFA) amount and composition and in TBARS were simultaneously determined in chicken breast and thigh muscles at intervals between 1 and 14 days of storage at 4°C (1, 3, 7, 10, 14,). The rates of lipid hydrolysis were fast in the first 3 days and then slowed until day 14; phospholipids showed the same pattern but hydrolysis of triacylglycerols was linear at least in thigh muscles. Oxidation increased linearly during storage (Alasnier, Meynier, 2000).

Changes in the Volatile Fraction of Cooked Chicken Meat during Chill Storage

For 24 or 48 at 4°C were examined; results obtained using an electronic nose were compared to those gained by GC-MS and GC olfactometry (using comparative aroma extract dilution analysis). Chill storage of cooked chicken meat produced large increases in concentration as well as in flavour dilution factors of typical lipid oxidation products such as saturated and unsaturated aldehydes as well as alkylated furans, especially within the first 24h (Siegmund, 1999).

Weight Loss during Freezing and the Storage of Frozen Meat

Weight loss and changes in sensory properties of beef and pork sides and quarters during long-term storage under different freezing and storage conditions were investigated. Meat samples from recently slaughtered animals were subjected to a range of chilling and packaging methods, including freezing while hot and packaging in polyethylene bags with or without chilling. The following experimental treatments (temp. and air flow velocity for freezing, and temp. and mode of storage, respectively) were investigated: A (- 20°C and 0.7 m/s during freezing, and - 13°C and 0.4 m/s during on-shelf storage); B (- 24°C and 0.79 m/s during freezing, and - 10°C and 0.4 m/s during storage); C (- 20°C and 0.8 m/s during freezing, and storage on hooks in 2 pipe cooled stores at – 13 and - 18°C); and D (- 25 to - 30°C and 3 m/s during freezing, and 18°C and 5 m/s pallet storage). Meat samples were weighed before and after freezing and at 1-month intervals during storage for 6 months. Results were statistically analysed by a multiple step-by-step regression method and sensory quality of meat after 6 months of frozen storage was assessed by a panel of judges and compared with non-frozen meat. Overall, wt. loss in meat was reduced at lower storage temp. meat from treatment C showed lower wt. loss than samples from A, B and D. Increasing air velocity increased wt. loss in unpackaged samples. Packaging samples in polyethylene reduced wt. loss by e"50 per cent; this effect was more pronounced in beef than in pork. No significant differences in sensory properties were detected between non-frozen meat and samples frozen for 6 months. Mendez Bustabad (1999).

The bone-darkening effect observed in young birds (dark discoloration around the bone, which becomes obvious when cooked). Bone darkening is caused by the leaching of hemoglobin from bone marrow. Leaching only occurs in young birds because the bones are not completely calcified and porous. Eating quality do not change. Removing the bone marrow or cooking prior to freezing will eliminate this defect. As a result, young birds such as broilers destined to be sold raw are not commonly frozen in carcass form but are deep chilled (- 2°C) instead.

Microbial Aspects of Poultry Meat

Poultry requires a freezing process that is rapid enough to minimize surface dehydration during freezing, avoid the chemical changes that can occur at temperatures just below the freezing point, and decrease drip losses during thawing. Rapid surface freezing generates a smooth chalky white surface, which is considered ideal for poultry. Rapid processes resulting in smaller ice crystals may also have the advantage of less thaw drip without affecting consumer eating quality significantly. Cryogenic freezing (- 196°C) with liquid nitrogen has been shown to improve color and reduce drip 3 per cent in frozen chicken thighs. Immersion freezing at -29°C has been found to produce surface color similar to that achieved by air blast freezing at -73°C. In addition, the desirable surface appearance in that study was well maintained during 20 weeks of storage at -29°C, but was maintained only 2 weeks at -7°C. When surface temperature exceeds - 7°C, the light surface appearance is lost. Despite differences in appearance, many reports indicate that the effects of typical freezing processes on the eating quality characteristics of poultry and poultry products are minor.

Effect of Antibacterial against Selected Bacteria

Bactericidal activity of Brifisol KRegistered was evaluated during chilling of broiler [chicken] carcasses. Brifisol KRegistered (1.5 per cent at 1°C for 60 min) significantly reduced Escherichia coli, coliforms and aerobic plate counts (APC) on postchill broilers and increased shelf life by 1 – 2 days when stored at 4.4°C. It is concluded that effective neutralization of all phosphate applications, whether the treatment is alkaline or acidic-based, is extremely important for accurate quantification of bactericidal efficacy Rathgeber and Waldroup (1995).

Wt. loss and aerobic bacterial counts were lower with rapid chilling than with slow chilling.

Effects of Ionizing Radiation on Microflora

Vacuum-canned commercial, mechanically deboned chicken meat was inoculated with either *clostridium botulinum* spores or Salmonella enteritidis and irradiation with 0, 1.5, and 3.0 kGy and storage at 5°C for 0, 2 and 4week. None of the samples stored at 5°C developed botulinum toxin however the sample kept at 28°C became toxic with in 18 hrs. Thayer ((DW), Boyd (G) and Huhtanen (CN)) (1995).

The Microbiological Profile of Chilled and Frozen Chicken

Effect of refrigeration and freezing temperature (4,0,-4,-12 and -18°C) on microbiological profile of 50 commercially processed chickens was determined. Results demonstrate that freezing chicken, either immediately after processing or after a period of refrigeration, will not improve its microbiological quality. Also, spoilage bacteria increased in processed chickens held at 4°C, but levels of salmonellae did not increase significantly. Bailey, J.S.; Lyon, B.G.; Lyon, C.E.; Windham, W.R. (2000).

Quality Evaluation of Refrigerated Chicken Wings Treated with Organic Acids

Effects of acetic acid, lactic acid or citric acid dipping on aerobic plate counts, Hunter on color values and sensory evaluation scores of chicken wings stored at 4°C were assessed. Treatment of chicken wings with 1 per cent AA is recommended over other acids due to greater antimicrobial effect and more favourable sensory results. Chang R. Kim; Marshall. D. L. (2000).

Microbial Cross-Contamination during Air Chilling of Poultry

Cross-contamination during air chilling is likely to be less that occurring at earlier stages of poultry processing when carcasses are more heavily contaminated. Cross-contamination was increased by use of water spray. Mead, G.C.; Allen, V.M.; Burton (2000).

Viruses, fungi, and parasites can cause microbiological problems in poultry. Spoilage organisms on poultry are similar to those found on red meats, including *Pseudomonas, Achromobacter, Micrococcus, Alcaligenes, Flavobacterium*, and others. The most common pathogen associated with poultry, however, is *Salmonella*.

Minimum temperatures for growth of various microorganisms vary from 10 to 10° C. Below - 10°C, microbial growth will not occur but microorganisms differ considerably in their sensitivity to freezing. Freezing and frozen storage has been demonstrated to reduce counts of most organisms on turkeys, including *Salmonella, Staphylococcus,* and *coliforms.* Reductions may be in the order of 97-99 per cent. Slow freezing appears to be more detrimental than rapid freezing to microbial survival, some orgainisms usually survive any freezing process. Effects of freezing on microbial populations are likely to be different at various locations within the same product.

Freezing and frozen storage damage to microbial cells is also increased by addition of salt and by a lowered pH.

Brown [69] concluded that the little work published did not agree on whether thawing contributed to any of the freezing-process damage observed in microbial cells. Systems involving heating under vacuum have been developed with claims of decreased drip and improved quality.

Consideration of the effects of freezing, frozen storage, and thawing on microbiological quality and safety clearly shows that the process is inurious to many microorganisms. However, there is also usually significant survival, other methods must be used to ensure elimination of pathogenic organisms from frozen poultry.

Sensory Aspects of Poultry Meat

Effect on Colour

Cryogenic of freezing (-196°C) with liquifed Nitrogen has shown to improve colour.

Effect on Appearance

The desirable surface appearance is well maintained during 20 weeks of storage at -29°C, but is maintains only 2 week at -7°C. When surface temp. exceeds -7°C, light surface appearance is lost.

Effect on Eating Quality

The effect of refrigeration on the eating quality is minimum. Freshness of food is maintained during the frozen period.

Effect of Probiotic Feeding Packaging Method

Use of probiotic poultry feeds has been processed as an alternative to conventional drug treatments for increasing feed conversion efficiency and growth rates of poultry while improving product safety to consumers. On the basis of sensory scores, meat balls from different groups were judged acceptable for up to 14 days (Mahajan, P.; Sahoo, J.; Panda, P.C., 2000).

Quality Characteristics of Restructured Chicken Steaks as Influenced by Packaging during Frozen Storag

Chemical, microbiological and sensory attributes of restructured chicken steak samples, packaged in vacuum (polyester/Al foil/polypropylene laminate) or in LDPE (250 gauge), were evaluated at regular intervals for up to 60 days during frozen storage. Vacuum-packaged products were rated higher in colour, flavour, juiciness, texture and overall acceptability during frozen storage. ***Bhoyar, A. M.; Pandey, N. K.; Anand (1998).***

References

1. Potter, N.N. and Hotchkiss, J.H., 1996. Food Science. 5th ed. Chapman and Hall, London, New York. ch(9). pp. 165-199.
2. Mountney, George.J; 1981. Poultry Products Technology,2nd ed. AVI Publication Westport, Connecticut. CH. Refrigerated storage pp.172-176.

3. Jeremiah, Lester E; 1996. Freezing effects of food Quality. Mareel Dekker. Inc. ch(Poultry and Poultry Products) pp. 85-108.
4. Alasnier(C), Meynier (A), Viau (M) and Gandemer(G).2000. Hydrolytic and oxidative changes in the lipids of chicken breast and thigh muscles during refrigated storage. Journal of Food Science.65(1); 2000; 9-14
5. Thayer (DW), Boyd (G) and Huhtanen (CN). 1995. Effects of ionizing radiation and anaerobic refrigerated storage on indigenous microflora. Journal of Food Protection 58(7); 752-757.
6. Rathgeber (BM) and Waldroup (AL). 1995. Antibacterial activity of a sodium acid pyrophosphate product in chiller water against selected bacteria. Journal of Food Protection 58(5); 530-534.
7. Siegmund, B; Pfannhauser, W. 1999. Changes of the volatile fraction of cooked chicken meat during chill storing: results obtained by the electronic nose in comparison to GC-MS and GC olfactometry. European Food Research and technology 208 (5/6) 336-341.
8. Mendez Bustabad, O. 1999. Weight loss during freezing and the storage of frozen meat. Journal of Food Engineering 41 (1) 1-11.
9. Borzuta. K. 1997 Effects of the fast chilling on some quantity and quality traits of beef meat. Journal of food Science and technology.
10. Erickson. M.C.1999. Flavour quality implications in chlorination of poultry chiller water. Food Research International 32 (9) 635-641.
11. Mahajan, P.; Sahoo, J.; Panda, P.C. 2000. Effect of probiotic feeding, packaging methods and seasons on the microbial and organoleptic qualities of chicken meat balls during refrigerated. Journal of Food Science and Technology, India 37 (1) 67-71.
12. Don Kim; Young-Ki Chang; Ki-Hwan Park; Young-Chun Lee. 2000. Effects of sub-freezing systems on the freshness of pork loin beef loin and tuna. Journal of Food Science and Technology 32 (2) 341-348.
13. Bhoyar, A.M.; Pandey, N.K. Anand, S.K. Verma, S.S. 1998. Quality characteristics of restructured chicken steaks as influenced by packaging during frozen storage. Indian Journal of Poultry Science 33 (1) 56-60.
14. Bailey, J.S.; Lyon, B.G.; Lyon, C.E.; Windham, W.R. 2000. The microbiological profile of chilled and frozen chicken. Journal of Food Protection 63 (9) 1228-1230.
15. Chang R. Kim; Marshall, D.L. 2000. Quality evaluation of refrigerated chicken wings treated with organic acids. Journal of Food Quality 23 (3) 327-335.
16. Mead, G.C.; Allen, V.M.; Burton, C.H.; Corry, J.E.L. 2000. Microbial cross-contamination during air chilling of poultry. Journal of British Poultry Science 41(2) 158-162.

Advances in Meat Preservation by Ionizing Irradiation

Introduction

Food irradiation is the process of exposing food to controlled levels of ionizing radiation to kill harmful bacteria, pests, or parasites, or to preserve its freshness. The process of food irradiation is often called *cold pasteurization*, because it kills harmful bacteria without heat. It has limited success in the past decade due to off-flavour and the requirement for sufficient toxicology testing. In 1989,36 countries approved the marketing of irradiation foods. The use of irradiation on medical products is increasing; economic and reliable sterilizing agent. Irradiation is a lethal agent against microorganisms.

Description of Radiation Energy

Radiation can be classified in two groups: 1) electromagnetic and 2) particle radiation.

Electromagnetic Radiation

Various types of ionizing radiation in the electromagnetic spectrum produce bacterial effects by transferring the energy of photon into characteristic ionizations in or near a biological target. In addition to creating pairs of positive and negative electron, ion can also produce free radicals and activated molecules, without any appreciable rise in temperature ("cold sterilization").Suggested irradiation: microwave, ultraviolet gamma, X rays, and electrons.

1. The lethal action of microwave is due to a thermal effect.
2. X radiation and Gamma radiation; identical in nature but have different origins.

Particle Radiation

The particles usually considered of importance in radiation biology are alpha and beta neutron, meson, positron and neutrino. The currently applicable particles to sterilization is Beta particle or electron. Alpha particles have limited penetrating ability. Neutrons is unacceptable since induces radioactivity. Mesons and protons are produced only by expensive, high energy machines.

Lethal Effects of Irradiation on Microorganisms

Intercellular Effects

- ☆ Lesion caused by the direct action of ionizing irradiation on a target molecules are the result of energy being transferred within the target molecule itself. Indirect action due to diffusion of radicals produced in the adjacent volume. Indirect effects, in a sense, are still within an organism, but inactive the organism by diffusion to, and by reacting with, a sensitive target site. An environmental effect caused by radicals and other radiation-produced compounds form extracellular and still can be lethal to a cell.

☆ Ionizing radiations can cause a wide variety of physical and biochemical effects in microorganisms. The primary cellular target that governs the lost of viability is the DNA molecule of the cell related to the chromosome volume. The larger volume, the more sensitive the biologic unit was to ionizing radiation.

Environmental Effects

One may consider those lethal effects that originate in the menstruum as a type of indirect effect. The influence of the menstruum can be altered by: 1) using dried preparations in order to restrict the moisture content only to that closely associated with the cell, 2) freezing the menstruum and cells to minimize the migration of free radicals, 3) varying the temperature during irradiation and 4) varying the concentration of the solute or organic material under consideration. To decrease or eliminate the microbial population from a surface or within a material by ionizing radiation involves additional considerations. The microbial contaminants will consist of mixed micro flora, distributed in a manner characteristic of the material. Microorganisms growing as a dense mass in restricted area, or diffuse when dispersed in liquid, will be destroyed at different rates. The physiological state of the organism will vary, and the composition of the menstruum surrounding the microorganism may also vary from that of an inert substance to a plant and animal tissue of high complexity.

Application of Ionizing Radiation for Destruction of Microorganisms:

Two approaches:

1. Partial or selective destruction (radiation pasteurization)
2. Complete destruction (radiation sterilization)

Radiation Sterilization of Food

If the intent is to produce a sterile food product, certain conditions must be met.For maximal shelf life stability, not only microorganisms but tissue enzymes should be inactivated. The food should be capable of possessing a long storage life without needing refrigeration. Enzyme requires a higher irradiation dosage for inactivation than microorganisms; therefore, a sub sterilization thermal treatment may be required to supplement radiation. The radiation tolerance of a material should be considered. The material will act as a shield, will also deter the extent of the penetration of beta and alpha rays.

Radiation Pasteurization of Food

The dose employed are considerably lower for pasteurization. Less off-flavour development. The most numerous organisms decreased, and the spoilage pattern, it is expected, altered and inhibited.

Radio pasteurization can extend the shelf life of a variety of fresh food products if certain factors are considered.

1. The initial number of microorganisms must be reasonably low.

2. The irradiated product should be maintained at a refrigeration temperature as low as possible.
3. The packaging must be the proper type
4. Recontamination after irradiation must be minimal
5. The dosage should be low enough to preserve the characteristic odor and flavour of the fresh product,

Chemical Effects of Ionizing Radiations

Capable initiating a vast array of chemical changes; gaseous, liquid and solid system. Ionizing radiation split or "radiolyze " water. Since many biological systems as well as most foods are aqueous systems, this effect on water is of key importance.

- ☆ Excited water
- ☆ Free radicals
- ☆ Ionized water molecules
- ☆ Hydrated electron
- ☆ The species then react among themselves or with other components of the system. In pure water and in the presence of air they produce in particular the following:
  - Hydrogen gas
  - Hydrogen peroxide
  - Water
  - Hydronium ion
  - Hydroxide ion

Preservation of Meat

The amount of energy absorbed by meat is expressed in rad unit. For unrefrigerated storage 4.5 megarad dose is required. Radiation Pasteurization- Use of les sterlising dose to extend shelf life.It is helpful in rendering Pork free of *Trichinella spiralis.*USFDA has regulated upto 1kGy for pork radiation. Lambert *et al.,* found that pork lion irradiated with 1kGy and packed under nitrogen has a shelf life of 26 days, which is 21 days more than stored at 5°C. Pork and poultry are the only meat approved for radiation in USA. High dosage causes undesirable chemical and physical change. Irradiation level up to 4 megarad produces characteristic of sulfur compound. Pork and chicken develop little irradiated flavour whereas beef develop strong irradiated flavour.

Significant Dates in Food Irradiation History

- ☆ 1895 – First paper published with the idea of irradiating food
- ☆ 1920 – Discovery that irradiation could be used to preserve food
- ☆ Early 1950s – "Atoms for Peace" studies performed
- ☆ 1957 – First commercial use to kill insects and insect eggs in spices in Germany

- ☆ 1963 – Approved to eliminate insect infestation for wheat and wheat flour
- ☆ 1964 – Approved to prevent sprouting in potatoes
- ☆ 1970s – NASA uses irradiated food for astronauts
- ☆ 1895 – First paper published with the idea of irradiating food
- ☆ 1920 – Discovery that irradiation could be used to preserve food
- ☆ Early 1950s – "Atoms for Peace" studies performed
- ☆ 1957 – First commercial use to kill insects and insect eggs in spices in Germany
- ☆ 1963 – Approved to eliminate insect infestation for wheat and wheat flour
- ☆ 1964 – Approved to prevent sprouting in potatoes
- ☆ 1970s – NASA uses irradiated food for astronauts

References

Lambert A D, Smith J P, Dodds K L. 1992. Physical, chemical and sensory changes in irradiated fresh pork packed in modified atmosphere. *J. Food Science* 57: 1294-9.

JOSEPHSON, *et al.*, 1978.

Blumenthal, D. 1990. *Food Irradiation: Toxic to Bacteria, Safe for Humans*; FDA Consumer.

JOSEPHSON E. S, THOMAS M. H., CALHOUN W. K. *Nutritional Aspects of Food Irradiation: An Overview*. Journal of Food Processing and Preservation. Volume 2, Issue 4, Date: September 1978, Pages: 299-313.

www.fda.gov/

Lee, P.R. 1994. Irradiation to prevent foodborne illness. J. Am. Med. Assoc. 272(4): 261.

Spoilage of Fish and its Detection Methods

Freshwater fish and salted water fish including other sea food products invariably undergoes spoilage changes by bacterial action, oxidation as well as autolysis. All fishes are rich in proteins while they are deficient in carbohydrate. Fat content of fish is rather variable depending on species. It is generally assumed that internal flesh of fish is sterile; however it undergoes very rapid decomposition due to inherent autolytic enzymes and because of less acid reaction of fish flesh that favours microbial growth. Fresh iced fish are invariably spoiled by bacteria; while salted and dried fish are more likely undergo fungal spoilage.

The spoilage of salt and freshwater fish appears to occur in essentially the same manner, with the chief differences being salt water fish contain more non-protein nitrogenous compouns like amino acids, ammonia, trimethylamine, creatine, taurine, uric acid, anserine, carnitine, carnosine and histamine. Bacteria that exist on fresh fish are generally found in three places- the outer slime, the gills, and the intestines of feeding fish. The most susceptible part of fish is the gills, so earlier sings of organoleptic spoilage may be noted by examining the gills for the presence of off-odours. If feeding fish is not eviscerated immediately, intestinal bacteria soon make their way through the intestinal walls and into the flesh of the intestinal cavity. This process is aided by the proteolytic enzymes, or enzymes of bacterial origin from the inside of the intestinal canal, or both. The skin of fish is rich in collagen and the scales are composed of scleroprotein (keratin group) which cannot be utilized by the bacteria so that these are among the last parts of fish to be decomposed.

Crustaceans differ from other fish in having about 0.5 per cent carbohydrate. Shrimp has been reported to have a higher content of free amino acids than fish and to contain cathepticlike enzymes that rapidly breakdown proteins. Crustacean muscle contains over 300 mg of nitrogen per 100g of meat, which is considerably higher than that of fish. The presence of higher quantities of free amino acids in particular and higher quantities of nitrogenous extractives in crustacean meats in general makes them quite susceptible to rapid attack by the spoilage flora. Initial spoilage of crustacean meats is accompanied by the production of large amounts of volatile base nitrogen, much as in the case with fish. Some of the volatile base nitrogen arises from the reduction of trimetylamine oxide present in crustacean shellfish. Creatine is lacking in shellfish, both crustacean and molluscan, and argining is prevalent.

Method of Quality Evaluation of Fish and Fishery Products

Quality can be judged by evaluating sensory quality, physical, chemical and microbiological quality as well as by statistical method.

1. Sensory Methods

Sensory methods denote scientific way of evaluation of fish and fish products by using human senses sight, smell, taste, touch and hearing. Sensory methods have the advantage of being simple, cheap and rapid. The spoiled fish shows opaque eye, darker gills and even with pressing with finger tips on the body of the fish makes depression and never return to their original position. However, they can be very subjective, as they are based on the assessment of individuals, their likes and dislikes. The senses of smell and taste are often used in combination, since the sense of taste is somewhat limited by itself. These senses are very powerful tolls in determining quality but require proper training and the use of proper descriptors and structured scaling.

2. Physical Methods

There is number of instruments available that quickly and easily measures the degree of spoilage of chilled fish. Some instruments are also effective in determining moisture content, properties of protein and fat, pH, texture and even electrical properties of fish. Changes in the electrical properties of the skin and underlying tissue are means of measuring the freshness in whole chilled fish. A decrease in meter reading indicates loss of freshness.

3. Chemical Methods

The chemical method of quality assessment of fish relied on the measurement of chemical constituents like water content, protein fat, ash content, salt, acidity and ammonia. A new method for determining the freshness of shrimp involves measuring the ammonia produced when shrimp is placed into a bag with water and sodium hydroxide. Several metabolites produced during storage of fish are good indicators of fish freshness. Indole production indicates the amount of decay in the product.

The measurement of TMA as a measure of freshness in marine fish, the test will not work for freshwater fish. Trimethylamine is produced from enzymatic and microbial action on the compound TMAO, and the in the increase in TMA is an indication of the progress of spoilage in the fish. The most widely used chemical test is Total volatile bases (TVB), which measures the content of trimethylamine (TMA), dimethylamine, ammonia and other basic nitrogenous compounds. The determination of TVB is much easier than TMA, and since both TMA and TVB contain nitrogen, their concentrations are represented in mg of nitrogen per 100 g of fish flesh. The upper limits of TVB compound vary greatly from 30mg/100g for frozen tuna to 100 to 200 mg for certain salted and dried fish. An analysis of hypoxanthine (Hy) also indicates spoilage in fish.

Other tests like peroxide value (PV), thiobarbituric acid (TBARS) value, nucleotide catabolites (known as the per cent K-value) also determine spoilage of fish. The K or "freshness" index gives an indication of fish freshness during the early stages after capture. Oxidative rancidity is measured by evaluating the peroxide value (PV) during the early stages when oxygen reacts with the unsaturated fats in fatty fish while the thiobarbituric acid-related substances (TBARS) is a measure of further reaction during later stages. Chemical methods are rapid, quantitative and reproducible. However, no one test is capable by itself of providing a picture of the full spectrum of changes that take place in fish and lead to its spoilage.

4. Microbiological Methods

Microbial examination of fish aims at evaluating hygienic quality of fish, including temperature abuse, and the possible presence of pathogenic microorganisms in the fish. They consist in the measurement of standard (SPC), total coliforms, various pathogens etc. They should be kept to the minimum as they are time consuming, costly and require technical skills. Several new rapid methods are being developed and marketed. They are based on immunological reactions (ELISA, monoclonal antibodies) or genetic engineering (PCR, DNA-probes).

5. Statistical Methods

Statistical methods are largely in process control that is in obtaining the correct number, size and kind of sample. The size of the sample can be determined using statistical principles which fix the number and kind of sample to be taken.

– Chapter 30 –

Cooking Methods and Preparation of Further Processed Poultry and Fish Products

I. Cooking Methods and Non-Meat Ingredients

Introduction

Meat and poultry dishes became popular with the affluent society during Moslem rule and later on during the British Raj when dishes like tikkia were created. In northern India, which covers Punjab, Kashmir, Uttar Pradesh and Delhi, meat and poultry are widely eaten and from these areas all the tandoori and moghlai dishes originate. So many meat dishes are prepared in different regions of which the most popular are described here.

Methods of Cooking Meat

Cooking

Background: meat, including poultry has been cooked or heat processed in some manner since before recorded history. The benefits of heat were probably obvious, perhaps consumers were sick less frequently with cooked as compared to raw meat due to destruction of pathogens. In addition the meat lasted longer before spoilage and the palatability was changed. Cooking can also negatively affect meat quality due to potential loss of some nutrients and potential formation of mutagenic compounds. But, marination prior to cooking may decrease mutagen levels of cooked poultry meat.

Cooking Methods

The medium used to apply heat to poultry products (air, steam, oil, or water) is one method of categorizing the different methods of cooking. The commercial processor typically utilizes in-line ovens or fryers whenever possible to maximize throughputs of products adaptable to these methods. Other products require batch processing under different conditions, such as canned items, kettle cooked whole birds and smoked or cured products. In general, for commercially processed poultry products, the in-line ovens and fryers are the preferred methods for many of the mass-processed poultry items marketed at retail and to restaurant or food service customers.

Dry heat cooking methods such as grilling produce drier product with lower yield than moist heat cooking methods such as baking. Likewise, higher heat rapid methods such as frying or searing can yield moisture product by rapidly cooking the surface and sealing in the juice. Marination is a common approach to reduce these cooking losses, thereby increasing yield and quality. The end point temperature required by law for pasteurization of poultry products labeled as fully cooked are 71°C (USDA standard for commercial cookers) or 74°C (FDA standard for retailer cooking). However, processors generally cooked to a slightly higher temperature (75 to 77°C) for a safety margin against process or product variations.

Ovens

Ovens are widely used in the industry. Ovens are usually designed as linear pass through where horizontal space in a plant is not limited, or as spiral pass through where horizontal space is limited but vertical space is available. Heat sources for these ovens are usually direct gas jets heating air inside the oven, gas jets heating air away from the product which is then transferred to the oven, or indirect heat from hot mineral oil heated externally and transferred to the oven to heat the internal air. Indirect heat sources are utilized to prevent the development of pink or red discoloration of some poultry products exposed to gases from the direct heat gas jet. Ovens may also utilized steam to cooked instead of or in addition to the previous methods of heating. Some ovens use impingement, where internal blowers force the heated air onto the product surface at high velocities. All these types of ovens have controls and sensors to monitor temperature and humidity to effectively and efficiently cook a variety of products. Products cooked under this include grilled, baked or roasted poultry items and many fried and fully cooked items are now partially cooked in a fryer but then finished in an oven in order to maximize yield.

Fryers

Commercial fryers are long vats built to contain heating frying oil, where the product passes through the oil on a continuous stainless steel conveyor belt. Heat was traditionally applied directly to the internal walls of the fryer through open flame gas jets, but safety concerns have limited its use. Nowadays, indirect heat fryers, utilizing hot mineral oil are used. Oils normally used to cooked products are food grade vegetables, typically soybean, corn, canola or blends. Oil quality is critical to good fried product quality as oil problems translate into poor appearance, flavour and odor of finished product. Fried products are usually battered and breaded items such as nuggets and patties.

Other Methods

Other cooking methods are available but are less widely used. A griddle oven has hot plates above and below product on a conveyor that can heat or cook thin items. Commercial microwave ovens are not widely used due to initial cost, potential for inconsistent heating and because of their batch mode of operation. A different method of cooking procedure utilizes an oven for a prepackaged product, in a method similar to canning, but with a flexible package. Cooked poultry is also freeze-dried to produce light and nutritious items with a long shelf life.

In general many types of cooking methods are available to produce ready to eat poultry products and a number of different methods are necessary to supply the variety of cooked products sought by consumers. Cooking generally improves the quality of the product although concerns are occasionally expressed over mutagens and loss of vitamins. The use of marination may somewhat alleviate these problems, and continuing research on cooking methods may also provide partial resolution.

- ☆ **Braising** - is a moist heat cooking method recommended for less tender cuts of meat.
  - Braising is an excellent method for cuts with high amounts of connective tissue making them succulent and tender.
  - For braising, meat is usually cut into serving-size portions rather than just cubes (as in stew).
- ☆ **Grilling and Barbecuing-**Grilling is a fast, dry method of cooking tender cuts with radiant heat directed from below or above the meat.
  - Char-grilling or barbecuing, and fan-grilling are variations on this method.
  - Beef and lamb cuts that are best for grilling are suitable for char-grilling, barbecue cookery and pan-grilling; most are also suitable for pan-frying.
- ☆ **Pan-grilling-** is another fast, dry heat method suitable for tender cuts, but the meat is cooked directly on the heated surface - usually a heavy cast-iron pan, ridged griddle pan, or on a metal hot-plate.
  - The cooking surface may be lightly greased, but minimal fat or oil is used.
- ☆ **Pot-roasting-** is the term applied to cooking larger joints or cuts in a similar way to braising.
  - It is carried out in a deep covered pot without any, or with barely any liquid.
- ☆ **Pan-frying (shallow frying)-** is a fast cooking method for small, tender cuts in a pan containing a small quantity of hot fat, oil, butter or clarified butter.
- ☆ **Roasting-** is a dry heat method that may use a small amount of fat or oil as a baste.
  - The meat is cooked in an oven or on a rotating spit over a fire, gas flame or electric grill bars.

- ☆ **Microwave cooking-** can be used for cooking or reheating meat.
- ☆ **Steaming-** is a moist heat cooking process.
  - The meat does not come into contact with the cooking liquid but instead is cooked by surrounding steam, sometimes under pressure.
  - Steaming results in tender, well flavoured, juicy meat with minimum weight loss or shrinkage.
  - Steaming under pressure is fast and easy, saves on energy and provides accurate meat portioning and cost control.
- ☆ **Simmering-** is a slow, gentle, moist method of cooking in liquid or stock, usually in a deeper pan than that used for poaching.
  - Liquid is heated to just below boiling point, approximately 95 to 99°C, higher than that used for poaching, with slightly more movement in the cooking liquid.
- ☆ **Stewing-**In stewing, meat cut into smaller pieces or cubes is cooked gently in liquid to completely cover it, and the vegetables are included.
  - A stew can be simmered in a pot on the stove top or cooked in a covered casserole in the oven.
  - Stewing is suitable for the least tender cuts of meat that become tender and juicy with the slow moist heat method.
- ☆ **Poaching-** is a very gentle, moist heat method of cooking using a minimum amount of reduced liquid or stock that is kept at just below simmering point, approximately between 90 to 94°C.
  - Poaching temperatures are lower than those used for simmering, and poaching times are shorter.
  - Tender cuts with lower amounts of connective tissue are best, for poaching.

Non-Meat Ingredients

Categories of non meat ingredients- Can be categorized by source

- ☆ Chemical substances
- ☆ Plant origin
- ☆ Animal origin

The functional properties of non-meat ingredients include their impact on:

- ☆ Taste
- ☆ Flavour
- ☆ Appearance
- ☆ Colour
- ☆ Texture
- ☆ Water binding

- Counteracting fat separation
- Preservation

Most substances have double or even multiple effects. Therefore, in order to provide an overview of the most common substances used as non-meat ingredients, they are listed below according to their origin, namely *chemical, animal,* or *plant origin*

a) Chemical Substances Used as Ingredients

There are various chemical substances approved for the different kinds of food processing, but in the specific case of **meat processing** the number of approved chemical substances is rather limited in most countries. The following are of significance:

- *Salt* (for taste, impact on meat proteins, shelf-life)
- *Nitrite* (for curing colour, flavour, shelf-life)
- *Ascorbic acid* (to accelerate curing reaction)
- *Phosphates* (for protein structuring and water binding)
- *Chemical preservatives* (for shelf-life)
- *Antioxidants* (for flavour and shelf-life)
- *Monosodium glutamate MSG* (for enhancement of flavour)
- *Food colouring substances* (synthetic and of plant origin)

b) Non-meat Ingredients of Animal Origin

Ingredients of animal origin are not commonly applied but may be useful for specific meat preparations. They all have functional properties (except whole milk), in particular improvement of water binding and prevention of fat separation during heat treatment. Apart from their functional properties, some of them can also be considered meat extenders, as mentioned below.

- *Milk caseinate* (90 per cent protein; used in small quantities (2 per cent); have functional water and fat binding properties)
- *Whole milk* or *non-fat dried milk* (=skim milk) (sometimes used in indigenous meat preparations as a protein extender)
- *Gelatine* (binding properties and meat extender)
- *Blood plasma* (predominantly binding properties)
- *Eggs* (extender and binding ingredient for meat pieces and fried sausages)
- *Transglutaminase* (exclusively binding properties)

c) Ingredients of Plant Origin

The most commonly used substances are:

- *Isolated soy protein* (90 per cent protein) and
- *Wheat gluten* (80 per cent protein) and, less importantly, protein isolates from other legumes.

- A third group of ingredients of plant origin are used as *meat extenders* (if rich in proteins) or *fillers* (if rich in carbohydrates) for meat product and sausage formulations. The purpose is to replace expensive meat for lower- or medium-grade products by cheaper ingredients of plant origin for cost reduction and volume increase.

Meat extenders/Plant products with high protein content are

- ***Soy flour*** (50 per cent protein)
- ***Soy concentrate*** (70 per cent protein)
- Other food legumes (***beans, peas, lentils***), used for special products only.
- *Cereal flours* from wheat, rice and corn
- *Starches* from wheat, rice, corn, potato and cassava
- *Breadcrumbs*
- *Rusk* (derived by mixing and baking wheat flour)
- **Cereals** to be added without milling, *e.g.* rice, corn
- *Roots* and *tubers, e.g.* cassava, sweet potato
- *Vegetable* and *fruits, e.g.* onions, bell pepper, carrots, green vegetables, bananas
- *Polysaccharides* (Hydrocolloids):
    - *Carrageenan:* It is the only hydrocolloid product of this group popular in meat processing, added in quantities of max. 1 per cent, improves sliceability and cohesiveness). The substance can be considered both *binder* and *filler*.

Important Non-Meat Ingredients in Meat Processing and their Properties

Key characteristics of non-meat ingredients used in the meat industries are provided below for guidance. They are listed by highlighting some of the most commonly used substances first with the rest roughly grouped in the order of frequency of use on meat processing.

Common Salt (Sodium Chloride)

Levels used: 1.5 – 3.0 per cent

Salt is the main agent used in meat processing and it contributes to basic taste characteristics of the final product. In processed meat products it usually ranges from 1.5 to 2.2 per cent. Apart from improving the taste, salt in combination with water assists in opening up the structure of proteins (solubilises myofibrillar proteins). These proteins gel upon heating and by entrapping moisture and fats give form, structure and firmness to the finished product. Salt used at the above levels also improves the water holding capacity of meat.

Seasonings (Spices)

Seasonings are indispensable for the manufacture of processed meat products.

Water

Water is the main component of meat (up to 80 per cent in lean meat).

Therefore typically all meat products contain lower or higher amounts of "natural" water. Besides its "natural" presence, water is used in many processed meat products also as an ingredient. However, the assumption by some consumers that water is added to meat products only to increase product weight and manufacturers' profits is incorrect. In fact, there are many types of meat products where the addition of water is needed *for technical reasons* or to *compensate for cooking losses.* The addition of water is essential during the manufacture of raw-cooked meat batters (meat loaves, frankfurter sausages etc). In this case, water acts together with salt and phosphates to solubilize muscle proteins, thus creating a strong protein network structure holding the product together after heat-treatment. In the case of precooked-cooked meat mixes, water is added to compensate for the cooking loss, as precooking of raw meat materials generates cooking losses of approximately 30 per cent. In order not to make the final products too dry, water losses are supplemented in the final meat mix. Care must be taken that no excess water is added, as this could lead to fat and jelly separation in the final product. Water is also needed as a *substrate* for curing substances or other non meat ingredients and for *re-hydration* of meat extenders. For cured cooked products, solutions of curing salt, which may also contain spices, phosphates and other ingredients, are injected into larger meat pieces for quick and equal distribution. In these cases the volume of the product will be increased by the injection of the curing brine, but will be reduced again during subsequent cooking. Technologies such as tumbling in combination with addition of phosphates and other substances make it possible to increase the yield further. Ideally, cooking losses are equivalent to the water previously injected. However, in the specific cases of cheaper cured-cooked reconstituted ham, tumbling in combination with addition of phosphates and binders can make it possible to retain higher amounts of water in the product.

Sodium Nitrite

Levels used: 0.01 – 0.03 per cent

The addition of relatively small quantities of sodium nitrite produces the development of the desired colour "pickling red" in processed meat products. Without nitrite meat products turn grey in colour when heated. Of special importance for canned meat products is the potential of nitrite to inhibit microbial growth. Furthermore, it retards the oxidative rancidity by stabilizing fats. The common commercial form of nitrite is ***"nitrite curing salt"*** or "pickling salt", a mixture of 0.5 - 0.6 per cent nitrite and 99.4 - 99.5 per cent sodium chloride.

Ascorbic Acid, Sodium Ascorbate, Erythorbate

Level used: 0.03 per cent

Ascorbic acid is perhaps better known as vitamin C. Its more stable salt form is sodium ascorbate or the chemically equivalent but cheaper sodium erythorbate. These so-called ***"cure accelerators"*** are used in curing-salt for processed meats because of their reducing properties.

These substances accelerate the reaction of nitrite with the red muscle pigments resulting in the development of the red curing colour. Meat products to be heat-treated during manufacture instantly develop a uniform red colour, which can be intensified in the presence of cure accelerators.

Phosphates

Levels used: 0.05 – 0.5 per cent

Phosphates have a wide application in the meat processing industry and improve binding and texture in processed meat products. They directly *increase the water-holding capacity* by raising the pH as their own pH is alkaline (above 7.0). Phosphates also stabilize the texture of meat products by *increasing protein solubility* in connection with salt and *reduce lipid oxidation/rancidity* and hence the occurrence of negative flavours. Phosphates have also shown the ability to *reduce microbial growth*. The most common phosphates used in meat processing are:

Sodium tri-poly-phosphate STPP (pH 9.8)

Sodium di-phosphate SDP (pH 7.3)

Milk Protein

Similar to isolated soy protein, **milk protein** (milk caseinate) has the ability to interact with meat proteins or complement deficits in meat protein available in extended meat mixes. Due to the small amount required (2 per cent) and its relatively high price, milk protein is primarily not a meat extender for volume increase but a functional ***binder*** to increase water holding and fat binding and reduce cooking losses.

Gelatine

Gelatine is an edible jelly composed of collagen proteins extracted from animal tissues (mainly skins, also bones) through boiling. Commercially available gelatine is a dry powder of various granule sizes, which is first dispersed in cold water and then completely solubilized in water of 50-60°C. The protein molecules of the gelatine absorb water and form a gel when cooling down. If meat pieces are mixed with the liquid gelatine, the cohesive properties, which are gradually strengthened with lowering the temperature, result in a solid, elastic and sliceable product.

Blood Proteins

Blood is not used everywhere for human food. Where its consumption is accepted, a great variety of meat products is possible, where whole blood is one of the major components. If the solid parts (blood cells) are separated from the blood, the liquid fraction called blood plasma remains, which is rich in protein (8- 9 per cent). Such a protein solution can play a valuable role in meat processing. In many locations, specialized enterprises produce blood plasma by centrifugation of hygienically obtained blood in slaughterhouses immediately after slaughter. Due to its hygienically sensitive nature, the blood plasma is best frozen or freeze-dried immediately after centrifugation. Flakes of ***plasma ice*** are the ideal form for further processing in meat products. This form of plasma is particularly suitable for ***raw-cooked meat products*** (frankfurter, hot dog, meat loaves etc.).

Carrageenan

Carrageenan is a hydrocolloid (often known as "gum") derived from aquatic plants (seaweed). Carrageenan is available as a refined powder, which is water soluble and has strong *water-binding and gelling* properties. Upon cooling it forms an elastic gel which remains stable during refrigerated storage. Carrageenan, needed only in small quantities of up to 1 per cent and added as a dry powder, can provide improved cooking yield and better sliceability and cohesiveness.

Transglutaminase

This is an enzyme needed in living animal organisms to repair lesions of body tissues and create stable structures by extensively cross-linking protein molecules. The recently introduced synthetic form of this substance develops similar effects in meat. It has the capacity to *form bonds* between superficial protein structures of individual smaller or larger muscle meat pieces. This effect can be used in various meat processing phases, from tumbling and reconstituting cooked hams to creating protein network structures in raw-cooked meat products. The substance is expected to have an impact on specific meat processing technologies, for example, tumbling procedures could be considerably shortened or the utilization of phosphates and other binding substances in raw-cooked or cured-cooked products reduced or completely substituted.

Vegetable Oil

Vegetable oil can be used to ***replace animal fat***, particularly in pork. Vegetable oil can be considered a meat extender as it replaces part of the animal tissue. It also assumes the function of the animal fat to make the meat mix soft and juicy after heat treatment. Thus the oil has also functional properties. Vegetable oil is added in the same way as animal fat to comminuted meat batters. It is important that the oil be cooled down (+1°C) before adding in order to keep the temperature of the meat mixes low. Best results can be achieved with vegetable oils displaying a pasty structure at this temperature.

Sugars

Levels used: 0.5 - 4.0 per cent

Sugars (sucrose, dextrose or corn syrup) may be added to meat products to provide specific flavour and counteract salty taste, *lower the* a_w *value*, which may be important for dried and canned products, and act in dry fermented sausages and raw hams as a nutrient source for microbes, which convert sugars into organic acids (lactic, acetic) resulting in souring.

Flavour Enhancer

They are intended to intensify flavour characteristics in specific meat preparations. Food proteins such as soy, milk or blood proteins or yeast extracts are partially hydrolyzed, *i.e.* broken down to simpler components (mainly peptides) which may have meat flavour or the property to strengthen meat flavours. One well known substance to strengthen meat flavour is monosodium glutamate (MSG). It is particularly popular in Asia where it is widely used in most meat dishes but also in many processed meat products (0.5 per cent or higher).

Food Colourings

Changing the colour of fresh and processed meats by means of food colourings is *not* common practice. Colourings may be derived from *natural sources* (*e.g.* orange yellow beta-carotene from green plants, red oleoresin from paprika, red colour from red beet juice). Others are made *synthetically* (also beta carotene derives now mainly from synthetic sources). Many of them are restricted for use only in particular food products.

II. Traditional Indian Poultry Products

Some of the common traditional poultry products are tandoori chicken, chicken sheek kabab, chicken curry, chicken kofta, chicken tikka, chicken samosa etc. other products like barbeque, chicken patties, chicken sausages etc also have a good market in urban areas.

1. Tandoori Chicken

Ingredients

1. 8 no: Large Chicken pieces
2. 11/4 cup: Yogurt
3. 2 tbs: Lime Juice
4. ½ quantity: Chopped Onion
5. 3-4: Dried Red Chillies
6. 2 tsp: Coriander Seeds
7. 2 cloves
8. Crushed Garlic
9. 1" piece: Grated Ginger
10. 1-2: Clove
11. 2 tsp: Garam Masala
12. 2 tsp: Chilli powder
13. Salt to taste

Method

Make slits in the flesh of the chicken pieces and rub lime juice and salt over them. Keep aside for half an hour.

Grind dried chillies, coriander seeds, ginger, garlic and clove together. Mix the paste with garam masala and chilli powder.

Heat a pan and sauté the masala. Add onions and fry. Pour yogurt and stir well. Remove the pan from fire.

Arrange chicken pieces in a dish and pour over the yogurt mixture. Refrigerate the marinade overnight or at least for 4-6 hours.

Arrange the chicken on a broiler tray cook it in a pre-heated oven for 20-30 minutes or brush oil over the chicken pieces and cook in a gas stove turning over till both sides are done.

Keep pouring oil and masala over the chicken pieces in between.

2. Chicken Barbeque

Ingredients

1. 4 seeded and sliced Red chili (Lal Mirchi)
2. 2 chopped Garlic cloves (Lasun)
3. 5 small Onion (Pyaj)
4. 2 tsp crushed Brown Sugar (Cheeni)
5. 1/2 cup Coconut Cream (Nariyal Malai)
6. 2 tsp Fish Sauce
7. 1 tblsp Tamarind Water (Imli Ka Pani)
8. 4 boneless Chicken Breast
9. As required Basil Leaves (Tulsi)
10. As required Coriander Leaves (Dhania Patta)
11. As required Salt (Namak)

Method

1. Grind chilies, garlic and onion to make a paste like mixture.
2. Combine sugar, coconut cream, fish sauce, tamarind water and salt.
3. Stir continuously.
4. Make cut 4 slashes in chicken breast.
5. Place chicken in a shallow dish.
6. Pour over spice mixture.
7. Turn to coat.
8. Cover dish.
9. Place it aside for 1 hour.
10. Place chicken on a piece of foil.
11. Grill chicken for about 4 minutes a side.
12. Bast occasionally till cooked thoroughly.
13. Garnish with basil or coriander leaves.

3. Chicken Seekh Kababs

- ✰ Culled or spent chicken meat can be utilized for making kababs.
- ✰ Lean meat is minced through 8mm plate of meat grinder.
- ✰ Wheat flour (3 per cent) and whole egg liquid(5 per cent) should be incorporated as binders to provide sufficient strength to the mince.
- ✰ Fat, salt and dry spices are added as per consumers preference.
- ✰ The mince is pasted around specially made iron bars(seekh) and cooked over moderate and uniform heat.
- ✰ Turning and basting with vegetable oil from time to time is done till doneness with brown colour is achieved.

4. Chicken Shami Kababs

- ✰ In preparation of shami kababs, meat chunks and water soaked black gram dal simmered in water for nearly 15 minutes before grinding.
- ✰ It is seasoned with salt, dry spices and condiment paste
- ✰ Egg liquid can also be added to the mince.
- ✰ It is made into round cakes which are then shallow fried with edible oil on a girdle till both sides are brown.

5. Chicken Kofta

Ingredients for Kofta

1. 2 pound chicken
2. 1 tbsp. turmeric paste or powder
3. 4 green chili - chopped
4. 11/2 tbsp. garlic paste or powder
5. ½ tbsp. garam masala paste
6. Ginger 1" – grated
7. 1 cup chopped onion
8. Chopped cilantro
9. Ghee or oil
10. Salt to taste

Ingredients for Gravy

1. 1 spoon turmeric paste or powder
2. ½ spoon red chilli paste or powder
3. 11/2 spoon garlic paste or powder
4. 11/2 spoon coriander paste or powder
5. ½ garam masala paste or powder
6. ½ spoon ginger paste or powder

7. 1 cup chopped onion
8. Bay Leaves – 3
9. Dry red chili - 2
10. Ghee or oil

Procedure

1. Boil the chicken in a pressure cooker half-filled with water for about half an hour.
2. De-bone the chicken once cooled off and then mash it nicely.
3. Add chopped cilantro, grated ginger, garlic paste, turmeric paste, garam masala and salt to the mashed
4. Chicken and knead them with fingers for about 10 minutes or until smooth.
5. Make small balls of the mashed chicken meat and deep fry them on ghee or cooking oil on medium to low heat until golden brown.
6. Drain excess oil and set aside.
7. Fry chopped onion in cooking oil or ghee in a frying pan until golden brown. Add ginger paste, garlic paste, turmeric paste, red chili paste, coriander paste, bay leaves, dry red chili to the oil and fry it for another 2-3 minutes.
8. Add two cups of water and bring it to a boil, turn down the heat, add the chicken balls in the gravy, cover and simmer for five minutes.
9. Serve garnished with cilantro leaves.
10. Serve with hot roti, paratha, nan

6. Poultry Pickle

- ☆ Dressed chicken is trimmed off excess fat and deboned.
- ☆ Now meat is cut into 2.5cm cubes,applied with 2 per cent salt and pressure cooked for 8 to 10 minutes.
- ☆ Cooked meat is taken out and fried at medium heat in mustard oil to get brown colour.
- ☆ Oil is decanted from the fried cubes and green curry stuff is fried in the same oil to get golden brown colour.
- ☆ Then it is followed by addition of dry spices,remaining 2 per cent salt and fried meat continuing frying for another 3-4minutes.
- ☆ After some cooling it is mixed with 10 per cent vinegar.
- ☆ The product has a shelf life of 100 days at an ambient temperature without any appreciable loss of quality attributes.

Formulation

Ingredients	*Quantity*
Lean meat	1 kg
Salt	40g
Spice mix	30g
Green curry stuff (onion, ginger and garlic paste)	50g
Citric acid (0.4 per cent)	5ml
Vinegar	100ml
Mustard oil	500g

Precautions

1. Handle the meat with thoroughly washed and cleaned hands.
2. Fry the green curry carefully so that they are not burnt.
3. Pack the pickle after cooling.
4. Always ensure the covering of contents in preheated and cooled mustard oil.

7. Chicken Samosa

- ☆ Lean chicken is minced through 5mm plate of a meat grinder.
- ☆ Condiments are fried in vegetable oil to get a golden brown and dry spices along with salt are added towards the end.
- ☆ Minced meat and cooked mashed potatoes are mixed with the fried spices and heating is continued for another 4-6minutes.
- ☆ The fried stuff is ready for filling.
- ☆ Dough portion of about 30g rolled out and divided into two halves.
- ☆ Each half is moulded into a triangular pouch and the fried stuff (20-25g) is filled in.
- ☆ The pouch is closed and samosas are deep fried in vegetable oil at medium heat to obtain a crispy product.

8. Chicken Sausage

The though meat from spent hens can be utilized for the preparation of chicken sausages. Deboned chicken meat is minced once through 9mm and then through 4mm plate of a meat grinder. Fat is minced separately through 4mm plate. Lean meat, ice flakes(10), salt and sodium nitrite are run along with fat in a bowl chopper to prepare a fine emulsion. Other ingredients like spices, condiments etc. are added in the final run for a min. meat emulsion is fill into casings with the help of a sausage filler and suitable links are made. The sausages may be cooked in water at 80°C for 15 to 20 min or steam cooked. Smoking along with cooking stabilizes the colour and imparts a characteristics flavour to the product.

9. Chicken Patties

Raw deboned chicken meat and fat are minced twice through a meat grinder. Other ingredients like wheat flour or texturised soy protein, salt, condiments, spices etc. are mixed to the ground meat in an electrically operated meat mixer. The blended mass is divided into 100g portions and moulded into patties. These are broiled in hot air oven at 180°C for 15 min and then turned upside down and again cooked for another 10 min to get a core temperature of about 72 °C. Hot patties may be used to prepare burgers or chilled in a refrigerator for later use.

10. Chicken Tikka

Dedoned chicken is minced in a meat grinder. Forty percent of the mince is pressure cooked for 2 min. Besides, peeled and shredded potatoes are partially cooked separately in boiling water. Minced meat (60 raw:40 cooked), shredded potatoes, rice powder, bread crumbs, salt, spices and condiments are thoroughly mixed in an electrically operated meat mixer. The blended mass is divided into 70g portions and moulded into tikkas. These are shallow fat fried in a girdle to achieve an internal temp of 70 °C. The product has a unique texture and is consumed as a hot snack.

11. Chicken Loaf

Chicken loaf is produced worldwide and there are a huge variety of products sold under this name. A high quality chicken loaf is made from chicken breast meat at 30-50 per cent. Extension and the finished product product is white in clour. Commonly no nitrite is added to such white products. The breast meat is minced with 20mm blade so that large pieces of meat are visible in the finished product. Amount and type of additives vary greatly but in most cases phosphate carrageenam and some starch is used. Proteins are not normally added in this extension unless food laws dictate a certain level of protein in the finished product. Phosphates and carrageen are added at the rate of 4-5 g and 2-5 g per kg of total mass depending on the desired level of extension. Products that extended around 50 per. Require 10-30g of starch per kg of total mass to prevent water separation if a waterproof casing is used. Starch and whey protein protein lighten the colour of the product and whey protein complements the flavour of chicken meat as well. High quality chicken loaf is also sometimes tumbled instead of being mixed. Tumbling lasts for around 3000-5000 rev. depending on level of extension and type of baffles inside the tumbler. Waterproof casings are most common, but fibrous casings can also be used for chicken loaf. Products in waterproof casings are cooked with steam or in hot water bath at 76-80°C until tem of 70-72 °C is reached. Fibrous casings may have a layer of smoke on the inside. Products in fibrous casings are dried at 60-65 °C for 30-60 minutes, smoked at 65-70 °C until the desired smoke colour is obtained and finally cooked in steam or a water bath at 76-80 °C. Drying and smoking add a distinctive appearance and taste to chicken loaf.

An economy chicken loaf typically uses chicken MDM, chicken emulsion and some thigh or breast meat as the raw material. In extreme cases the chicken loaf is made predominantly from chicken MDM and chicken skin emulsion and hardly any real meat is used. Amount and type of additives used for economy chicken vary greatly and many different combinations are possible. In general the amount of salt is 16-20 g per kg of finished product, soy protein 20-40 g and starch 40-120 g per kg of finished product. Nitrite is occassionally introduced in economy chicken products. The processing technology for economy chicken loaf is different from higher quality chicken loaf in that sometimes the MDM, chicken skin emulsion and around 30 per cent of the total brine are mixed together in a bowl cutter at slow knife speed to eliminate all possible lumps of MDM and skin emulsion. This slurry is then added to the mixer with the other minced meat and remaining brine and mixed. Mixture is then filled in waterproof casings and cooked at 76-80°C. In extreme cases all the raw materials are placed in the bowl cutter and all the brine is added at a slow knife speed. Once all the brine is added and the desired degree of comminution reached, the total mass is removed and placed in a mixer. Mixing takes place under vacuum and is followed by filling, cooking, cooling and packing.

12. Chicken Sausage with Oil

Chicken sausages such as hot dogs or frankfurters are commonly made from a mixture of chicken thigh and breast meat. If a white non cured product is desired, then most of the meat used must be chicken breast, which adds considerable cost. Cured sausages, where a pink red curing colour is desired, can contain thigh meat and some MDM meat besides breast meat. Low cost products are produced with thigh and MDM meat only.

Processing

The technology of working with oil is very similar to the lean meat method. Lean meat is cut at a medium speed with additives (phosphates, salt, nitrite and spices) and around 70 per cent of the total water and ice. The temperature drops to around 0°C when the water and ice is added and the knife speed is switched to fast. When the temp has risen to around 4-6°C, the remaining 30 per cent of water and ice is added, bringing the tem back to 0°C. After cutting at a fast speed for a short while and once the temp starts to rise again, the chilled oil is added gradually while cutting continues. The oil is not added all at once because the solubilized protein has to act on a very large surface area to emulsify the oil and this takes time. Adding the oil gradually to the activated protein ensures that it is emulsified properly. The oil should be added at such a speed that all the oil has been added by the time that the tem of the sausage reaches around 3-5°C. Starch or other fillers are added (if applied) once the added oil is fully emulsified which is visible at around 6-10°C. During emulsification of the oil, the sausage mass changes visibly from being sloppy and darkish into a firm and light coloured mass. It is essential that chilled oil around 1-4 dc, is used in the process to keep the temperature down and to allow the oil to be effectively worked into the sausage mass. The emulsion is usually filled into collagen casings of around 22-26 mm dm. after filing the product is steamed at 76-80°C until a core temp of 70°C is reached; it is then showered, cooled in a blast chiller, placed in a chiller and vacuum packed. Occasionally the filled product is smoked prior to moist heat treatment or smoked flavour is added to the emulsion to obtain a frankfurter type product.

13. Meat Balls

Ingredients	*Percentage*
Meat	75 per cent
Water	10 per cent
Additives	10 per cent (phosphates, salt and spices)
Starch	5 per cent

Meat balls are eaten in soup, in sauce and as part of many rice and noodle dishes, particularly in Asia. The quality, size and flavour of meatballs vary greatly according to local eating habits. Meatballs can be made from beef, pork or chicken. High quality meatballs use 85 per cent CL grade meat and contain around 70-75 per cent meat, 10-15 per cent water and ice and around 10 per cent powdered additives such as phosphates, salt and spices together with 6-10 per cent starch. The combination of a fairly high meat content, a moderate amount of added water and high levels of starch results in a spongy-firm product, which is most often desired. Low quality meat balls contain less meat, more water and fat and often additives such as soy protein to increase the firmness and sponginess. The fine emulsion is usually made using the all in method and balls of different sizes are formed from the fine emulsion and dropped into containers of hot water at 80-90°C. Meatballs are cooked in hot water and then either sold directly to consumers on the same day at wet markets (daily markets) without being packed, or they are cooled, vacuum packed and sold under refrigeration in shops. Meatballs that are not packed are occasionally dipped into a solution containing benzoate or sorbate, which coats the surface and acts as a preservative.

14. Nihari

- ☆ This meat dish is very much popular in Delhi.
- ☆ In its preparation meat is deep fried and then mix salt, chili powder, turmeric, coriander powder, pepper and ginger paste.
- ☆ Then add a little water and some flour and heat to boil this mixture.
- ☆ Add spice mix and 3-4 cups water then cove to tenderize it.
- ☆ It will take about 5 - 6 hours for chicken and more if using beef.
- ☆ Fry some onion slices in oil until golden brown. Garnish the Nihari with it.
- ☆ Fresh coriander, ginger and green chilies can also be used for garnishing.

Conclusion

The list of convenience meat products is on the increase. These ready to eat products have a bright scope in India. These have already become quite common at the fast food corners and restaurants in the urban areas. With the vast availability of different meat animals comminuted meat are likely to surpass other food products.

References

1. Alan R. Sams (2001). Poultry Meat Processing, Department of poultry Science, Texas A and M university.
2. Gerhard Fischer (2006). Meat Products Handbook (Practical Science and Technology).
3. Shai Barbut (2001). Poultry Products Processing: An Industry Guide.
4. Sharma B.D. (1999). Jaypee brothers medical publishers, Meat and Meat Products Technology(Including Poultry Products Technology),Indian meat industry,PP.1-7,Processing of some convenience poultry products, pp. 111-115.
5. Susan E. Gebhardt and Robin G. Thomas (2002). Nutritive Value of Foods, USDA, Agricultural Research Service Home and Garden Bulletin Number 72.
6. Internet source (Indian chicken recipe.com, surf India.com, Patna daily.com)
7. www.nopr.niscair.res.in/bitstream
8. http://www.indobase.com/recipes
9. http://www.bestgoadeals.com

III. Processing Technology of Some Major Poultry Products

Introduction

Poultry meat is consumed all over the world and over the last few decades has increased in popularity in many countries. Among the reasons for this increased consumption are the relatively low costs of production, the rapid growth rate of poultry, the high nutritional value of the meat and the introduction of many new further processed products. Overall the poultry industry has changed dramatically over the past 50 years. Today the poultry industry is highly integrated and managed by a number of large corporations. The internet and e-commerce are starting to play a major role in marketing. For eg. In the summer of 2000 some of the major North American meat processors created on-line business of business marketing for poultry meat. Within the last couple of decades, many new processed poultry products have been introduced in the market. The poultry industry has taken the initiative to develop fresh, marinated and fully cooked products and has adopted some red meat recipes. All have helped to increase consumption and move away from seasonal demand. In the past items such as whole turkeys were primarily sold in north America prior to thanksgiving and Christmas. Such a pattern significantly limited the increase in sales of poultry meat. After the industry realizes this limitations and started to market smaller cut up portions and further processed products, the situation improved. In the beginning red meat recipes were modified to manufacture poultry products eg. Frankfurters and later new technologies were developed exclusively for poultry eg. Chicken nuggets. Overall the poultry industry successfully responded to consumer demand for more convenient food items including semi and fully prepared items. Today consumers can choose meat products from a wide variety consisting of a few hundred different different products to assist the consumer, various systems have been suggested for classifying meat products.

One of the most common ways to classify products is to group them into six categories:

- ☆ Fresh *e.g.* Fresh poultry breakfast sausage
- ☆ Uncooked and smoked *e.g.* Italian sausage
- ☆ Smoked and cooked *e.g.* Bologna and Frankfurters
- ☆ Pre-Cooked eg. Liver sausage and blood sausage
- ☆ Dry/semi dry or fermented *e.g.* Dry salami
- ☆ Cooked meat specialities *e.g.* Luncheon meat and loaves

In addition, the development of new technologies represent two additional categories:

- ☆ Restructured meat products, such as cutlets, where small bits and pieces of meat are made into a whole muscle fillet- like product by using freezing, high pressure and hydrocolloid gums.
- ☆ Surimi like products, such as special chicken rolls where minced meat is washed to remove pigments and enzymes and extruded to obtain a fiber muscle like texture.

Examples of Major Processed Poultry Products

Products	*Comments*
Smoked turkey breast	Whole muscle or restructured
Poultry roll	White and dark meat
Turkey ham	Cured dark meat
Summer sausage	Fermented product
Poultry frankfurter	Fine emulsion in small diameter casings
Poultry bologna	Fine emulsion in small diameter casings
Poultry patties	Hamburger type not cured
Breakfast sausage	Ground product, sold fresh or frozen
Chicken nuggets	Whole muscle or restructured
Fried chicken	Battered and breaded (uncooked or precooked)
Roasted, barbecued chicken	Prepared with dry heat, crisp skin
Jellied chicken loaf	Cooked meat held in a gelatin matrix
Turkey bacon	Layers of light and dark meat

1. Flavoured Turkey Roast (30 per cent pump)

Ingredients

Meat: 100.0 kg boneless, skinless turkey breast

Brine: 30.0 kg

The brine is made by mixing:

21.8 kg cold water

3.8 kg ice flakes

4.0 kg brine and cure unit (salt, sugar, phosphate, erythorbate, nitrite)

0.4 kg roast seasonings (natural roast flavour, spices)

Spice rub: 6 g roast-flavoured rub mixed with 18 ml of water, per 1 kg of umbled roast.

Processing

Inject the turkey breast meat with 30 per cent brine. Tumble (preferentially under vacuum) for 4 hours at 12 - 15 rpm; start immediately after injecting. Rest overnight and tumble for 1 - 2 hours at 12 - 15 rpm. Combine two turkey breasts (thick end over thin end) and wrap with collagen film before stuffing into a ham net #22 - 3 (*i.e.*, a net with 22 squares around the circumference, made up of three stitches between squares). Clip both ends of the net. Mix five parts of roast-flavoured rub together with three parts of water until a thick paste has been formed, and rub the roasts evenly. Place roasts on smoke screens, place in an oven and cook. Dry cook at 90°C for 1 hour or until the surface is completely dry. Steam cook at 78°C to an internal temperature of 71°C. Shower with cold water to cool down quickly.

2. Smoked Turkey Breast

Ingredients

Turkey breast

Brine solution (water, salt, spices and sometimes gums)

Whey proteins

Lactate

Hydrocolloid gums

Processing

Smoked turkey breast is a premium product produced either whole breast muscle or its portions. A brine solution (*i.e.* Water, salt, spices and sometimes gums) is added to the muscle often by direct injections, prior to smoking and cooking. The meat is massaged or tumbled after brine injection to assist in moisture absorbing and achieving an even distribution of the non meat ingredients within the muscle. The latter is important in the processing of any meat product, as an uneven distribution of salt etc can cause serious flavour, colour and textural problems. Hydrocolloid gums such as carrageenans are often added to assist in holding the injected brine that can reach 30-50 percent. Non meat proteins *e.g.* whey proteins can also be added for the same purpose. Additives such as lactate are sometimes added for preservation. The breast muscle is then stuffed into a netting (the muscle can be covered with skin), smoked and cooked in a smoke house until an internal temperature of at least 70°C is reached.

3. Turkey Ham

Turkey ham is typically manufactured from turkey thigh meat. The product is usually linear than the traditional pork ham. In the initial manufacturing step, a brine solution (water, salt, phosphates, flavourings and nitrite) is added either by injection or marination of small meat pieces. Tumbling is commonly used when when brine is used as a marinating solution to help achieve maximum absorbtion, even distribution of curing ingredients and extraction of salt soluble proteins to the surface, which is important for binding the muscle chunks together during later heating. Meat is then stuffed into fibrous casings that determine the shape of the final product and size. The ham is smoked or smoke flavourings are added to the raw batter and cooked to at least 68°C.

4. Summer Sausage

It represents a group of fermented meat products where commonly a lactic acid bacteria culture is added. The product can be made from dark poultry meat, skin and fat, but usually some pork meat and fat are included. Lactic Acid Bacteria lowers the pH of the product from 5.7 to 4.8 and also to add unique flavour. Industry mainly uses commercial starter cultures with a known composition of microorganisms (mainly LAB). Recently a lot of progress has been made in the field of starter cultures, mainly through the use of genetic engineering. The use of a starter culture is highly recommended because it ensures that LAB dominates the fermentation, suppresses pathogens and produces the desired flavours. After the fermentation, the product is either smoked, cooked or only dried. The dry product is usually shelf stable due to its low pH and low water activity.

5. Frankfurters and Bologna

They are examples of finely comminuted meat products that have homogenous appearances. Leg meat, trimmings, skin and mechanically deboned meat are usually used as raw materials. When lean leg meat is used, fat and skin are added. Meat is finely chopped in a bowl chopper or an emulsion mill that efficiently chops the meat particles and emulsifies the meat. Salt is added to extract the meat proteins. Nitrite is added to inhibit *Clostridium botulinum* growth and provide the typical cured meat colour. The meat batter is then stuffed into cellulose casings, smoked and cooked in a smokehouse. Low microbial contamination and refrigerated temperatures are important in prolonging the shelf life, where some manufacturers guarantee a shelf life of 50 days.

6. Chicken Hot Dogs/Bologna

Ingredients

Meat: 86.0 kg mechanically deboned chicken meat

Ice: 14.0 kg

Spices and Additives Binder unit 8.70 kg (salt, soy/whey proteins, spices, erythorbate)

Curing salt 0.3 kg

Phosphate 0.3 kg

Processing

Chop the slightly frozen meat with about 5 kg of flaked ice in a bowl chopper for a few revolutions. Add the binder unit, salt and phosphate and chop at the high speed setting while adding the rest of the ice until the temperature reaches 8–10°C. Remove the batter from the chopper. Stuff into easy-peel hot dog casings and link to desired size. Place the product on a smokehouse tree.

Smoke and Cook

Dry cook for 5 minutes or as required at 55°C. Hot smoke at 55°C and 25 per cent relative humidity for 20–30 minutes. Steam cook at 75°C to an internal temperature of 71°C. Shower with cold water for 10 minutes. Refrigerate overnight prior to peeling the casings.

Note: for bologna, use the same formulation and procedure, and then stuff into large-diameter cellulose or fibrous casings. The heat process should be lengthened to achieve a 71°C internal temperature.

7. Chicken Nuggets

Chicken nuggets are one of the most successful poultry products introduced in the 1980's. originally the product was prepared from a single piece of slightly marinated breast meat that was battered and breaded. Later nuggets made from trimmings, dark meat, skin, mechanically deboned meat and their combinations started to appear in the market. The product is usually prepared by marinating and mixing the meat pieces with a brine solution (water, salt and flavourings) until all the solution is absorbed. The meat is then put through a forming machine that creates the product's desired shape (square or oval), followed by battering, breading and deep fat frying. Frying is done to preserve the product shape, assure breading adherence and to provide the typical crispy texture of the breading.

8. Jellied Turkey Roll

Ingredients

Meat: 45 kg white turkey roast (see White Turkey Roast recipe)

Vegetables: 15 kg broccoli heads and/or canned mushrooms

Gelatin: 40 kg gelatin solution (7 kg seasoned gelatin powder plus water)

Processing

Dice the turkey roast into 1 x 1 x 1 cm cubes. Rinse the broccoli (and/or mushrooms) with hot water and mix with the diced meat. Completely dissolve the dry gelatin powder in hot water (80°C). You can add a little bit of oil to the hot water to avoid foaming. Fill clear plastic casings (*e.g.*, 12 cm diameter) with the diced meat and vegetable mix. Add the proper amount of gelatin solution into the casings and remove all air bubbles prior to clipping. Cool in a cold water bath.

IV. Shelf Stable Chicken Meat Products

As meat products are highly perishable commodity due to favourable conditions for growth of micro-organisms and lipid oxidation, many processing techniques have been standardized for several meat products, but most of them have limited shelf-life at ambient temperature. So it is now challenging tasks for the meat technologists to adopt newer techniques which could combat microbial growth and lipid oxidation on the developed products. Development of low moisture or dehydrated meat products could be one of the better options to combat the present problems. In this direction hurdle technology is of paramount importance. Several hurdles or processes are used minimally in optimum combination for development of shelf-stable meat products which can stored without or with minimum refrigeration. So research innovations in this area is undoubtably more important in tropical countries like India. Recent advances in processing and preservation technology of shelf stable meat products was reported by Sahoo *et al.*, 2013.

1) Chicken Snack Sticks Incorporated with Oat Meal and Ragi Flour

Research investigation was undertaken to develop and extend the shelf life at room temperature of a health oriented functional based chicken snack sticks (CSS) by standardizing the level of oat meal or ragi flour alone or in combination and thereafter incorporating antimicrobial agents (Nisin and Potassium sorbate) and antioxidants (Sodium ascorbate and Tocopherol acetate) and vacuum packaging of CSS. It was observed that the optimum level of oat meal and ragi flour was 4.2 per cent and 8.4 per cent, respectively while developing CSS with better physico-chemical and sensory quality. Further it was noticed that the combined effect of oat meal and ragi flour at their optimum level was synergistic in improving the physico-chemical quality and sensory attributes in respect of crispiness, AT, MFI and OA and enriching crude fibre and ash content of CSS. Finally, vacuum packaged CSS treated with above mentioned antimicrobial agents and antioxidants greatly improved oxidative stability (TBARS value, PV, FFA per cent), significantly ($p<0.05$) lowered SPC (log 2.20 cfu/g) and enhanced sensory quality during the storage period of two months at a room temperature of 25±2°C with 60±3 per cent relative humidity (Kale *et al.*, 2009a,b, Kale *et al.*, 2010a,b).

2) Health Oriented Chicken Meat Biscuits

Studies were conducted for the development and quality evaluation of health oriented functional based chicken meat biscuits (CMB) using hurdle technology. Meat level, baking temperature and baking time were optimized by Box-Behnken design of Response surface methodology (RSM). 50 per cent meat level, 140°C baking temperature and 45 minutes baking time conditions were selected as best responses taking target for texture and colour profiles, moisture, baking yield, water activity and sensory characteristics. The optimized product was tested for the selection of best natural antioxidant (AO) among clove powder, nutmeg powder, caraway powder and cinnamon powder and best natural antimicrobial (AM) among eugenol, peppermint oil, orange oil and thymol crystals. Among all the natural antioxidants studied, 0.2 per cent clove powder was found superior in its AO activity with respect to DPPH and ABTS activity, TBARS number, FFA content and peroxide value while in case of natural antimicrobials, 0.3 per cent eugenol was having highest antimicrobial effect with respect to standard plate count and also for odour score. The selected level of clove powder and eugenol at different proportions were incorporated in CMB for storability study at room temperature (35 ±2 °C, 70 per cent R.H.) under modified atmosphere packaging with 50 per cent N_2 and 50 per cent CO_2. When control aerobic and control modified atmosphere packaged and treated MAP samples were compared, the combination of natural preservatives and MAP was found to be more effective in preserving the quality of CMB for a storage period of 60 days with respect to moisture per cent, hydratability, water activity, TBARS number, peroxide value and FFA contents besides having positive effect on the colour and texture profiles, microbiological and sensory quality. Also the proximate composition of CMB at the end of the storage did not differ significantly from that of before storage (Singh *et al.*, 2011).

3) Functional Chicken Noodles

Shelf-stable chicken meat noodles (CMN) were developed with spent hen and refined wheat flour for their profitable utilization and sustained consumers demand to meet their protein needs in diet. Meat level and processing conditions were optimized with a three-factor (meal levels, steaming time and drying time) three levels (-1, 0 and +1) central composite experimental design of Response Surface Methodology following preparation of 20 different varieties of chicken meat noodles. The optimum processing conditions standardized were adopted for development of CMN along with chitosan, EDTA, eugenol and peppermint essential oil for selecting best preservative which was then used for storage stability study at ambient temperature (35±2°C, 70 per cent RH) under aerobic and modified atmosphere (MAP) packaging conditions. Results indicated that on the basis of different responses analyzed (product yield, moisture content, pH, protein, fat, water solubility index, hardness, adhesiveness, total colour changes and overall acceptability scores), 60 per cent meat level, 9 hrs drying time and 12 min steaming time was found to be optimum for development of CMN. Amongst the all preservatives eugenol treatment exhibited powerful antioxidant activity, higher lipid stability and overall acceptability but lower microbial count in developed CMN. When control and eugenol treated products were compared in storability studyat ambient temperature (35±2°C, 70 per cent RH) under different packaging conditions, water activity (a_w) was significantly lowered in modified atmospheres (50 per cent N_2 + 50 per cent CO_2) packaged samples than that of aerobic control and eugenol treatments. Water absorption index (WAI) or water solubility index (WSI) however did not vary significantly amongst the treatments but noodles with eugenol treatment and kept under modified atmospheric condition showed lower peroxide value, lipid oxidation and FFA contents besides their positive impacts on antioxidant activities, colour and texture profiles, microbial quality and sensory attributes. All noodles stored at ambient temperature (35±2°C, 70 per cent RH)under aerobic and MAP packaging conditions were well acceptable up to 90 days (Khare *et al.*, 2013).

4) Chicken Meat Caruncles with Natural Preservatives

Studies were conducted to develop shelf stable chicken meat caruncles using spent hen meat, starches, flours, natural preservatives along with modified atmosphere packaging for safety and benefit of the consumers. The process of development of chicken meat caruncles was optimized using three factor three level Box-Behnken design of response surface methodology. Three levels of meat (60 per cent, 65 per cent and 70 per cent), oil level (2.5 per cent, 5 per cent and 7 per cent) and cooking time (3, 4 and 5 mins) were considered for which 17 different runs were conducted. The process was standardized at 65 per cent meat level, 5 per cent oil level and at 4min cooking time. The flours and starches were used successfully to increase the cooking yield and to improve the sensory attributes. Developed chicken meat emulsion with 60 per cent tapioca starch along with 0.2 per cent clove powder produced better results in terms of physico-chemical characteristics, oxidative stability and microbiological parameters than 3 per cent ginger and 2 per cent garlic paste during the period of refrigeration storage at 4±1°C for 9 days. Chicken meat caruncles prepared by using 0.2 per cent clove powder along with 50 per cent CO_2:50 per cent N_2 modified atmosphere packaging produced better acceptability of the product by improving the sensory attributes, decreasing the microbial load and inhibiting the lipid peroxidation (FFA, PV, TBARS number, DPPH per cent inhibition and ABTS per cent inhibition) and thus maintained freshness of quality better than their control counterparts up to a storage period of 60 days at room temperature (35±2°C and 70 per cent R.H) (Singh et al.2012a,b,c; 2013a,b).

5) Hurdle Treated Restructured Chicken Meat Slices

A series of experiments were conducted to develop and extend shelf life of hurdle technology restructured chicken meat slices (RCMS) in aerobic and MAP conditions. Among the three different humectants, *viz.* 0.5 per cent carboxymethyl cellulose (CMC), 5 per cent texturized soy protein (TSP) and 3 per cent skim milk powder (SMP) used while developing the RCMS, SMP 3 per cent was superior to others as it had significantly reduced water activity (a_w), increased emulsion stability and cooking yield, had lower standard plate count (SPC) and improved sensory quality of the RCMS. Amla powder 0.75 per cent (T_1) as acidulant was superior to mango powder 0.5 per cent (T_2) and L-ascorbic acid 0.4 per cent (T_3) in respect of colour and texture profiles, microbiological quality and sensory attributes of RCMS. Aloe vera gel 3 per cent (T_1) as a natural preservative was found superior to cinnamaldehyde 0.25 per cent (T_2) and aloe vera gel 1.5 per cent plus cinnamaldehyde 0.1 per cent (T_3) as it showed significantly lower pH, better a_w, significantly lower TBARS number, higher superoxide anion scavenging activity (SASA) and total phenolic content, improved hardness and chewiness character and lower SPC of RCMS. Addition of chitosan 1 per cent further improved the quality of RCMS during the refrigerated storage (4±1°C) conditions. The shelf life of RCMS in MAP (CO_2:N_2, 50:50) under refrigerated condition was found to be 30 days against only 15 days in the aerobic packaged samples. Based on different physico-chemical, microbiological, colour and texture profiles and sensory parameters hurdle treatment along with chitosan incorporation and MAP storage was found to be the most preferred RCMS (Jimomi *et al.*, 2012a,b, Jimomi *et al.*, 2013).

6) Hurdle Treated Chicken Meat Croquettes

A series of experiments were conducted to develop and extend shelf life of hurdle treated chicken meat croquettes in aerobic and MAP conditions. Among the three different humectants, *viz.* 5 per cent texturized soy protein (TSP), 0.5 per cent carrageenan and combination of 5 per cent texturized soy protein (TSP) + 0.5 per cent carrageenan used while developing the chicken meat croquettes, combination of 5 per cent texturized soy protein (TSP) + 0.5 per cent carrageenan was superior to others as it had significantly reduced water activity (a_w), increased emulsion stability and cooking yield and improved sensory quality of the chicken meat croquettes. Emulsion pH of 5.6 (T_2) was found to be better than other emulsion pH of 6.0 (T_1) and 5.2 (T_3) with the addition of lactic acid in respect of physico-chemical parameters, colour and texture profiles, and sensory attributes of chicken meat croquettes. Eugenol 0.05 per cent (T_2) as a natural preservative was found to be better as compared to chitosan 1 per cent (T_1) as it showed significantly ($P<0.05$) lower pH, a_w, TBARS number and higher SASA, ABTS and DPPH and higher score for all sensory attributes of chicken meat croquettes. The shelf life of chicken meat croquettes in MAP (CO_2:N_2, 50:50) under refrigerated condition was found to be 45 days against 30 days in the control aerobic packaged samples. Based on different physico-chemical, oxidative stability, microbiological quality, colour and texture profiles and sensory attributes, hurdle treatment along with MAP storage was found to be the most preferred for improvement in quality and extending shelf life of chicken meat croquettes (Sharma *et al.*, 2012, Sharma *et al.*, 2013).

7) Hurdle Treated Chicken Sausages

Study was conducted to develop hurdle technology based chicken sausages (HTCS) with extended storage life by employing multiple hurdles such as control of water activity (a_w), acidity level (pH), incorporation of natural antioxidant/ antimicrobial substances and packaging conditions. The hurdles were optimized *viz.* a_w with the humectants (Carrageenan, Texturized soy protein; combination), pH (lactic acid, L-ascorbic acid; combination), antimicrobials and antioxidants (chitosan, honey and eugenol) and packaging conditions (Aerobic and Modified atmosphere packaging; MAP). The efficacy of different hurdles was assessed on the basis of physico-chemical (water activity, pH, emulsion stability, cooking yield, titratable acidity), oxidative stability [Thiobarbituric acid reacting substances (TBARS) number, 2-2-azinobis-3-ethylbenthiazoline-6-sulphonic acid radical cation ($ABTS^+$) activity, 2, 2 diphenyl-1picrylhydrazyl (DPPH) radical scavenging activity, superoxide anion scavenging activity (SASA), total phenolic content], instrumental colour and texture profile, sensory and microbiological parameters. The combination of 50 per cent CO_2 + 50 per cent N_2 was used in MAP. Minimum level of water activity (0.945) was achieved with the addition of combination of 0.5 per cent Carrageenan + 5 per cent TSP as humectants in HTCS. The desired pH of 5.6-5.7 was achieved by incorporation of 2M L-ascorbic acid within acceptable sensory quality. The synergistic effect of chitosan, honey and eugenol exhibited stronger antioxidant activity. HTCS were stable up to 20 days and 35 days at 4±1°C under aerobic and MAP packaging conditions, respectively with acceptable physico-chemical, sensory and microbiological quality (Thakur *et al.*, 2012a,b,c).

8) Chicken Meat Waddi

Three different batches of chicken meat waddi containing black gram flour + saboodana flour in 50:50 ratio (T1), 75:25 ratio (T2) and 100:00 ratio (T3) in the formulation were prepared. Minced chicken meat and flour combination were used in 30: 70 ratio. In the formulation other ingredients like refined soybean oil, salt, polyphosphate, sodium ascorbate, sodium nitrite, spice mix, baking powder, carragenan and chilled water were used to make meat emulsion in a dough maker. The meat emulsion about 15g each was made into small balls or waddis of uniform size. Cooking was done in a pre-heated oven at 175°C first for 30min., then after turning again cooked for another 15 min. The waddis were cooled after cooking, packed in LDPE bags and kept at room temperature.

The emulsion pH of waddis significantly ($P<0.05$) decreased with the increase in the quantity of black gram flour, the lowest pH being observed in T3 batch. The cooked product pH (5.90) was significantly higher in T3 batch as compared to T1 and T2 waddis. Cooking yield per cent was also increased significantly with the increase in black gram flour and decrease in saboodana flour. The moisture per cent in waddis was significantly higher in T2 batch, whereas the protein and fat per cent were significantly higher in T3 batch containg 100 per cent black gram flour. There was a significant linear decrease of water activity in order of T1(0.714) >T2(0.695) >T3(0.520). The colour profile studies indicated no significant variation in L*value, a*value and b*value. On texture profile analysis (TPA) of waddis it was found that there was no significant variation of different textural characteristics such as hardness, sringiness, stringiness, cohesiveness, chewiness, gumminess and resilience among the T1, T2 and T3 batches of waddis. The microbiological assay of the samples showed that coliform count and staphylococcus count were absent in all the batches. There was no significant difference of standard plate count and yeast and mould count among the three different batches of waddis which ranged from log 1.36 to log 1.50 and log 0.33 to log 0.43 cfu/g, respectively. The sensory evaluation of waddis indicated that there was no significant variation in any of the sensory attributes such as colour and appearance, flavour, texture, juiciness and overall acceptability among T1, T2 and T3 batches. Based on the above findings it is concluded that black gram flour and saboodana flour in the ratio of 50:50, 75:25 and 100:00 can successfully be used in preparation on chicken waddis with 100 per cent black gram flour in the formulation of waddis is most preferable (Sahoo *et al.*, 2012b,21012d).

V. Manufacture and Quality of Convenient Egg Products

Introduction

The term egg products refers to processed and convenience forms of eggs for commercial, foodservice, and home use. For many years, eggs were marketed primarily as shell eggs, but in recent years egg consumption in the form of egg products has increased.

Consumption of Egg Products

Consumption of egg products in 1984 was 15 per cent of the total eggs produced, or 25.6 million cases of shell eggs further processed. By 2003, the numbers increased to about 30 per cent of the total egg production, or 60.9 million cases of shell eggs broken into egg products. Today, the production of frozen eggs has leveled out, some growth is noted in dried egg production, and production of refrigerated liquid eggs has greatly increased.

Global egg consumption has tripled in the past 40 years with consumer quality expectations increasing just as fast. Consumer research has shown that egg yolk-influenced color of foods (such as bakery products, egg pasta, etc.) is important for consumers.

Many new convenience forms of egg products are reaching the marketplace, both in the home and through foodservice and commercially processed foods. In fact, tremendous growth of the use of egg products has occurred in the foodservice industry, particularly in breakfast menu items and in the utilization of hard-cooked eggs on salad bars.

Natural Egg Products

Five main products come from an egg breaking plant

1. Liquid white
2. Liquid yolk
3. Liquid whole egg
4. Shells
5. Inedible liquid

Liquid Egg White

The solids content of liquid egg white is usually very close to 12 per cent. The only way to change this is to vary the breaking stock and, even then, the potential variation should be within ±1 per cent. Eggs that have lost considerable moisture (*i.e.*, those with large air cells) or smaller pullet eggs with high interior quality will cause the solids level to be higher. Fresh eggs from older birds have lower solids levels. However weather and respiratory diseases may also decrease the egg-white solids.

The pH of egg white can range from 7.6 – 9.3. This increase is strictly a function of the amount of CO_2 lost from the egg. Most commercial white will have a pH of 8.4-9.1. CO_2 loss depends on the temperature of the egg, the amount of CO_2 in the environment, and the degree of egg shell sealing (oiling).

The bacterial quality of liquid egg white (which is usually very good) is strictly a function of the quality of the egg being broken, the sanitation in the plant, handling practices. Also, small amount of yolk will cause bacteria to grow much faster in egg white after processing. Egg yolk inactivates lysozymes and supplies nutrients not present in egg white.

Liquid Egg Yolk

The solids content of pure egg yolk from fresh eggs is about 51.9±0.1 per cent. It is very constant. Age of the egg, meeting the amount of water migration from the white, the only major factor affecting the initial egg-yolk solids. The solids level in egg yolk produced by egg breaking machines can be affected by many things. Usually this solids level is in the 44 to 48 per cent range, depending on the amount of egg white adhering to the yolk. However, most "Plain" egg yolk is standardized by the addition of egg white to 43 to 44 per cent solids level. Why this solids level? There is a large transitional change in the viscosity of egg yolk between the 45 to 48 per cent solids level, which is easy to see when preparing egg yolk with different solids levels.

Liquid Whole Egg

This is a blend of egg white and yolk. In natural proportions, it may range between 23 and 25 per cent egg solids, yet, even without the addition of egg white, lower solid levels are possible. This standard has change over a period of many years. If whole egg is formed by blending liquid egg white and yolk, the solids level must be standardized to 24.2 per cent (USDA regulations). Generally, this many require the addition of more yolk than is present in natural proportions in the liquid from shell eggs. The pH of liquid whole egg can vary from 7.0 to 7.6, usually 7.2, depending on the history of the egg. Like egg white, the pH of whole egg within this range, is a function of the amount of CO2 in the shell eggs at the time of breaking.

The bacterial quality of raw liquid whole egg may not be as good as raw white or yolk. Yet, it is much better than many food products that have a high reputation for low total plate counts.

Egg Shells

There are 3 common methods for the disposal of egg shell from breaking plants.

1. As fertilizer
2. As a feed stuff.
3. As a waste product to be taken to municipal dumps.

At least 4 dehydrators have been installed for this purpose in the world.

Inedible Eggs

By law, at least in the United States, certain types of eggs are classed as inedible or unfit for human consumption. Most of these products are derived from leakers, eggs with blood or meat spots, and egg white from centrifuged egg shells. Solids content of inedible may vary between that for egg white to whole egg. There are no standards for this product except that it should be denatured, usually with a green dye.

Growing Market

The dramatic growth in global egg consumption and associated world trade with eggs means that quality control of production and processing has never been more important. There are increases in demand worldwide for convenience foods because homemakers have less time to prepare meals in their own kitchens. As a result, more eggs are traded and transported in a liquid form to meet processors' requirements. This offers many advantages with regards to disease control and hygiene. Going down this road, however, demands strict monitoring of quality and marketing criteria.

International egg trade now amounts to over a million tonnes per year. The use of egg products in convenience foods is increasing just as rapidly, for instance for mayonnaise, pasta, biscuits and pastries.

Worldwide trade in liquid and powder egg products has a lot more behind it than just saving labour in the home or in the catering industry. The food safety consideration is a very large part of the development. Egg products are prepared in specialised plants under strict hygiene and safety regulations, such as ISO and HACCP. It therefore offers a safer and more convenient product through pasteurization and professional control.

Fueled by increasing consumer demand for more convenience food products, growth of the egg products industry is expected to continue.

Manufacture

The first step in producing an egg product is removal from the shell, followed by filtering and cooling to maintain quality while awaiting processing. Further processing may include the addition of non-egg ingredients, mixing or blending, stabilizing, pasteurizing, cooling, and packaging for freezing or subsequent to drying.

Egg products are processed in sanitary facilities under rigorous inspection by the United States Department of Agriculture.The first step in making egg products is breaking the eggs and separating the yolks and whites from the unwanted shells.Eggs are processed by automated equipment that move the eggs from flats, wash and sanitize the shells, break the eggs and separate the whites and the yolks or keeps them together for whole egg products. The liquid egg products is filtered, mixed, and then chilled prior to additional processing. This liquid egg product (in a pasteurized format) is obtained by re-hydrating powdered egg product. Powdered Eggs provide all the natural goodness of an egg in a convenient, non-perishable package. From here the egg product is pasteurized. The law requires that all egg products distributed for consumption be pasteurized. This means they must be rapidly heated and held at a minimum required temperature for a specified time. This process destroys Salmonella and any other bacteria, but does not cook the egg or affect the color, flavour, or nutritional value.

Quality Control

For suppliers of egg products, it is desirable to extend the shelf life of an egg product, such that the purchaser can store the product for several weeks and reliably use the product without the product having developed unacceptable levels of harmful microbes or undesirable taste and/or flavour properties during storage, (*e.g.*, rotten smell or sour taste).

Egg products intended for consumption are often stored and/or treated by one or more methods in order to increase the shelf life of the egg product. For example, egg products are typically stored at about 4° C to hinder the growth of microbes, which typically grow best at higher temperatures. By storing the egg product at cool temperatures, the shelf life of the egg product can be extended for several weeks. The shelf life of the stored egg product is typically assessed by determining the concentration of bacteria in the product and subsequently evaluating organoleptic properties of the product.

In addition, the egg product may also be treated by one or more methods to decrease or eliminate harmful microbes from the egg product before storage. In particular, the egg products may be pasteurized (*e.g.*, heat-treated).

Electromagnetic radiation may also be used to reduce or eliminate the number of harmful microbes present in the egg product. For example, the egg product may be treated with radio waves and/or gamma irradiation. These methods of pasteurization may be useful in extending the shelf life of processed egg products by several weeks. Anti-microbial agents may also be used to extend the shelf life of egg products. For example, anti-microbial agents can extend the shelf life of egg products by killing microbes (*i.e.* cidal agents) or by keeping microbes from growing (*i.e.* static agents). Antibiotics may be used occasionally, but eggs from treated hens are removed from the market for a specified period of time in accordance with applicable regulations.

However, present commercial methods of storing and/or treating egg products only increase the shelf life of the product by several weeks. For suppliers and users of egg products, a method of further extending the shelf life of egg products is desirable.

The USDA-approved pasteurization methods assure food manufacturers that they're using high-quality, safe egg products. The companies involved in producing egg products conduct thousands of quality assurance tests to be sure harmful bacteria are destroyed during the pasteurization process.

Although pasteurized refrigerated eggs may have a limited shelf life of a few weeks, both frozen and dried egg products, when properly stored, will maintain a stable shelf life for months.

Microbial Quality

The risk of contamination by microorganisms, and mostly by Salmonella, is a major concern in the sectors of egg production and egg product manufacturing. Under healthy breeding conditions, the egg content is generally sterile. However, it can be contaminated by a diversified microbiota containing food spoilage microorganisms and sometimes pathogenic bacteria. The egg has however remarkable self-defence properties intended to preserve the embryo of any microbial invasion during its development. Egg breaking systematically involves the contamination of egg white and egg yolk through contact with the spoiled shells, thus giving rise to highly perishable egg products. The control of their microbiological quality is required, in particular when they are integrated in raw or undercooked food.

Nutritional Quality

1. High quality protein

   Require more protein per kg than younger adults.

   Eggs least expensive source of high quality protein.

2. Vitamins and minerals

   Two large eggs provide:

30 per cent riboflavin, 12 per cent vitamin A, 16 per cent vitamin $B_{12,}$ 12 per cent folate. 12 per cent vitamin D, 16 per cent phosphorous, 8 per cent vitamin $B_{6'}$ 34 per cent selenium, 8 per cent iron, 8 per cent zinc, 6 per cent vitamin E

3. Carotenoids

   Studies indicate that dietary lutein and zeaxanthin help preserve the health of the aging eye against age-related macular degeneration and cataracts. Addition of 1.3 egg yolks per day to the diets of 11 middle-aged subjects: increased plasma lutein [38 per cent] and increased plasma zeaxanthin [128 per cent]

4. Choline

   Choline an essential nutrient

   - AI for men 550 mg/day
   - AI for women 425 mg/day

   Increased needs during pregnancy and lactation

   Choline supplements

   - increased new neurons
   - formation of memory centers
   - decreased programmed cell death
   - life-long changes in nerve growth factors and calretinin

Advantages

Quality

Most egg products are virtually indistinguishable from fresh eggs in nutritional value, flavour, and most functional properties. These qualities are well retained during proper storage.

Economy

Reduced handling, minimal shipping cost, and elimination of breakage results in reduced-cost formulations.

Safety

Egg products are pasteurized to destroy Salmonella and other bacteria

Minimal Storage Space

A 30-lb. can of frozen eggs is equivalent to about 22 dozen large shell eggs.

Stability

When properly stored according to their type, egg products will keep their quality over several months.

Uniformity

Egg products can be produced to definite specifications to assure the same performance in formulations time after time.

Convenience

Bulk quantities may be ordered and ingredients weighed and incorporated into formulas with less labor. Equipment needs are minimal, cleanup is simplified, and, except for packagings, there is no waste for disposal.

Other Advantages

Egg products are used widely by the food service industry and the commercial food industry. They are scrambled or made into omelets, or used as ingredients in egg dishes or other foods such as mayonnaise or ice cream. Food manufacturers use pasteurized egg products because of their convenience and ease in handling and storing. Because egg products are pasteurized, institutional foodservice operators, such as fast food chains, restaurants, hospitals, and nursing homes, use egg products to ensure a high level of food safety. Some egg products are sold in retail food stores.

Why Egg is Used for Manufacture of different Food Products?

The diverse roles of egg in the recipes occur due to :

their particularly high water solubility, excellent foaming and emulsification capacities, heat coagulability, and high nutritive values. They contribute structure to a product that contains egg. The quality of eggs is dependent upon the egg itself. For example, in hard cooked eggs the size of the air cell will impact whether it is oval egg or has an indentation on the end, a "less than perfect" egg for "hard boiled", deviled eggs. In custard sauces, the chalazae removal is thought, by the true chef, to improve the quality of the product. For these reasons, it is important to know the egg and factors which impact the quality of the egg and resulting products.

Eggs and egg whites have been used as a clarifier. The process is as it sounds, the clearing of a liquid. Master chefs use it to clarify stock to produce clear consommes. In the old "campfire coffee", egg white was added to coagulate around the coffee grounds and clarify it. It is of interest that clarification is used for other items. For example, many years ago we had a relative who would give us gallons of clarified butter. This was butter that had been carefully warmed to melt the butter fat. This fat was then drawn off and the milk solids removed. The hypothesis was that it would keep "fresh" longer. Actually, theory would support this antedoctal idea. With drawing off the fat, the water and salts, syngeristic components, would no longer be available to take part in the hydrolytic rancidity reaction.

Egg whites, egg yolks, whole eggs, and egg washes brushed on breads and other baked products add a rich, shiny glaze. The glaze is caused primarily by the protein and fat interaction. The simple glaze is generally made by adding a "little water" to the egg and brushing it on.

General Changes of Egg during Processing and Preparation Procedures

The coagulation of eggs is critical to many food products. Coagulation is simply the solidifying of the egg by the application of heat. In many instances, the egg in a formula will serve to glue the product together. For example, it is sometimes added to meat loaf or on the surface of okra, in both instances serving as a glue. Certainly, the coagulation of the white and yolk permits the "structure" of the product for deviled eggs. A large portion of the discussion of stirred and baked custard hinges on egg coagulation. It is of interest in the many products to know the coagulation mechanism of the yolk and the white. Following are the general temperatures at which various egg parts and egg products will coagulate: egg white 60-65°C, egg yolk 65-70°C, custard 82°C. Generally, whole egg begins to become opaque at around 60°C and increases in viscosity to 72°C. At 75°C it is a soft curd and increases in firmness up to 87°C. Certainly, heat is the critical factor in bringing about the denaturation of the egg protein and forming structure. However, heat has many other causative factors. It should be remembered that heating the egg product itself, if (liquid or dried form) has been done during the pasteurization of eggs. This heat will decrease the functional properties of these eggs. Again, one needs to be reminded that the rate of heating, the added ingredients, the concentration of the egg and other subtle factors will impact the range of temperature and the optimum endpoint. The work on model systems of eggs by Pawayal *et al.* (1946) essentially appears to indicate that there is a relationship between time and rate of heating. The faster the mixture heats the lower the point of increased viscosity. Practically speaking, what are the implications of the differing coagulation points of the various egg parts? When most consumers talk about egg products they likely are thinking about the whole shell eggs and the many different foods. Neff [Neff, J. 1998. Foods of Tomorrow. The Great Egg Breakthrough. Food Processing 59(1): 25.] indicates that in 1997 there were 6.443 million dozen eggs in the shell and 1.621 million dozen breaker eggs consumed. The per capita egg consumption was 171.5 shell eggs and 66.5 breaker eggs. However, there are other egg products used by the consumer, foodservice industry, and value-added portion of the food industry. Most consumers are well aware of the market for egg substitutes and egg replacers. Although one should review egg selling sites to get the latest on available products, some of the different egg products are as follows: Dried Eggs: (blends of whole egg and/or yolk with sugar or corn syrup) added, flake albumen, free-flowing whole egg or yolk solids, instant egg white solids, spray-dried egg white solids, stabilized whole egg yolk solids (glucose free), whole egg or yolk solids, Frozen Eggs: egg white, egg yolks, salted whole egg, salted yolks, sugared yolks, whole eggs, whole eggs with com syrup, whole eggs with added yolk (fortified), whole eggs with yolks and corn syrup, yolk and white blends w/wo sweeteners or salts Refrigerated Liquid Egg Products: egg whites, egg yolks and various mixtures of these. Speciality Products come in a wide variety of forms. Some of my favorites are the precooked egg yolks/whites and cooked egg white with a center tube of cooked yolk. There are boiled eggs available for purchase by institutions. One can order the "real egg" in about any form desired. There are many products that serve as egg substitutes or replacers. Eggs have also been used as substitutes for other ingredients. Neff reported the work of Dan Neumeister in developing a heat-denatured egg yolk to substitute for potassium bromate to improve the texture and outward appearance of bread.

What is the Effect of the Egg Product in a Custard?

Funk *et al.*, 1969 has plotted the heat penetration of custards as essentially rise steadily to 74°C and then slowing down in rate until approximately 82°C and rising again to above 87°C. They observed that the type of egg processing (foam-spray, frozen, freeze, spray-dried) did make a slight difference in the heating rate. Workers have hypothesized that the actual coagulation occurs as a two step process. The first step is the actual denaturation of the protein and the second step is the protein-protein interaction and the formation of a gel or increased viscosity. Lowe (1942) observed that forewarming of the milk may decrease curdling and shortening cooking time. However, it is important to remember that 0.75 per cent of the milk protein is heat coagulable.

Which of the Following are Egg Custards?

A custard is made of egg, milk, sugar and usually salt and flavouring. Through application of heat and manipulation, custards can become a viscous sauce or a semi-rigid gel. In each case, denaturation of the egg protein, ovalbumin, conalbumin, and ovoglobulin is primarily responsible for the thickening of the custard. Stirred custards are cooked on top of the range while gel type custards are usually baked. Custards may be altered by manipulation or ingredient variation. Because egg is the primary structural ingredient of a custard, some differences are seen when fresh, frozen, old, dried or egg substitutes are used. The egg source, for example duck or turkey, also influences custard quality. Milk, although not as structurally important as egg, contributes to the viscosity or gel strength of the finished product. Calcium ions present in the milk are needed in the formation of a thicker custard, as custards made with water will not gel or thicken. Differences in processing will also influence the custard quality. Nonhomogenized milk produces a baked custard with a thinner crust, more delicate browning and better sheen than those custards made with homogenized milk. For example, stirred custard usually is considered to have "more body". Sugar is also important to the viscosity and gel strength of custards. Sugar tends to increase the denaturation temperature of the egg proteins resulting in a less stiff product. Salt and flavouring have no appreciable affect on custard quality other than for taste. The proportion of ingredients is important to custard quality. The concentration of egg protein is proportional to the viscosity or gel strength of the custard. With increasing concentration, a custard sauce becomes more viscous and the gel strength of a baked custard firmer. Also, with increased egg protein, the product becomes more sensitive to end point temperature. End point temperature is the point at which optimum denaturation has occurred without curdling or syneresis. Milk serves to dilute the egg protein so less viscosity and gel strength are observed with increasing proportions of milk. Because sugar increases the denaturation temperature of egg proteins, increased sugar concentrations results in softer custards. At a 30 per cent sucrose oncentration, a custard will not gel at all. Producing a good quality custard depends on a number of factors. In addition to the proportion and ingredient variation, temperature and rate of cooking are important. A custard heated slowly begins to thicken at a lower temperature, thickens gradually over a wider temperature range and reaches doneness at a lower temperature. On the other hand, a custard heated rapidly must be heated to a higher temperature before thickening begins and overcooking, resulting in curd formation or porosity, occurs easily. Syneresis or weeping results as the curds separate from the serum. Slow cooking can be achieved by placing the baked custard mixture in a waterbath in the oven or by using a double boiler with a stirred custard. Endpoint is indicated when the stirred custard "coats the spoon", or when a knife inserted into the baked custard "comes out clean".

Which of the following custards was cooked the longest? Which of the following custards could represent the custard having the greatest amount of sugar? Which of the following custard could likely represent the custard having egg white substituted for the whole egg? When one turns to a recipe or formula and it lists eggs as an ingredient, it is usually understood to be whole chicken eggs. The egg itself and the method of processing of the food product it is in will make a difference in the reaction of cooking. The effect of ingredients in products will make a difference. Certainly it will vary depending upon the product and the function of the egg. Following are some affects.

Milk's contribution in egg products such as custards is underestimated. As early as 1942, Carr and Trout reported research that indicated the cooking time for custards made with homogenized milk took 15 to 20 minutes longer than custards made with nonhomogenized milk. Heat penetration was slower. Additionally, viscosity and gel strength was greater with homogenized milk. However, this webber has observed that milk's effect on egg gelation is not well documented. Milk contains electrolytes which will enhance viscosity and gel strength. Sugar will inhibit and delay denaturation of the egg proteins, depending upon the product. In a custard, it delays coagulation so that equivalent thickening (from the standard) will occur only at a higher temperature, if at all. In the production of foams, it has been shown that adding sugar will delay the formation of an egg white foam. However, once a foam is formed, it is more stable. A variety of factors may influence the pH of eggs. Shimada and Matsushita (1980) observed that pH and protein concentration affected coagulation of egg albumin. The net charge of egg albumin increased up to pH 8, plateauing up to pH 11 at which time no coagulation occurred. The charge would increase as concentration increased. This is due to the change of the proteins themselves. Certainly if one adds acid to a egg containing product it will coagulate faster. This effect is often utilized. For example, angelfood cake foam has lemon juice or cream of tartar added as a stabilizer. The amount, how it is processed and type of eggs makes a difference. The part of the egg will impact the functional properties within an egg product. Researchers have determined that egg yolk will also coagulate, beginning at ~65C, losing fluidity at 70°C and coagulating at 85°C. Woodward and Cotterill (1987) felt that the major denaturation occurred in egg yolk at 68°C to 70°C. Egg white will coagulate approximately 5C higher. As with egg white, there was significant pH-temperature interdependence. Other workers (Shimada and Matsushita, 1980) have observed that coagulation increased with increased protein level and concentration. This is of particular importance when using selected fluid or dried egg products. The method of processing the egg makes a difference. Research done by Funk *et al.*, in1969 plotted the heat penetration of custards, rising steadily to 74°C and then slowing down in rate until approximately 82°C and rising again to about 87°C. They observed that the type of egg (foam-spray, frozen, freeze, spray-dried) did make a slight difference in the heating rate. Another study conducted by Downs *et al.* (1970) observed hat spray-dried eggs tended to coagulate faster than frozen, freeze-dried and foam-spray-dried eggs.

Because they provide certain desirable functional attributes, egg products are widely used as ingredients in many food products. Different convenient value added egg products are given below:

1. Whole Eggs

Hard cooked eggs are well-known for their convenience, consistency, value and quality. Hard cooked eggs are ideal for slicing, wedging, chopping, serving whole or as a garnish. They are an attractive ingredient, and make for picture-perfect deviled eggs

2. Diced Eggs

Diced eggs can be used in any situation; regardless of venue, they save time, labor and storage space. Provides excellent eye appeal; holds up extremely well in salads.

- ✰ Unique processing techniques ensure tender whites and bright yellow yolks.
- ✰ pH balanced to resist greening and prolong product life

3. Deviled Eggs

Hard-cooked eggs are cut along the long axis. Yolk is removed and seasoned with soft salad mixture and put back to the hollow in egg few hours after preparation and is a popular dish in restaurants where they have moulds in the shape of egg-half into which albumen is poured and a ball of the size of yolk is lowered to create space for yolk. The mould is cooked by steam and later on, yolk-salad mix is filled mechanically or by hand followed by cryogenic freezing of deviled eggs.

4. Pickled Eggs

Pickling is an effective means of preserving and marketing quail eggs which weigh about 10g or small size(40-45g) chicken eggs as nutritious, ready-to-eat product. The product does not require refrigeration for storage, transport and marketing, unless intended for very long period of storage. Apart from fast food outlets, pickled eggs find an important place in mid day meal programme of school going children to improve their nutritional status.

Vinegar Based Pickled Eggs

Pickling requires eggs in solid form. For this, fresh eggs are held at room temperature for 24hours prior to hard cooking in simmering water for about 10minutes for quail eggs and 15minutes for chicken eggs. Immediately after the cooking, the hot water is poured out and eggs are cooled in running tap water for improved peeled appearance of eggs. The cooked eggs can be peeled manually or mechanically and washed to remove the shell particles and or shell membrane pieces, if any, adhering to the surface of solidified albumen. Only properly peeled eggs, free from any cracks torn albumen, shall be utilized for pickling. The egg showing damaged albumen can be used for salad dressing.

The process for preparation of vinegar based pickle consists of dipping hard cooked and peeled eggs in pickling solution(1:1 w/v) consists of 50 per cent vinegar, 8 per cent common salt, 2 per cent spice mix, 0.02 per cent tartrazine(permitted food color) and 2 per cent each of garlic and ginger. The solution is boiled for about 10minutes, filtered through clean muslin and the hot solution is poured over the cooled and peeled eggs in presterilized glass jars or food grade plastic jars. The jars are capped and the product is allowed to season for 2 days (quail eggs) and 4 days (chicken eggs) at ambient temperature after which it is ready for consumption.

Oil Based Pickled Eggs

For the preparation of domestic type oil-cum-spice based pickled eggs, hard cooking and peeling operations are the same as described earlier.

The spice mixes and condiments (garlic and ginger mince) are fried in refined mustard oil till light brown color. The pickle gravy, peeled eggs and acetic acid thoroughly mixed and the finished product is then packaged in either glass or plastic jars or more economically in HDPE pouches. In this process edible oil acts as an additional preservative. This pickle can be kept satisfactorily for 6 months and 12 months under ambient and refrigeration storage conditions respectively.

5. Egg Roll

This is cylindrical in shape. It is prepared by cooking a uniform layer of albumen around the centre of yolk in a tubular mould. This product is sliced and used in salad dressing. It looks like the central out of a normal hard-boiled egg.

6. Egg Nog

It is a nutritious egg based drink. It contains egg, milk, sugar and flavourings and can be served cold or hot.

7. Albumen Ring

This is a high protein, crispy snack food which looks like onion ring. This product is manufactured by cooking egg albumen in ring shaped moulds and then battering, breading and deep fat frying.

8. Mayonnaise

This is a semi-solid egg yolk based product. It is an emulsion of edible vegetable oil (80 per cent), yolk (10 per cent), vinegar and various seasonings in which yolk acts as an emulsifier for the uniform dispersions of oil in non-oily substances so as to stabilize the emulsion.

9. Angel Cake

This is prepared from egg albumen. A typical recipe and methods of its preparation are given below:

Ingredient	*Quantity (per cent)*
Liquid egg albumen	40
Powdered sugar	30
Cake flour	25
Wheat starch	3.8
Monocalcium phosphates	0.6
Common salt powder	0.5
Sodium bicarbonate	0.1

The egg albumen, monocalcium phosphate, salt and sugar are mixed and whipped by wire whip for 5 minutes at high speed in an electric mixer bowl. The other ingredients like cake flour, wheat starch and sodium bicarbonate are incorporated and blended into batter of uniform consistency prior to baking it in a hot air oven at 190°C for about 30 minutes. The finished product is delicious and has very soft texture.

10. Canned Egg Curry

This is ready-to-eat canned egg product. The hard boiled and peeled eggs are fried in edible oil to light brown color. The gravy is prepared by mixing and frying spices and condiments (garlic, ginger and onion) to suit salt. The peeled eggs and gravy are mixed in the ratio of 55:45(±5 per cent), filled in lacquered metal cans leaving 1.5cm head space, exhausted and hermetically sealed. The sealed cans are then subjected to retorting (1kg/cm^2 pressure for about 20minutes) to ensure sterilization of the product without burning or over cooking. The canned egg curry should have characteristic taste and flavour without any disintegration of eggs during one year of its storage life under ambient storage.

11. Scotch Eggs

Scotch eggs are hard-cooked peeled eggs wrapped in a layer of sausage which are deep-fat-fried. Yolk should be at the centre of the boiled eggs otherwise the sausage will not adhere properly to the surface. Recipe for sausage mix is dependent on local preferences; but usually contain soya protein, ground meat and seasonings. Hard-cooked peeled eggs are kept moist, then rolled in wheat flour and wrapped into formed sausage. Finally, they are again rolled in breading mix (consisting of corn flakes) and then subjected to deep-fat frying in oil at 177°C for 7 minutes. Such eggs have a shelf life of 30 days at 4°C.

12. Custards

Consist of cooked mixture of eggs, milk, sugar and flavourings. If the mixture is cooked on a stove to creamy pourable consistency, it is called stirred custard. It is eaten as a sauce poured over cake or fruit. If the mixture is cooked in a water bath in an oven to a firm gel-like consistency, it is called baked custard. It is a dessert itself but, can also be used as a base for toppings or sauces. The custards can be frozen for storage and distribution.

References

1. Stadelman, W.J. and Cotterill, O.J. 2002, Egg Science and Technology, 4th edition, CBS Publishers, New Delhi
2. http://www.google.com/url?sa=t and source=web and cd=1 and ved=0CB4QFjAA and url=http%3A%2F%2Fwww.fsis.usda.gov%2Ffact sheets%2FEgg_Products_and_Food_Safety
3. http://www.google.com/url?sa=t and source=web and cd=3 and ved=0CCsQFjAC and url=http%3A%2F%2Fusda.mannlib.cornell.edu% 2FMannUsda%2FviewDocumentInfo.do
4. http://www.google.com/url?sa=t and source=web and cd=2 and ved=0CCQQFjAB and url=http%3A%2F%2Fwww.georgiaeggs.org% 2Fpages%2Fegg products.html
5. http://www.google.com/url?sa=t and source=web and cd=14 and ved=0CGIQFjAN and url=http%3A%2F%2Fwww.foodsafety.gov%2 Fkeep%2Ftypes
6. http://www.google.com/url?sa=t and source=web and cd=17 and ved=0CEUQFjAGOAo and url=http%3A%2F%2Fwww.aeb.org%2Ffood-manufacturers
7. http://www.google.com/url?sa=t and source=web and cd=6 and ved=0CC0QFjAF and url=http%3A%2F%2Fen.wikipedia.org

VI. Manufacture and Quality of Dehydrated Egg Products

Introduction

Dehydration

The removal of water from food inhibits the growth of microorganisms and slows down the chemical reactions in the constituents of food and thus, preserved its quality. Dehydration is a successful way of preserving eggs, and the egg drying industry has developed over several years. Research has played a major role in solving problems which involve chemical, functional and microbiological properties of dried egg products. This principal of dehydration is applied in the production of dried egg products from albumen, yolk and whole egg separately depending on their usages in food and non food industries.

Advantages of Egg Dehydration

1. They can be stored at low cost under dry storage or refrigeration.
2. They require less space than shell or liquid eggs.
3. Low tranportation cost.
4. Easy to handle.
5. They are not susceptible to bacterial growth when held in storage.
6. They have good uniformity.

Preparation of Egg Melange

The process of conversion of shell eggs into dried egg products consists of washing of eggs and breaking them individually in cups by hand or machine, inspection for odour and blood spot etc, collection of contents as whole liquid, albumen or yolk, homogenisation, filtration, pasteurization, desugaring and dehydration of egg melange.

Different Pasteurization Methods

1. **Lactic acid aluminium sulfate pasteurisation method** : *In this method* one ounce of aluminium sulfate is well mixed in 1lb 25 per cent lactic acid and then added @ 6.5lb per 1000 lb liquid egg. The egg content is heated to a temperature of 62°C for 3.5 to 4 min.
2. **Heat in combination with H_2O_2 pasteurisation**: For this method, egg product pH is maintained at normal range before heated it 52-53°C for 1.5min to inactivate catalase enzyme. A 10 per cent solution of H_2O_2 is added into liquid egg at 0.075 to 0.10 per cent levels.The chemical reaction takes place for 2min and then they are cooled and catalase enzyme is added to destroy residual hydrogen peroxide.
3. **Heat cum vacuum pasteurisation**: Liquid whole egg is heated to 57C° for 3.5 min under low vacuum of 17-20".

Different Desugaring Methods

1. **Spontaneous bacterial fermentation:** Fermentation of liquid egg is generally accomplished by naturally contaminating bacterial species at 23.9-29.4°C for 6-7days.
2. **Controlled bacterial fermentation :** ***Streptococcus lactis*** @ 1 per cent by weight is used to desugaring of liquid whole eggs at 37°C for 0.5 to 2 hrs. This procedure of desugarization helps to reduce glucose level from 0.320 per cent to 0.0006 per cent.The pH is adjusted to 7-7.5.
3. **Yeast fermentation :** ***Saccharomyces cerevisae* (baker's yeast)** @0.2 to 0.4 per cent in weight at 22-23°C for 2 to 4 hrs at pH 6.0 ferment the reducing sugar present in egg.

4. **Enzyme fermentation :** This fermentation carried out using glucose oxidase from *Aspergillus niger* and *Penicillium glaucum.*

Drying Methods

1. Spray Drying
2. Pan Drying
3. Belt Drying
4. Freeze Drying

1. Spray Drying

The spray drying process enables removal of nearly all the water from a heat sensitive biological product like eggs in such a way that the valuable constituents are not only unaffected but even further refined. The basic feature of spray drying that enables this is the atomization of the liquid egg product into a spray of droplets that is dispersed into hot air. The spray has an extensive surface area and moisture evaporation is virtually instantaneous.

Flow Diagram for Preparation of Whole Egg Powder

Inspection and cleaning of egg

↓

(2 per cent detergent sanitizer at 40°C temperature for 3 min)

↓

Breaking and inspection
Homogenization and filtration

↓

Pasteurization at 62.5°C for 3.5 min

↓

Desugarization(Glucose-oxidase enzyme or Baker's yeast)

↓

Repasteurisation

↓

Spray drying (4-5 per cent moisture,Inlet air temperature 160°C and outlet temperature 60°C;atomizer speed at 2000rpm)

↓

Vacuum drying(in vacuum self dryer to reduce moisture content to 2 per cent at 60°C for 2-3hrs)

↓

Packaging in metal cans under nitrogen or flexible pouches

↓

Storage (6 months at room temperature without nitrogen and 12 months at room temperature with nitrogen)

2. Pan Drying

It is used for producing albumen flakes.A thin layer of liquid albumen is poured on shalow metal trays and dried at moderate temperature(54-56°C)in hot air oven or water gasket pan for uniform drying.

3. Belt Drying

It involves spreading of thin layer of liquid egg material on a continuous aluminium belt moving through a hot air steam.A modification of this method is foam drying in which liquid egg is beaten into foam which is subsequently dried in a thin layer on a perforated belt.This yields a granular egg product.

4. Freeze Drying

In freeze drying,water is removed from the product while it is in the frozen state.This is accomplished by freezing the product and then subjecting it to a very high vacuum.Heat must be supplied to the product while it is drying.On freezing yolk or whole egg liquid appear as thick,lumpy and tenacious mass.The amount of gelatin is more in frozen yolk than in frozen whole egg liquid.In order to overcome this problem,they are blended with 5-10 per cent salt or sugar.Enzymes such as 0.03 per cent pepsin or 0.5 per cent trypsin can also be used instead of salt or sugar to control gelatin.

Types of Dried Egg Products

1. Egg Powder

It is prepared from whole liquid egg by spray drying method as discussed earlier. Omelets can be prepared by mixing one part of egg powder with three parts of lukewarm water along with salt, spices and condiments to suit the taste.

BIS Specifications for Egg Powder

Characteristics	*Requirements*
Moisture(per cent), max	2.0
Protein(per cent) min	45.0
Fat(per cent), min	40.0
Solubility(per cent), min	85.0
Boric acid	Absent

Contd...

Contd...

Characteristics	*Requirements*
P_2O_5, (per cent) min	1.25
Total ash(per cent), max	3.6
Acid insoluble ash(per cent), max	0.10
Oxygen content(per cent), max	2.0
Total bacterial count/g, max	75,000
Coliform count/g, max	100
Yeast and mold count/g, max	50
Salmonella	Absent

2. Yolk Granules

The egg yolk is homogenised, filtered to remove vitelline membrane, pasteurised, whipped and then sprayed on a perforated belt passing through a heated chamber. The dried foam produced is then crushed to desired granulation. Removal of glucose from the yolk prior to drying results in more stable granular product. The product finds use in the manufacture of sponge cakes, doughnuts and cookies because of its excellent emulsifying properties.

3. Albumen Flakes

This is a dried crystalline product prepared from the albumen of egg by pan drying method. There are two types of albumen flakes; edible and inedible. The edible flakes are prepared from fresh,wholesome eggs. Low grade and damaged eggs can be utilised for manufacture of non edible albumen flakes.

BIS Specifications for Albumen Flakes

Characteristics	*Requirements*
Moisture(per cent), max	8
pH	5.5 – 6
Solubility(per cent), min	80
Glucose(per cent), max	0.10

4. Egg Omelete Mix

Omeletes are prepared by mixing one part of dehydrated omlete mix with three parts of water and stirring for about 3-4 times till uniform in consistency before frying.

The recipe for its preparation is given below:

Ingredients	*Quantity (per cent)*
Whole egg powder	74
Hydrogenated vegetable oil	5
Dehydrated onion rings	15
Dehydrated green chillies	2
Common salt powder	2
White pepper powder	2

5. Scrambled Egg Mix

Like omlete mix another ready to use convenient product,such as dehydrated scrambled egg mix has been formulated for quick preparation of the product.

Formulation for scrambled egg mix:

Ingredients	*Quantity (per cent)*
Whole egg powder	77.5
Whole milk powder	15.0
Common salt powder	2.0
White pepper powder	0.5
Hydrogenated vegetable oil	5.0

Quality

Eggs are low in saturated fat and are one of the best sources of vitamin D, a nutrient that is essential to the development of strong bones. In fact, eggs are a nutritional powerhouse. For only 75 calories you get high quality protein and varying amounts of 13 essential vitamins and minerals, including A, B_{12} and folate.

Powdered, dried eggs provide a convenient alternative to fresh eggs and add quality and consistent performance to the list of attributes. Dry egg products can be stored up to a year or longer under proper storage conditions. The risk of bacterial contamination due to improper handling is significantly reduced and the clean up time is reduced as well. For bakers, powdered egg products provide consistency from batch to batch and are always ready. Another great aspect of dried egg products is that you can choose from an assortment of finished products. It's time consuming and difficult to properly separate egg whites from egg yolks. With the powdered variations you can opt for whole dried eggs, powdered egg whites, and even dried egg yolks.

1. Microbiological Quality

Microbial growth usually occurs during the desugaring process.When the liquid eggs are dried they must be pasteurised. The only pathogen of concern is Salmonella. Pan dried albumen should be held at a temperature of 51.7°C for 5 days and until it is negative for salmonella(USDA 1980).The risk of post contamination exists in both liquid eggs and dried egg products. Dried egg products must be reconstituted before use in order to avoid growth and spoilage by Salmonella. Pasteurised egg products and heat dried egg whites shall be sampled and analysed for the presence of salmonella(USDA 1980).

Dehydrated egg products should be kept cool, less than 50°F (10°C), to maintain quality. Once containers of egg solids have been opened, they should be resealed tightly to prevent contamination and absorption of moisture. If dried eggs are combined with dry ingredients and held for storage, they should be sealed tightly in a closed container and stored in the refrigerator at 32° to 50°F (0° to 10°C). Reconstituted eggs should be used immediately.

2. Physico-chemical Quality

Chromatographic and electrophoretic studies have indicated that only minor changes occur in egg white protein when it is spray dried. The denaturation and coagulation of the proteins are considered to be the chemical changes involved during pasteurisation. Minute quantities of fats are changed from the contaminating yolk are probably changed from highly emulsified state to a free state during drying. These free fats could spread and coat the dried particles, thus reducing the foaming ability of the white when reconstituted. The presence of natural glucose in eggs can cause chemical changes during drying. The Maillard reaction is minimised by drying to a low moisture content.

The density of egg products is not affected by dehydration. When a dried egg product is reconstituted to its natural solids, it has about the same density as the liquid from which it was dried. Pan dried egg products are much higher in bulk density than their spray dried counterparts. Bulk density of a spray dried product can generally be increased by milling the material and decreased by injecting gas into the liquid before drying.

3. Functional Quality/Properties

Whipping

Eggs have the ability to incorporate air and form a relatively stable foam when beaten with a wire whip or other mechanical devices. Egg white usually has a loss of whipping properties when dried without pretreatment. This loss apparently results from a combination of the drying process itself and any physical treatment therein. The small amount of yolk that inadvertently contaminate egg white during egg breaking and separating can adversely affect the whipping properties of egg white.

Emulsifying

Egg yolk is rated four times as effective as egg white as an emulsifier, and whole egg is intermediate. The very excellent emulsifying properties of egg yolk are attributed to its lecithoproteins. In fact, drying actually enhances the emulsifying properties of whole egg(Chaplin,1951).

Coagulation

The ability of egg products to coagulate and bind pieces of food together is one of their most important functional properties. Egg proteins denature and coagulate over a wide range of temperatures. Under proper drying and storage conditions, dried egg products retain their heat coagulating properties quite well. However if drying conditions are too severe or if storage conditions are adverse, whole egg and yolk products can lose their heat coagulating properties as well as their solubility.

Flavour

Flavour of eggs can be changed by adverse drying conditions and also by storage. Almost all egg white products have the free glucose removed before drying. Thus,there is little, if any, change in flavour during dehydration. Any off-flavours noted in dried egg white are probably caused by the methods used for processing.

Nutrition

Drying of eggs under normal conditions causes little, if any,loss of nutritional properties of the eggs. Vitamin A, vitamins B, thiamine, riboflavin, pantothenic acid have been determined in dried whole egg and found to be essentially the same as that in the fresh egg product.

References

1. http://books.google.co.in
2. http://www.usaeggs.org
3. http://www.springerlink.com
4. http://www.unece.org/trade/agr/standard/eggs/e/63produc.pdf
5. http://pvj.com.pk/pdf-files/30_4/219-222.pdf
6. AOAC, 1990b. Egg and Egg Products. (Solids in Eggs). In K. Helrich (Ed.,), 15th Ed. Official methods of analysis. Arlington, Virginia, USA.
7. http://en.wikipedia.org/wiki/Egg
8. Stadelman,W.J. and Cotterill,O.J.2002.Egg Science and Technology,4th Ed, CBS Publishers, New Delhi.

Index

E

F

M

N

O

P

Q

R

S

Y

Z